IMMUNOLOGY

IMMUNOLOGY

Janis Kuby

*Professor of Biology,
San Francisco State University*

*Faculty,
Joint Medical Program,
University of California at Berkeley*

W. H. Freeman and Company
New York

Cover illustration of AIDS viruses budding from an infected T cell was provided by L. Montagnier/CNRI, Science Photo Library.

Library of Congress Cataloging-in-Publication Data

Kuby, Janis.
   Immunology / Janis Kuby.
      p.   cm.
   Includes bibliographical references and index.
   ISBN 0-7167-2257-7
   1. Immunology.   I. Title.
   [DNLM: 1. Immune System.   2. Immunity.   QW 504 K95i]
QR181.K83   1992
616.07'9 — dc20
DNLM/DLC   91-44429
for Library of Congress   CIP

Printed in the United States of America

2 3 4 5 6 7 8 9   RRD   9 9 8 7 6 5 4 3 2

To
my family, David, Rebecca, and Beth-Alisha,
whose love and encouragement made it possible to complete this book.

And to
my mentor, Leon Wofsy,
who instilled in me a love for immunology and teaching
and who taught me, by his example, to always put people first.

And to
all the support from friends, extended family, and the grace of God
that has seen me through an earthquake, a fire, and cancer
during the writing of this book!

Contents

Preface

As a teacher of immunology, I have had the pleasure of watching the field explode from an infusion of new information in the past decade. Each day, newspapers and magazines carry reports of the remarkable advances research in immunology brings to clinical medicine. These include the use of engineered monoclonal antibodies for tumor detection and killing; the use of tumor-infiltrating lymphocytes and melanoma cells engineered with the gene for tumor necrosis factor; the development of the SCID-human mouse as a model system for AIDS; the development of soluble CD4 immunoadhesions for the treatment of AIDS; the development of a successful gene therapy for the treatment of severe combined immunodeficiency; the use of cytokines as an intervention in hypersensitivity, infectious diseases, graft rejection, tumor growth, and AIDS; revolutionary developments in vaccine design based on the differences in B-cell and T-cell epitopes; the development of various new recombinant vaccines; and the role the MHC plays in our susceptability to disease. Until recently, the gap between basic research and its clinical application was so wide that these two endeavors were seen as quite separate and distinct. Now, this gap has narrowed dramatically. To better reflect this interface of basic research and clinical medicine, I have integrated discussions of important clinical advances throughout the text and especially in the chapters on cancer, AIDS, autoimmunity, hypersensitivity, transplantation, infectious disease, vaccines, and immunodeficiency.

However, it is the creative design of the experimental work that lies *underneath* these advances in immunology that stirs the imagination and makes this such an exciting field today. For this reason, I have sought to present immunology to students using an experimental approach, incorporating the landmark experiments that have formed the theoretical framework of immunology. Seeing how experiments develop enables students to witness the experimental process as it unfolds from simple curiosity or frustrating dilemma to resolution. I can imagine no better way for students to learn the basic concepts and methods of immunology.

Immunology is a beginning textbook for students who must develop an understanding of the subject whether they are in the sciences or in clinical medicine. It evolved from my fourteen years of teaching undergraduate and graduate students at San Francisco State University and, more recently, teaching in the joint medical program of the University of California at Berkeley. As a teacher I became aware of the need for a textbook that first, and foremost, gives students an appreciation of immunology as a field based solidly upon experimental results, and second, integrates research results along with their clinical applications within the pedagogical framework of the book.

The text begins with a detailed overview of the immune system, which is intended to give students an introduction to the subject, as well as provide a framework for more fully understanding the context of later chapters. Chapter 2 gives students the background they need to understand the important experimental systems and techniques that are currently used by immunologists and features discussions of the various recombinant DNA techniques, DNA transfection into cultured cells, and the production of transgenic mice. Each of these techniques is critical to the design of many of the most exciting experiments in the field today. The remainder of the book presents the theoretical evolution of immunology in the context of its experimental development and weaves into this approach frequent, up-to-date discussions of clinical applications. Chapters 3 through 16 describe the components and functioning of the immune system. Chapter 17 begins a series of clinically oriented chapters that describe vaccines, autoimmune diseases, infectious diseases, transplantation immunology, cancer, and AIDS. Many chapters are unique, but I would especially like to single out four: Chapter 21 on AIDS is especially comprehensive because basic research on the subject has greatly increased our understanding of the immune system. Chapter 7 on monoclonal antibodies discusses several new technologies including the engineering of monoclonal antibodies, the development of abzymes, and the production of monoclonal antibodies from combinatorial gene libraries. Chapter 8 on the major histocompatability complex provides up-to-date coverage on the genes and gene products of the MHC. New experiments utilizing site-directed mutagenesis, exon shuffling, and transfection of MHC genes are featured in the discussion of the structure and function of the MHC. The chapter also includes recent information on the regulation of expression of class I and class II MHC molecules. Finally, Chapter 8 includes an in-depth discussion of the MHC and antigen presentation, focusing on the segregation of class I and class II MHC molecules within different antigen processing pathways. In Chapter 18 on vaccines, many of the key concepts developed in earlier chapters have been applied to the production of effective vaccines. This chapter includes discussions of synthetic peptide vaccines and the new experimental vaccines, such as recombinant antigen vaccines and recombinant vector vaccines that promise to be the vaccines of the future.

Each chapter ends with practical teaching aids: study questions, chapter summaries, and research references. The study questions that appear at the end of each chapter have been used as exam questions at the University of California at Berkeley and at San Francisco State University. These questions serve as additional teaching tools while providing a challenging review for the students. Answers to the study questions, as well as a glossary, are provided at the back of the book. Chapter summaries highlight and review key concepts. The current research references will enable students to go to the primary literature within the relevant field for each topic.

In writing this book I have appreciated and tried to incorporate the suggestions of its many reviewers. I am especially grateful for the advice of Lisa Steiner, MIT; Walter Esselman, Michigan State University; Mark Davis, Stanford University; Nilabh Shastri, University of California at Berkeley; Susan Swain, University of California at San Diego; Diane Eardley, University of California at Santa Barbara; Pat Jones, Stanford University; John Nedrud, Case Western Reserve University; Anne Good, University of California at Berkeley; David Lubaroff, University of Iowa; Linda Bradley, University of California at San Diego; Robert Ellis, Colorado State University; Andrea Hubbard, University of Arizona; Marian Koshland, University of California at Berkeley; Joseph Goodman, University of California at San Francisco; David Raulet, MIT; Nora Sarvetnik, Scripps Research Institute; Kirk Johnson, Genentech Corporation; Wendy Havran, University of California at Berkeley.

I am grateful as well for the help and encouragement that I received from my many friends and colleagues. I especially want to thank my colleagues at San Francisco State University, my dean, James Kelley, my chairman,

Crellin Pauling, and my colleagues, William Wu, Remo Morelli, Ruth Doell, Mary Lucky, Michael Goldman, Bernard Goldstein, Dick Davis, Ann and Leigh Auleb, Rick Bernstein, Gregory Antipa, and Lisa Sardinia. I also want to thank my graduate student Amanda McNeese for her work on the index. Finally, I want to thank my secretary and good friend, Dotty Sims, who has been a constant source of support and encouragement along with Dennis and Jeanne Kuby.

I would also like to acknowledge my pleasure in working with the staff of W. H. Freeman and Company. In particular, I would like to thank Diane Maass for her expert editorial advice, for her attention to detail, for her direction of the manuscript and illustrations, and for her friendship and support during many stressful stages of the process. I would like to thank Nancy Singer for her outstanding work on the design and layout of this book. I also wish to acknowledge Mary Shuford and Gary Carlson who helped me during many critical times in this process. I am indebted to Armand Schwab for his many invaluable suggestions as a developmental editor; his many years of experience as managing editor of Scientific American Magazine brought clarity and breadth to my writing without altering its basic style. I am also grateful for Ruth Steyn's exceptional attention to detail. I would also like to thank Patrick Fitzgerald, who believed in me and started me on the road to this publication, and Kirk Jensen, who directed the early stages of the manuscript.

IMMUNOLOGY

Overview of the Immune System

The immune system is a remarkably adaptive defense system that has evolved in vertebrates to protect them from invading pathogenic microorganisms and cancer. It is able to generate an enormous variety of cells and molecules capable of specifically recognizing and eliminating an apparently limitless variety of foreign invaders. These cells and molecules act together in an exquisitely adaptable dynamic network whose complexity rivals that of the nervous system.

Functionally, an immune response can be divided into two interrelated activities—recognition and response. Immune recognition is remarkable for its specificity. The immune system is able to recognize subtle chemical differences that distinguish one foreign pathogen from another. At the same time, the system is able to discriminate between foreign molecules and the body's own cells and proteins. Once a foreign organism is recognized, the immune system enlists the participation of a variety of cells and molecules to mount an appropriate response, known as an effector function, to eliminate or neutralize the organism. In this way the system is able to convert the initial recognition event into different effector responses, each uniquely suited to eliminate a particular type of pathogen.

This chapter will present a broad overview of the cells and molecules that comprise the immune system and the mechanisms by which they protect the body against foreign invaders. As is always the case with an overview, the details have been simplified to reveal the essential structure of the immune system. Substantive discussions, experimental approaches, and in-depth definitions are left to the chapters that follow.

Historical Perspective

The discipline of immunology grew out of the observation that individuals who had recovered from certain infectious diseases were thereafter protected from the disease. The Latin term *immunis*, meaning exempt, is the source of the English word *immunity*. The concept of immunity can be traced back to 430 B.C. In describing a plague in Athens, Thucydides, the great historian of the Peloponnesian War, wrote that only those who had recovered from the plague could nurse the sick because they would not contract the disease a second time. Although the concept of immunity existed in folklore, it was almost two thousand years before the concept was successfully converted into a medically effective practice.

The first recorded crude attempts to induce immunity were performed by the Chinese and Turks in the fifteenth century. Various reports suggest that the dried crusts derived from smallpox pustules were either inhaled into the nostrils or inserted into small cuts in the skin (a technique called *variolation*). In 1718 Lady Mary Wortley Montagu, the wife of the British ambassador to Constantinople, observed the positive effects of variolation on the native population and had the technique applied to her own children. The technique was significantly improved by the English physician Edward Jenner in 1798. Jenner was intrigued by the fact that milkmaids who contracted cowpox (a mild disease) were subsequently immune to smallpox (a disfiguring and often fatal disease) and reasoned that it might be possible to protect people from smallpox by inoculating them with the fluid from a cowpox pustule. He tested his idea by

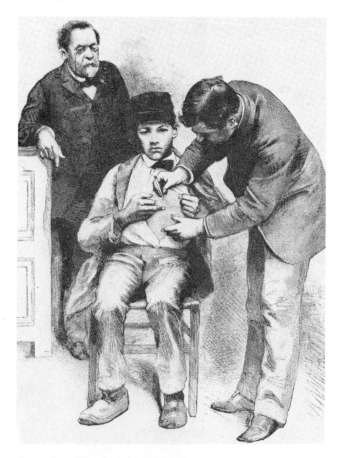

Figure 1-1   Wood engraving of Louis Pasteur watching Joseph Meister receive the rabies vaccine. [From *Harper's Weekly* **29**:836, 1885; courtesy of National Library of Medicine.]

inoculating an eight-year-old boy with fluid from a cowpox pustule and later intentionally infected the child with smallpox. The child did not develop smallpox. Nevertheless, one cannot help but question the ethical implications of such an experiment!

Jenner's technique of inoculating with cowpox to protect against smallpox spread quickly throughout Europe, but it was nearly 100 years before the technique was applied to other diseases by Louis Pasteur. As so often happens in science, serendipidity combined with astute observation provided the next major advance in immunology. Pasteur had been studying the bacterium that causes fowl cholera. He had succeeded in growing the organism in culture and had shown that it could induce cholera when injected into chickens. His studies were interrupted by his summer vacation, and when he returned, he used an old culture of the bacterium to inject into the chickens. The chickens became ill but—surprisingly—they recovered. Pasteur then grew a fresh culture of the bacterium. He intended to inject it into some fresh chickens, the story goes, but was low on chickens and therefore used the previously injected chickens. Much to his surprise, the chickens survived and were completely protected from the disease. Pasteur recognized that aging had weakened the virulence of the pathogen and that such an attenuated strain might be administered to protect against disease. He called this attenuated strain a *vaccine* (from Latin *vacca*, cow) in honor of Jenner's work with cowpox inoculation.

Pasteur extended these findings to other diseases, demonstrating that it was possible to attenuate, or weaken, a pathogen and administer the attenuated strain as a vaccine. In a now classical experiment at Pouilly-le-Fort in 1881, Pasteur vaccinated one group of sheep with heat-attenuated anthrax bacillus and then invited the public to watch as he challenged the sheep with a virulent culture of *Bacillus anthracis.* All the vaccinated sheep lived, whereas all unvaccinated animals died. These experiments marked the beginnings of the discipline of immunology. In 1885, Pasteur administered the first vaccine to a human, a young boy who had been bitten repeatedly by a rabid dog (Figure 1-1). The boy, Joseph Meister, lived and later became a custodian at the Pasteur Institute. In 1940, during the Nazi occupation of Paris, the Nazis asked Meister to give them the keys to Pasteur's crypt. Rather than surrender the keys to the Nazis, Meister took his own life.

Discovery of Humoral and Cellular Immunity

Although Pasteur proved that vaccination worked, he did not understand the mechanisms involved. The experimental work of Emil von Behring and Shibasaburo Kitasato in 1890 provided the first insights into the mechanism of immunity, earning von Behring the Nobel prize in medicine in 1901 (Table 1-1). Von Behring and Kitasato demonstrated that *serum* (the noncellular part of blood) from animals previously immunized to diph-

Table 1-1 Nobel prizes for immunologic research

Year	Recipient	Country	Research
1901	Emil von Behring	Germany	Serum antitoxins
1905	Robert Koch	Germany	Cellular immunity to tuberculosis
1908	Elie Metchnikoff Paul Ehrlich	Russia Germany	Work on immunity: phagocytosis (Metchnikoff) and antitoxins (Ehrlich)
1913	Charles Richet	France	Anaphylaxis
1919	Jules Bordet	Belgium	Complement mediated bacteriolysis
1930	Karl Landsteiner	U.S.A.	Discovery of human blood groups
1951	Max Theiler	South Africa	Developed yellow fever vaccine
1957	Daniel Bovet	Switzerland	Antihistamines
1960	F. Macfarlane Burnet Peter Medawar	Australia Great Britain	Discovery of acquired immunological tolerance
1972	Gerald Edelman Rodney Porter	U.S.A. Great Britain	Chemical structure of antibodies
1977	Rosalyn Yalow	U.S.A.	Developed radioimmunoassay
1980	George Snell Jean Dausset Baruj Benacerraf	U.S.A. France U.S.A.	Major histocompatibility complex
1984	Georges Koehler Cesar Milstein Niels Jerne	Germany Great Britain Denmark	Monoclonal antibody Immune regulatory theories
1991	E. Donnall Thomas Joseph Murray	U.S.A. U.S.A.	Transplantation immunology

theria could transfer the immune state to unimmunized animals. A serum antitoxin was suggested as the protective agent, and researchers spent the next decade characterizing the active component from immune serum. A serum component was shown to neutralize toxins, precipitate toxins, rupture (lyse) bacteria, and clump (agglutinate) bacteria—and it was named for each of these activities: antitoxin, precipitin, bacterolysin, and agglutinin. For some time it seemed that each of these activities might be due to a different serum component, and it was not until the 1930s that a single substance, called an *antibody*, was shown to be responsible for all of these activities. Because immunity was mediated by antibodies contained in body fluids (known at the time as *humors*) it was called *humoral immunity*.

Paralleling the discovery of serum antibody was the discovery by Elie Metchnikoff, in 1883, that cells also contribute to the immune state of an animal. Metchnikoff had observed that certain white blood cells were able to engulf microorganisms. He named these cells *phagocytes* in reference to their ability to ingest foreign ma-

terial. Metchnikoff observed that phagocytic cells were more active in immunized animals and hypothesized that cells, rather than antibodies, were the major effector of immunity. A controversy developed between those who held to the concept of humoral immunity and those who agreed with Metchnikoff's concept of *cell-mediated immunity*. The controversy foreshadowed the interrelated roles of humoral and cellular activities, both of which were later shown to be necessary for the immune response. In the 1950s the lymphocyte was identified as the cell responsible for both cellular and humoral immunity.

Early Theories of Immunity

One of the greatest enigmas about the antibody molecule is its specificity for foreign material, or *antigen*. Two major theories were proposed to account for this specificity: the *selective* theory and the *instructional* theory (Figure 1-2). The earliest conception of the selective

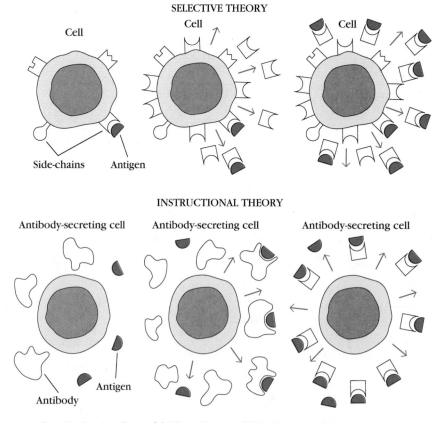

Figure 1-2 Early theories of antibody specificity. (a) The selective theory suggested that an antigen selects and binds to a specific side-chain receptor (antibody), which causes the cell to produce and release side-chains with the same specificity. The antigens bind to the side-chains in a lock and key arrangement. (b) The instructional theory suggested that a particular antigen would serve as a template around which the selected antibodies would enfold.

theory dates to Paul Ehrlich in 1900. In an attempt to explain the origin of serum antibody, Ehrlich proposed that cells expressed a variety of "side-chain" receptors that could react with infectious agents. Binding of an infectious agent to a side-chain receptor was envisioned as a complementary lock-and-key type of interaction. Ehrlich suggested that the interaction between an infectious agent and a cell's side-chain receptor would result in the release of the side chain and would induce the cell to produce and release more side-chain receptors with the same specificity. Ehrlich's theory was a selective theory: the side-chain specificity was determined prior to antigen exposure and antigen selected the appropriate side chain.

In the 1930s and 1940s the selective theory was replaced by various instructional theories. According to these theories, antigen played a central role in determining the specificity of the antibody molecule. The instructional theories suggested that a particular antigen would serve as a template around which antibody would fold. The antibody would thus assume a configuration complementary to that of the antigen template. Such concepts, first postulated by Friedrich Breinl and Felix Haurowitz and later popularized by Linus Pauling, made sense within the limitations of scientific knowledge at that time. But as new information emerged about the structure of DNA, RNA, and protein, the instructional theories were shown to be wrong.

In the 1950s, selection theories resurfaced and, through the insights of Niels Jerne, David Talmadge, and Macfarlane Burnet, were refined into a theory that came to be known as the *clonal-selection theory.* According to this theory, individual lymphocytes express membrane receptors that are specific for distinct antigens. Each lymphocyte expresses a unique receptor specificity, which is determined prior to the appearance of antigen. Binding of an antigen to a specific receptor activates the cell, resulting in its proliferation into a clone of cells, each with the same immunologic specificity as the original parent cell. The clonal-selection theory has been further refined and is now accepted as the underlying paradigm of modern immunology. This theory will be examined in more depth later in the chapter.

Innate (Nonspecific) Immunity

Immunity—the state of protection from infectious disease—has both nonspecific and specific components. Innate, or nonspecific, immunity refers to the basic resistance to disease that a species possesses. Innate immunity can be envisioned as comprising four types of defensive barriers: anatomic, physiologic, endocytic and phagocytic, and inflammatory.

Anatomic Barriers

Physical and anatomical barriers that tend to prevent the entry of pathogens are an organism's first line of defense against infection. The skin and the surface of mucous membranes, for example, provide an effective barrier to the entry of most microorganisms. Intact skin physically prevents the penetration of most pathogens; it also limits most bacterial growth because of its low pH, which results from its content of lactic and fatty acids. In order to gain entry, then, most pathogens need to colonize and penetrate the mucous-membrane barrier, but such colonization and penetration is inhibited by a number of innate defenses: Ciliated epithelial cells sweep entering microorganisms from the respiratory and gastrointestinal tracts. Saliva, tears, and mucous secretions may wash away potential invaders and contain antibacterial and antiviral proteins that destroy pathogens. If a pathogen eludes these anatomic defenses, it still must evade the other types of innate defenses.

The importance of anatomic barriers was highlighted by a recent study which showed that mice appeared to differ in their susceptibility to infection by a schistosome, a parasitic helminth that causes schistosomiasis, a chronic and debilitating disease in humans. After the mice were infected with the schistosome, some of the mice appeared to eliminate the schistosome before its life cycle could be completed whereas other mice were not able to do so. The group that eliminated the schistosome was thought to be immune and was considered to be a potential animal model for investigating new ways of treating the disease in humans. After a great deal of research funding was poured into this mouse model, it was discovered that its ability to clear the schistosome had nothing to do with a specific immunological response; instead, it was due to anatomical differences in the blood vessel architecture of the lungs and liver in these two groups of mice. The study cautioned against advancing immunological explanations before simple anatomical or physiological mechanisms have been investigated.

Physiologic Barriers

Physiologic barriers include temperature, pH, oxygen tension, and various soluble factors. Many species are not susceptible to certain diseases simply because their body temperature inhibits pathogen growth. Chickens, for example, display innate immunity to anthrax because their high body temperature inhibits the growth of this pathogen. Gastric acidity also provides an innate physiologic barrier to infection; indeed, few ingested microorganisms can survive the low pH of the stomach. A variety of soluble factors also contribute to nonspecific immunity. Among these soluble proteins are lysozyme, interferon, and complement. *Lysozyme*—a hydrolytic enzyme found in mucous secretions—is able to cleave the peptidoglycan layer of the bacterial cell wall. *Interferons* are a group of proteins produced by virus-infected cells. Among their many functions is the ability to bind to nearby cells and induce a generalized antiviral state. *Complement* is a group of serum proteins that circulate in an inactive proenzyme state. These proteins can be activated by a variety of specific and nonspecific immunologic mechanisms that convert the inactive proenzymes into active enzymes. The activated complement components participate in a controlled enzymatic cascade that results in membrane-damaging reactions, which destroy pathogenic organisms.

Endocytic and Phagocytic Barriers

Another important innate defense mechanism is the ingestion of extracellular macromolecules through either *endocytosis* or *phagocytosis.* In endocytosis, the macromolecules contained within the extracellular tissue fluid are internalized by cells. This internalization occurs as small regions of the plasma membrane invaginate, or fold inward, forming small (approximately 0.1 μm) endocytic vesicles. Endocytosis occurs through one of two processes: *pinocytosis* or *receptor-mediated endocytosis* (Figure 1-3). In pinocytosis, macromolecules are internalized through nonspecific membrane invagination. Because pinocytosis is nonspecific, the internalization of macromolecules occurs in proportion to their concentration. In receptor-mediated endocytosis, macromolecules are selectively internalized after binding to specific membrane receptors.

Following internalization by either process, the endocytic vesicles fuse with each other and are delivered to *endosomes.* The endosomes, acidic compartments within the cell, serve a sorting function. Their acid environment facilitates dissociation of the receptor from its ligand. The remaining macromolecules contained within the endosome are routed along a different pathway, where they fuse with *primary lysosomes,* to form structures known as *secondary lysosomes.* Primary ly-

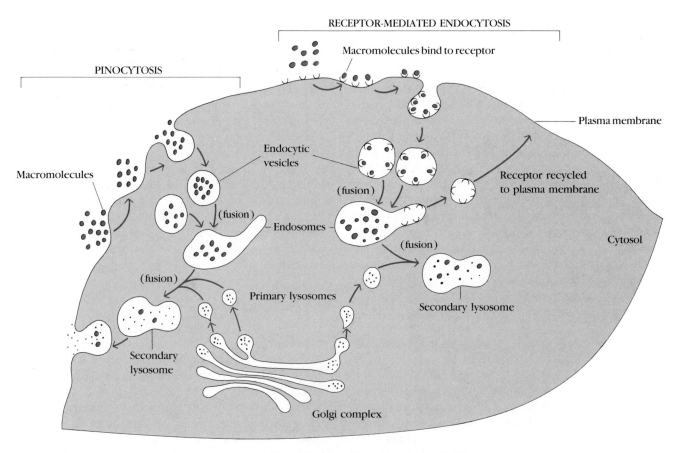

Figure 1-3   Endocytosis—the internalization of macromolecules within the extracellular fluid—occurs by pinocytosis or receptor-mediated endocytosis. In both processes, the ingested material is degraded via the endosomal processing pathway.

sosomes are derived from the golgi complex and contain large numbers of degradative enzymes, including proteases, nucleases, lipases and other hydrolytic enzymes. Within secondary lysosomes, the ingested macromolecules are then digested into small breakdown products (e.g., peptides, nucleotides, and sugars) in the *endosomal processing pathway*.

Phagocytosis involves the ingestion of particulate material, including whole pathogenic microorganisms (Figure 1-4). In phagocytosis, which differs from endocytosis in several ways, the plasma membrane expands around the particulate material to form large vesicles called *phagosomes*. These vesicles are roughly 10-to-20 times larger than endocytic vesicles. The expansion of the membrane in phagocytosis requires participation of microfilaments, which do not take part in endocytosis. Only specialized cells are capable of phagocytosis, whereas endocytosis is carried out by virtually all cells. The specialized phagocytic cells include blood monocytes, neutrophils, and tissue macrophages (see Chapter 3). Once particulate material is ingested into phagosomes, the phagosomes fuse with lysosomes and the ingested material is then digested in the endosomal processing pathway by a process similar to that seen in endocytosis.

Barriers Created by the Inflammatory Response

Tissue damage caused by a wound or by invasion by a pathogenic microorganism induces a complex sequence of events collectively known as the *inflammatory response*. Many of the classic features of the inflammatory response were described as early as 1600 B.C. in Egyptian papyrus writings. In the first century A.D., the Roman physician Celsus described the "four cardinal signs of inflammation" as *rubor* (redness), *tumor* (swelling), *calor* (heat), and *dolor* (pain). In the second century A.D., another physician, Galen, added a fifth cardinal sign: *functio laesa* (loss of function).

The cardinal signs of inflammation reflect three major events that occur in an inflammatory response: (1) increased blood flow, (2) increased capillary permeability, and (3) influx of phagocytic cells. The increase in blood flow to the affected area occurs as the blood vessels that carry blood away from the area constrict, resulting in engorgement of the capillary network. The engorged capillaries produce tissue redness (*erythema*) and an increase in tissue temperature. An increase in capillary permeability facilitates an influx of fluid and cells from the engorged capillaries into the surrounding tissue. The fluid that accumulates (*exudate*) has a much higher protein content than fluid normally released from the vasculature. Accumulation of exudate contributes to the tissue swelling. The increased capillary permeability also

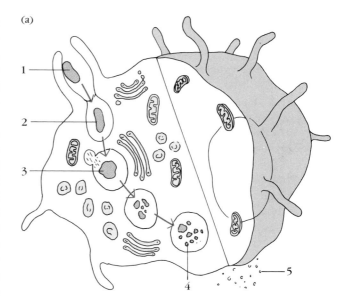

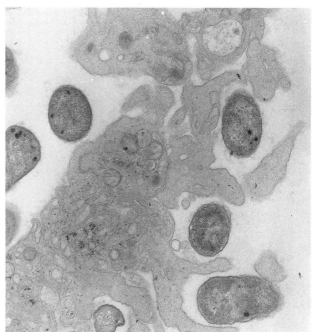

Figure 1-4 (a) The steps in phagocytosis: 1) attachment of the bacteria to long membrane evaginations, called pseudopodia, 2) ingestion into phagosomes, movement of the phagosome toward the lysosome, 3) fusion of the lysosome with the phagosome, releasing the enzyme contents of the lysosome into the phagosome, 4) digestion and 5) elimination of the ingested material. (b) Transmission electron micrograph of a phagocytic cell (neutrophil) showing pseudopods engulfing *E. coli* bacteria. (Calibration mark = 1 micron.) [Part (b) courtesy of Dr. Joseph R. Goodman, Dept. of Pediatrics, University of California at San Francisco.]

facilitates the migration of various white blood cells from the capillaries into the tissues. Phagocytic cells are the major type of white blood cell to emigrate. The emigration of phagocytes involves several steps: first, the phagocytes adhere to the endothelial wall (*margination*); then, they move between the capillary endothelial cells into the tissue (*diapedesis*); and finally, they migrate through the tissue to the site of the wound or infection (*chemotaxis*) (Figure 1-5).

The events in the inflammatory response are initiated by a complex series of interactions involving several chemical mediators; whose interactions are still only partially understood. Some of these mediators are derived from invading microorganisms, some are released from damaged tissue, some are generated by several plasma enzyme systems, and some are products of various white blood cells participating in the inflammatory response. Among the chemical mediators released in response to tissue damage are various serum proteins called *acute-phase proteins*. The concentrations of these proteins increase dramatically in tissue-damaging infections. *C-reactive protein* is a major acute-phase pro-

tein produced by the liver in response to tissue damage. C-reactive protein binds to the C-polysaccharide cell-wall component found on a variety of bacteria and fungi and activates the complement system, resulting in increased clearance of the pathogen either by complement-mediated lysis of the pathogen or by complement-mediated increases in phagocytosis.

Four enzyme systems in blood plasma participate in the inflammatory response: the clotting system, the kinin system, the fibrinolytic system, and the complement system. These four enzyme systems generate factors that induce constriction of the blood vessels, increased capillary permeability, diapedesis, chemotaxis, and clearance of the pathogen. These systems are discussed in more detail in Chapter 11.

Acquired (Specific) Immunity

Acquired, or specific, immunity reflects the presence of a functional immune system that is capable of specifically recognizing and selectively eliminating foreign micro-

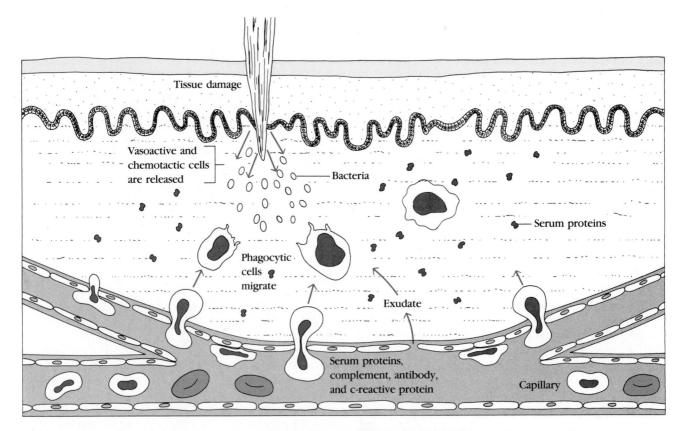

Figure 1-5   The inflammatory response. A bacterial infection causes tissue damage with release of various vasoactive and chemotactic factors. These factors induce increased blood flow to the area, increased capillary permeability, and influxes of white blood cells, including phagocytic and lymphocytes, from the blood into the tissues. The serum proteins contained in the exudate have anti-bacterial properties and the phagocyte will begin to engulf the bacteria.

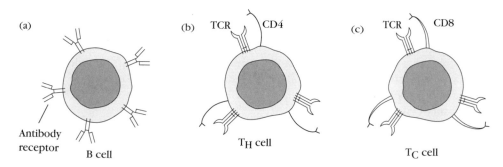

Figure 1-6 The membrane receptors for antigen on B cells and T cells. (a) B cells have about 10⁵ molecules of membrane-bound antibody receptor per cell. Each antibody molecule possesses identical specificity for antigen and can interact directly with antigen. (b) T lymphocytes have about 10⁵ molecules of the antigen-binding T-cell receptor per cell, each with identical specificity. T cells bearing CD4 always recognize antigen associated with class II MHC, and generally function as T helper cells. (c) T cells bearing CD8 always recognize antigen associated with class I MHC, and generally function as T cytotoxic cells.

organisms and molecules. Unlike innate immunity, acquired immunity displays *specificity, diversity, memory,* and *self/nonself recognition.* These four features characterize all immune responses.

The specificity of the immune system can be seen in its capacity to distinguish subtle differences among antigens. In some cases a single mutation, resulting in a single amino acid substitution, is all that is necessary for an antigen to escape an effective immune response. The immune system is capable of generating tremendous diversity in its recognition molecules, allowing it to specifically recognize billions of uniquely different structures on foreign antigens. Once the immune system has responded to an antigen, it exhibits memory; that is, a second encounter with the same antigen induces a heightened state of immune reactivity. Because of this attribute, the immune system can confer life-long immunity to many infectious agents. Finally, the ability of the immune system to respond only to foreign antigens indicates that the immune system is capable of distinguishing self from nonself. It is essential that the immune response be limited to nonself-antigens, for the consequence of an inappropriate response to self-antigens can be a fatal autoimmune disease.

Acquired immunity does not occur independently of innate immunity. Cells of the phagocytic system, most notably macrophages, are intimately involved in activation of the specific immune response. At the same time, various soluble factors, produced during a specific immune response, have been shown to augment the activity of these phagocytic cells. As an inflammatory response develops, for example, soluble mediators are produced that attract cells of the immune system. The immune response will, in turn, serve to regulate the intensity of the inflammatory response. Through the carefully regulated interplay of acquired and innate immunity, the two systems work together to effectively eliminate a foreign invader.

The Cells of the Immune System

Generation of an effective immune response involves two major groups of cells: *lymphocytes* and *antigen-presenting cells.* Lymphocytes are one of many types of white blood cells produced in the bone marrow during the process of hematopoiesis (see Chapter 3). Lymphocytes leave the bone marrow, circulate in the blood and lymph system, and reside in various lymphoid organs. The attributes of specificity, diversity, memory, and self/nonself recognition are mediated by the lymphocytes. Lymphocytes are able to recognize antigens by means of membrane receptors specific for the foreign material. There are two major populations of lymphocytes: the B lymphocytes (B cells) and the T lymphocytes (T cells).

B Lymphocytes

B lymphocytes mature within the bone marrow and leave the marrow expressing a unique antigen-binding membrane receptor (Figure 1-6a). The B-cell receptor is an *antibody molecule,* a membrane-bound glycoprotein. The basic structure of the antibody molecule consists of two identical heavy polypeptide chains and two identical light polypeptide chains. The chains are held together by disulfide bonds. The amino-terminal ends of each heavy-and light-chain pair form a cleft within which antigen binds. When a B cell encounters the antigen for which its membrane-bound antibody is specific, the cell begins to divide rapidly; its progeny differentiate into *memory B cells* and effector cells called *plasma cells.* Memory B cells have a longer lifespan and continue to express membrane-bound antibody with the same specificity as the original parent cell. Plasma cells do not produce membrane-bound antibody but instead produce the antibody in a form that can be secreted. Plasma cells live for only a few days but they secrete enormous amounts of antibody during this time. It has been estimated that a single plasma cell can secrete more than 2000 molecules of antibody per second. Secreted antibodies are the major effector molecule of humoral immunity.

T Lymphocytes

T lymphocytes also arise from hematopoietic stem cells in the bone marrow. Unlike B cells, which mature within the bone marrow, T cells migrate to the thymus gland to mature. During its maturation within the thymus, the T cell comes to express a unique membrane receptor for antigen. The *T-cell receptor* is a heterodimer, composed of two protein chains, either alpha and beta ($\alpha\beta$) or gamma and delta ($\gamma\delta$), which are linked by disulfide bonds. The amino-terminal ends of the two chains fold together to form the antigen-binding cleft of the T-cell receptor. Unlike B-cell receptors, which can recognize antigen alone, T-cell receptors can recognize antigen only in association with cell-membrane proteins known as *major histocompatibility complex (MHC) molecules.* When a T cell encounters antigen associated with a MHC molecule on a cell, the T cell proliferates and differentiates into *memory T cells* and various effector T cells.

There are two subpopulations of T cells: *T helper (T_H) cells* and *T cytotoxic (T_C) cells.* A third type of T cell, called a *T suppressor cell* has been postulated, but recent evidence has led many researchers to question whether its lineage is distinct from the T_H and T_C subpopulations (see Chapter 14). The T helper and T cytotoxic cells can be distinguished by their display of one of two membrane glycoproteins, either CD4 or CD8 (see Figure 1-6b). The T cells displaying CD4 generally function as T_H cells, whereas those displaying CD8 generally function as T_C cells (see Chapter 3). In response to the recognition of antigen and MHC, a T_H cell secretes various growth factors known collectively as *cytokines* or, more specifically, *lymphokines.* As a T_H cell is activated, it becomes an effector cell secreting various lymphokines. These lymphokines play an important role in activating B cells, T_C cells, phagocytic cells, and various other cells that participate in the immune response. Changes in the pattern of lymphokines produced by T_H cells results in qualitative changes in the type of immune response that develops. Under the influence of T_H-derived lymphokines, when the T_C cell recognizes antigen together with MHC molecules, the T_C cell proliferates and differentiates into an effector cell called a *cytotoxic*

T lymphocyte (CTL). In contrast to the T_H cell, the CTL generally does not secrete many lymphokines and instead acquires cytotoxic activity. The CTL has a vital function in monitoring the cells of the body and eliminating any that display antigen, such as virus-infected cells, tumor cells, and cells of a foreign tissue graft.

Antigen-Presenting Cells

Activation of both the humoral and cell-mediated branches of the immune system requires lymphokines produced by T_H cells. It is essential that activation of T_H cells be carefully regulated because an inappropriate T_H-cell response to self-components can have fatal autoimmune consequences. To ensure careful regulation, the T_H cell can be activated following antigen recognition only when the antigen is displayed together with MHC on the surface of specialized cells called *antigen-presenting cells (APCs)*. Antigen-presenting cells, which include macrophages, B cells, and dendritic cells, are distinguished by their expression of a particular type of MHC molecule. These specialized cells internalize antigen, either by phagocytosis or by endocytosis, and then re-express a part of that antigen, together with the MHC molecule, on their membrane. The T_H cell then recognizes the antigen associated with the MHC molecule on the membrane of the antigen-presenting cell.

Functions of Humoral and Cell-Mediated Immune Responses

As mentioned earlier, immune responses can be divided into humoral and cell-mediated responses. The term *humoral* is derived from the Latin *humor*, meaning body fluid; thus humoral immunity refers to immunity that can be conferred on a nonimmune individual by administration of serum antibodies from an immune individual. The humoral branch of the immune system involves interaction of B cells with antigen and their subsequent proliferation and differentiation into antibody-secreting plasma cells (Figure 1-7). The antibody functions as an effector molecule of the humoral response by binding to antigen and neutralizing it or facilitating its elimination. When an antigen is coated with antibody, it can be eliminated in several ways. For example, antibody can cross-link the antigen, forming clusters that are more readily ingested by phagocytic cells. Binding of antibody to the antigen also can activate the complement system, resulting in lysis of the foreign organism. Antibody can also neutralize toxins or viral particles by coating them and preventing their subsequent binding to host cells.

Effector T cells generated in response to antigen are responsible for cell-mediated immunity (Figure 1-7). Unlike humoral immunity, which can be transferred by

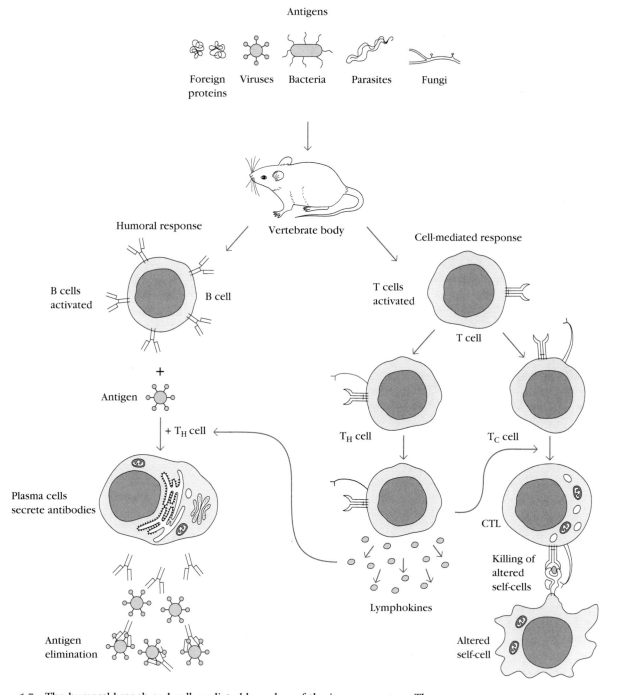

Figure 1-7 The humoral branch and cell-mediated branches of the immune system. The humoral response involves interaction of B lymphocytes with antigen and their differentiation into antibody-secreting plasma cells. The secreted antibody binds to the antigen and facilitates its clearance from the body. The cell-mediated response involves various subpopulations of T lymphocytes that recognize antigen presented on self-cells. T_H cells respond to antigen with the production of lymphokines and cytotoxic T lymphocytes (CTL) mediate killing of cells that have been altered by antigen (e.g., virus-infected cells).

serum antibody, cell-mediated immunity can only be transferred by immune T cells. Both T_H and CTLs serve as effector cells in cell-mediated immune reactions. Lymphokines secreted by T_H cells can activate various phagocytic cells, enabling them to phagocytose and kill microorganisms more effectively. This type of cell-mediated immune response is especially important in host defense against intracellular bacteria. Activated cytotoxic T lymphocytes participate in cell-mediated immune reactions by killing altered self-cells; they play an important role in the killing of virus-infected cells and tumor cells.

Recognition of Antigen by B and T Lymphocytes

Antigens, which are generally very large and complex, are not recognized in their entirety by T or B lymphocytes. Instead, both T and B lymphocytes recognize discrete sites on the antigen called antigenic determinants, or *epitopes*. Epitopes are the immunologically active regions on a complex antigen, the regions that actually bind to a B- or T-cell's receptor. The most important difference in antigen recognition by T lymphocytes and B lymphocytes is that B cells can recognize an epitope alone, whereas T cells can recognize an epitope only when it is present on the surface of a self-cell in association with a MHC molecule. The two branches of the immune system are therefore uniquely suited to recognize antigen in different milieus. The humoral branch (B cells) recognizes an enormous variety of epitopes;

those displayed on the surface of bacteria or viral particles, as well as those displayed on soluble proteins or glycoproteins that have been released from invading pathogens. The cell-mediated branch (T cells) recognizes epitopes displayed together with molecules of the major histocompatibility complex on self-cells. As noted previously, the cell-mediated branch of the immune response is uniquely suited to recognize altered self-cells, such as virus-infected self-cells and cancerous cells.

Four related but distinct cell-membrane molecules are responsible for antigen recognition by the immune system: membrane-bound antibodies on B cells; heterodimeric T-cell receptors (either $\alpha\beta$ or $\gamma\delta$); class I MHC molecules present on all nucleated cells; and class II MHC molecules present on antigen-presenting cells. Each of these molecules plays a unique role in antigen recognition, ensuring that the immune system can recognize and respond to different types of antigen.

Generation of B-Cell and T-Cell Specificity and Diversity

The specificity of each B cell is determined by the specificity of its membrane-bound antigen-binding receptor (i.e., antibody) expressed by that cell. The antibody receptor on a B cell can recognize different epitopes with incredible precision. Even protein antigens that differ by only a single amino acid can often be discriminated from each other. Each mature B cell's distinct antibody specificity is generated by random rearrangements of a series of gene segments encoding the anti-

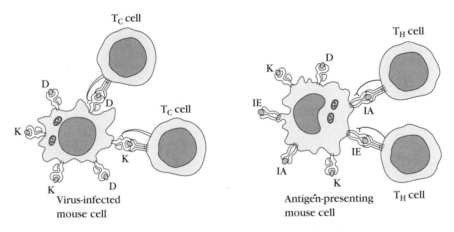

Figure 1-8   Class I and class II MHC molecules are encoded by different loci within the MHC complex. The class I MHC molecules are encoded by the K and D loci in mice or the A, B, and C loci in humans and are expressed on nearly all nucleated cells. The class II MHC molecules are encoded by the IA and IE loci in mice or the DP, DQ, and DR loci in humans and are only expressed on antigen presenting cells. T helper cells generally recognize antigen expressed together with the class II MHC molecule and are class II restricted, T cytotoxic cells are generally class I restricted, recognizing antigen together with class I MHC molecules.

body molecule as the B cell matures in the bone marrow (see Chapter 8). As a result of this combinatorial process, the B cell comes to express a single gene arrangement for the antibody's heavy and light chains, so that each B lymphocyte synthesizes a single antibody molecule. The lymphocyte displays some of these molecules as receptors on its membrane; all 10^5 antibody molecules on a given B lymphocyte have identical specificity, giving each B lymphocyte, and the clone of daughter cells to which it gives rise, a distinct specificity for antigen. The mature B lymphocyte is therefore said to be *antigenically committed.*

The fine specificity of the antibody molecule is coupled to an enormous diversity. The random gene rearrangements that occur during B-cell maturation generate an enormous number of antibody specificities. The resulting B-cell population consists of individual B cells, each expressing a distinct antibody specificity, that collectively expresses enormous diversity—estimated to exceed 10^8 different antibody specificities.

The attributes of specificity and diversity that characterize the antibody molecule of the B cell also apply to the $\alpha\beta$ or $\gamma\delta$ heterodimers of the T cell. As in B-cell maturation, the process of T-cell maturation also involves random rearrangements of a series of gene segments encoding the cell's antigen receptor (see Chapter 10). Each T lymphocyte expresses about 10^5 receptors per cell, and all 10^5 receptors on a cell and its clonal progeny have identical specificity for antigen. The process of random rearrangement of the genes encoding the T-cell receptor is capable of generating enormous diversity—on the order of 10^{15} unique receptor specificities. Unlike the antibody receptor of the B cell, the enormous potential diversity of the T-cell receptor is later diminished through a process of selection in the thymus—a process ensuring that only T cells with receptors capable of recognizing antigen associated with MHC molecules will be able to mature (see Chapter 10).

Role of the Major Histocompatibility Complex

The major histocompatibility complex (MHC) is a large genetic complex with multiple loci. The MHC loci encode two major classes of membrane molecules: class I and class II MHC molecules (see Figure 1-8). The class I molecules are glycoproteins found on the membrane of nearly all nucleated cells, always in association with a small protein called β_2-microglobulin. There are three class I loci in humans (A, B, and C) and two in mice (K and D). Each of the class I MHC loci has a large number of different *alleles,* that is, different forms of the same gene. A person inherits one allele from each parent for each locus and therefore expresses multiple class I MHC

molecules on each of his or her nucleated cells. Class II MHC molecules are glycoproteins expressed by the various specialized cells that function as antigen-presenting cells. There are three class II loci in humans (DR, DP, and DQ) and two in mice (IA and IE). Each class II locus has two genes, an α gene and a β gene, which respectively encode the α and β chains of the class II MHC molecule. As in the case of the class I MHC, there are a large number of different alleles for each class II locus. Because a person inherits one allele from each parent for each locus, the surface of the antigen-presenting cell has multiple class II MHC molecules.

MHC molecules also function as antigen-recognition molecules, but unlike the B- or T-cell receptors, MHC molecules do not posses fine specificity for antigen; instead, MHC molecules bind to a broader spectrum of molecules than do antibodies and T-cell receptors. Both class I and class II MHC molecules have a structure in which the distal region (farthest from the membrane) of different alleles display wide variation in their amino acid sequences. These distal regions form a cleft within which the epitope sits. With the epitope thus bound, the class I and class II MHC molecules present the foreign antigen to T lymphocytes. Because the structure of the epitope-binding cleft is determined by differences in the allelic form of the genes encoding class I and class II molecules, the ability of an individual to present an antigen to T lymphocytes is influenced by the particular set of alleles that they have inherited.

Processing and Presentation of Antigens

In order for a foreign protein antigen to be recognized by a T cell it must be degraded into small peptides that form physical complexes with a class I or class II MHC molecule. This conversion of proteins into MHC-associated peptide fragments is called *antigen processing.* Whether an antigen will be processed and presented together with class I MHC or class II MHC molecules appears to be determined by the route that the antigen takes to enter a cell (Figure 1-9).

Exogenous antigen is produced outside of the host cell and enters the cell by endocytosis or phagocytosis. Antigen-presenting cells, such as macrophages and B cells, process the exogenous antigen into peptide fragments within the endosomal processing pathway. Experiments suggest that the class II MHC molecules are expressed within the endosomal processing pathway and that peptides produced during antigen processing bind to the cleft within the class II MHC molecule. The MHC molecule bearing the peptide is then exported to the cell surface. Since class II MHC expression is limited to antigen-presenting cells, expression of exogenous peptide/MHC complexes will be limited to these cells.

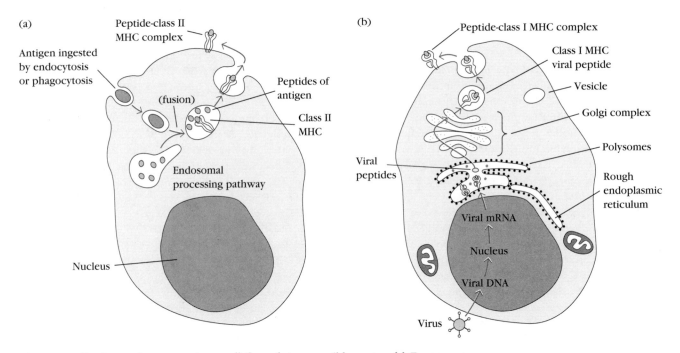

Figure 1-9 Foreign antigen can enter a cell through two possible routes. (a) Exogenous antigen, ingested by endocytosis or phagocytosis, is thought to enter the endosomal processing pathway. Here, within an acidic environment, the antigen is digested into small peptides which are then expressed with class II MHC molecules on the membrane of the antigen-presenting cell. (b) Endogenous antigen, which is produced within the cell itself, as in a virally-infected cell, will be processed within the cytoplasm and expressed with class I MHC membrane molecules.

T cells displaying CD4 recognize antigen associated with class II MHC and are said to be *MHC class II restricted.* These cells generally function as T helper cells.

Endogenous antigen is produced within the host cell itself. Two common examples are viral proteins synthesized within virus-infected host cells and unique proteins synthesized by cancerous cells. Endogenous antigens are thought to be degraded into peptide fragments that bind to class I MHC molecules within the endoplasmic reticulum. The peptide-MHC complex is then transported to the cell membrane. Since all nucleated cells express class I MHC molecules, all cells producing endogenous antigen will use this route to process the antigen. T cells displaying CD8 recognize antigen associated with class I MHC and are said to be *MHC class I restricted.* These cells generally function as T cytotoxic cells.

Clonal Selection

A mature immunocompetent animal contains a large number of antigen-reactive clones of T and B lymphocytes; the specificity of each of these clones is determined by the specificity of the antigen-binding receptor on the membrane of the clone's lymphocytes. *The specificity of each T and B lymphocyte is determined prior to contact with the antigen.* As described previously, during maturation of each T and B cell, its specificity is determined by the random gene rearrangements of the membrane receptor genes. The role of antigen becomes critical when it interacts with and activates mature, antigenically committed T and B cells, bringing about the

Figure 1-10 Maturation and clonal selection of B lymphocytes. Maturation, which occurs in the absence of antigen, produces antigenically committed B cells, each of which expresses antibody with a single antigenic specificity (shown here as W, X, Y, and Z). Clonal selection occurs when a given antigen binds to a B cell whose membrane-bound antibody molecules are specific for epitopes on that antigen. Clonal expansion of the selected antigen-reactive B cells leads to a clone of memory B cells and effector cells, called plasma cells; all cells in the expanded clone are specific for the original antigen. The plasma cells secrete antibody reactive with the activating antigen. Similar processes occur in the T-lymphocyte population resulting in clones of T memory and effector cells; the latter include T$_H$ cells, which secrete lymphokines, and cytotoxic T lymphocytes (CTL).

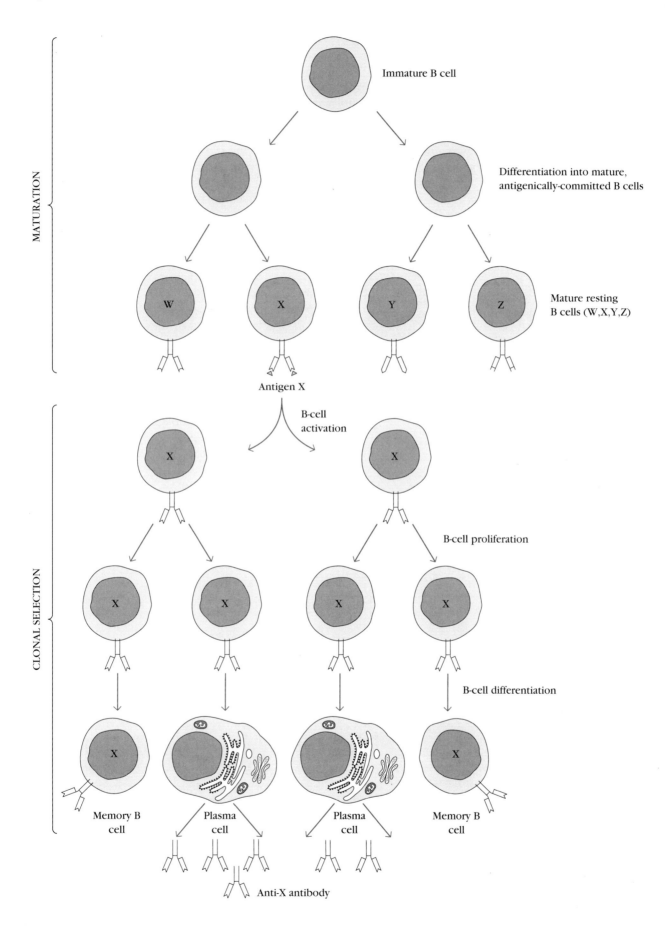

MATURATION

Immature B cell

Differentiation into mature, antigenically-committed B cells

Mature resting B cells (W,X,Y,Z)

Antigen X

CLONAL SELECTION

B-cell activation

B-cell proliferation

B-cell differentiation

Memory B cell

Plasma cell

Plasma cell

Memory B cell

Anti-X antibody

expansion of the population of cells with a given antigenic specificity. In this process of clonal selection, an
antigen binds to and stimulates a particular cell to
undergo mitosis and develop into a clone of cells with
the same antigenic specificity as the original parent cell
(Figure 1-10).

Clonal selection provides a framework for understanding three aspects of acquired immunity: specificity,
memory, and self/nonself recognition. Specificity is

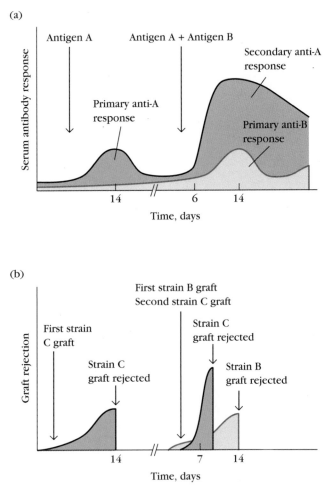

Figure 1-11   Differences in the primary and secondary response to injected antigen (humoral response) and to skin
graft (cell-mediated response) reflect the phenomenon of
immunologic memory. (a) When an animal is injected with
an antigen, it produces a primary serum antibody response
of low magnitude and relatively short duration, peaking at
about 10–17 days. A second immunization with the same
antigen results in a secondary response that is greater in
magnitude, peaks in less time (2–7 days), and lasts longer
(months to years) than the primary response. (b) When skin
from a strain B mouse is grafted onto a strain A mouse, the
graft is rejected in about 10–14 days. If a second strain A
graft is grafted onto the same mouse, it is rejected much
more vigorously and rapidly than the first graft.

shown because only lymphocytes whose receptors are
specific for a given epitope on an antigen will be clonally
expanded and thus mobilized for an immune response.
Memory is displayed by the larger number of antigen-
reactive lymphocytes present after clonal selection.
Many of these lymphocytes appear to have a longer
lifespan and are referred to as memory cells. The initial
encounter of an antigen-specific lymphocyte with an
antigen induces a *primary response*; a second contact
with antigen will induce a more rapid and heightened
secondary response (Figure 1-11). The amplified memory-cell population accounts for the more rapid and
intense response that characterizes a secondary response and distinguishes it from the initial primary response. Self/nonself discrimination is accomplished by
the clonal elimination, during development, of lymphocytes bearing self-reactive receptors or by the functional
suppression of these cells in adults.

Clonal selection occurs within both the humoral and
cell-mediated branches of the immune system. In the
humoral branch, antigen induces the clonal proliferation
of B lymphocytes into antibody-secreting plasma cells
and B memory cells. In the cell-mediated branch, the
recognition of an antigen-MHC complex by a specific
T lymphocyte induces clonal proliferation into various
T cells with effector functions, such as T helper and T
cytotoxic cells, and into T memory cells.

Cellular Interactions Required for Generation of an Immune Response

Both the humoral and the cell-mediated branches of the
immune system require interaction among several different types of cells to induce a specific immunologic
response. These cells include various antigen-presenting
cells, T_H cells, and either B cells for induction of humoral
immunity or T_C cells for induction of cell-mediated immunity. Both branches require that antigen be processed
and presented with a class II MHC molecule on the
membrane of appropriate antigen-presenting cells, in
particular macrophages, which also secrete a cytokine
called interleukin 1 (IL-1).

Activation and Proliferation of T Helper Cells

The generation of both humoral and cell-mediated immune responses depends on the activation of T_H cells.
This process begins when a T_H cell, whose membrane
receptor is specific for processed antigen, and its associated class II MHC molecule interact with an antigen-
presenting cell (Figure 1-12). This interaction, together
with IL-1, induces a series of membrane changes in the
T_H cell, leading to its activation. The activation of the
T_H cell induces secretion of another cytokine, interleu-

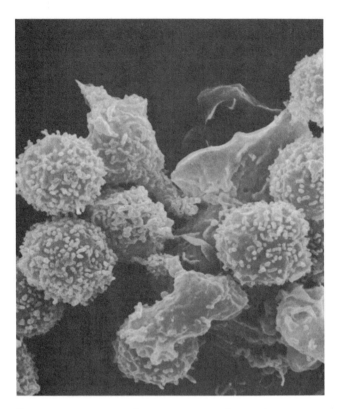

Figure 1-12 Scanning electron micrograph reveals numerous T lymphocytes interacting with a single macrophage. The macrophage presents processed antigen associated with class II MHC molecules to the T cells. [From William E. Paul, ed., 1991, *Immunology: Recognition and Response*, W. H. Freeman and Company, New York; courtesy of Morten H. Nielsen and Ole Werdelin.]

kin 2 (IL-2), and the expression on the cell of a high-affinity membrane receptor for IL-2. The secreted IL-2 binds to the newly expressed receptor and autostimulates T_H-cell proliferation. The clonally expanded population of antigen-specific T_H cells can now play a role in the activation of the B and T lymphocytes that generate the humoral and cell-mediated responses, respectively.

Generation of the Humoral Response

Mature antigen-committed B lymphocytes are seeded out from the bone marrow to circulate in the blood or lymph or to reside in various lymphoid organs. The lifespan of the B cell is only a few days unless antigen interacts with the cell, thereby triggering further differentiation and maturation. The events leading to B-cell activation require antigen crosslinkage of the B cell's membrane-antibody receptor and growth factors secreted by macrophages and T_H cells (Figure 1-13). The interaction with the antigen-specific T_H cell is facilitated by the B cell itself, which serves as an antigen-presenting cell for the T_H cell. Unlike the macrophage, which is

nonspecific, the B cell specifically captures antigen with its membrane antibody receptor and then internalizes some of that antigen, which is processed and re-presented on the membrane with a class II MHC molecule. The antigen-specific T_H cell binds to this antigen-MHC complex and thereupon secretes a number of cytokines, including interleukin 2 (IL-2), interleukin 4 (IL-4), interleukin 6 (IL-6), and interferon gamma (IFN-γ), which serve to activate various stages of B-cell division and differentiation. Interleukin 1 secreted by macrophages also acts as a growth factor for the B lymphocyte. The activated B lymphocyte undergoes a series of cell divisions over approximately a 5-day period differentiating into a population of both antibody-secreting plasma cells and memory cells.

Generation of the Cell-Mediated Response

The cell-mediated response is generated by various subpopulations of T lymphocytes. As in the case of the humoral response, a clonally expanded population of antigen-specific activated T_H cells is required. These T_H cells serve to activate various T effector cells that generate cell-mediated responses. The T_C cell, for example, recognizes processed antigen associated with class I MHC on the membrane of self-cells. In the presence of IL-2 secreted by the T_H cell, the T_C cell becomes a cytotoxic T lymphocyte (CTL), which mediates membrane damage to the altered self-cell leading to cell lysis (Figure 1-13).

The cytokines secreted by activated T_H cells also regulate the proliferation and differentiation of a number of nonspecific effector cells that play various roles in cell-mediated immune responses. These nonspecific effector cells do not possess the immunologic attributes of specificity and memory, and so the regulation of their activity depends on the activity of the antigen-specific T_H cell. Various cytokines, such as interleukin 2 and interferon gamma, have been shown to activate macrophages, for example. These *activated macrophages* exhibit enhanced phagocytic activity and enhanced ability to kill ingested pathogens. In addition, these activated macrophages have been shown to be capable of killing certain tumor cells and cells infected by parasites. The *natural killer (NK) cell* is another nonspecific effector cell whose activity is enhanced by interleukin 2 and interferon gamma produced by activated T_H cells. The NK cell is a large, granular lymphocyte that lacks the membrane markers of the T- and the B-cell lineages. NK cells have been shown to kill tumor cells; however, how these cells recognize a tumor cell is unclear, given that they lack the specific antigen-binding receptors of either B or T cells.

In some cases antibody molecules produced during the humoral response can influence the cell-mediated

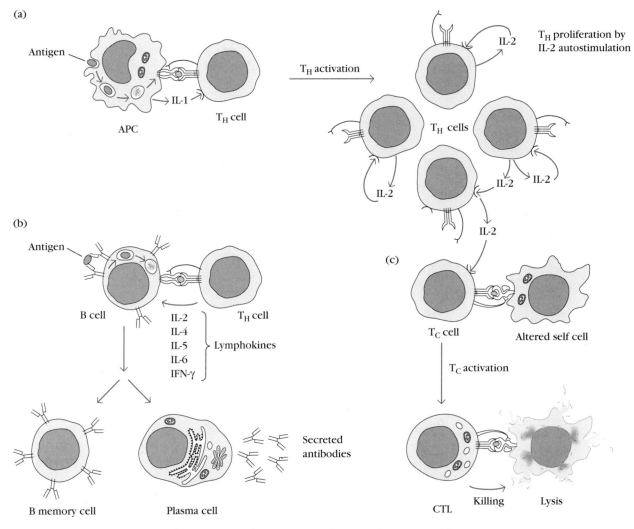

Figure 1-13 Cellular interactions (colored arrows) involved in induction of immunity. (a) Generation of both humoral and cell-mediated immune responses requires activation and proliferation of T$_H$ cells. The T$_H$ cell recognizes processed antigen associated with a class II MHC molecule on the membrane of an antigen presenting cell. This interaction, together with interleukin-1, will activate the T$_H$ cell. Activation of the T$_H$ cell causes the cell to begin to secrete IL-2 and express a membrane receptor for IL-2. The secreted IL-2 binds to the IL-2 receptor autostimulating T$_H$ proliferation. (b) Generation of the humoral response begins with antigen crosslinkage of the B cell membrane antibody receptor. Some of the antigen is internalized, processed in the endosomal processing pathway and expressed on the B cell membrane together with class II MHC molecules. The T$_H$ cell recognizes the antigen together with the class II MHC on the B cell membrane and secretes various lymphokines that activate the B cell to proliferate and differentiate into antibody-secreting plasma cells and B memory cells. (c) Generation of the cell-mediated response to, for example, a virus-infected cell begins when a T$_C$ cell recognizes processed viral antigen associated with class I MHC on the membrane of the infected cell. This recognition together with the growth factor, IL-2, secreted from the T$_H$ cell leads to activation of the T$_C$ cell into a cytotoxic T lymphocyte (CTL) capable of lysing the infected self-cell.

response to a foreign cell. Both macrophages and some NK cells, for example, have membrane receptors that can bind the carboxyl-terminal end of an antibody molecule. The amino-terminal end of an antibody molecule contains the antigen-binding site. Thus, an antibody may bind both to the foreign cell and to NK cells or macrophages, forming a bridge that allows these cells to interact with the foreign cell. In this process, referred to as *antibody-dependent cell-mediated cytotoxicity (ADCC)*, antibody provides the specificity, but killing is mediated by the nonspecific macrophage or NK cell.

References

ADA, G. L., and G. NOSSAL. 1987. The clonal selection theory. *Sci. Am.* **257**(2):62.

GREY, H. M., A. SETTE, and S. BUUS. 1989. How T cells see antigen. *Sci. Am.* **261**(5):56.

MARRACK, P., and J. KAPPLER. 1986. The T cell and its receptor. *Sci. Am.* **254**(2):36.

TONEGAWA, S. 1985. The molecules of the immune system. *Sci. Am.* **253**(4):122.

Study Questions

1. Indicate to which branch(es) of the immune system—the humoral or cell-mediated—each of the following statements applies by placing an X in the appropriate column. Some statements may apply to both branches.

Statement	Humoral	Cell-mediated
a. Involves class I MHC molecules		
b. Most likely responds to viral infection		
c. Involves T helper cells		
d. Involves processed antigen		
e. Most likely responds to an organ transplant		
f. Involves T cytotoxic cells		
g. Involves B cells		
h. Involves CD8		
i. Most likely responds to bacterial infection		
j. Involves secreted antibody		

2. Name three features of a secondary immune response that make it different from a primary immune response.

3. How does clonal selection contribute to memory in the immune response?

4. Interleukin 2 is a nonspecific growth factor that stimulates growth of T_H cells during the immune response. In view of this nonspecificity of IL-2, what mechanism assures that only those T_H cells specific for a given antigen are activated and that all other T_H cells are not activated.

5. Compare and contrast the four antigen-recognition molecules utilized by the immune system—membrane-bound antibody, T-cell receptor, class I MHC molecules, and class II MHC molecules—in terms of (a) their specificity for antigen, (b) their cellular expression, and (c) the types of antigen they recognize.

Experimental Systems

Experimental systems, in which well-defined populations of lymphocytes can be studied, are used to unravel the complex cellular interactions involved in the immune response. The choice of experimental system influences the kinds of data that can be generated and places certain limitations on the interpretation of those data: In vivo systems, which involve the whole animal, provide the most natural experimental conditions. However, due to their complexity, in vivo systems have a myriad of unknown and uncontrollable cellular interactions that add ambiguity to the interpretation of data. At the other extreme are in vitro systems, in which defined populations of lymphocytes are studied under controlled and consequently repeatable conditions; in vitro systems can be simplified to the extent that individual cellular interactions can be studied effectively. Yet in vitro systems have their own limitations, the most notable of which is their artificiality. One must ask whether a cellular response observed in vitro reflects reality or is a product of the unique conditions generated by the in vitro system itself. In this chapter some of the experimental systems routinely used by immunologists to study the immune system are described. The chapter also includes a discussion of some of the techniques provided by recombinant DNA technology that have revolutionized the study of the immune system in the past decade or so.

Experimental Animal Models

The study of the immune system in vertebrates is dependent on suitable animal models. The choice of an animal depends on its suitability for attaining a particular research goal. If large amounts of antiserum are sought, a rabbit, goat, sheep, or horse might be an appropriate experimental animal. If the goal is development of a protective vaccine, the animal chosen must be susceptible to the infectious agent so that the efficacy of the vaccine can be assessed. In many cases mice or rabbits will serve for vaccine development, but if growth of the

Table 2-1   Some inbred mouse strains commonly used in immunology

Strain	Abbreviation	Common substrains	Characteristics
A	A	A He A J A WySn	High mammary tumor incidence in some substrains
AKR	AK	AKR J AKR N AKR Cum	High incidence of leukemia. AKR Cum carries Thy 1.2 allele while others carry Thy 1.1; this gene encodes a surface protein of T cells
BALB c	C	BALB c*j* BALB c AnN BALB cBy	Sensitive to radiation
CBA	CBA	CBA J CBA H CBA N	CBA J carries *rd* gene causing retinal degeneration CBA N carries *xid* gene causing X-linked immunodeficiency
C3H	C3	C3H He C3H HeJ C3H HeN	Carries *rd* gene causing retinal degeneration. Many substrains have a high mammary tumor incidence because they carry a mammary tumor virus that is passed via maternal milk to offspring
C57BL 6	B6	C57BL 6J C57BL 6By C57BL 6N	
C57BL 10	B10	C57BL 10J C57BL 10ScSn C57BL 10N	Very closely related to B6, but differs in at least two loci. Often used as a partner when preparing congenic mice
C57BR	BR	C57BRcd*j*	Frequent pituitary and liver tumors
C57L	L	C57L J C57L N	Susceptible to experimental autoimmune encephalomyelitis (EAE). Frequent pituitary and reticular cell tumors

infectious agent is limited to humans and primates, vaccine development may require the use of monkeys, chimpanzees, or baboons. The use of primates for research purposes must be carefully regulated to ensure that each species is protected from extinction. For most basic research in immunology, mice have been the experimental animal of choice. They are easy to handle, are genetically well characterized, and have a rapid breeding cycle. Of all species, the immune system of the mouse has been the most extensively characterized. The value of basic research in the mouse system is highlighted by the enormous impact this research has had on clinical intervention in human disease.

Inbred Strains

To control experimental variation caused by differences in the genetic backgrounds of experimental animals, immunologists often work with *inbred strains*—that is, genetically identical animals produced by inbreeding. The rapid breeding cycle of mice makes them particularly well suited for the production of inbred strains, which are developed by repeated inbreeding between brother and sister littermates. In this way the heterozygosity of alleles that is normally found in randomly outbred mice is replaced by homozygosity at all loci. Usually repeated inbreeding for 20 generations yields an

Strain	Abbreviation	Common substrains	Characteristics
C58	C58	C58 J C58 LwN	High leukemia incidence
DBA 1	D1	DBA 1J DBA 1N	Very active
DBA 2	D2	DBA 2J DBA 2N	Very active. Low response to pneumococcal polysaccharide type II
HRS	HRS	HRS J	Carries *hr* (hairless) gene, usually in a heterozygous state
NZB	NZB	NZB BINJ NZB N	High incidence of autoimmune hemolytic anemia, lupus-like nephritis. When crossed with NZW the mice develop an autoimmune disease that appears to be the counterpart of systemic lupus erythematosus (SLE)
NZW	NZW	NZW N	When crossed with NZB the F1 develops autoimmunity (SLE)
P	P	P J	High leukemia incidence
SJL	S	SJL J	High level of aggression and severe fighting to the point of death, especially among males. Susceptible to the development of certain autoimmune diseases
SWR	SWR	SWR J	Susceptible to development of several autoimmune diseases
I29	I29	I29 J I29SvJ	High incidence of spontaneous teratocarcinoma

SOURCE: Adapted from Federation of American Societies for Experimental Biology, 1979, *Biological Handbooks*, Vol. III: Inbred and Genetically Defined Strains of Laboratory Animals.

inbred strain whose progeny are homozygous at more than 98% of all loci. There are currently over 150 different inbred strains of mice, which are designated by a series of letters and/or numbers (Table 2-1). Most of these strains are purchased by immunologists from such suppliers as Jackson Laboratory in Bar Harbor, Maine. Inbred strains have also been produced in rats, guinea pigs, hamsters, rabbits, and domestic fowl.

Since inbred animals are genetically identical (*syngeneic*), they make it possible to study the immune response in the absence of variables that can be introduced by genetic differences among animals. Once inbred strains became available, immunologists could isolate lymphocyte subpopulations from one animal and inject them into another animal of the same strain. It was with this type of experimental system that immunologists were first able to show that lymphocytes from an antigen-primed animal could transfer immunity to an unprimed syngeneic recipient.

Adoptive-Transfer Systems

In some cases it is important to eliminate the immune responsiveness of the syngeneic host so that the response of only the transferred lymphocytes can be studied in isolation. In adoptive-transfer experiments this is achieved by inactivating the immune cells of the syngeneic recipient. Inactivation can be achieved by exposure to x-rays, to which lymphocytes have been shown to be extremely sensitive. Subjecting a mouse that will serve as host to sublethal doses of x-rays (650–750 rads) can kill 99.99% of its lymphocytes, after which the lymphocytes from the spleen of a syngeneic donor can be studied without interference. In some adoptive-transfer experiments higher x-ray levels are used (900–1000 rads) to eliminate the entire hematopoietic system. This is sometimes necessary if the recipient's hematopoietic cells might influence the adoptive-transfer experiment. The x-irradiated mice will die unless reconstituted with bone marrow from a syngeneic donor.

The adoptive-transfer system has enabled immunologists to study the development of injected lymphoid stem cells in various organs of the recipient. Adoptive-transfer experiments have also facilitated the study of various populations of lymphocytes and of the cellular interactions required to generate an immune response. For example, it was through such experiments that immunologists were first able to show that a T helper cell is necessary for B-cell activation in the humoral response.

Cell-Culture Systems

The complexity of the cellular interactions that generate an immune response has led immunologists to rely heavily on various types of in vitro cell-culture systems. A variety of cells can be cultured including primary lymphoid cells, cloned lymphoid cell lines, and hybrid cells.

Primary Lymphoid Cell Cultures

Primary lymphoid cell cultures can be obtained by isolating lymphocytes directly from blood or lymph or from various lymphoid organs by tissue dispersion. The lymphocytes can then be grown in a chemically defined basal medium containing saline, sugars, amino acids, vitamins, trace elements, and various other nutrients, to which various serum supplements are added. Because in vitro culture techniques require from 10- to 100-fold fewer lymphocytes than typical in vivo techniques, they have enabled immunologists to assess the functional properties of minor subpopulations of lymphocytes. It was by means of cell-culture techniques, for example, that immunologists were first able to define the functional differences between CD4$^+$ T helper cells and CD8$^+$ T cytotoxic cells.

Cell-culture techniques have also been used to identify various cytokines involved in the activation, growth, and differentiation of various cells involved in the immune response. Early experiments showed that media conditioned by the growth of various lymphocytes or antigen-presenting cells would support the growth of other lymphoid cells. Many of the individual cytokines that characterized various conditioned media have subsequently been identified and purified, and in many cases the genes encoding them have been cloned. The soluble growth factors elaborated by monocytes and macrophages are called *monokines*, and the ones elaborated by lymphocytes are called *lymphokines*. These cytokines, which play a central role in the activation and regulation of the immune response, are discussed more fully in Chapter 11.

Cloned Lymphoid Cell Lines

Primary lymphoid cell cultures comprise a heterogeneous group of cells which can be propagated only for a limited time. This heterogeneity complicates interpretation of experiments aimed at understanding the molecular and cellular mechanisms by which lymphocytes generate an immune response. To avoid these problems immunologists use cloned lymphoid cell lines and hybrid cells.

Normal mammalian cells generally have a finite lifespan in culture; that is, after a number of population doublings characteristic of the species and cell type, the cells stop dividing. Tumor cells or normal cells transformed with chemical carcinogens or viruses, however, can be propagated indefinitely in tissue culture. (they are said to be immortal). Such cells are referred to as *cell lines.* The first cell line—the mouse fibroblast L cell—was derived in the 1940s from cultured mouse subcutaneous connective tissue by exposing the cultured cells to a chemical carcinogen, methylcholanthrene, over a 4-month period. In the 1950s another important cell line, the HeLa cell, was derived by culturing human cervical cancer cells. Since these early studies, hundreds of cell lines have been established. Various techniques can be used to ensure that a cell line is derived from a single parent cell. Such a cloned cell line consists of a population of genetically identical cells which can be grown indefinitely.

A variety of cell lines are used in immunologic research. Table 2-2 list some of these lines and describes some of the properties of the cells. (Many of the properties described will not have meaning for the reader at this stage, but later chapters refer to some of these lines, so the table can serve as a helpful summary.) Some of these cell lines were derived from spontaneously occurring tumors of lymphocytes, macrophages, or other accessory cells involved in the immune response. In other cases the cell line was induced by transformation of normal lymphoid cells with viruses such as Abelson's murine leukemia virus (A-MLV), simian virus 40 (SV-40), Epstein-Barr virus (EBV), and human T-cell leukemia virus (HTLV-1). The lymphoid cell lines differ from primary lymphoid cell cultures in several important ways: They survive indefinitely in tissue culture, they show various abnormal growth properties, and they often have an abnormal number of chromosomes. Cells with more

Table 2-2   Cell lines commonly used in immunologic research

Cell line	Description
L-929	Mouse fibroblast cell line often used in DNA transfection studies
SP2/0	Nonsecreting mouse myeloma often used as a fusion partner for hybridoma secretion
P3X63-Ag8.653	Nonsecreting mouse myeloma often used as a fusion partner for hybridoma secretion
MPC 11	Mouse IgG_{2a}-secreting myeloma
P3X63 Ag 8	Mouse IgG_1-secreting myeloma
MOPC 315	Mouse IgA-secreting myeloma
J558	Mouse IgA-secreting myeloma
ABE-8.1/2	Mouse pre-B cell lymphoma
7OZ/3	Mouse pre-B lymphoma used to study early events in B-cell differentiation
BCL 1	Mouse B-cell lymphoma that expresses membrane IgM and IgD and can be activated with mitogen to secrete IgM
LBRM-33	Mouse T-cell lymphoma that secretes high levels of IL-2 after mitogen activation
CTLL-2	Mouse T-cell line whose growth is dependent on IL-2; it often is used to assay IL-2 production
C6VL	Mouse thymoma expressing CD3 and CD4
PU 5-1.8	Mouse monocyte-macrophage line
P338 D1	Mouse monocyte-macrophage line that secretes high levels of IL-1
WEHI 265.1	Mouse monocyte line
P815	Mouse mastocytoma cells often used as targets to assess killing by cytotoxic T lymphocytes (CTLs)
YAC-1	Mouse lymphoma cells often used as targets for NK cells
COS-1	African green monkey kidney cells transformed by SV40 that often are used in DNA transfection studies

or less than the normal diploid number of chromosomes for a species are said to be *aneuploid*. The big advantage of cloned lymphoid cell lines is that they can be grown for extended periods in tissue culture, enabling immunologists to obtain large numbers of homogeneous cells in culture.

Until the late 1970s immunologists had not succeeded in maintaining normal T cells in tissue culture for extended periods. In 1978 a serendipitous finding led to the observation that conditioned medium containing a T-cell growth factor was required. The essential component of the conditioned medium turned out to be interleukin 2 (IL-2). By culturing normal T lymphocytes with antigen in the presence of IL-2, clones of antigen-specific T lymphocytes could be isolated. These individual clones could be propagated and studied in culture and even frozen for storage. After thawing, the clones continued to grow and express their original antigen-specific functions.

By using cloned lymphoid cell lines immunologists have been able to study a number of events that would have been impossible to examine without large numbers of homogeneous cells. For example, the study of the molecular events involved in lymphocyte activation by antigen was hampered by the low frequency of antigen-specific B and T lymphocytes because molecular changes occurring in one responding cell could not be detected against a background of 10^3–10^6 nonresponding cells. T- and B-cell lines with known antigenic specificity have provided immunologists with clonal populations in which to study the membrane and intracellular events involved in antigen recognition. Similarly, the molecular-level genetic changes corresponding to different maturational stages can be studied in cell lines that appear to be "frozen" at different stages of differentiation. Cell lines have also contributed to understanding of soluble factors produced by lymphoid cells. The value of some cell lines lies in their ability to secrete large quantities of various monokines or lymphokines; other lines have proved to be valuable because they express membrane receptors for particular monokines or lymphokines. These cell lines have been used by immunologists to purify and eventually to clone the genes of various lymphokines and their receptors.

There are, however, a number of limitations with lymphoid cell lines. Variants arise spontaneously in the course of prolonged culture, necessitating frequent subcloning to limit the cellular heterogeneity that can develop. If variants are selected in subcloning, it is possible that two subclones derived from the same parent clone may represent different subpopulations. Moreover, any cell line derived from tumor cells or transformed cells may have unknown genetic contributions characteristic of the tumor or of the transformed state, so that caution is called for when one extrapolates from results obtained with cell lines to the normal situation in vivo. Nevertheless, transformed cell lines have made a major contribution to the study of immunology, and a number of molecular events discovered in experiments with transformed cell lines have later been shown to take place in normal lymphocytes.

Hybrid Lymphoid Cell Lines

In somatic-cell hybridization, immunologists fuse normal B or T lymphocytes with tumor cells, obtaining a heterokaryon; after random loss of some chromosomes, a *hybridoma* is formed containing a single nucleus with chromosomes from each of the fused cells. Historically, cell fusion was promoted with Sendai virus, but now it is generally done with polyethylene glycol. Normal antigen-primed B cells for example, can be fused with cancerous plasma cells, called myeloma cells (Figure 2-1). The hybridoma thus formed continues to express the antibody genes of the normal B lymphocyte but is capable of unlimited growth, a characteristic of the myeloma cell. Such B-cell hybridomas have revolutionized immunology because hybridoma clones can be propagated that secrete antibody with a single antigenic specificity, called *monoclonal antibody* in reference to its derivation from a single clone. Chapter 7 discusses this process in detail.

T-cell hybridomas can also be obtained by fusing T lymphocytes with cancerous T-cell lymphomas. Again, the resulting hybridoma continues to express the genes of the normal T cell but acquires the immortal-growth properties of the cancerous T lymphoma cell. Immunologists have generated a number of stable hybridoma cell lines representing T helper and T cytotoxic lineages. These T-cell hybridomas have two major disadvantages: (1) the cells tend to be unstable, since they are aneuploid as a result of random chromosome loss and (2) the tumor-cell fusion partner contributes some unknown genetic components to the hybrid cells.

Recombinant DNA Technology

The techniques developed in recombinant DNA technology have had an impact on every area of study in immunology. Genes can be cloned, DNA can be sequenced and recombinant protein products can be produced, providing immunologists with defined components with which to study the structure and function of the immune system. Some of the recombinant DNA techniques commonly employed in immunologic research are briefly described in this section; many of these techniques are referred to in subsequent chapters.

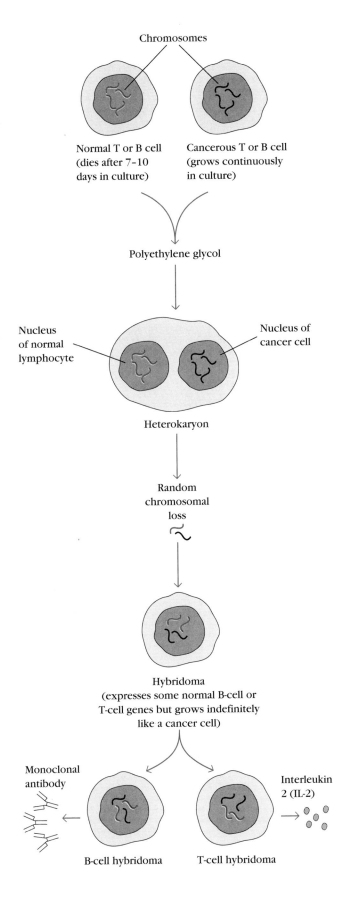

Chromosomes

Normal T or B cell
(dies after 7–10
days in culture)

Cancerous T or B cell
(grows continuously
in culture)

Polyethylene glycol

Nucleus
of normal
lymphocyte

Nucleus of
cancer cell

Heterokaryon

Random
chromosomal
loss

Hybridoma
(expresses some normal B-cell or
T-cell genes but grows indefinitely
like a cancer cell)

Monoclonal
antibody

Interleukin
2 (IL-2)

B-cell hybridoma

T-cell hybridoma

Restriction-Endonuclease Cleavage of DNA

A variety of bacteria produce enzymes, called *restriction endonucleases*, that degrade foreign DNA (e.g., bacteriophage DNA) but spare the bacterial cell DNA, which is protected by methylation. The discovery of these bacterial enzymes in the 1970s opened the way to a major technological advance in the field of molecular biology. Before the discovery of restriction endonucleases, double-stranded DNA (dsDNA) could be cut only with DNases. These enzymes do not recognize defined sites and therefore randomly cleave DNA into a variable series of small fragments, which are impossible to order. In contrast, restriction endonucleases recognize and cleave DNA at specific sites, called *restriction sites*, which are short double-stranded sequences containing four to eight nucleotides (Table 2-3). A restriction endonuclease cuts both DNA strands at a specific point within its restriction site. Some enzymes, like *Hpa*I, cut on the central axis and thus generate blunt-ended fragments. Other enzymes, such as *Eco*RI, cut the DNA off-center from the central axis of the recognition site, producing staggered cleavage products. These staggered fragments have a short single-stranded DNA extension, called a *sticky end*, extending from one of the strands of the double-stranded fragment. When two DNA molecules are cut with the same restriction enzyme, the sticky ends will be complementary, so that the two molecules can be joined by base pairing to generate a recombinant DNA molecule (Figure 2-2). Several hundred different restriction endonucleases have been isolated and many are available commercially, allowing researchers to purchase enzymes that cut DNA at defined restriction sites.

Restriction Mapping of DNA

The DNA fragments generated with restriction endonucleases can be separated according to size by means of agarose gel electrophoresis. The smaller DNA fragments move faster than the larger fragments, generating a series of bands that can be detected with ethidium bromide dye, which binds to DNA. The molecular weight

Figure 2-1 Production of B-cell or T-cell hybridomas by somatic-cell hybridization. The resulting hybridomas continue to express some of the genes of the fused B or T cell but now have the immortal-growth properties of the tumor cell. This procedure is used to produce B-cell hybridomas secreting monoclonal antibody or T-cell hybridomas secreting various growth factors.

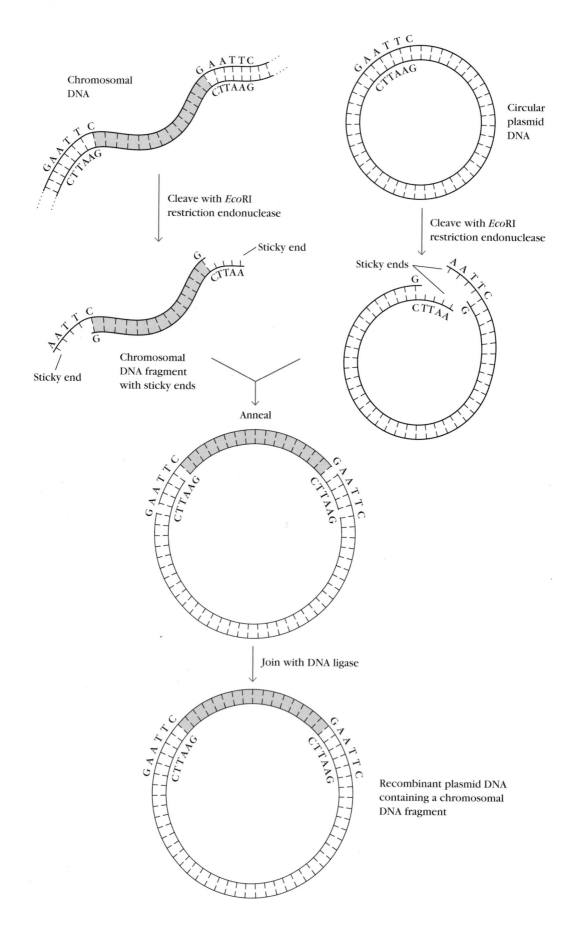

Table 2-3 Some restriction enzymes and their recognitions sequences

Microorganism source	Abbreviation	Sequence* 5′ → 3′ 3′ → 5′
Bacillus amyloliquefaciens H	*Bam*HI	G G A T C C C C T A G G
Brevibacterium albidum	*Bal*I	T G G C C A A C C G G T
Escherichia coli RY13	*Eco*RI	G A A T T C C T T A A G
Haemophilus aegyptius	*Hae*II	Pu G C G C Py Py C G C G Pu
Haemophilus aegyptius	*Hae*III	G G C C C C G G
Haemophilus haemolyticus	*Hha*I	G C G C C G C G
Haemophilus influenzae Rd	*Hind*II	G T Py Pu A C C A Pu Py T G
Haemophilus influenzae Rd	*Hind*III	A A G C T T T T C G A A
Haemophilus parainfluenzae	*Hpa*I	G T T A A C C A A T T G
Haemophilus parainfluenzae	*Hpa*II	C C G G G G C C
Providencia stuartii 164	*Pst*I	C T G C A G G A C G T C
Streptomyces albus G	*Sal*I	G T C G A C C A G C T G
Xanthomonas oryzae	*Xor*II	C G A T C G G C T A G C

* Vertical arrows indicate locations of single-strand cuts within the restriction site. Enzymes that make off-center cuts produce fragments with short, single-stranded extensions at their ends.

SOURCE: J. D. Watson, J. Tooze, and D. T. Kurtz, 1983, *Recombinant DNA: A Short Course*, W. H. Freeman and Company.

Figure 2-2 Formation of recombinant DNA molecules. A restriction endonuclease that produces fragments with sticky ends is used to cleave two different DNA molecules (in this case, a circular plasmid DNA and a linear chromosomal DNA). The complementary sticky ends of the two different fragments anneal and can be joined permanently with DNA ligase. In this example a recombinant plasmid DNA molecule is formed.

(a)

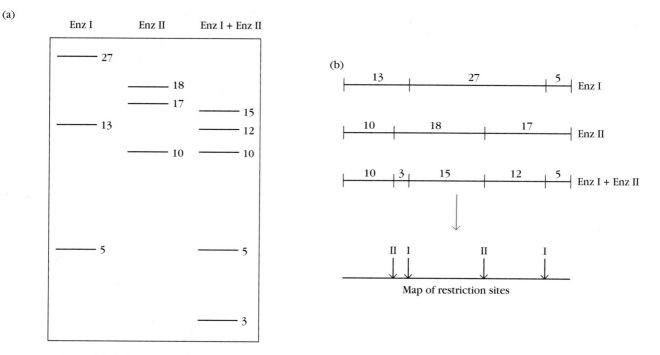

Figure 2-3   A simplified illustration of restriction enzyme mapping. (a) Cloned DNA is digested with two restriction endonucleases (Enz I and Enz II) alone and in combination,
and the resulting fragments are separated by gel electrophoresis. The numbers in the diagram refer to the length of each fragment in kilobases. (b) Comparison of the sizes of the
fragments produced in the three digests permits ordering of the restriction sites relative
to each other. In this example, the DNA sample contained two sites for Enz I and two
sites for Enz II.

of each DNA fragment can be determined from standard curves obtained by electrophoresing DNA fragments of known size in parallel. By cleaving a DNA sample with two or more restriction endonucleases (alone and in combination), it is possible to determine the location of the restriction sites and the relative distances between them. This procedure is called *restriction mapping* (Figure 2-3).

Cloning of DNA Sequences

The development of DNA cloning technology in the 1970s provided a means of amplifying a given DNA fragment to such an extent that unlimited amounts of identical DNA fragments could be produced. In DNA cloning a given DNA fragment is inserted into an autonomously replicating DNA molecule, called a cloning *vector*, so that the inserted DNA is replicated with the vector. Most often the vector is a bacteriophage or *plasmid* (a small circular, extrachromosomal molecule that can replicate independently in a host cell); the most common host is the bacterium, *Escherichia coli.* The DNA fragments to be cloned are usually obtained from one of two sources: genomic DNA or complementary DNA (cDNA).

Cloning of Complementary DNA

Complementary DNA is prepared by isolating messenger RNA (mRNA) from cells and transcribing it into complementary DNA (cDNA) with the enzyme reverse transcriptase, which can be isolated from certain RNA viruses. Reverse transcriptase copies mRNA by adding nucleotides to a primer, forming a mRNA-cDNA hybrid; in the production of cDNA, a poly-T primer is used, since most mRNAs have a poly-A tail. Double-stranded cDNA can be obtained from the mRNA-cDNA hybrid in a number of ways. In one method, the hybrid is treated with alkali, which destroys the RNA strand but not the DNA

Figure 2-4   cDNA cloning using a plasmid vector. (*Left*) formation of double-stranded cDNA is outlined. (*Right*) plasmid DNA containing an ampicillin-resistance gene is cut with a restriction endonuclease that produces blunt ends. Following addition of a poly-C tail to the 3′ ends of the cDNA and a poly-G tail to the 3′ ends of the cut plasmid, the two DNAs are mixed, annealed, and joined by DNA ligase, forming the plasmid vector. The vector is transferred into *E. coli* cells, which are grown in the presence of ampicillin to select cells containing the vector.

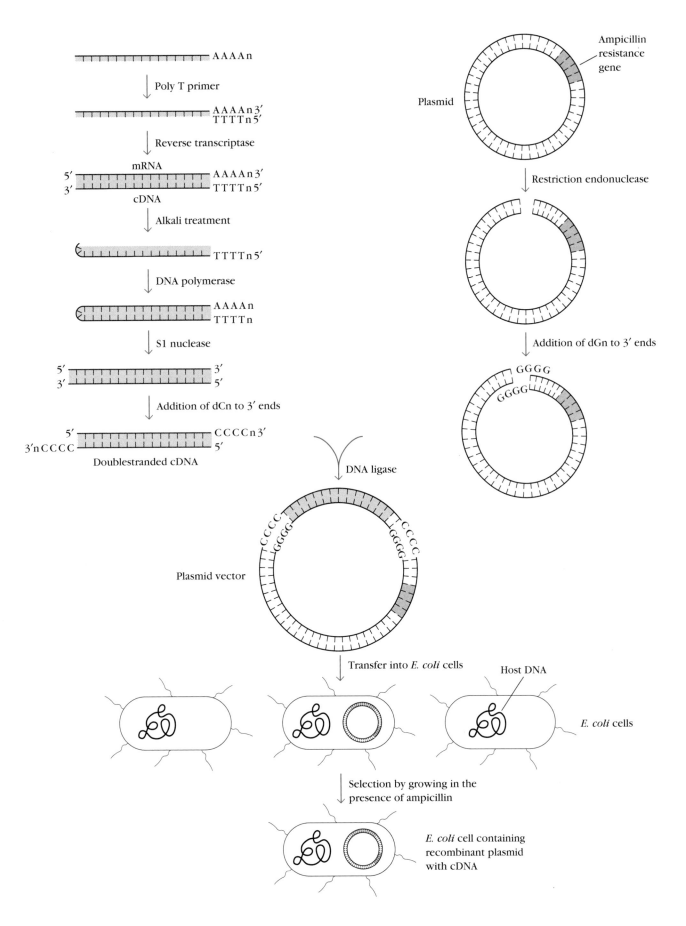

strand. The resulting single-stranded cDNA forms a small hairpin at its 3′ end, which serves as a primer for the synthesis by DNA polymerase of a complementary strand. After synthesis of the second strand, the hairpin is cleaved with S1 nuclease to generate a conventional double-stranded cDNA (Figure 2-4).

The cDNA can be cloned by inserting it into a plasmid vector carrying a selectable gene conferring resistance to the antibiotic ampicillin. The circular plasmid is cut with a restriction endonuclease that produces double-stranded blunt ends. The cDNA and the plasmid can be joined by several methods. In one method, called *tailing*, a terminal deoxynucleotidyl transferase enzyme adds short stretches of poly C to the 3′ ends of the cDNA molecule and short stretches of poly G to the 3′ ends of the plasmid DNA. When the plasmid DNA and cDNA are then mixed, the poly-G tail of the vector molecule anneals with the poly-C tail of the cDNA molecule. Following ligation, the recombinant plasmid DNA is subsequently transferred into specially treated *E. coli* cells by one of several possible techniques; this transfer process is called *transformation*. The ampicillin-resistance gene on the plasmid serves as a selectable marker for identifying bacterial cells containing the plasmid DNA because only those cells are able to grow in the presence of the antibiotic (see Figure 2-4). A collection of DNA sequences within plasmid vectors representing all the mRNA sequences derived from a cell or tissue is called a *cDNA library*.

Cloning of Genomic DNA

Genomic DNA fragments are obtained by cleaving chromosomal DNA with restriction endonucleases that produce sticky ends. The genomic DNA can be cloned using bacteriophage λ as the vector (Figure 2-5). Bacteriophage λ DNA is 48.5 kilobases (kb) long and contains a central section of about 15 kb that is not necessary for λ replication in *E. coli* and can therefore be replaced with foreign genomic DNA. Generally, the λ DNA is treated with a restriction enzyme that cuts the DNA on both sides of the central 15-kb section, and this section is removed. Then the genomic DNA is cut with the same restriction enzyme. The single-stranded sticky ends of the λ DNA and the genomic DNA can be annealed and ligated to form a recombinant phage. Sometimes the genomic DNA is cut with another restriction enzyme that does not produce sticky ends complementary to those on the λ DNA fragments. In these cases, short DNA duplexes that include a restriction site, called linkers, are added to the genomic DNA fragments, enabling the fragments to anneal with the sticky ends on the λ fragments. As long as the recombinant DNA does not exceed the length of the original λ phage DNA by more than 5%, it can be packaged into the λ phage head and can

be propagated in *E. coli*. This means that one can clone somewhat more than 1.5×10^4 base pairs in one λ phage particle. It has been calculated that about 1 million different recombinant λ phage particles would be needed to form a complete *genomic DNA library* representing the entire haploid genome of a mammalian cell, which contains about 3×10^9 base pairs.

Often the 15- to 20-kb stretch of DNA that can be cloned in bacteriophage λ is not long enough to include the regulatory sequences that lie outside the 5′ and 3′ ends of the direct coding sequences of a gene. However, much larger genomic DNA fragments—between 30 and 50 kb in length—can be cloned in a *cosmid vector*, which is a plasmid that has been genetically engineered to contain the *cos* sites of λ DNA as well as an antibiotic-resistance gene. The *cos* sites are DNA sequences that allow packaging into the λ phage head of any DNA up to 50 kb in length. A recombinant cosmid vector, although not a fully functional bacteriophage, can infect *E. coli* and replicate as a plasmid, generating a *cosmid library*. Even larger DNA fragments, approaching a megabase in length, can be cloned in yeast artificial chromosomes, which are linear DNA segments that can replicate in yeast cells.

Identification of DNA Clones

Once a cDNA or genomic DNA library is prepared, it must be screened to identify a particular DNA fragment. This is accomplished by a process called in situ hybridization. The cloned bacterial colonies, yeast colonies, or phage plaques containing the recombinant DNA are transferred onto nitrocellulose or nylon filters by a process called replica plating (Figure 2-6). The filter is then treated with NaOH, which both lyses the bacteria and denatures the DNA, allowing single-stranded DNA (ssDNA) to bind to the filter. The filter with bound DNA then is incubated with a radioactive probe specific for the gene of interest. The probe will hybridize with the colonies or plaques on the filter that contain the sought-after gene, and they can be identified by autoradiography. The position of the positive colonies or plaques on the filter shows where the corresponding clones can be found on the original agar plate.

Various radioactive probes can be used to screen a library. In some cases radiolabeled mRNA or cDNA serves as the probe. When the protein encoded by the gene of interest has been purified, it is possible to work backward from the amino acid sequence, using the genetic code, to determine the probable nucleotide sequence of the corresponding gene. A known sequence of five or six amino acid residues is all that is needed to synthesize radiolabeled oligonucleotide probes with which to screen a cDNA or genomic library for a particular

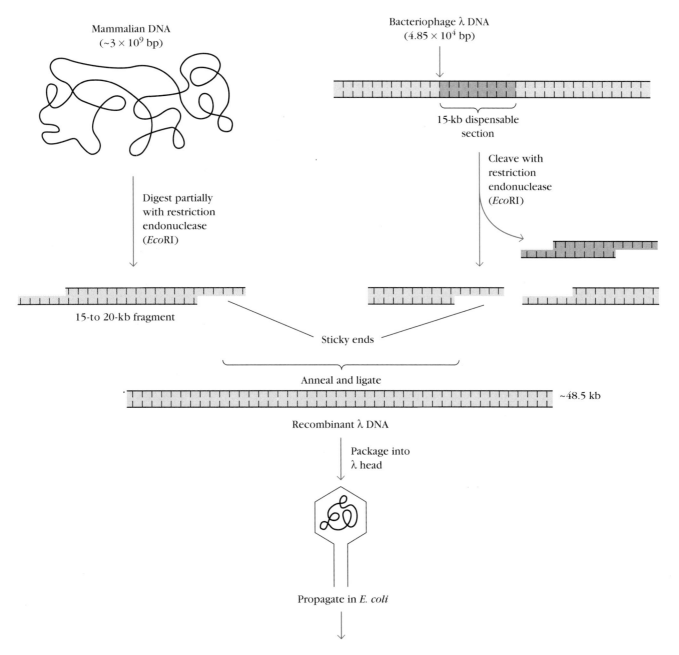

Figure 2-5 Genomic DNA cloning using bacteriophage λ as the vector. Genomic DNA is partially digested with *Eco*RI, producing fragments with sticky ends. The central 15-kb region of the λ phage DNA is cut out with *Eco*RI and discarded. The sticky ends of the genomic and λ DNA fragments are then annealed and ligated. After the resulting recombinant λ DNA is packaged into a phage head, it can be propagated in *E. coli*.

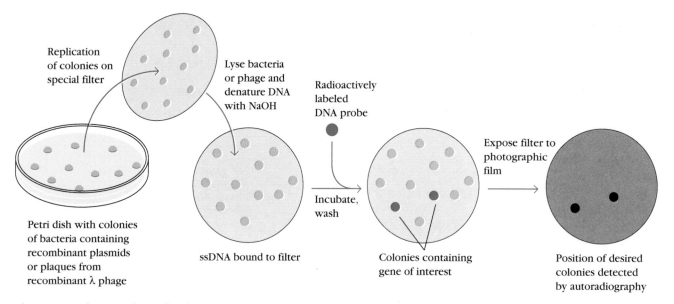

Figure 2-6   Selection of specific clones from cDNA or genomic DNA library by in situ hybridization. A nitrocellulose or nylon filter is placed against the plate to pick up the bacterial colonies or phage plaques containing the cloned genes. The filter is then placed in a NaOH solution and heated, so that the denatured ssDNA becomes fixed to the filter. A radioactive probe specific for the gene of interest is incubated with the filter. The position of the colonies or plaques containing the desired gene is revealed by auto-radiography.

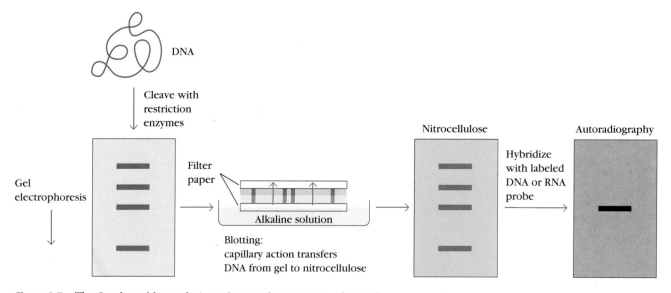

Figure 2-7   The Southern blot technique detects the presence of specific sequences in DNA fragments. The DNA fragments produced by restriction-enzyme cleavage are separated by size by agarose gel electrophoresis. The agarose gel is overlaid with a nitocellulose or nylon filter and a thick stack of paper towels. The gel is then placed in an alkaline salt solution, which denatures the DNA. As the paper towels soak up the moisture, the solution is drawn through the gel into the filter, transferring each ssDNA band to the filter. This process is called blotting. After heating, the filter is incubated with a radiolabeled probe specific for the sequence of interest; DNA fragments that hybridize with the probe are detected by autoradiography. [Adapted from James Darnell, Harvey Lodish, and David Baltimore, 1990, *Molecular Cell Biology*, 2d ed., Scientific American Books.]

gene. To cope with the degeneracy of the genetic code, peptides incorporating amino acids encoded by a limited number of codon sequences are usually chosen. Oligonucleotides representing all possible codon sequences for the peptide are synthesized and used as probes to screen the library.

Southern Blotting

As noted already, DNA fragments generated by restriction-endonuclease cleavage can be separated on the basis of length by agarose gel electrophoresis. An elegant technique developed by E. M. Southern can be used to

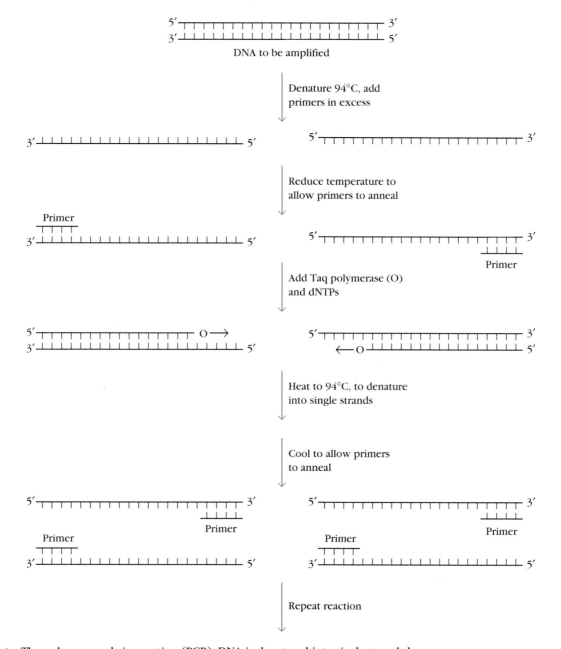

Figure 2-8 The polymerase chain reaction (PCR). DNA is denatured into single strands by a brief heat treatment and is then cooled in the presence of an excess of oligonucleotide primers complementary to the DNA sequences flanking the desired DNA segment. Taq polymerase, a heat-resistant DNA polymerase obtained from a thermophilic bacterium, is used to copy the DNA from the 3' ends of the primers. Because all of the reaction components are heat stable, the heating and cooling cycle can be repeated many times, resulting in alternate DNA melting and synthesis, and rapid amplification of a given sequence. [Adapted from James Darnell, Harvey Lodish, and David Baltimore, 1990, *Molecular Cell Biology*, 2d ed., Scientific American Books.]

identify any fragment band containing a given gene sequence (Figure 2-7). In this technique called *Southern blotting*, DNA is cut with restriction enzymes and the fragments are separated according to size by electrophoresis on an agarose gel. Then the gel is soaked in NaOH to denature the dsDNA, and the resulting ssDNA fragments are transferred onto a nitrocellulose or nylon filter by capillary action. After transfer, the filter is incubated with an appropriate radiolabeled probe specific for the gene sequence of choice. The probe hybridizes with the ssDNA fragment of interest, and the position of the fragment band is determined by autoradiography. Southern blot analysis played a critical role in unraveling the mechanism by which diversity is generated for the immunoglobulin molecule and T-cell receptors.

Polymerase Chain Reaction

The *polymerase chain reaction* (*PCR*) is a powerful technique for amplifying specific DNA sequences even when they are present at extremely low levels in a complex mixture (Figure 2-8). The procedure requires that the DNA sequences flanking the desired DNA sequence be known, so that short oligonucleotide primers can be synthesized. The DNA mixture is denatured into single strands by a brief heat treatment. The DNA is then cooled in the presence of an excess of the oligonucleotide primers, which hybridize with the complementary ssDNA. A temperature-resistant DNA polymerase (called Taq polymerase) is then added, together with the four deoxyribonucleoside triphosphates, and each strand is copied. The newly synthesized DNA duplex is separated by heating and the cycle is repeated. In each cycle there is a doubling of the DNA sequence; in only 25 cycles the desired DNA sequence can be amplified about a million-fold. The DNA amplified by PCR can be further characterized by Southern blotting, restriction-enzyme mapping, and direct DNA sequencing. The PCR has enabled immunologists to amplify genes encoding important molecules of the immune response, such as MHC proteins, T-cell receptor, and immunoglobulins.

Gene Transfer into Mammalian Cells

A variety of genes involved in the immune response have been isolated and cloned by use of the techniques described in the previous section. The expression and regulation of these genes has been studied by introducing the cloned gene into cultured cells and, more recently, into the germ line of animals.

Transfer of Cloned Genes into Cultured Cells

Diverse techniques have been developed for transfecting genes into cells. A common technique involves the use of a retrovirus in which a viral structural gene has been replaced with the cloned gene to be transfected. The altered retrovirus is then used as a vector for introducing the cloned gene into cultured cells. Because of the properties of retroviruses, the recombinant DNA integrates into the cellular genome with a high frequency. In an alternative method, the cloned gene of interest is complexed with calcium phosphate. The calcium phosphate–DNA complex is slowly precipitated onto the cells and the DNA is taken up by a small percentage of them. In another transfection method called *electroporation*, an electric current creates pores in cell membranes through which the cloned DNA is taken up. In both of these latter methods, the transfected DNA integrates, apparently at random sites, into the DNA of a small percentage of treated cells. Generally the cloned DNA being transfected is engineered to contain a selectable marker gene, such as one coding for resistance to neomycin. Following transfection the cells are cultured in the presence of neomycin. Because only the transfected cells are able to grow, the relatively small number of transfected cells in the total cell population can be identified and selected.

Transfection of cloned genes into cells has proved to be a highly effective technique in immunologic research. By transfecting genes involved with the immune response into cells lacking those genes, the product of a specific gene can be studied apart from other interacting immune-gene products. For example, transfection of MHC genes into mouse L cells has enabled immunologists to study the role of MHC molecules in antigen-presentation to T cells. Transfection of the gene encoding the T-cell receptor has provided information about the antigen-MHC specificity of the T-cell receptor.

Transfer of Cloned Genes into Germ-line Cells

Transgenic mice are produced by injecting foreign cloned DNA (referred to as the *transgene*) into a fertilized egg (Figure 2-9). In the technically demanding process of producing transgenics, fertilized mouse eggs are held under suction at the end of a pipet and the transgene is micro-injected into one of the pronuclei with a fine needle. The transgene integrates into the chromosomal DNA of the pronucleus and is passed on to the daughter cells of eggs that survive the process. The eggs are implanted in the oviduct of "pseudopreg-

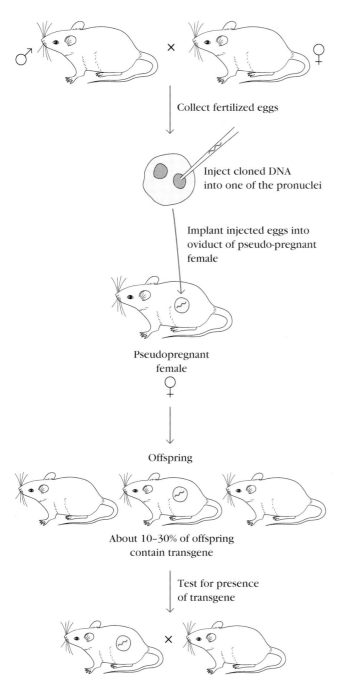

Figure 2-9 General procedure for producing transgenic mice. Fertilized eggs are collected from a pregnant female mouse. Cloned DNA (referred to as the transgene) is microinjected into one of the pronuclei of the fertilized egg. The eggs are then implanted into the oviduct of pseudopregnant foster mothers (obtained by mating a normal female with a sterile male). About 10–30% of the offspring will have the transgene incorporated into their chromosomal DNA and will express the transgene in all of their somatic cells. By linking tissue-specific promoters to the transgene, it is also possible to achieve tissue-specific expression of the transgene.

Collect fertilized eggs

Inject cloned DNA into one of the pronuclei

Implant injected eggs into oviduct of pseudo-pregnant female

Pseudopregnant female

Offspring

About 10–30% of offspring contain transgene

Test for presence of transgene

Breed transgenics

nant" females, and transgenic pups are born after 19 or 20 days of gestation. In general the efficiency is low, with only one or two transgenic mice produced for every 100 fertilized eggs collected.

With transgenic mice immunologists have been able to study the expression of a given gene in a living animal. Although all the cells in a transgenic animal contain the transgene, differences in the expression of the transgene in different tissues has shed light on mechanisms of tissue-specific gene expression. By constructing a transgene with a particular *promoter* (the DNA segment to which RNA polymerase binds to begin transcription), one can control the expression of a given transgene. For example, the metallothionein promoter is activated by zinc. Transgenic mice carrying a transgene linked to a metallothionein promoter can therefore be induced to express the transgene at a particular time by addition of zinc to their water supply. Other promoters, such as the insulin promoter, are tissue-specific. By producing transgenics carrying a transgene linked to the insulin promoter, one can limit expression of the transgene to pancreatic cells.

Summary

1. Inbred strains allow immunologists to work routinely with syngeneic, or genetically identical, mice. With these strains, aspects of the immune response can be studied uncomplicated by unknown variables that could be introduced by genetic differences between animals.

2. In adoptive-transfer experiments, lymphocytes are transferred from one mouse to a syngeneic recipient mouse that has been exposed to a sublethal (or potentially lethal) dose of x-rays. The irradiation inactivates the immune cells of the recipient, so that one can study the response of only the transferred cells.

3. With in vitro cell-culture systems, populations of lymphocytes can be studied under more defined conditions than are possible with in vivo animal systems. Such systems include primary cultures of lymphoid cells, cloned lymphoid cell lines, and hybrid lymphoid cell lines. Unlike primary cultures, cell lines are immortal and homogeneous. With cell lines, the intracellular events and cell products associated with individual subpopulations of lymphocytes can be investigated. Such studies are difficult, if not impossible, with the heterogeneous populations typical of primary cultures.

4. The ability to identify, clone, and sequence immune-system genes, using recombinant DNA techniques, has revolutionized the study of all aspects of the immune response. Both cDNA, which is prepared by transcribing mRNA with reverse transcriptase, and genomic DNA can be cloned. Generally, cDNA is cloned using a plasmid vector; the recombinant DNA containing the gene to be cloned is propagated in *E. coli* cells. Genomic DNA can be cloned with bacteriophage λ as the vector or with cosmid vectors, both of which are propagated in *E. coli*. Larger genomic DNA fragments can be cloned within yeast artificial chromosomes, which can replicate in yeast cells.

5.   Cloned genes can be transfected, or transferred, into cultured cells by several methods. Commonly, immune-system genes are transfected into cells that do not express the gene of interest. For example, the role of different MHC proteins in antigen presentation to T cells has been established by transfection of specific MHC genes into cells that do not express those genes.

6.   DNA also can be introduced into the germ-line cells of animals, after which the transgene is replicated in all the somatic cells of the animal. Studies with transgenic mice have shed light on the tissue-specific expression of immune-system genes.

References

BARINAGA, M. 1989. Making transgenic mice: is it really that easy? *Science* **245**:590.

BELL, J. 1989. The polymerase chain reaction. *Immunol. Today* **10**:351.

BERGER, S. L., and A. R. KIMMEL (eds.). 1987. Guide to molecular cloning techniques. *Methods Enzymol.* **152**:(entire volume).

BURKE, D. T., G. F. CARLE, and M. V. OLSO, 1987. Cloning of large segments of exogenous DNA into yeast by means of artificial chromosome vectors. *Science* **236**:806.

CAMPER, S. A. 1987. Research applications of transgenic mice. *Biotechniques* **5**:638.

DENIS, K. A., and O. N. WITTE. 1989. Long-term lymphoid cultures in the study of B cell differentiation. In *Immunoglobulin Genes.* Academic Press, p. 45.

DEPAMPHILIS, M. L., S. A. HERMAN, E. MARTINEZ-SALAS et al. 1988. Microinjecting DNA into mouse ova to study DNA replication and gene expression and to produce transgenic animals. *Biotechniques* **6**(7):622.

KAVATHAS, P., and L. A. HERZENBERG. 1986. Transfection for lymphocyte cell surface antigens. In *Handbook of Experimental Immunology.* Vol. 3: Genetics and Molecular Approaches to Immunology. D. M. WEIR, ed. Blackwell Scientific Publications, p. 91.1.

MORRISON, S., and V. T. OI. 1986. Lymphoid cell gene trans-

fer. In *Handbook of Experimental Immunology.* Vol. 3: Genetics and Molecular Approaches to Immunology. D. M. WEIR, ed. Blackwell Scientific Publications, p. 92.1.

OLD, R. W., and S. B. PRIMROSE. 1985. *Principles of Gene Manipulation: An Introduction to Genetic Engineering.* Blackwell Scientific Publications.

SAIKI, R. K., D. H. GELFAND, S. STOFFEL et al. 1988. Primer-directed enzymatic amplification of DNA with a thermostable DNA polymerase. *Science* **239**:487.

SCHLESSINGER, D. 1990. Yeast artificial chromosomes: tools for mapping and analysis of complex genomes. *Trends Genet.* **6**(8):254.

WATSON, J. D., J. TOOZE, and D. T. KURTZ. 1983. *Recombinant DNA: A Short Course.* W. H. Freeman and Company.

Study Questions

1.   Explain why the following statements are false.
    a.   The amino acid sequence of a protein can be determined from the nucleotide sequence of a genomic clone encoding the protein.
    b.   Transgenic mice can be prepared by microinjection of DNA into a somatic-cell nucleus.
    c.   Primary lymphoid cultures can be propagated indefinitely and are useful in studies on specific subpopulations of lymphocytes.

2.   The gene diagrammed below contains one leader (L), three exons (E), and three introns (I). Illustrate the primary transcript, mRNA, and the protein product that could be generated from such a gene.

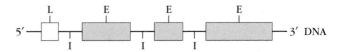

3.   What would be the result if you failed to include a selectable marker gene in a transfection experiment?

4.   What would be the result if a transgene were injected into one cell of a four-cell mouse zygote rather than into a fertilized mouse egg before it divides?

5.   A circular plasmid was cleaved with *Eco*RI, producing a 5.4 kb band on a gel. A 5.4 kb band was also observed when the plasmid was cleaved with *Hin*dIII. Cleaving the plasmid with both enzymes simultaneously resulted in a single band 2.7 kb in size. Draw a possible restriction map of this plasmid.

6.   Explain briefly how you might go about cloning a gene for interleukin 2. Assume that you have available a monoclonal antibody to IL-2.

Cells and Organs of the Immune System

The immune system consists of many structurally and functionally diverse organs and tissues that are widely dispersed throughout the body. These organs can be classified on the basis of functional differences as *primary* and *secondary* lymphoid organs. The primary organs provide appropriate microenvironments for lymphocyte maturation. The secondary organs are uniquely suited to trap antigen from defined tissues or vascular spaces and provide sites where mature lymphocytes can interact effectively with that antigen. The blood vasculature and lymphatic systems interconnect these organs, uniting them into a functional whole. Carried within the blood and lymph and populating the various lymphoid organs are the cells that participate in the immune response. The central cell of the immune system is the lymphocyte, which accounts for roughly 25% of the white blood cells and 99% of the nucleated cells in the lymph. There are approximately 10^{12} lymphocytes in humans, the equivalent in cellular mass to that of the brain or liver! These lymphocytes continuously recirculate between the blood and lymph and the various lymphoid organs, thereby providing a high degree of cellular integration to the immune system as a whole.

Cells of the Immune System

A variety of white blood cells, or *leukocytes*, participate in the development of an immune response (Table 3-1). Of these cells, only the lymphocytes possess the attributes of diversity, specificity, memory, and self/nonself recognition, the hallmarks of an immune response. All the other cells play accessory roles, serving either to activate lymphocytes or to increase the effectiveness of antigen clearance by phagocytosis or by secretion of various immune effector molecules.

Hematopoiesis

In humans, *hematopoiesis*, the formation and development of red and white blood cells from stem cells, begins in the yolk sac in the first weeks of embryonic development. Here yolk sac stem cells differentiate into primitive erythroid cells containing embryonic hemoglobin. In the third month of gestation, the stem cells migrate from the yolk sac to the fetal liver and then to the spleen; these two organs have major roles in hematopoiesis from the third to the seventh months of gestation. As gestation continues, the bone marrow becomes the major hematopoietic organ; by the time of birth hematopoiesis has ceased within the liver and spleen.

It is remarkable that every functionally specialized mature blood cell is derived from a common *stem cell*. In contrast to a unipotent cell, which differentiates into a single cell type, a hematopoietic stem cell is *pluripotent*, able to differentiate along a number of pathways and thereby generate erythrocytes, granulocytes, monocytes, mast cells, lymphocytes, and megakaryocytes. These stem cells are few in number, occurring with a frequency of one stem cell per 10^4 bone marrow cells. The study of stem cells has been hampered by the low frequency of these cells and the fact that they cannot yet be maintained in tissue culture. As a result, little is

Table 3-1   Normal adult blood cell counts

Cell type	Cells/mm^3	%
Red blood cells	5.0×10^6	
Platelets	2.5×10^5	
Leukocytes	7.3×10^3	
Neutrophil		50–70
Lymphocyte		20–40
Monocyte		1–6
Eosinophil		1–3
Basophil		< 1

known about the regulation of their proliferation and differentiation. By virtue of their capacity for self-renewal, stem cells are maintained at homeostatic levels throughout adult life; however, when there is an increased demand for hematopoiesis, stem cells display an enormous proliferative capacity. This can be demonstrated in mice whose hematopoietic systems have been completely destroyed by a lethal dose (950 rads) of x-rays. Such irradiated mice will die within 10 days unless they are infused with normal bone marrow cells from a syngeneic, or genetically identical, mouse. Whereas a normal mouse has 3×10^8 marrow cells, infusion of only 10^4–10^5 donor bone marrow cells (i.e., 0.01–0.1% of the normal level) is sufficient to completely restore the hematopoietic system, demonstrating the enormous proliferative and differentiative capacity of the few stem cells in the donor bone marrow.

Early in hematopoiesis, a pluripotent stem cell differentiates along one of two pathways, giving rise to either a *lymphoid stem cell* or a *myeloid stem cell* (see Figure 3-2). Subsequent differentiation of lymphoid and myeloid stem cells generates committed *progenitor cells* for each type of mature blood cell. Progenitor cells have lost the capacity for self-renewal and are committed to a given cell lineage. The lymphoid stem cell generates T and B progenitor lymphocytes. The myeloid stem cell generates progenitor cells for erythrocytes, neutrophils, eosinophils, basophils, monocytes, mast cells, and platelets. Progenitor commitment depends on the acquisition of responsiveness to particular growth factors. When the appropriate growth factors are present, these progenitor cells proliferate and differentiate, giving rise to the corresponding type of mature red or white blood cells. The particular microenvironment within which a progenitor cell resides influences the quality and quantity of growth factors, thus controlling differentiation.

In adult bone marrow, the hematopoietic cells grow and mature on a meshwork of stromal cells, which are nonhematopoietic cells that support the growth and differentiation of the hematopoietic cells. Stromal cells include fat cells, endothelial cells, fibroblasts, and macrophages. Stromal cells influence hematopoietic stem-cell differentiation by providing a hematopoietic-inducing microenvironment consisting of a cellular matrix and either membrane-bound or diffusable growth factors. As hematopoietic stem cells differentiate in this microenvironment, their membranes acquire deformability, allowing the mature cells to pass through the sinusoidal wall into the sinuses of the bone marrow, from whence they enter the circulation.

Spleen Colony-Forming Assay

The earliest evidence proving that the various cell lineages in the bone marrow originate from pluripotent hematopoietic stem cells came from a classic experiment of J. E. Till and E. A. McCulloch in 1961. Their examination of mice lethally irradiated with x-rays revealed extensive cellular loss specifically in the hematopoietic organs; especially noticeable were changes in the spleen, whose structure after x-irradiation showed an absence of cellular mass except for the network of reticular connective cells. When Till and McCulloch injected low numbers of syngeneic bone marrow cells into these irradiated mice, some of these cells were carried to the spleen, where they formed visible nodules on the surface of the spleen, called *colony-forming units–spleen (CFU-S)*. The nodules resulted from clonal expansion of either a single pluripotent stem cell or progenitor cell. Dissection of these nodules revealed that some contained mixtures of differentiated cells: erythrocytes, granulocytes, monocytes, and megakaryocytes. The actual proof that these differentiated cells were clonal progeny of a single stem cell was obtained by modifying this experiment. Low-level x-irradiation (700 rads) can induce random, nonlethal chromosomal damage in some cells; such chromosomal alteration can serve as a marker because all clonal progeny will express the same chromosomal alteration, which is visible by karyotype analysis. Till and McCulloch repeated their experiment, this time injecting low numbers of marked 700-rad x-irradiated bone marrow into the lethally irradiated mice.

Examination of the resulting nodules revealed that all the cell types exhibited the identical chromosomal alteration, proving that all the cells were descendants of the same stem cell. Although lymphocytes were not present in the splenic nodules, they were found scattered throughout the spleen and also carried the same chromosomal alteration exhibited by the nodular colonies, proving that they also were derived from a common pluripotent stem cell.

Hematopoietic Growth Factors

Development of cell-culture systems that can support the growth and differentiation of lymphoid and myeloid stem cells led to the identification of numerous hematopoietic growth factors. In these in vitro systems, bone-marrow stromal cells are cultured to form a layer of adherent cells; freshly isolated bone-marrow hematopoietic cells placed on this layer will grow and produce large visible colonies (Figure 3-1). If the cells are cultured on semisolid agar, the clonal progeny will be immobilized and can be analyzed for cell types. Colonies containing stem cells can be replated, producing mixed colonies containing a number of differentiated cell types; progenitor cells, which cannot be replated, produce lineage-restricted colonies.

(a)

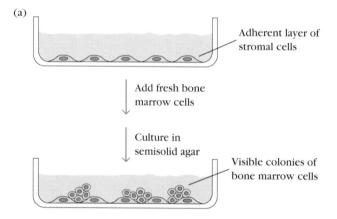

(b)

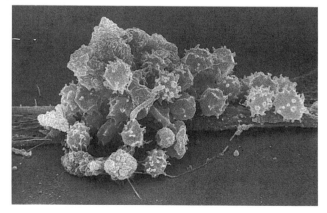

Figure 3-1 (a) Experimental scheme for culturing bone-marrow hematopoietic cells. Such systems have been used to study the role of various growth factors in hematopoiesis. (b) Scanning electron micrograph of cells in a long-term culture of human bone marrow. Adherent stromal cells form a matrix on which the hematopoietic cells proliferate. Cells can be transfered to semisolid agar for colony growth. The colonies can then be analyzed for differentiated cell types. [From M. J. Cline and D. W. Golde, 1979, *Nature* **277**:180.]

Various growth factors have been shown to be required for the survival, proliferation, differentiation, and maturation of hematopoietic cells in culture. These growth factors, or cytokines, were originally detected in serum or in conditioned medium from in vitro cell cultures and were defined on the basis of their ability to stimulate the formation of hematopoietic cell colonies in bone marrow cultures. Among the cytokines detected by this method was a family of acidic glycoproteins, the *colony-stimulating factors (CSFs)*, named for their ability to induce the formation of distinct hematopoietic cell lineages. Four distinct colony-stimulating factors have been identified: multilineage colony-stimulating factor (multi-CSF), also known as interleukin 3 (IL-3); granulocyte-macrophage colony-stimulating factor (GM-CSF); macrophage colony-stimulating factor (M-CSF); and granulocyte colony-stimulating factor (G-CSF). Another important hematopoietic cytokine detected by this method is a glycoprotein produced by the kidney, called *erythropoietin*, that induces terminal erythrocyte development and regulates red blood cell production. Other cytokines involved in hematopoiesis include interleukin 4 (IL-4), interleukin 5 (IL-5), interleukin 6

(IL-6), interleukin 7 (IL-7), interleukin 8 (IL-8), and interleukin 9 (IL-9). Many of these cytokines are secreted by bone-marrow stromal cells, activated T helper (T_H) cells, and activated macrophages.

Biochemical purification of the hematopoietic growth factors was initially hampered by their extremely low physiologic concentrations, with biological activities present at concentrations as low as 10^{-12} *M*. A major breakthrough in the study of these cytokines came when the genes encoding them were cloned, allowing the gene to be transfected into cultured cells. The cloned cytokine gene products have been shown to induce the proliferation and differentiation of hematopoietic progenitor cells in culture (Table 3-2). The colony-stimulating factors act in a stepwise manner, inducing proper maturation of the hematopoietic cells. Multi-CSF (IL-3) acts early in differentiation, possibly even at the level of the pluripotent stem cell, to induce formation of all the nonlymphoid blood cells, including erythrocytes, monocytes, granulocytes (neutrophils, eosinophils, and basophils), and megakaryocytes. GM-CSF acts at a slightly later stage, but it also induces formation of all the nonlymphoid blood cells. M-CSF and G-CSF act

Table 3-2   Effect of cytokines on hematopoietic cells

Target cells acted on in bone marrow	Cytokines										
	Multi-CSF (IL-3)	GM-CSF	G-CSF	M-CSF (CSF-1)	IL-4	IL-5	IL-6	IL-7	IL-8	IL-9	EPO
Pluripotent stem cell	+	+	−	−	−	−	−	−	−	−	−
Myeloid stem cell	+	+	−	−	−	−	+	−	−	−	−
Granulocyte-monocyte progenitor	+	+	+	+	−	−	−	−	−	−	−
Monocyte progenitor	+	+	−	+	−	−	−	−	−	−	−
Neutrophil progenitor	+	+	+	−	−	−	−	−	+	−	−
Eosinophil progenitor	+	+	−	−	−	+	−	−	−	−	−
Basophil progenitor	−	+	−	−	+	−	−	−	−	−	−
Mast cell	+	+	−	−	+	−	−	−	−	+	−
Megakaryocyte	+	+	−	−	−	−	−	−	−	−	+/−
Erythroid progenitor	+/−	+/−	−	−	−	−	−	−	−	−	+
Lymphoid stem cell											
B progenitor	−	−	−	−	+	−	−	+	−	−	−
T progenitor (thymus)	−	−	−	−	−	−	−	+	−	−	−

Key: (+) = indicates cytokine acts on the indicated target cell to stimulate its proliferation and differentiation; (−) = no effect of the cytokine on the indicated cell. See Figure 3-2 for the position of the various target cells in the overall pathway of hematopoiesis.

still later to promote the formation of monocytes and neutrophils, respectively. The commitment of a progenitor cell to a given differentiation pathway has been shown to be associated with the expression on the cell of membrane receptors that are specific for particular cytokines. The macrophage progenitor cell, for example, bears specific receptors for M-CSF; the binding of M-CSF to these receptors stimulates cellular proliferation and differentiation in a concentration-dependent manner.

Regulation of Hematopoiesis

Hematopoiesis is a continuous process that generally maintains a steady state in which the production of mature blood cells equals their loss (principally as the cells age). The average erythrocyte has a lifespan of 120 days before it is phagocytosed and digested by macrophages in the spleen. The various white blood cells have lifespans ranging from days for the neutrophils to as long as 20–30 years for some of the T lymphocytes. It is estimated that to maintain steady-state levels the average human must produce 3.7×10^{11} blood cells per day. The process of hematopoiesis must, of necessity, involve complex regulatory mechanisms to achieve homeostasis of the individual cell types. These regulatory mechanisms must provide steady-state levels of the various red and white blood cells and yet have enough built-in flexibility to allow for rapid increases in production by ten- to twentyfold to meet the demands of infection or hemorrhage. Steady-state levels of hematopoiesis are maintained by controlled cytokine production by the bone-marrow stromal cells. These cells have been shown to produce GM-CSF, M-CSF, G-CSF, IL-4, IL-6, and IL-7. Although multi-CSF (IL-3) is the earliest-acting cytokine, it has not been detected in stromal cells, but only in activated T_H cells. It is thought that some other, as yet unidentified, cytokine must be produced by bone-marrow stromal cells to maintain steady-state levels of the pluripotent stem cells.

In response to infections, localized influxes of white blood cells generate an inflammatory reaction that can limit the infection. The hematopoietic system is capable of rapid expansion and maturation of specific cell lineages to provide the necessary cells for this localized inflammatory response. This inducible hematopoietic activity is regulated by activated T_H cells and activated macrophages, which secrete a number of cytokines that stimulate proliferation and differentiation of different white blood cells involved in the immune response. Among these cytokines are the colony-stimulating factors GM-CSF, G-CSF, and M-CSF, discussed previously, and the following interleukins: IL-3 (multi-CSF), IL-5, and IL-6, which stimulate early hematopoietic progenitor cells; IL-4, which stimulates the B progenitor and mast cell progenitor; IL-8, which enhances neutrophil activity;

and IL-9, which promotes mast cell growth. The concerted actions of these factors induce localized hematopoietic activity to meet the needs of the immune system to fight infection (Figure 3-2).

Production of different hematopoietic lineages can be regulated either by changes in the local concentrations of cytokines or by altered expression of the receptors for different cytokines on different lineages. Expression of the M-CSF receptor, for example, varies significantly among different hematopoietic lineages. Cells of the erythroid, lymphoid, eosinophilic, and megakaryocytic lineages lack M-CSF receptors, cells of the neutrophilic lineage express low levels of M-CSF receptors, and cells of the monocyte-macrophage lineage express high levels of M-CSF receptors. Since the level of receptor expression governs the responsiveness of a lineage to M-CSF concentrations, only cells of the monocyte-macrophage lineage respond to low concentrations of M-CSF, while cells of the neutrophil lineage require much higher concentrations of M-CSF to induce a response; the other hematopoietic lineages do not respond to M-CSF at all.

The binding of a CSF to its receptor causes some of the receptors to be internalized by the cell; internalization serves to down-modulate receptor expression on the cell. With fewer receptors on its membrane, the cell becomes progressively less responsive to the CSF, and proliferation of the lineage slows down. This down-modulation of CSF-receptor expression can even be induced by the binding of unrelated CSFs to their receptors. For example, when GM-CSF binds to its receptor, it induces the cell to down-modulate the expression of G-CSF and M-CSF receptors as well. This down-modulation of G-CSF and M-CSF receptors causes the lineages bearing these receptors to become less responsive to these CSFs.

Hematopoiesis can also be regulated by degradation of the CSF following binding to the CSF receptor. Experiments suggest that binding of M-CSF to the receptor results in degradation of the cytokine. As the monocyte numbers increase, there is an increase in M-CSF receptors, which results in increased M-CSF degradation. The concentration of M-CSF would be expected to fall as cell numbers increase, thereby slowing further proliferation and differentiation of this lineage as long as the number of monocytes remains high.

Role of Hematopoietic Growth Factors in Leukemia

Regulatory abnormalities in the expression of hematopoietic cytokines or their receptors may result in some leukemias. Colony-stimulating factors are secreted by a limited number of cells, including activated T lymphocytes, macrophages, endothelial cells, and bone-marrow stromal cells. As mentioned above, each factor induces

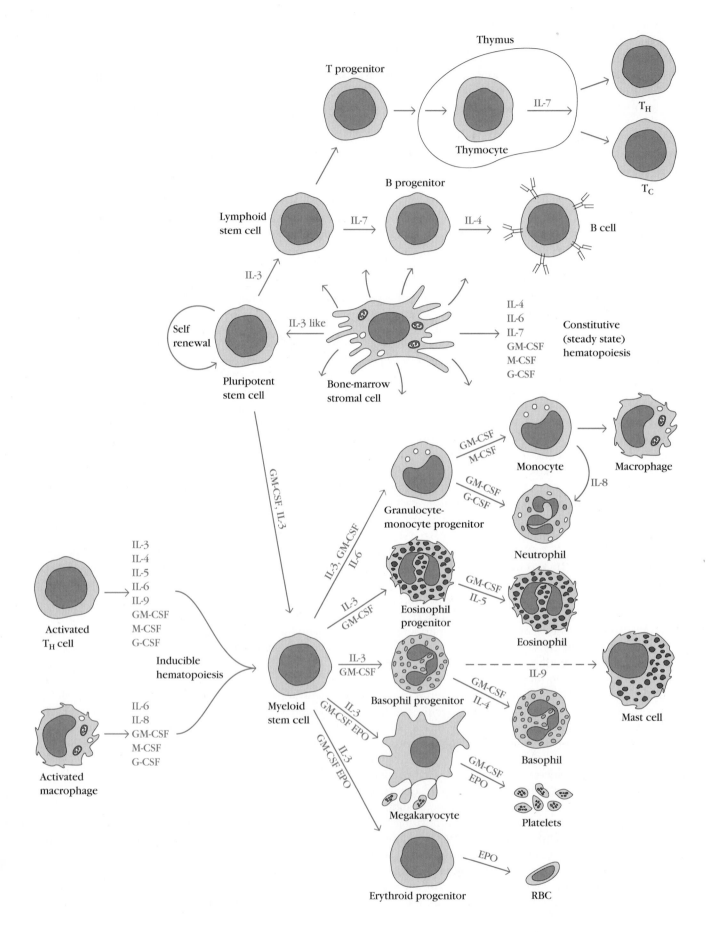

Figure 3-2 Regulation of hematopoiesis by cytokines that stimulate the proliferation and/or differentiation of various hematopoietic cells. In the absence of infection, bone-marrow stromal cells are the major source of hematopoietic cytokines. In the presence of infection, cytokines produced by activated macrophages and T$_H$ cells induce additional hematopoietic activity, resulting in the rapid expansion of the WBC population that is necessary for fighting infection.

the proliferation and differentiation of only those hematopoietic stem cells that bear a receptor. By limiting receptor expression to certain cells and growth factor secretion to other cells, hematopoiesis can be controlled. Expression of the receptor for a growth factor appears to be linked to cellular differentiation following proliferation induced by earlier-acting growth factors. A defect in regulation of expression of either the growth factor or its receptor could lead to unregulated cellular proliferation. Failure to down-modulate receptor expression following GM-CSF activation may lead to a leukemic state (Figure 3-3a). The binding of GM-CSF

induces down-modulation of both G-CSF and M-CSF receptors on normal hematopoietic cells but not on leukemic cells. This failure of GM-CSF to down-modulate the G-CSF or M-CSF receptors on leukemic cells may allow leukemic cells to respond to low levels of CSFs that would not induce the proliferation of normal down-modulated hematopoietic cells.

Inappropriate expression of a hematopoietic cytokine by a cell bearing a receptor for that cytokine could also lead to unregulated cancerous proliferation. Some findings suggest that this phenomenon occurs in some leukemias. For example, leukemic cells from some patients with acute myeloid leukemia have been shown to secrete GM-CSF, whereas normal myeloid cells do not secrete this growth factor (see Figure 3-3b). Similarly, when normal myeloid cell lines bearing receptors for GM-CSF are transfected with cloned GM-CSF cDNA, they autostimulate their own growth in the absence of added GM-CSF (see Figure 3-3c); if these transfected cells are injected into mice, the animals develop leukemias. Per-

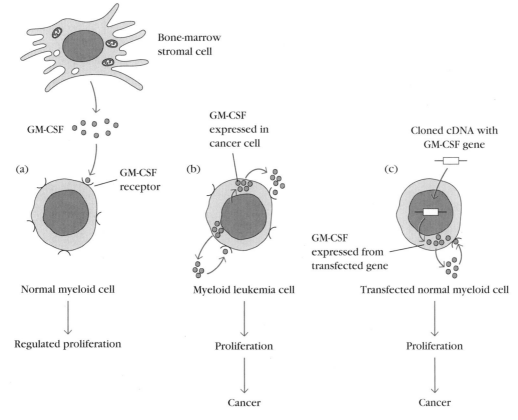

Figure 3-3 (a) Hematopoietic cells express membrane receptors for particular colony-stimulating factors secreted by bone-marrow stromal cells. Proliferation of the hematopoietic cell is therefore regulated, in part, by the local concentration of growth factor. (b) Inappropriate secretion of GM-CSF by some myeloid leukemia cells leads to auto-stimulation. (c) Transfection of GM-CSF cDNA into normal myeloid cell lines will lead to unregulated proliferation of the transfected cells. Injection of these transfected cells into mice results in leukemia.

haps the strongest evidence that such abnormal auto-stimulation can lead to cancerous proliferation comes from the human adult T-cell leukemia associated with the HTLV-I retrovirus, which infects human T cells and transforms them into leukemic cells. HTLV-I–infected T cells begin to express the IL-2 receptor in the absence of previous antigen activation. Secretion of IL-2 by these same cells allows unregulated cellular proliferation resulting in leukemia. The molecular basis for this transformation is discussed in detail in Chapter 11.

Enrichment of Hematopoietic Stem Cells

I. L. Weissman and colleagues developed a novel way of enriching pluripotent stem cells from the bone marrow of mice where it constitutes a mere 0.05% of all bone marrow cells. They began by taking advantage of the fact that the various progenitor cells and mature red and white blood cells bear specific differentiation antigens. They could remove these differentiated cells from the bone marrow by reacting them with fluorescent monoclonal antibodies specific for the differentiation antigens and then removing the labeled cells by flow cytometry using a fluorescence-activated cell sorter (Figure 3-4a). After each sorting, the remaining cells were assayed for their ability to restore hematopoiesis in a lethally x-irradiated mouse. As long as fewer and fewer cells could restore hematopoiesis in this system, it indicated that the pluripotent stem cell was being progressively enriched. By removing those hematopoietic cells expressing known differentiation antigens, these researchers were able to obtain a 50- to 200-fold enrichment in

pluripotent stem cells. To further enrich the pluripotent stem cell, the remaining cells were incubated with various monoclonal antibodies raised against cells likely to represent early differentiation stages in hematopoiesis. One of these monoclonal antibodies recognized a dif-

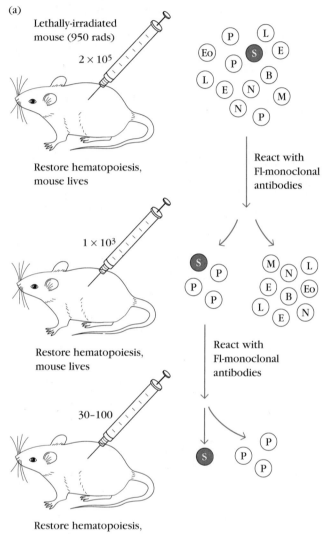

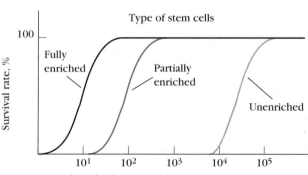

Figure 3-4   Enrichment of the pluripotent stem cell has been achieved by using monoclonal antibodies specific for membrane molecules expressed on differentiated lineages but absent on undifferentiated lineages. (a) Removal of differentiated hematopoietic cells with monoclonal antibody: M = monocyte, N = neutrophil, L = lymphocyte, Eo = eosinophil, E = erythrocyte, B = basophil. The remaining cells were enriched in stem cells (S) and progenitor cells (P). In each successive enrichment fewer and fewer cells were able to reconstitute the lethally x-irradiated mouse. (b) Assays of stem-cell preparations based on their ability to restore hematopoiesis to lethally irradiated mice. Only animals in which hematopoiesis occurs will survive. Progressive enrichment of stem cells is indicated by the decrease in the number of injected cells needed to restore hematopoiesis. The fully enriched preparation was obtained by treating the partially enriched preparation with monoclonal antibody against Sca-1, an early differentiation antigen. A total enrichment of about 1000-fold is possible by this procedure.

ferentiation antigen called stem cell antigen-1 (Sca-1). This monoclonal antibody allowed the pluripotent stem cell to be enriched by flow cytometry to such a degree that between 30 and 100 of these cells could restore hematopoiesis in a lethally x-irradiated mouse in contrast to a requirement of $1-3 \times 10^4$ nonenriched bone marrow cells (Figure 3-4b).

If similar techniques to enrich pluripotent stem cells can be developed in humans, it might be possible to use enriched stem-cell preparations in a variety of clinical

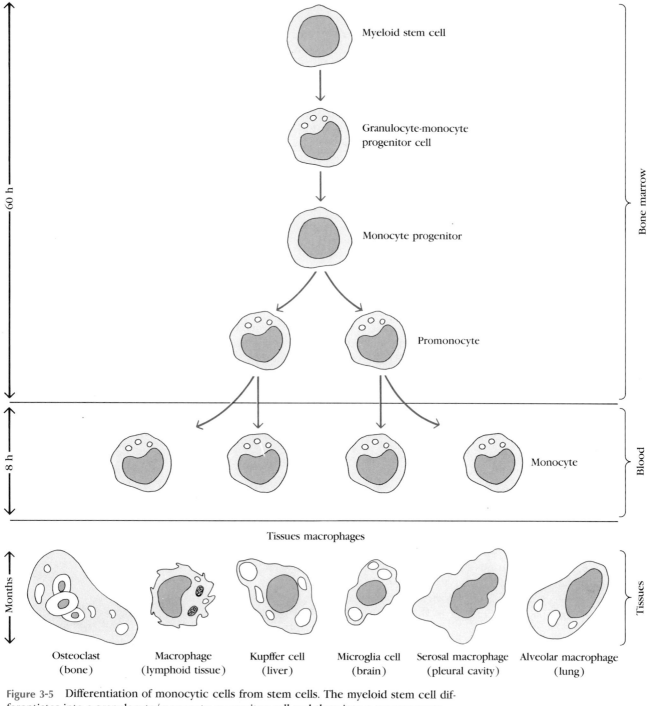

Figure 3-5 Differentiation of monocytic cells from stem cells. The myeloid stem cell differentiates into a granulocyte/monocyte progenitor cell and then into a promonocyte within the bone marrow. Promonocytes enter the blood and differentiate into the mature monocyte. The monocytes circulate in the blood for about 8 h and then migrate into the tissues where the cell differentiates into specific tissue macrophages. [Adapted from E. R. Unanue and P. M. Allen, 1987, *Hosp. Pract.* (April 15): 88.]

treatments. Currently individuals with various immunodeficiency diseases, certain cancers, or radiation damage require bone marrow transplants for survival. The ability to transplant stem cells rather than whole bone marrow might increase the acceptance of the foreign cells and decrease the incidence of a fatal complication, called graft-versus-host disease, in which lymphocytes in the donor bone marrow begin to attack the recipient's cells. With advances in genetic engineering it may soon be possible to transfer good genes into stem cells removed from individuals with known genetic blood-cell disorders, such as sickle cell anemia and thalassemia, and then reinject the engineered stem cells back into the individual. In the first attempt at gene therapy, lymphocytes from a young girl born with a severe combined immunodeficiency disease (SCID) were genetically engineered to replace a defective gene. The genetically altered lymphocytes were then infused back into the girl. However, since lymphocytes are not capable of self-renewal, the process needs to be repeated at periodic intervals. When the pluripotent stem cell is finally isolated in humans, it will make it possible to restore the defective gene in a self-renewing population.

Mononuclear Cells

The mononuclear phagocytic system consists of circulating monocytes in the blood and macrophages in the tissues. During hematopoiesis in the bone marrow, myeloid progenitor cells differentiate into promonocytes, which leave the bone marrow and enter the blood, where they differentiate further into monocytes. As they circulate in the bloodstream for about 8 h, the monocytes enlarge and then migrate into the tissues as they differentiate to become macrophages. The differentiation involves a number of changes: the cell enlarges, its intracellular organelles increase in both number and complexity, and it acquires increased phagocytotic ability and secretes a variety of soluble factors (Figure 3-5). Macrophages serve different functions in different tissues and are named to reflect their tissue location. For example, liver macrophages are called *Kupffer cells*, lung macrophages are called *alveolar macrophages*, brain macrophages are called *microglial cells*, and splenic macrophages are called *lymphoid macrophages*.

Functions of Monocytes and Macrophages

Monocytes and macrophages were initially thought to function simply as phagocytic cells. Recently, however, it has become clear that their phagocytic function is only the beginning of their functional role in the immune response. Following phagocytosis, these cells serve a

vital function both as antigen-presenting cells and as secretory cells. As the monocyte differentiates into the macrophage, many of these functional activities increase. The three primary biological functions of these cells are examined in this section, with the emphasis on macrophage activity.

Phagocytosis. Macrophages are actively phagocytic cells capable of ingesting and digesting exogenous antigens such as whole pathogenic microorganisms, insoluble particles, injured and dead host cells, cellular debris, and activated clotting factors. In the first step in phagocytosis, macrophages are attracted by and move toward a variety of substances generated in an immune response; this process is called *chemotaxis*. The next step in phagocytosis involves *attachment* of the antigen to the macrophage cell membrane. (Complex antigens, such as whole bacterial cells or viral particles, tend to adhere well and are readily phagocytosed; isolated proteins and

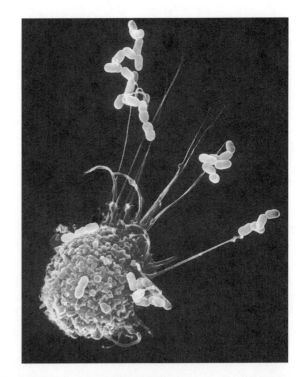

Figure 3-6 Scanning electron micrograph of a macrophage showing the first step of phagocytosis, in which a macrophage contacts a bacterium by extending long pseudopodia. The pseudopodia then draw the bacteria to the macrophage membrane. Lennart Nilsson [Boehringer Ingelheim International GmbH, photo.]

encapsulated bacteria tend to adhere poorly and are less readily phagocytosed.) Attachment induces membrane protrusions called *pseudopodia* to extend around the attached material (Figure 3-6). The pseudopodia fuse and the material is then contained within a membrane-bound structure called a *phagosome*, which then enters the endosomal processing pathway. In this pathway, a phagosome moves toward the cell interior, where it fuses with a *lysosome*, to form a *phagolysosome*. The contents of the lysosome include hydrogen peroxide, oxygen free radicals, peroxidase, lysozyme, and various hydrolytic enzymes, which contact the ingested material and digest it. The digested contents of the phagolysosome are then eliminated in a process called *exocytosis* (Figure 3-7).

Most phagocytosed microorganisms are killed as the contents of the lysosome are released into the phagosome. There are, however, some microorganisms that can survive and multiply within the phagosome of macrophages. These intracellular pathogens include *Listeria monocytogenes*, *Salmonella typhimurium*, *Neisseria gonorrhoea*, *Mycobacterium avium*, *Mycobacterium tuberculosis*, *Mycobacterium leprae*, *Brucella abortus*, and *Candida albicans*. Some of these pathogens prevent fusion of the lysosome with the phagosome and are able then to proliferate within the phagosomes; others have cell-wall components that render them resistant to the contents of the lysosome; and still others survive within the macrophage by escaping from the phagosome and proliferating within the cytoplasm of the infected macrophage. These intracellular pathogens, which have developed a clever defense against the nonspecific phagocytic defense system, are shielded from a specific immunologic response. A unique cell-mediated immunologic defense mechanism, called delayed hypersensitivity, that combats such pathogens is discussed in Chapter 13.

Antigen Processing and Presentation. Not all of the antigen ingested by macrophages is degraded and eliminated by exocytosis. Experiments with radiolabeled antigens have demonstrated the presence of radioactive antigen components on the macrophage membrane after most of an antigen has been digested and eliminated. As discussed in Chapter 1, phagocytosed antigen is metabolically converted within the endosomal processing pathway into peptides that associate with a class II MHC molecule. These peptide–MHC II complexes then move to the macrophage membrane, where the processed antigenic peptides are presented to T_H cells (see Figure 3-7a). The presentation of antigen in association with class II MHC molecules is a critical requirement for the activation of T_H cells (see Figure 1-13). As

Chapter 9 will make clear, this presentation is central to development of both the humoral and the cell-mediated immune responses.

Secretion of Factors. A number of important proteins central to development of the immune response are secreted by the macrophage (Table 3-3). When macrophages phagocytose antigen, they are activated and begin to secrete interleukin 1 (IL-1), which acts on T_H cells and is required for their cellular activation following antigen recognition (see Figure 1-13). Interleukin 1 also affects vascular endothelial cells, thus influencing the inflammatory response, and affects the thermoregulatory center in the hypothalamus, leading to the fever re-

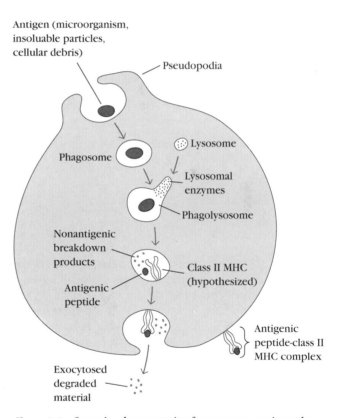

Antigen (microorganism, insoluable particles, cellular debris)

Pseudopodia

Lysosome

Phagosome

Lysosomal enzymes

Phagolysosome

Nonantigenic breakdown products

Class II MHC (hypothesized)

Antigenic peptide

Antigenic peptide-class II MHC complex

Exocytosed degraded material

Figure 3-7 Steps in phagocytosis of exogenous antigens by macrophages. Following adherence to the macrophage membrane the active membrane of the macrophage extends long pseudopodia around the attached material. The pseudopodia fuse drawing the material into the cell enclosed in a membrane-bound organelle called a phagosome. The lysosome fuses with the phagosome, releasing its contents into the phagolysosome. Most of the ingested material is digested and eliminated through exocytosis. Some of the digested peptides are thought to interact with the class II MHC molecule. The antigenic peptide–class II MHC complex then moves to the cell surface, where it can be recognized by a T_H cell.

Table 3-3 Some factors secreted by activated macrophages that function in the immune response

Factor	Function
Interleukin 1 (IL-1)	Costimulatory factor: induces activation of T_H cells following antigen/MHC activation, promotes inflammatory response and fever
Complement proteins	Promotes elimination of pathogens and inflammatory response
Hydrolytic enzymes	Promotes inflammatory response
Interferon alpha (IFN-α)	Activates cellular genes resulting in the production of proteins that confer an antiviral state on the cell
Tumor necrosis factor (TNF-α)	Kills tumor cells
Interleukin 6 (IL-6) GM-CSF G-CSF M-CSF	Each promotes inducible hematopoiesis

sponse. Activated macrophages also secrete a variety of other factors involved in the development of an inflammatory response. These include a group of serum proteins, called *complement*, that assist in the elimination of foreign pathogens and in the ensuing inflammatory reaction. The *hydrolytic enzymes* contained within their lysosomes can also be secreted by activated macrophages. The buildup of these enzymes within the tissues contributes to the inflammatory response and can, in some cases, lead to extensive tissue damage. Activated macrophages also secrete soluble factors, such as *tumor necrosis factor* α (*TNF-α*), which can kill a variety of cells. The secretion of these *cytotoxic factors* has been shown to contribute to tumor destruction by macrophages. Finally, as discussed earlier, activated macrophages secrete a number of cytokines that stimulate inducible hematopoiesis.

Enhancement of Macrophage Function

Macrophage activity can be enhanced by certain molecules elaborated during an immune response. The macrophage membrane possesses receptors for certain classes of antibody and for certain complement components. When an antigen (e.g., a bacterium) is coated with the appropriate antibody or complement component, it is more readily bound to the macrophage membrane and phagocytosis is enhanced. Antibody and complement serve as *opsonins* (from Latin *opsonium*, relish) and the entire process is called *opsonization*. In one study the rate of phagocytosis of an antigen was increased 4000-fold in the presence of specific antibody to the antigen. Macrophage activity can also be increased by agents that increase the number of macrophages at a given site of infection. Monocytes and macrophages are summoned to the site of an immune reaction by a variety of *chemotactic factors*. Among these factors are factors secreted by activated T cells, various complement components, and certain components of the clotting system.

Although phagocytosis of antigen initially activates macrophages, their activity can be further enhanced by various activating factors. For example, interferon gamma (IFN-γ) secreted by activated T cells binds to receptors on macrophages and activates them. Because such activated macrophages develop increased phagocytic activity and higher levels of lysosomal enzymes, their ability to ingest and eliminate potential pathogens is enhanced. In addition, these activated macrophages secrete cytotoxic proteins (e.g., TNF-α) that help them eliminate a broader range of pathogens, including virus-infected cells, tumor cells, and intracellular bacteria. Activated macrophages also express higher levels of class II MHC molecules, allowing them to function more effectively as antigen-presenting cells. Thus macrophages and T_H cells exhibit an interacting relationship during the immune response with each facilitating activation of the other.

Granulocytic Cells

The granulocytes are classified as *neutrophils*, *eosinophils*, or *basophils* on the basis of cellular morphology and cytoplasmic staining characteristics. The neutrophil, which has a granulated cytoplasm that stains with both acid and basic dyes, is often called a *polymorphonuclear leukocyte* for its multilobed nucleus. The eosinophil has a bilobed nucleus and a heavily granulated cytoplasm that stains with the acid dye eosin Y (hence its name). The basophil has a lobed nucleus and heavily granulated cytoplasm that stains with the basic dye methylene blue. Both neutrophils and eosinophils are phagocytic, whereas basophils are not. Neutrophils, which constitute 50–70% of the circulating white blood cells, are much more numerous than eosinophils (1–3%) or basophils (<1%).

Neutrophils

Neutrophils are produced in the bone marrow during hematopoiesis. They are released into the peripheral blood and circulate for 7–10 h before migrating into the tissues, where they have a 3-day lifespan. Observation of neutrophil migration reveals that the cell first adheres to the vascular endothelium and then penetrates the gap between the endothelial cells lining the blood vessel wall. Adherence to the vascular endothelial cell is by means of various membrane receptors. From there the cell passes through the vascular basement membrane and out into the tissue spaces. A number of substances generated in an inflammatory reaction serve as chemotactic factors that promote a buildup of neutrophils at the site of inflammation. Among these chemotactic factors are some of the complement components, components of the blood-clotting system, and products secreted by activated T cells. The process of phagocytosis by neutrophils is similar to that described for macrophages, except that neutrophils lack lysosomes. Instead neutrophils contain lytic enzymes and bactericidal substances within primary and secondary granules. These granules fuse with the phagosome, whose contents are then digested and eliminated much as they are in macrophages.

Eosinophils

Eosinophils, like neutrophils, are motile, phagocytic cells that can migrate from the blood into the tissue spaces. Their phagocytic role is significantly less important than that of neutrophils, and it is thought that their major role is in defense against parasitic organisms. The secretion of the contents of eosinophilic granules results in damage to the parasite membrane.

Basophils

Basophils are not phagocytic and function by releasing pharmacologically active substances contained within their cytoplasmic granules. They have a major role in allergic responses during which they release the contents of their granules. Basophils are discussed in detail in Chapter 16 in the section on type I hypersensitive reactions.

Mast Cells

Mast cell precursors, which are formed in the bone marrow during hematopoiesis, are released into the blood as undifferentiated precursor cells and do not differentiate until they leave the blood and enter the tissues. Mast cells can be found in a wide variety of tissues including the skin, connective tissues of various organs, and mucosal epithelial tissue of the respiratory, genitourinary, and digestive tracts. Like circulating basophils, these cells have large numbers of cytoplasmic granules containing histamine and other pharmacologically active substances. These cells, together with blood basophils, play an important role in the development of allergies and are discussed in more detail in Chapter 16.

Dendritic Cells

The dendritic cell acquired its name because it is covered with a maze of long membrane processes resembling dendrites of nerve cells (Figure 3-8). Dendritic cells have been very difficult to study because conventional procedures for isolating lymphocytes or other accessory immune-system cells tend to damage the long dendritic processes, so that the cells fail to survive. Recently gentler dispersion techniques using enzymes have facilitated isolation of these cells for in vitro study. In addition to their unusual dendritic shape, dendritic cells share several structural and functional features. They express high levels of class II MHC molecules and function as important antigen-presenting cells for T-cell activation. After capturing antigen in the tissues, dendritic cells migrate to various lymphoid organs where they present the antigen to lymphocytes. Dendritic cells are found in nonlymphoid organs and tissues, in lymphoid organs, and in the blood and lymph (Table 3-4).

The nonlymphoid dendritic cells include Langerhans cells of the epidermis and the interstitial dendritic cells

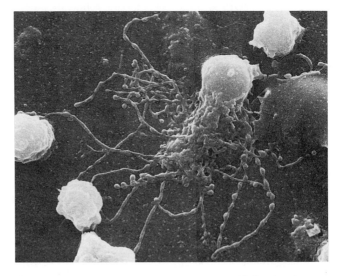

Figure 3-8 Scanning electron micrograph of follicular dendritic cells showing long "beaded" dendrites. The beads are coated with antigen-antibody complexes. The dendrites emanate from the cell body [From A. K. Szakal et al., 1985, *J. Immunol.* **134**: 1353. © 1985 American Association of Immunologists. Reprinted with permission.]

Table 3-4   Dendritic cells

Distribution	Cell type
Nonlymphoid organs	
Skin	Langerhans cells
Organs	Interstitial dendritic cells
Lymphoid organs	
T-cell areas	Interdigitating dendritic cells
B-cell areas	Follicular dendritic cells
Circulation	
Blood	Blood dendritic cells
Lymph	"Veiled" cells

that populate most organs (e.g., heart, lungs, liver, kidney, gastrointestinal tract). The nonlymphoid dendritic cells capture antigen and carry the antigen to regional lymph nodes. As these nonlymphoid dendritic cells enter the blood and lymph, they change morphologically and become "veiled" cells. In the blood these cells account for <0.1% of leukocytes. In organ transplants, resident populations of nonlymphoid dendritic cells may migrate from the transplanted organ to regional lymph nodes where they serve to activate recipient T cells against the foreign antigens of the transplanted organ. This process will be discussed more fully in Chapter 22.

The lymphoid dendritic cells include the interdigitating dendritic cells and the follicular dendritic cells. The interdigitating dendritic cells are found in T-cell–rich regions of lymphoid organs including the spleen, lymph nodes, and thymus. T cells and interdigitating dendritic cells form large multicellular aggregates, which may enhance the likelihood of effective antigen-MHC presentation to T cells. Follicular dendritic cells were named for their exclusive location in organized structures of the lymph node called lymph follicles. These lymph follicles are rich in B cells, and the follicular dendritic cells are thought to trap antigen, facilitating B-cell activation. The follicular dendritic cells express high levels of membrane receptors for antibody and complement. Circulating antibody-antigen complexes bound to these receptors have been shown to be retained on the dendritic cell membrane for very long periods of time, ranging from weeks to months. An electron-dense layer of antigen-antibody complexes can be seen covering the dendritic processes of these cells in Figure 3-8. The presence of antigen-antibody complexes on the membrane of the follicular dendritic cells is thought to play a role in the development of memory B cells within the lymph follicle.

The dendritic cells in each of these locations have morphologic and functional differences but may arise from a common progenitor cell and may represent various stages of a single lineage. Until the dendritic progenitor is identified, the relationship of each of the different dendritic cells to one another remains unresolved.

Lymphoid Cells

Lymphocytes are the white blood cells responsible for the immune response. Their characteristics account for the immune system's attributes of diversity, specificity, memory, and self/nonself recognition. Lymphocytes, which constitute 20–40% of the body's white blood cells, circulate in the blood and lymph and are capable of migrating into the tissue spaces and lymphoid organs. The lymphocytes can be broadly subdivided on the basis of function and cell-membrane components into three populations: B cells, T cells, and null cells. All three cell types are small, motile, nonphagocytic cells, which cannot be distinguished morphologically. B and T lymphocytes that have not interacted with antigen are said to be resting lymphocytes in the G_0 phase of the cell cycle. Such resting cells, known as *small lymphocytes*, are only about 6 μm in diameter, and their cytoplasm forms a barely discernible rim around the nucleus. These resting cells have densely packed chromatin, few mitochondria, and a poorly developed endoplasmic reticulum and Golgi apparatus. Interaction of a B or T lymphocyte with antigen, in the presence of other factors to be discussed later, induces the lymphocyte to enter the cell cycle, progressing from G_0 into G_1, S, G_2, and M (Figure 3-9).

As it progresses through the cell cycle, the lymphocyte enlarges into a 15-μm-diameter *blast cell*, called a *lymphoblast*, which has an increased cytoplasm-to-nucleus ratio and more organellar complexity. The lymphoblasts further differentiate into either various effector cells or into a population of memory cells. The effector cells have short lifespans, generally ranging from a few days to a few weeks. Plasma cells are the effector cell of the B-cell lineage. These cells have a characteristic cytoplasm developed for active secretion with abundant endoplasmic reticulum arranged in concentric layers and many Golgi vesicles (Figure 3-9). The effector cells of the T-cell lineage include the T_H cell and the CTL. The memory cells are long-lived cells that reside in the G_0 phase of the cell cycle until activated by a secondary encounter with antigen.

Different lineages or maturational stages of lymphocytes can be distinguished by their expression of membrane molecules recognized by particular monoclonal antibodies. At first each membrane molecule identified by a particular monoclonal antibody was named by the individual researchers. This led to a plethora of desig-

(a)

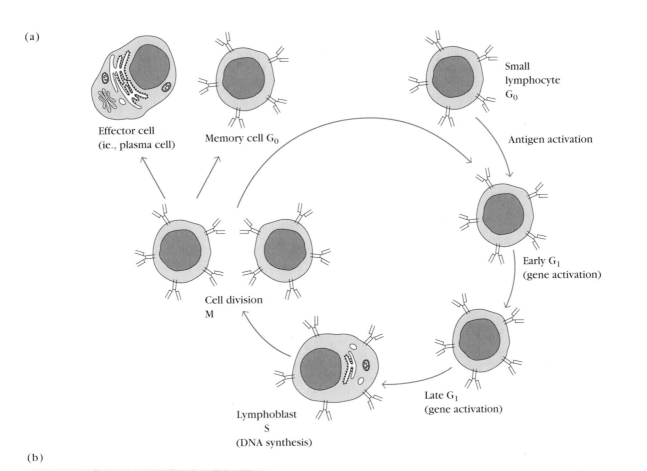

(b)

Figure 3-9 (a) As lymphocytes progress through the cell cycle they undergo morphologic changes. A small resting (unprimed) lymphocyte resides in the G_0 phase of the cell cycle. At this stage, B and T lymphocytes cannot be distinguished morphologically, although they have distinctive surface markers by which they can be identified. Following antigen activation the B or T cell enter the cell cycle and progress from G_1 into the S phase where DNA is replicated. The cell at this stage enlarges into a lymphoblast cell. Following mitosis both memory and effector cells are generated. (b) Electron micrographs of a small lymphocyte showing condensed chromatin indicative of a resting cell, an enlarged lymphoblast showing decondensed chromatin, and a plasma cell showing abundant endoplasmic reticulum arranged in concentric layers. The three cells are shown at the same magnification. [Part (b) courtesy of Dr. Joseph R. Goodman, Dept. of Pediatrics, University of California at San Francisco.]

nations for the same membrane molecule. In 1982 the
First International Workshop on Human Leukocyte Differentiation Antigens was held to develop a uniform
nomenclature for leukocyte membrane molecules. The
outcome of this workshop was to group all of the monoclonal antibodies that reacted with a particular membrane molecule as a *cluster of differentiation* or *CD*.
New monoclonal antibodies that recognize leukocyte
membrane molecules are analyzed to determine if they
fall within a given CD designation or are given a new
CD designation if they identify a new membrane molecule. Although the CD nomenclature was originally developed for human leukocyte membrane molecules, the
homologous membrane molecules found in other species, such as mice, are commonly referred to by the
same CD designations. Table 3-5 lists some of the CD
designations of human leukocytes.

   The general characteristics and functions of B and T
lymphocytes were discussed in Chapter 1 and are re-
viewed briefly in the following sections. These central
cells of the immune system are examined in more detail
in later chapters.

B Lymphocytes

The B lymphocyte derived its name from its site of
maturation in the bursa of Fabricius in birds; the name
turned out to be apt, for its major site of maturation in
mammals is the bone marrow (see Figure 3-2). Mature
B cells can be distinguished from other lymphocytes by
the presence of membrane-bound immunoglobulin (antibody) molecules, which serve as receptors for antigen.
There are approximately 1.5×10^5 molecules of antibody on the membrane of a single B cell, with each
molecule having an identical binding site for antigen.
Appropriate interaction between antigen and the antibody receptor on a B cell, together with T-cell and
macrophage interactions, induces clonal selection of the
B cell, involving cell division and differentiation and generating a population of plasma cells and memory cells
(see Figure 1-10). The plasma cells lack membrane-
bound antibody; instead they actively secrete one of five
classes of antibody. All clonal progeny from a given B
cell secrete antibody molecules with the same antigen-
binding specificity.

Table 3-5   Cluster of differentiation (CD) antigens on human cells

CD Designation	Synonyms	Main cellular expression	Function
CD1a CD1b CD1c	T6, Leu-6, OK-T6	Thymocytes, dendritic cells	?
CD2	T11, LFA-2, E-receptor	T cells, NK cells	Adhesion molecule, receptor for LFA-3 and sheep RBC's
CD3	T3, OKT3, Leu 4	T cells	Signal transduction element of TCR
CD4	T4, OKT4, Leu3	T cell subset (class II MHC restricted)	Adhesion molecule: binds to class II MHC
CD5	T1, OKT1, Leu-1	T cells, B cell subset	?
CD6	T12	T cell and B cell subset	?
CD7	—	T cell subset	?
CD8	T8, Leu-2, Lyt2	T cell subset (class I MHC restricted)	Adhesion molecule: binds to class I MHC
CD9	—	Monocytes, pre-B cells, platelets	?
CD10	J5, CALLA, BA-3	Pre-B cells	Neural endopeptidase
CD11a	LFA-1 & chain	Leukocytes	Adhesion molecule: binds to ICAM-1
CD11b	Mac-1, CR3 α chain	Monocytes, NK cells, granulocytes	Adhesion molecule: iC3b receptor

Table 3-5 Continued

CD Designation	Synonyms	Main cellular expression	Function
CD11c	p150, 95, CR4 α chain	Monocytes, NK cells granulocytes	Adhesion molecule: iC3b receptor
CDw12	—	Monocytes, granulocytes	?
CD13	—	Monocytes, granulocytes	Aminopeptidase
CD14	MO2	Monocytes	?
CD15	—	Granulocytes	?
CD16	FcRIII	NK cells, granulocytes	Low affinity receptor for γ Fc
CD17	—	Granulocytes, monocytes, platelets	?
CD18	LFA-1 family β chain	Leukocytes	β chain for CD11a, CD11b, CD11c
CD19	B4	B cells	?
CD20	B1	B cells	? (part of Ca^{2+} channel)
CD21	CR2, C3d receptor	B cells	Receptor for C3d, Epstein-Barr virus receptor
CD22	—	B cells	?
CD23	FcεRIIb	Activated B cells, macrophages, eosinophils	Low affinity Fcε receptor
CD24	—	B cells granulocytes	?
CD25	p55 low affinity IL-2 receptor (TAC)	Activated T and B cells	IL-2 receptor β chain
CD26	—	Activated T and B cells, activated macrophages	Serine peptidase
CD27	—	T cells, plasma cells	?
CD28	Tp44	T cells	Receptor for costimulator molecules
CD29	β chain of VLA adhesion molecules	Leukocytes	Adhesion molecule
CD30	Ki-1	Activated T and B cells, Reed-Sternberg cells	?
CD31	gpIIa	Monocytes granulocytes, platelets	?
CDw32	FcRII	Monocytes, macrophages, granulocytes, activated B cells	Fc receptor for IgG
CD33	—	Monocytes, myeloid progenitor cells	?
CD34	—	Myeloid progenitor cells	?

Table 3-5 Continued

CD Designation	Synonyms	Main cellular expression	Function
CD35	CR1; C3b receptor	Granulocytes, erythrocytes, B cells erythrocytes	CR1 receptor for C3b and C4b
CD36	gpIIIb	Monocytes, platelets	Platelet adhesion
CD37	—	B cells	?
CD38	T10	B cells, thymocytes, activated T cells	?
CD39	—	Mature B cells	?
CD40	—	B cells	Possible role in memory cell formation
CD41	gpIIb/IIIa	Platelets	Platelet aggregation
CD42	gpIX	Platelets, megakaryocytes	Platelet adhesion
CD43	—	Leukocytes	?
CD44	Pgp-1, Hermes	Leukocytes, erythrocytes	Homing receptor
CD45	T200, leukocyte common antigen	Leukocytes	Role in signal transduction
CD45R	Restricted T200		Role in signal transduction
CD45RO		Memory cells	
CD45RA		Naive T cells	
CD45RB		B cells	
CD46	Membrane cofactor protein (MCP)	Leukocytes, epithelial cells,	Regulator of complement activation
CD47	—	Leukocytes	?
CD48	—	Leukocytes	?
CDw49a	VLA α1 chain	T cells, monocytes	Associates with CD29 forming VLA-1 (β1 integrin), adhesion molecule
CDw49b	VLA α2 chain	Platelets, activated T cells, monocytes	Associates with CD29 forming VLA-2 (β1 integrin), adhesion molecule
CDw49c	VLA α3 chain	T cells, some B cells	Associates with CD29 forming VLA-3 (β1 integrin), adhesion molecule
CDw49d	VLA α4 chain	Monocytes, T cells, B cells	Associates with CD29 forming VLA-4 (β1 integrin), Peyers patch homing receptor
CDw49e	VLA α5 chain	T cells, some B cells and monocytes	Associates with CD29 forming VLA-5 (β1 integrin), adhesion to fibronectin

Table 3-5   Continued

CD Designation	Synonyms	Main cellular expression	Function
CDw49f	VLA α6 chain	Platelets	Associates with CD29 forming VLA-6 (β1 integrin), adhesion molecule
CDw50	—	Leukocytes	?
CD51	Vitronectin α chain	Platelets	Adhesion molecule
CDw52	—	Leukocytes	?
CD53	—	Leukocytes	?
CD54	ICAM-1	Broad cellular distribution	Adhesion molecule, binds to LFA-1
CD55	Decay accelerating factor	Broad cellular distribution	Involved in complement regulation
CD56	Leu-19	NK cells	Adhesion molecule
CD57	HNK-1	NK cells, subset of T and B cells	?
CD58	LFA-3	Leukocytes	Adhesion molecule, ligand for CD2
CD59	MIRL	Broad cellular distribution	Regulation of MAC formation
CDw60	—	Platelets, subset of T cells	?
CD61	Vibronectin β chain, gpIIIa	Platelets	Adhesion receptor
CD62	GMP-140	Platelets, endothelial cells	Adhesion to endothelium
CD63	—	Activated platelets; monocytes, macrophages	?
CD64	FcRI	Monocytes, macrophages	High-affinity Fcv receptor; role in phagocytosis, ADCC, macrophage activation
CDw65	—	Granulocytes	Possible role in neutrophil activation
CD66	—	Granulocytes	?
CD67	—	Granulocytes	?
CD68	—	Monocytes, macrophages	?
CD69	—	Activated B and T cells, macrophages, NK cells	?
CD70	—	Activated T and B cells	?

Table 3-5   Continued

CD Designation	Synonyms	Main cellular expression	Function
CD71	T9, transferrin receptor	Activated T and B cells, macrophages, proliferating cells	Transferrin receptor
CD72	—	B cells	?
CD73	—	Subsets of T and B cells	Ecto-5′-nucleotidase
CD74	Class II MHC invariant (v) chain; Ii	B cells, monocytes, macrophages; other class II⁺ cells	Associated with newly synthesized class II MHC molecules within the cell
CD75	—	Mature B cells	?
CD76	—	Mature B cells, subset of T cells	?
CD77	—	Follicular center B cells	?
CD78	Ba	B cells	?

SOURCE: Adapted from Leukocyle Typing IV. White Cell Differentiation Antigens, W. Knapp, B. Dorken, W. R. Gilks, et al. eds. Oxford University Press, 1989.

T Lymphocytes

T lymphocytes derive their name from their site of maturation in the thymus. Like B lymphocytes, these cells have membrane receptors for antigen. The T-cell receptor for antigen is structurally distinct from immunoglobulin but does have some structural features in common with the immunoglobulin molecule, most notably in the structure of its antigen-binding site. What distinguishes the T-cell receptor from membrane-bound antibody on B cells is that it recognizes antigen only when the antigen is associated with a self-molecule encoded by genes within the major histocompatibility complex (MHC). The T cell recognizes antigen associated with self-MHC, which is also called *altered self.* This points to a fundamental difference between humoral and cell-mediated branches of the immune system. Whereas the B cell is capable of binding soluble antigen, the T-cell system is restricted to binding antigen displayed on self-cells. This antigen may be expressed together with MHC molecules on the surface of antigen-presenting cells or on virus-infected cells, cancer cells, and grafts. The T-cell system has developed to eliminate these altered self-cells, which pose a threat to the normal functioning of the body.

T-cell subpopulations can be distinguished by the presence of one or the other of two membrane molecules, CD4 and CD8. T cells that express CD4 recognize antigen associated with class II MHC molecules, whereas T cells expressing CD8 recognize antigen associated with class I MHC. Thus the expression of CD4 versus CD8 corresponds to the MHC restriction of the T cell. In general, expression of CD4 and of CD8 also defines two major functional subpopulations of T lymphocytes. The CD4⁺ T cells generally function as T helper (T_H) cells and are class II restricted; CD8⁺ T cells generally function as T cytotoxic (T_C) cells and are class I restricted. T_H cells proliferate extensively following antigen/class II MHC recognition on an antigen-presenting cell. T_H cells secrete a variety of cytokines, commonly called *lymphokines*, which play a central role in the activation of B cells, T_C cells, and a variety of other cells that participate in the immune response. The T_C cell is activated by interaction with an antigen-MHC complex on the surface of an altered self-cell (e.g., virus-infected cell) in the presence of appropriate lymphokines (see Figure 1-13). Activated T_C cells, called *cytotoxic T lymphocytes* (*CTL*), mediate the killing of the altered self-cells. By determining the number of CD4-bearing and CD8-bearing T cells, the ratio of T_H to T_C cells can be ascertained. This ratio is approximately 2:1 in normal human peripheral blood. In certain diseases, such as immunodeficiency diseases or autoimmune diseases, this ratio may show significant alterations.

Another subpopulation of T lymphocytes—called *T suppressor* (T_S) cells—has been postulated. It is clear that some T cells mediate suppression of the humoral and the cell-mediated branches of the immune system, but no actual T_S cell has been isolated and cloned; it is therefore not known whether T_S cells make up a separate subpopulation or whether the observed suppression is simply the result of suppressive activities of the T_H and T_C subpopulations. The T suppressor cell is examined in more detail in Chapter 14.

The classification of CD4$^+$, class II–restricted cells as T_H cells and CD8$^+$, class I–restricted cells as T_C cells is not absolute. Instead, some functional T_H cells have been shown to express CD8 and recognize antigen associated with class I MHC, and some functional T_C cells are class II restricted and express CD4. Even the functional classification is not absolute. For example, many T_C cells have been shown to secrete a variety of lymphokines and exert effects on other cells comparable to that exerted by T_H cells. The distinction between T_H and T_C cells, then, is not always clear; there can be ambiguous functional activities. However, because these ambiguities are the exception and not the rule, the general description of T helper cells as being CD4$^+$ and class II restricted and of T cytotoxic cells as being CD8$^+$ and class I restricted is adhered to, unless otherwise specified, throughout this text.

Null Cells

A small group of peripheral-blood lymphocytes, called null cells, fail to express the membrane molecules that distinguish T and B lymphocytes. These cells also fail to display antigen-binding receptors of either the T- or B-cell lineage and therefore lack the attributes of immunologic specificity and memory. One functional population of null cells called *natural killer (NK)* cells are large, granulated lymphocytes, which constitute 5–10% of the peripheral-blood lymphocytes in humans. The natural killer cell was first described in 1976, when it was shown that certain null cells display cytotoxic activity against a wide range of tumor cells in the absence of any previous immunization with the tumor. NK cells were subsequently shown to play an important role in host defense against tumor cells. Killing of tumor cells appears to be mediated by a cytotoxic factor secreted by natural killer cells. NK cells can interact with tumor cells in two different ways. In some cases, an NK cell makes direct membrane contact with a tumor cell in a nonspecific, antibody-independent process. Some NK cells, however, possess membrane receptors for the carboxyl-terminal end of the antibody molecule. These NK cells can bind to antitumor antibodies bound to the surface of tumor cells and subsequently destroy the tumor; this specific process is called *antibody-dependent cell-mediated cytotoxicity*. The exact mechanism of tumor-cell killing by NK cells, the focus of much current experimental study, is discussed further in Chapter 13.

In humans, a disease called Chédiak-Higashi syndrome is associated with an absence of NK cells and an increased incidence of lymphomas. In mice, a correlation also exists between an absence of NK cells and susceptibility to tumor growth. Mice with an autosomal recessive mutation called *beige* lack NK cells and show an increased susceptibility to tumor growth when they are injected with live tumor cells. These findings strongly suggest that NK cells play an important role in host defense against tumors.

Organs of the Immune System

A number of morphologically and functionally diverse organs have various functions in the development of an immune response. These organs can be divided on the basis of function into the primary (or central) and secondary (or peripheral) lymphoid organs (Figure 3-10). Immature lymphocytes generated during the process of hematopoiesis in the bone marrow mature and become committed to a particular antigenic specificity within the primary lymphoid organs. Only after the lymphocyte has matured within the primary lymphoid organ is the cell immunocompetent (i.e., capable of mounting an immune response). In mammals, the primary lymphoid organs are the bone marrow, where B-cell maturation occurs, and the thymus, where T-cell maturation occurs.

A variety of peripheral lymphoid organs exist, each uniquely suited to trap antigen from defined tissues or vascular spaces and provide sites where mature, immunocompetent lymphocytes can interact effectively with that antigen. The lymph nodes function to collect antigen from the intracellular tissue fluids, whereas the spleen filters blood-borne antigens. The respiratory and gastrointestinal tracts have their own set of mucosal-associated lymphoid tissue (MALT)—including Peyer's patches, tonsils, adenoids, and the appendix—which trap antigens entering through various mucous membrane surfaces.

Primary Lymphoid Organs

Thymus

T-cell progenitors formed in the course of hematopoiesis enter the thymus gland as immature *thymocytes* and mature there to become antigen-committed, immunocompetent T cells. The thymus is a flat, bilobed organ situated above the heart. Each lobe is surrounded by a capsule and is divided into lobules, which are separated from each other by strands of connective tissue called trabeculae. Each lobule is organized into two compartments: the outer compartment, or *cortex*, is densely packed with thymocytes, whereas the inner compartment, or *medulla*, is sparsely populated with thymocytes. The actual maturation sequence within the

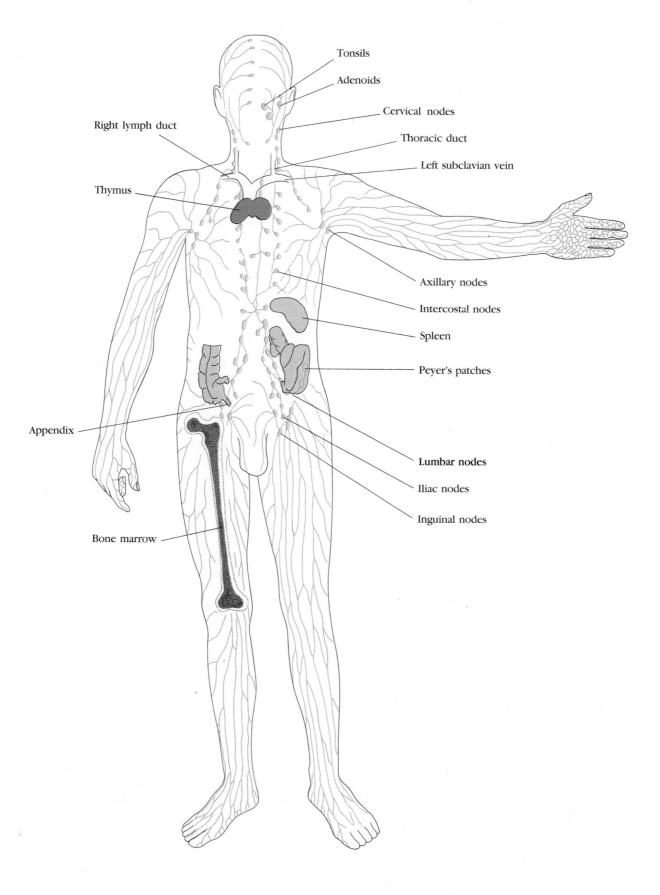

Figure 3-10 The human lymphoid system. The primary organs (bone marrow and thymus) are shown in dark red; the secondary organs and tissues, in light red. These structurally and functionally diverse organs and tissues are interconnected by the blood vessels and lymph vessels (gray). Only one bone is shown, but all major bones contain marrow and are thus part of the lymphoid system [Adapted from N. K. Jerne, 1973, The immune system. *Sci. Am.* (**229**):54.]

thymus is not known. Generally it is thought that progenitor T cells enter the thymus and begin to multiply within the cortex. Here there is rapid proliferation of thymocytes coupled to an enormous rate of cell death.

A small subset of more mature thymocytes are then thought to migrate from the cortex to the medulla where they continue to mature and finally leave the thymus via postcapillary venules. There appear to be exceptions to this sequence, with some studies showing that a small subpopulation of cortical thymocytes can mature and leave the thymus without ever entering the medulla.

Both cortex and medulla are crisscrossed by a three-dimensional network of stromal cells composed of epithelial cells, interdigitating dendritic cells, and macrophages, which make up the framework of the thymus and contribute to thymocyte maturation. Many of these stromal cells physically interact with the developing thymocytes (Figure 3-11). Some thymic epithelial cells in

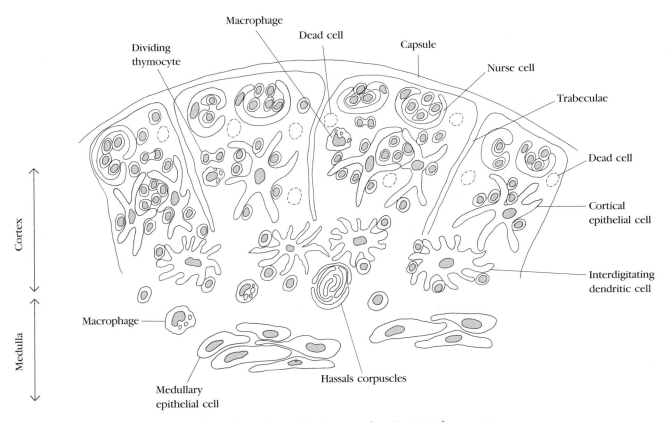

Figure 3-11 Diagrammatic cross section of a portion of the thymus, showing several lobules separated by connective tissue strands (trabeculae). Progenitor T cells produced in the bone marrow during hematopoiesis enter the thymus as immature thymocytes and mature into functional T-cell subpopulations. The outer cortex is densely populated and is thought to contain immature thymocytes, which undergo rapid proliferation coupled with an enormous rate of cell death. The medulla is sparsely populated and is thought to contain more mature thymocytes. During their stay within the thymus, thymocytes interact with a three-dimensional network of stromal cells (composed of epithelial cells, interdigitating dendritic cells, and macrophages). These cells produce thymic hormones and express high levels of class I and class II MHC molecules. Several unique cells are also found in the thymus including the thymic "nurse" cell, an epithelial cell which engulfs up to 50 thymocytes with its long membrane processes and Hassall's corpuscles containing concentric layers of degenerating epithelial cells. [Adapted from W. van Ewijk, 1991, *Annu. Rev. Immunol.* **9**:591.]

the outer cortex, called "nurse" cells, have long membrane processes that surround as many as 50 thymocytes, forming large multicellular complexes. Other cortical epithelial cells have long interconnecting cytoplasmic processes that form a network and have been shown to interact with numerous thymocytes as they traverse the cortex. At the junction of the cortex and the medulla bone marrow-derived interdigitating dendritic cells are located. These cells also have long processes that have been shown to interact with developing thymocytes.

Maturation and Selection of T Lymphocytes. Thymic epithelial cells secrete hormonal factors necessary for the differentiation and maturation of T lymphocytes. Four hormonal factors have been characterized: α_1-thymosin, β_4-thymosin, thymopoietin, and thymulin. When bone marrow cells are cultured with these factors, T-cell lineage membrane molecules have been shown to appear, although the role of each of these factors on T-cell maturation within the thymus remains unknown. Thymic stromal cells have also been shown to secrete a cytokine, IL-7, which also plays a role in T-cell maturation within the thymus.

In the course of thymocyte maturation within the thymus, the antigenic diversity of the T-cell receptor is generated by a series of random gene rearrangements (see Chapter 10). As discussed, mature T cells can recognize antigen only when it is associated with either a class I MHC molecule or a class II MHC molecule. Thus, once cells expressing antigen-binding receptors are formed in the thymus, they must be subjected to a selection process, so that only T cells recognizing antigenic peptides in the context of self-MHC molecules are released from the thymus. Thymic stromal cells play a role in this selection process. Both cortical and medullary epithelial cells and the interdigitating dendritic cells at the corticomedullary junction express high levels of class I and class II MHC molecules. It is thought that developing thymocytes are exposed to these MHC molecules as the thymocyte matures within the thymus. Those T cells bearing receptors that recognize foreign peptides associated with self-MHC will be selected and allowed to mature; this process is called *positive selection.* Any developing thymocytes that are unable to recognize MHC molecules are not selected and are thought to be eliminated by a process called *programmed cell death or apoptosis.* Included among the positively selected thymocytes will be some cells that recognize self-antigen associated with self-MHC. These cells are potentially self-reactive and must therefore be eliminated by negative selection. In *negative selection* any thymocyte with a high-affinity receptor for self-MHC alone or self-antigen + self-MHC is eliminated.

By means of positive and negative selection in the thymus, potentially self-reactive T cells are eliminated and only those cells are allowed to mature whose re-

ceptor recognizes MHC plus foreign antigen. It is estimated that 95–99% of all thymocyte progeny die within the thymus without ever maturing. It is speculated that this high rate of death reflects the elimination of thymocytes whose receptors cannot recognize foreign antigenic peptides displayed by self-MHC or whose receptors recognize self-peptides displayed by self-MHC. The process of positive and negative selection in the thymus is discussed more fully in Chapter 10.

Relationship between Thymic Function and Immune Function. The first evidence implicating the thymus in immune function came from experiments involving neonatal thymectomy in which the thymus was surgically removed from newborn mice. These thymectomized mice showed a dramatic decrease in circulating lymphocytes of the T-cell lineage and an absence of cell-mediated immunity. A congenital birth defect in humans (DiGeorge syndrome) and in certain mice (nude mice) that involves failure of the thymus to develop provides further evidence. In both cases there is an absence of circulating T cells and of cell-mediated immunity and an increase in infectious disease.

Evidence suggests that the decline in immune functions that accompanies aging, leading to an increase in infections, autoimmunity, and cancer, results primarily from changes in the T-cell component of the immune system. The thymus reaches its maximal size at puberty and then atrophies, with a significant decrease in both cortical and medullary cells and an increase in the total fat content of the organ. Whereas the average weight of the thymus is 70 g in infants, its average weight is only 3 g in the elderly. This thymic involution, with the associated decrease in cortical size, medullary size, and hormonal production, precedes the decrease in immune function that is seen with aging. A number of experiments have been designed to look at the effect of age on the immune function of the thymus. In one experiment the thymus from a 1-day-old or 33-month-old mouse was grafted into thymectomized adult littermates. Mice receiving the newborn thymus graft showed a significantly larger improvement in immune function than mice receiving the 33-month-old thymus.

Bone Marrow

In birds a lymphoid organ called the bursa of Fabricius is the primary site of B-cell maturation. There is no bursa in mammals and no single counterpart to it as a primary lymphoid organ. Instead, regions of the bone marrow and possibly of other lymphoid tissues serve as the "bursal equivalent" where B-cell maturation occurs. Because B-cell development in mammals does not take place in a single anatomic structure, it is difficult to study B-cell development in mammals, and much remains unknown about this process.

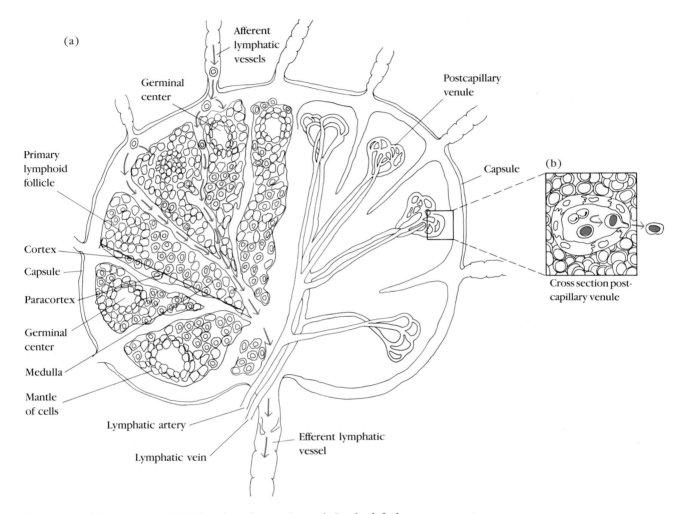

Figure 3-12 (a) Two views of the lymph node are pictured. On the left the arrangement of reticulum and lymphocytes in the cortex, paracortex, and medulla is depicted. Following antigenic challenge, antigen is trapped by macrophages and dendritic cells within the cortex and paracortex. T cells are concentrated within the paracortex and are activated by antigen presented by dendritic cells or macrophages. The activated T_H cells migrate to the cortical lymphoid follicles and serve to activate B cells. As B cells are activated, the primary follicle develops into a secondary follicle consisting of a ring of tightly packed cells surrounding a germinal center. B cells mature into plasma cells and memory cells within the germinal centers. The resulting antibody-secreting plasma cells migrate to the medulla. Lymphocytes circulating in the lymph system are carried into the node through the afferent lymphatics. These lymphocytes can enter the reticular matrix of the node or can pass through the node and leave via the efferent lymphatic vessel. The right side of the diagram depicts the lymphatic artery, lymphatic vein, and postcapillary venule. The postcapillary venules are organized around the lymphoid follicles and germinal centers. (b) Lymphocytes can also enter the lymph nodes from the venous system by passing through specialized capillary endothelial cells in the postcapillary venules. This process is called extravasation and is important in allowing recirculating lymphocytes to pass through the lymph node where they can contact antigen which has been trapped by the node.

Secondary Lymphoid Organs

Lymph Nodes

Lymph—a pale, watery, proteinaceous tissue fluid—flows from the intercellular tissue spaces into lymphatic capillaries and then into a series of larger collecting vessels called lymphatics (see Figure 3-10). During passage of the lymph from the tissues to the lymphatics, it becomes progressively enriched in lymphocytes. The lymphatics carry the lymph through regional lymph nodes, where it filters through a cellular network containing phagocytic cells and reticular dendritic cells, which trap antigen carried by the lymph. The largest lymphatic vessel, the thoracic duct, empties into the left subclavian vein near the heart, connecting the lymph system with the blood system, so that lymphocytes circulate from the lymphatics into the blood.

Lymph nodes are encapsulated bean-shaped structures containing a reticular network packed with lymphocytes, macrophages, and dendritic cells. They are found clustered at junctions of the lymphatics and serve as the first organized structure to encounter most antigens. Morphologically, a lymph node can be divided into three roughly concentric regions: cortex, paracortex, and medulla (Figure 3-12). The outermost layer, the cortex, contains lymphocytes (mostly B cells) and macrophages arranged in poorly defined clusters called *primary follicles*. Following antigenic challenge, the primary follicle becomes a larger *secondary follicle*, a ring of concentrically packed lymphocytes surrounding a center (the *germinal center*) in which large proliferating lymphoblasts and plasma cells are interspersed with macrophages and follicular dendritic cells. The germinal centers are sites of intense B-cell activation and differentiation into plasma and memory cells. (In children with B-cell deficiencies, the cortex lacks primary follicles and germinal centers.) Beneath the cortex is the paracortical region, which is populated with T lymphocytes. The paracortex also contains dendritic cells thought to have migrated from tissues to the node. These cells have large numbers of the class II MHC molecules necessary for activation of T$_H$ cells by antigen. Lymph nodes taken from neonatally thymectomized mice show a severe depletion of cells from the paracortical region; the paracortex is therefore sometimes referred to as a thymus-dependent area in contrast to the cortex, which is thymus-independent. The innermost layer, the medulla, is more sparsely populated with lymphocytes, but many of these are plasma cells actively secreting antibody molecules.

Afferent lymphatic vessels pierce the capsule of a lymph node at numerous sites and empty lymph into the subcapsular sinus. Lymph coming from the tissues percolates slowly inward through the cortex, paracortex, and medulla, allowing phagocytic cells and reticular dendritic cells to trap any bacteria or particulate material carried by the lymph. Following infection or introduction of other antigens to the body, the lymph leaving a node through its single efferent lymphatic vessel is enriched with antibodies newly secreted by medullary plasma cells and also has a 50-fold higher concentration of lymphocytes than the afferent lymph. The increase in lymphocytes is due in part to lymphocyte proliferation within the node in response to antigen, but most of the increase represents blood-borne lymphocytes that migrate into the node by passing between specialized endothelial cells lining the postcapillary venules of the node. Estimates are that 25% of the lymphocytes leaving a lymph node have migrated across this endothelial layer and entered the node from the circulation. Because antigenic stimulation within a node can increase this migration tenfold, the concentration of lymphocytes in nodes involved in an active immune response can increase greatly, resulting in visible swelling of the nodes. As is discussed later in this chapter, it is thought that factors released in lymph nodes during antigen stimulation facilitate this increased lymphocyte migration.

Spleen

The spleen is a large, ovoid secondary lymphoid organ situated high in the left abdominal cavity. Unlike lymph nodes, which are specialized to trap localized antigen from regional tissue spaces, the spleen is adapted to filtering blood and trapping blood-borne antigens: it thus responds to systemic infections. The spleen is surrounded by a capsule, which sends a number of projections called trabeculae into the interior to form a compartmentalized structure. The compartments are of two types, called red pulp and white pulp, with a diffuse marginal zone between them (Figure 3-13). The splenic red pulp consists of a network of sinusoids populated with macrophages and numerous erythrocytes; it is the site where old and defective red blood cells are destroyed and removed. Many of the macrophages within the red pulp contain engulfed red blood cells or iron pigments from degraded hemoglobin. The splenic white pulp surrounds the arteries, forming a periarteriolar lymphoid sheath (PALS) populated mainly by T lymphocytes. Clusters of B lymphocytes in the PALS form primary follicles occupying a more peripheral position. Upon antigenic challenge, these primary follicles develop into characteristic secondary follicles containing germinal centers (like those in the lymph nodes) where rapidly dividing B lymphoblasts and plasma cells are surrounded by dense clusters of concentrically arranged lymphocytes.

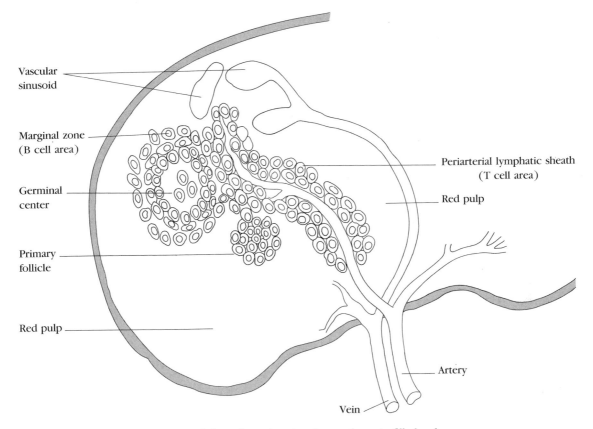

Figure 3-13 Diagrammatic representation of the spleen showing the erythrocyte-filled red pulp interspersed with the lymphocyte-rich white pulp. The spleen does not contain lymphatic vessels. The arterial blood supply pierces the splenic capsule at the hilus and divides into progressively smaller arterioles ending in vascular sinusoids that drain back into the splenic vein. The white pulp of the spleen forms a sleeve around the splenic arterioles called the periarteriolar lymphoid sheath (PALS). The PALS contains numerous T lymphocytes. Closely associated with the PALS is a B-cell–rich area, called the marginal zone, containing lymphoid follicles that can develop into germinal centers. As with the lymph node, the germinal centers of the spleen are also sites of intense B-cell proliferation into plasma cells and memory cells.

Unlike the lymph nodes, the spleen is not supplied by afferent lymphatics draining the tissue spaces. Instead, blood-borne cells and antigens are carried into the spleen through the splenic artery, which empties into the marginal zone. As antigen enters the marginal zone, it is trapped by dendritic cells, which carry the antigen to the periarteriolar lymphoid sheath. Lymphocytes entering via the blood enter the marginal zone in the sinuses and migrate to the periarteriolar lymphoid sheath. Experiments with radioactively labeled lymphocytes show that more recirculating lymphocytes daily pass through the spleen than through all the lymph nodes combined. The effects of splenectomy on the immune response depends on the age at which the spleen is removed. In children, splenectomy often leads to an increased incidence of bacterial sepsis caused primarily by *Pneumococcus*, *Meningococcus*, and *Hemophilus influenzae*. Splenectomy in adults has less adverse effects, although it leads to some increase in blood-borne bacterial infections, or bacteremia.

Mucosal-Associated Lymphoid Tissue (MALT)

A variety of lymphoid tissues are found at various locations along mucous membrane surfaces. Some of these tissues are thought to take part in B-cell development within the bone marrow. Their major role, though, appears to be as secondary lymphoid tissue. They play an important role in trapping antigens that have gained entry through the epithelial mucous membrane surface of the respiratory and gastrointestinal tracts and provide localized sites for lymphocyte interaction with that antigen. Structurally these tissues range from loose clusters of lymphoid cells with little organization in the lamina propria mucosa of the intestinal villi to organized structures such as the tonsils, appendix, and Peyer's patches (see Figure 3-10).

The tonsils are found in three locations: lingual at the base of the tongue; palatine at the side of the back of the mouth; and nasopharyngeal (adenoids) in the roof of the nasopharynx. All three tonsil groups are nodular structures consisting of a meshwork of reticular cells and fibers interspersed with lymphocytes, macrophages, granulocytes, and mast cells. Follicles and germinal centers are present and, as in the lymph nodes, represent sites of active B-cell proliferation. Surrounding the germinal centers are regions showing T-cell activity. The tonsils play a role in defense against antigens entering through the nasal and oral epithelial routes.

Peyer's patches consist of 30–40 lymphoid nodules on the outer wall of the intestines. These structures also contain follicles from which germinal centers develop upon antigenic stimulation. The follicles, which are very close to the intestinal mucosal epithelium, are thought to be the sites where antigens penetrate the intestinal epithelium, thus facilitating accumulation of antigen within organized lymphoid structures.

Lymphocyte Recirculation

Lymphocytes are capable of a remarkable level of recirculation, continuously moving through the blood and lymph to the various lymphoid organs (Figure 3-14). James Gowans demonstrated this capacity for recirculation in 1964 by isolating lymph from a thoracic duct of a rat and radiolabeling the lymphocytes and then transfusing them into normal animals. By monitoring the location of the labeled cells at various time intervals, Gowans found that the lymphocytes spent 2–12 h in the blood before appearing in the lymph or lymphoid organs. As lymphocytes recirculate, they make contact with antigens presented on the surface of antigen-presenting cells in the peripheral lymphoid organs. This feature allows maximal numbers of antigenically committed lymphocytes to encounter and interact with antigen. Since only about one in 10^3–10^6 lymphocytes can recognize a particular antigen, it would appear that a large number of antigen-committed T or B cells must contact antigen on a given antigen-presenting cell within a relatively short period of time in order to generate a specific immune response. The odds of the small percentage of lymphocytes committed to a given antigen actually making contact with that antigen when it is present are greatly increased by the extensive recirculation of lym-

phocytes. Experiments have shown that when a particular antigen is injected, T cells specific for that antigen disappear from the circulation within 48 h, suggesting that all the specific T cells encounter the antigen in peripheral lymph organs and cease recirculating within that time period.

In order for recirculating lymphocytes to enter various lymphoid organs or inflammatory-tissue spaces, the lymphocytes must adhere to and pass between the endothelial cells lining the walls of blood vessels by a process called *extravasation*. This process occurs most readily in regions of vascular endothelium that possess specialized cells with a plump, cuboidal ("high") shape; such regions are called *high endothelial venules* (*HEVs*) (Figure 3-15a and b). Each of the secondary lymphoid organs, with the exception of the spleen, contains HEVs. When frozen sections of lymph nodes, Peyer's patches, or tonsils are incubated with lymphocytes and washed to remove unbound cells, over 85% of the bound cells are found adhering to HEVs, even though HEVs account for only 1–2% of the total area of the frozen section (Figure 3-15c).

The expression of HEVs in lymphoid organs is influenced by antigenic activation of lymphocytes. When animals are raised in a germ-free environment HEVs fail to develop. The need for antigenic activation of lymphocytes in maintaining the expression of HEVs can be demonstrated by surgically blocking the afferent lymphatic vasculature to a node so that antigen entry to the node is blocked. Within a short period of time the HEVs show impaired function and eventually revert to a more flattened morphology.

The endothelial cells of HEVs express on their surface special molecules called *cell-adhesion molecules* (*CAMs*). As an immune response develops, lymphokines produced at the site activate these endothelial cells to increase their expression of CAMs, thereby facilitating leukocyte extravasation to tissue sites where activation of immune-system cells occurs. Recirculating lymphocytes, monocytes, and granulocytes bear adhesion-molecule receptors by means of which the recirculating cells bind to CAMs on endothelial cells in the HEV. One group of cell-surface receptors that bind adhesion molecules is the *integrin receptor family*. These receptors are heterodimeric proteins that facilitate cell-to-cell interactions within the immune system as well as leukocyte adherence to vascular endothelial cells.

Different integrins are expressed by different populations of leukocytes, allowing for the selective interaction of different leukocytes with CAMs expressed on other cells or along the vasculature (Table 3-6). For example, the integrin LFA-1, expressed by all leukocytes, recognizes an adhesion molecule called ICAM, which is expressed by a variety of cells, including activated vascular endothelium. The integrin VLA-4 is specific to T lymphocytes and recognizes an adhesion molecule called VCAM. The importance of integrin molecules in extravasation is demonstrated by the autosomal recessive disease, leukocyte-adhesion deficiency (LAD), characterized by recurrent bacterial infections and impaired healing of wounds. The deficiency stems from abnormal synthesis of one chain of the integrin receptor present on leukocytes. The absence of these receptors on lymphocytes, monocytes, and granulocytes prevents their extravasation from the blood vessels to the tissues. As a result, the immune-system cells cannot interact with antigens in the tissues, and affected individuals have

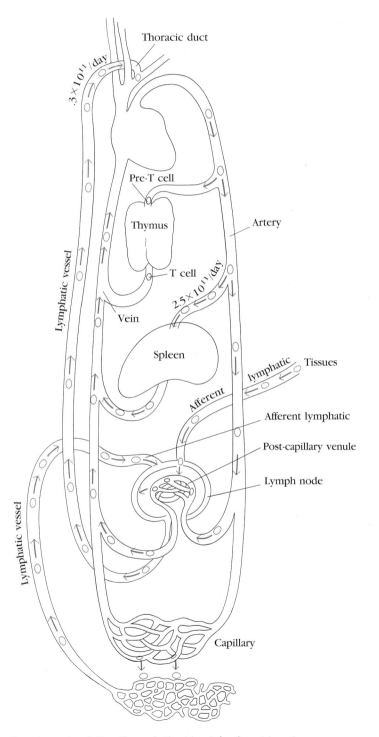

Figure 3-14   Diagram of lymphocyte recirculation through the blood (red) and lymph vasculature (gray) to the major organs of the lymphatic system.

(a)

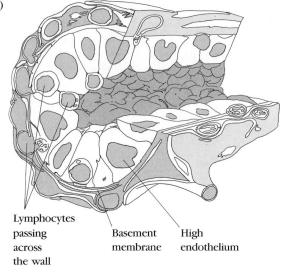

Lymphocytes
passing
across
the wall

Basement
membrane

High
endothelium

(b)

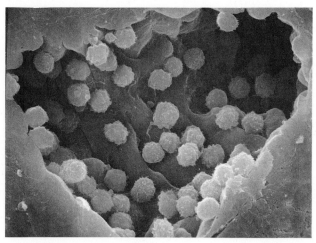

(c)

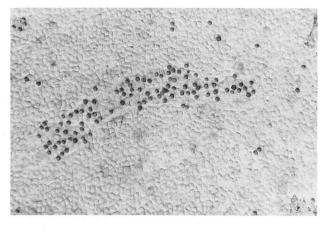

an increase in the frequency and severity of bacterial infections.

Some vascular adhesion molecules are distributed in a tissue-specific manner. These tissue-specific adhesion molecules have been called *vascular addressins* (*VAs*) because they serve to direct the extravasation of different populations of recirculating lymphocytes to particular peripheral lymphoid organs. The tissue-specific distribution of these addressin molecules can be demonstrated by tissue-specific differences in binding of monoclonal antibodies to HEVs. For example, some monoclonals bind only to vascular addressins in the HEVs of Peyer's patches, whereas other monoclonals bind only to vascular addressins in the HEVs of lymph nodes. Mature recirculating lymphocytes have cell-surface receptors that recognize the tissue-specific vascular addressins. Because these receptors direct the circulation of various populations of lymphocytes to particular tissues, they have been called *homing receptors*. Recent evidence suggests that different populations of lymphocytes bear homing receptors that recognize different vascular addressins and thus are directed to (or home in on) particular lymphoid organs (Figure 3-16). For example, B lymphocytes show preferential homing to mucosal-associated lymphoid tissues, whereas T lymphocytes home to lymph nodes.

The actual process of extravasation is thought to involve two steps: a homing step and an integrin-mediated adhesion step (Figure 3-17). In the first step, the homing receptor on a lymphocyte interacts with a tissue-specific vascular addressin on a HEV. In the second step, cellular adhesion is strengthened by binding of an integrin receptor on the lymphocyte with a CAM on the HEV. This latter interaction, for example, might involve the integrin LFA-1 and ICAM or the integrin VLA-4 and VCAM (see Table 3-6).

Figure 3-15 (a) Schematic diagram showing a cross section of a lymph node postcapillary venule with high endothelium. Lymphocytes are shown in various stages of attachment to the HEV, and extravasation also shown across the wall into the cortex of the node. (b) Scanning electron micrograph showing numerous lymphocytes bound to the surface of a high endothelial venule. (c) Incubation of lymphocytes (darkly stained) with frozen sections of lymphoid tissue reveals that 85% of the lymphocytes are bound to HEVs (cross sections) which comprise only 1–2% of the total area of the tissue section. [Part (a) adapted from A. O. Anderson and N. D. Anderson, 1981, in *Cellular Functions in Immunity and Inflammation*, J. J. Oppenheim, D. L. Rosenstreich, and M. Potter, eds. Elsevier, North-Holland; part (b) from S. D. Rosen and L. M. Stoolman, 1987, *Vertebrate Lectins*, Van Nostrand Reinhold; part (c) from S. D. Rosen, 1989, *Current Opinion in Cell Biology* 1:913.]

Table 3-6 Some receptors involved in lymphocyte homing and recirculation

Receptor	Type	Cellular distribution	Function
LFA-1 (CD11a)	Adhesion receptor	Leukocytes	Binds to ICAM-1 and ICAM-2 on vascular endothelial cells
VLA-4 (CDW49d)	Adhesion receptor	Leukocytes	Binds to VCAM-1 on vascular endothelial cells
ELAM-1	Adhesion receptor	Vascular endothelium	Binds to unidentified receptor on neutrophils
HCAM	Homing receptor	Lymphocytes, increased on B cells	Binds to vascular addressins on MALT HEVs
MEL-14	Homing receptor	Lymphocytes, neutrophils increased on T cells	Binds to vascular addressins on peripheral lymph node HEVs
LPAM-1	Homing receptor	Lymphocytes	Binds to vascular addressins on Peyer's patches HEVs

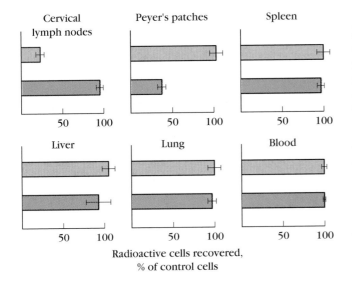

Figure 3-16 Experimental demonstration of tissue-specific lymphocyte homing. Radiolabeled lymphocytes were incubated with either monoclonal antibody A.11 (gray) or I.B2 (red), which are specific for different homing receptors. The lymphocytes were then transferred to syngeneic recipients and the accumulation of radioactivity in various organs was measured after 2 h. The radioactivity recovered was expressed as a percentage of that recovered with control lymphocytes not treated with antibody. Binding of antibody to a homing receptor inhibits interaction of the receptor with its vascular addressin. The results thus indicate that one homing receptor (reactive with antibody A.11) directs lymphocytes to cervical lymph nodes, whereas the other homing receptor (reactive with antibody I.B2) directs lymphocytes to Peyer's patches. [From J. J. Woodruff, L. M. Clark, and Y. H. Chen, 1987, *Annu. Rev. Immunol.* **5**:201.]

Recirculation and homing of lymphocytes are regulated by the immune system in several ways. Expression of adhesion molecules, including CAMs and VAs, is influenced by certain lymphokines generated early in an immune response. For example, IL-1, IFN-γ, and TNF-α, all of which are secreted by activated macrophages, have been shown to increase expression of ICAMs by nearby endothelial cells. This increase in ICAM expression following macrophage activation by antigen leads to an increase in the extravasation of lymphocytes, monocytes, and neutrophils to sites of immune activation. Lymphocyte homing is also influenced by the state of activation of the lymphocytes. T and B lymphocytes often lose their homing receptors following activation by antigen. This loss of homing receptors ensures that lymphocytes that have encountered antigen will stay at the site where antigen is present rather than continue to recirculate.

Experiments suggest that the acquisition of tissue-specific homing receptors by T lymphocytes occurs in the course of the maturation of the T lymphocytes within the thymus gland. Pre-T cells seeded out from the bone marrow during hematopoiesis preferentially adhere to thymic endothelial cells and migrate into the thymus gland for T-cell maturation. As thymocytes mature within the thymus, they acquire homing receptors that direct their migration into peripheral lymphoid organs. One such homing receptor, recognized by a monoclonal antibody called MEL-14, has been shown to be present at high levels on most peripheral circulating T cells but to be present at low levels on most thymocytes. However, a small population (1–3%) of cortical thy-

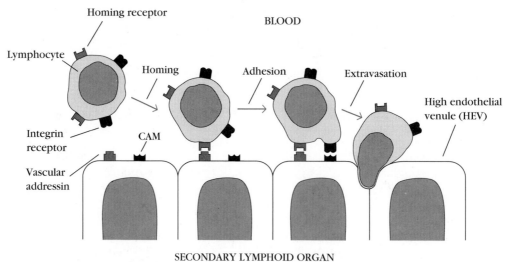

Figure 3-17   Model of lymphocyte homing and extravasation in secondary lymphoid organs containing high endothelial venules (HEVs). HEV cells possess two types of adhesion molecules: tissue-specific vascular addressins, which are present in certain lymphoid organs, and cell-adhesion molecules (CAMs), which are expressed by various cells and are not tissue-specific. A recirculating lymphocyte has homing receptors that are specific for a given addressin. Binding of the lymphocyte to the vascular addressin is followed by integrin-mediated adhesion to a CAM, allowing the lymphocyte to adhere to the HEV and extravasate into the lymphoid organ. [Adapted from A. Duijvestijn and A. Hamann, 1989, *Immun. Today* **10**:26.].

mocytes express high levels of this receptor; these cells also express other surface molecules characteristic of mature T cells. Thus the acquisition of the MEL-14 receptor appears to correlate with T-cell maturation within the thymus.

In addition to their role in lymphocyte adhesion to vascular endothelial cells, many of the adhesion molecules also serve to increase the strength of the functional interactions between cells of the immune system. Various adhesions molecules have been shown to contribute to the T_H–APC, T_H–B cell, and CTL–target cell interactions. We will discuss these interactions more fully in Chapters 10, 12, and 13.

Summary

1.   The cells that participate in the immune response are white blood cells, or leukocytes, all of which develop from a common pluripotent stem cell during hematopoiesis.

2.   Various hematopoietic growth factors (cytokines) induce proliferation and differentiation of the different blood cells. This process is closely regulated to assure steady-state levels of each of the different types of blood cells.

3.   The lymphocyte—the central cell of the immune system—is the only cell to possess the attributes of specificity, diversity, memory, and self/nonself recognition.

4.   The monocyte, macrophage, and neutrophil are accessory immune-system cells whose primary function is to phagocytose and eliminate antigen. Phagocytosis is facilitated by opsonins such as antibody and complement, which increase the attachment of antigen to the membrane of the phagocyte.

5.   In addition to phagocytosis, the macrophage plays an important role in T-cell activation by processing and presenting antigen in association with a class II MHC molecule and by secreting interleukin-1.

6.   The primary lymphoid organs provide sites where lymphocytes mature and become antigenically committed. The T lymphocytes mature within the thymus, and B lymphocytes mature within the bursa of Fabricius in birds and largely in the bone marrow in mammals.

7. The secondary lymphoid organs function to capture antigen and to provide sites where lymphocytes interact with that antigen and undergo clonal selection.

8. Lymphocytes undergo constant recirculation between the blood, lymph, lymphoid organs, and tissue spaces. Homing receptors on lymphocytes, which interact with tissue-specific adhesion molecules on high endothelial venules, direct lymphocyte recirculation in a tissue-specific fashion.

References

BERG, E. L., L. GOLDSTEIN, M. A. JUTILA, et al. 1989. Homing receptors and vascular addressins: cell adhesion molecules that direct lymphocyte traffic. *Immunol. Rev.* **108**:5.

DEXTER, T. M., and E. SPOONCER. 1987. Growth and differentiation in the hemopoietic system. *Ann. Rev. Cell Biol.* **3**:423.

DORSHKIND, K. 1990. Regulation of hematopoiesis by bone marrow stromal cells and their products. *Annu. Rev. Immunol.* **8**:111.

DUIJVESTIJN, A., and A. HAMANN. 1989. Mechanisms and regulation of lymphocyte migration. *Immunology Today* **10**:23.

DUSTIN, M. L., and T. A. SPRINGER. 1991. Role of lymphocyte adhesion receptors in transient interactions and cell locomotion. *Annu. Rev. Immunol.* **9**:27.

GALLATIN, M., T. P. ST. JOHN, M. SIEGELMAN, et al. 1986. Lymphocyte homing receptors. *Cell* **44**:673.

KAUSHANSKY, K. 1987. The molecular biology of the colony stimulating factors. *Blood Cells* **13**:3.

MOORE, M. A. S. 1991. The clinical use of colony stimulating factors. *Annu. Rev. Immunol.* **9**:159.

SPANGRUDE, G. J., S. HEIMFELD, and I. WEISSMAN. 1988. Purification and characterization of mouse hematopoietic stem cells. *Science* **241**:58.

SPRINGER, T. A. 1990. Adhesion receptors of the immune system. *Nature* **346**:425.

STEINMAN, R. M. 1991. The dendritic cell system and its role in immunogenicity. *Annu. Rev. Immunol.* **9**:271.

TUSHINSKI, R. J., I. T. OLIVER, L. J. GUILBERT, et al. 1982. Survival of mononuclear phagocytes depends on a lineage-specific growth factor that the differentiated cells selectively destroy. *Cell* **28**:71.

VAN EWIJK, W. 1991. T-cell differentiation is influenced by thymic microenvironments. *Annu. Rev. Immunol.* **9**:591.

WOODRUFF, J. J., L. M. CLARKE, and Y. H. CHIN. 1987. Specific cell-adhesion mechanisms determining migration pathways of recirculating lymphocytes. *Annu. Rev. Immunol.* **5**:201.

YEDNOCK, T. A., and S. D. ROSEN. 1989. Lymphocyte homing. *Adv. Immunol.* **44**:313.

Study Questions

1. For the following situations, indicate where in the lymph node you would expect to see large numbers of rapidly proliferating cells:

   a. Normal mouse immunized with a protein antigen.

   b. Normal mouse with a viral infection.

   c. Neonatally thymectomized mouse immunized with a protein antigen.

   d. Neonatally thymectomized mouse immunized with a thymus-independent antigen (bacterial lipopolysaccharide, LPS), which is capable of activating B cells without requiring T_H cells.

2. Do monocyte progenitor cells secrete M-CSF or have receptors for M-CSF? What would be the consequences to the cell if both M-CSF and the receptor for M-CSF were expressed?

3. List the primary lymphoid organs and summarize their functions in the immune response?

4. List the secondary lymphoid organs and summarize their functions in the immune response.

5. List two important functions of the epithelial cells in the thymus.

6. What is antigenic commitment and what is clonal selection? Where do these processes take place? How do these processes contribute to specificity and memory in the immune response?

7. Inflammatory mediators, including interferon gamma, interleukin 1, and tumor necrosis factor, cause induction of ICAM on a wide variety of tissues. What effect might this have on the localization of immune cells?

8. In Weissman's method for enriching pluripotent stem cells, why is it necessary to use lethally irradiated mice?

9. What effect does thymectomy have on an adult mouse? On a neonatal mouse? Why should there be any difference?

10. How could you determine whether T cells and B cells tend to populate different areas of the secondary lymphoid organs?

11. In order to study the mechanism of lymphocyte homing, you are trying to find mice with homing defects. After an exhaustive search you identify two mice (designated A and B) whose lymphocytes fail to home to their own cervical lymph nodes, although they do home to other lymphoid tissue such as Peyer's patches. To determine the nature of these defects, you isolate lymphocytes from mouse A, mouse B, and a normal control mouse of the same strain, radiolabel these cells, and then inject samples of all three labeled cell preparations into all three mice. You then determine the presence $(+)$ or absence $(-)$ of the labeled lymphocytes in the cervical lymph nodes of each animal. The results, shown in the table below, indicate whether homing occurs.

Source of labeled lymphocytes	Presence ($+$) or absence ($-$) of labeled cells in cervical lymph node		
	Mouse A	Mouse B	Control mouse
Mouse A	$-$	$+$	$+$
Mouse B	$-$	$-$	$-$
Normal control mouse	$-$	$+$	$+$

a. What kind of membrane defect might mouse A have?

b. What kind of defect might mouse B have?

c. Design an experiment to test your hypothesis.

CHAPTER

4

Antigens

Antigens are substances able to induce a
specific immune response. The molecular properties of antigens and the way in
which these properties ultimately contribute to
immune activation is central to our understanding of the immune system. Some of the molecular features of antigens recognized by B or T
cells are described in this chapter. The contribution made by the biological system to immunogenicity also is explored, since it is ultimately the
biological system that determines whether a
molecule, capable of binding to a B or T cell's
antigen-binding receptor, can thereupon induce
an immune response. Fundamental differences
in the way T and B lymphocytes recognize antigen determine which molecular features of an
antigen are recognized by each branch of the
immune system. These differences also are
examined in this chapter and illustrated by typical viral and bacterial antigens.

Immunologic Properties of Antigens

Antigens can be defined on the basis of four immunologic properties: immunogenicity, antigenicity, allerogenicity, and tolerogenicity. *Immunogenicity* is the ability to induce either a humoral or cell-mediated immune response:

> B cells + antigen → plasma cells + memory cells
>
> T cells + antigen → T effector cells + memory cells

In this context, an antigen is more appropriately called an *immunogen. Antigenicity* is the ability to combine specifically with the final products of the above responses (i.e., antibodies and/or cell-surface receptors). Although all molecules possessing the property of immunogenicity also possess the property of antigenicity, the reverse is not true. Some small molecules, referred to as *haptens,* possess the property of antigenicity but are not capable, by themselves, of inducing a specific immune response. In other words, they lack immunogenicity.

Allerogenicity is the ability to induce various types of allergic responses. *Allergens* are immunogens that tend to activate specific types of humoral or cell-mediated responses having allergic manifestations. *Tolerogenicity* is the capacity to induce specific immunologic nonresponsiveness in either the humoral or the cell-mediated branch. Tolerogenicity and allerogenicity are discussed in Chapters 13 and 15, respectively.

Factors That Influence Immunogenicity

In order to provide protection against infectious disease, the immune system must be able to recognize bacteria, bacterial products, fungi, parasites, and viruses as immunogens. Closer analysis has shown that the immune system actually recognizes particular macromolecules of an infectious agent, generally either proteins or polysaccharides. Proteins function as the most potent immunogens, with polysaccharides ranking second. In contrast, lipids and nucleic acids of an infectious agent generally do not serve as immunogens unless they are complexed to proteins or polysaccharides. Immunologists tend to use soluble proteins or polysaccharides as immunogens in most experimental studies of humoral immunity (Table 4-1). For cell-mediated immunity, only proteins serve as immunogens. These proteins are not recognized directly; instead they must first be processed into small peptides and then presented in association with MHC molecules on the membrane of a cell before they can be recognized as immunogens.

Immunogenicity is not an intrinsic property of a macromolecule but rather is a condition dependent on a

Table 4-1   Molecular weight of some common experimental antigens used in immunology

Antigen	Approx. molecular weight (Da)
Bovine gamma globulin (BGG)	150,000
Bovine serum albumin (BSA)	69,000
Flagellin (monomer)	40,000
Hen egg-white lysozyme (HEL)	15,000
Keyhole limpet hemocyanin (KLH)	>2,000,000
Ovalbumin (OVA)	44,000
Sperm whale myoglobin (SWM)	17,000
Tetanus toxoid (TT)	150,000

number of interrelated factors involved in the total biological system. For example, the common experimental antigen bovine serum albumin (BSA) is not immunogenic when reinjected into a cow, but it can serve as an excellent immunogen when injected into a rabbit. Generally, then, a macromolecule must be foreign to the animal exposed to it to exhibit immunogenicity. With a given foreign macromolecule, differences in the biological system can influence immunogenicity. This is illustrated most dramatically by comparisons of the immune response of different inbred strains of mice to peptide fragments of a complex protein such as sperm whale myoglobin. A peptide of sperm whale myoglobin that is immunogenic in one inbred strain may not be immunogenic in another inbred strain. The properties that most immunogens share in common and the contribution the biological system makes to the expression of immunogenicity are discussed in the next two sections.

Contribution of the Immunogen to Immunogenicity

Immunogenicity is determined, in part, by four properties of the immunogen: its foreignness, molecular weight, chemical composition and complexity, and ability to be degraded by macrophage enzymes.

Foreignness

In order to elicit an immune response, a molecule must be recognized as nonself. It is thought that the recognition of self occurs early in fetal development as the immature lymphocyte is exposed to self-components.

Any molecule not seen during this critical period is seen as nonself, or foreign, by the immune system. When an antigen is introduced into an organism, the degree of its immunogenicity depends on the degree of its foreignness. Generally, the greater the phylogenetic distance between two species, the greater the genetic (and therefore the antigenic) disparity between them. For example, the antigen BSA would be expected to exhibit greater immunogenicity in a chicken than in a more closely related species such as a goat. There are some exceptions to this rule: Some macromolecules (e.g., collagen and cytochrome *c*) are conserved evolutionarily and therefore display very little immunogenicity across diverse species lines. Conversely, some self-components (e.g., corneal tissue and sperm) are effectively sequestered from the immune system, so that if these tissues are injected even into the animal from which they originated, they will serve as immunogens.

Molecular Size

There is a correlation between the size of a macromolecule and its immunogenicity. The best immunogens tend to have a molecular weight approaching 100,000 daltons (Da). Generally substances smaller than 5000–10,000 are poor immunogens; however, in a few instances substances with a molecular weight of less than 1000 Da have proved to be immunogenic (see Table 4-1).

Chemical Composition and Heterogeneity

Size and foreignness are not, by themselves, sufficient for determining immunogenicity; other properties are needed as well. For example, synthetic homopolymers (polymers composed of a single amino acid or sugar) tend to lack immunogenicity regardless of their size. Synthesis of copolymers made up of different amino acids has shed light on the contribution of chemical complexity to immunogenicity. Copolymers of sufficient size, containing two or more amino acids, are immunogenic. The addition of aromatic amino acids, such as tyrosine or phenylalanine, has a profound effect on the immunogenicity of these synthetic polymers (for an example of copolymer structure, see Figure 4-4). For example, a synthetic copolymer of glutamic acid and lysine requires a minimum molecular weight of 30,000–40,000 Da for immunogenicity. The addition of tyrosine to the copolymer reduces the minimum size required for immunogenicity to between 10,000 and 20,000, whereas the addition of both tyrosine and phenylalanine reduces the minimum molecular weight for immunogenicity to 4000. All four levels of protein organization—primary, secondary, tertiary, and quaternary—contribute to the structural complexity of a protein and hence affect its immunogenicity (Figure 4-1).

Degradability

The development of both humoral and cell-mediated immune responses requires interaction of T_H cells with antigen that has been phagocytosed, processed, and presented in association with MHC on the surface of macrophages or other antigen-presenting cells (see Figure 3-7). Therefore, macromolecules that cannot be degraded and processed by antigen-presenting cells are poor immunogens. This can be illustrated by synthesizing polymers of D-amino acids. D-amino acids are stereoisomers of L-amino acids. Because the degradative enzymes within macrophages can only degrade proteins containing L-amino acids, not their stereoisomers, polymers of D-amino acids cannot be processed by macrophages. As a result, D-amino acids are poor immunogens.

In general, large, insoluble macromolecules are more immunogenic than small soluble ones because they are more readily phagocytosed and processed. Intermolecular chemical cross-linking, heat aggregation, and attachment to insoluble matrices have been routinely used to increase the insolubility of macromolecules, facilitating their phagocytosis and increasing their immunogenicity.

Contribution of the Biological System to Immunogenicity

Even when the foreignness, size, complexity, and degradability of a macromolecule are sufficient to make it immunogenic, the development of an immune response will depend on certain properties of the biological system that the antigen encounters.

Genotype of the Recipient Animal

The genetic constitution of an immunized animal influences the type of immune response the animal manifests, as well as the degree of the response. For example, Hugh McDevitt showed that two different inbred strains of mice exhibited very different responses to a synthetic polypeptide immunogen. Following exposure to the immunogen, one strain produced high levels of serum antibody, whereas the other strain produced low levels. When the two strains were crossed, the F_1 generation showed an intermediate response to the immunogen. By backcross analysis, the F_1 gene controlling immune responsiveness was mapped to a subregion of the major histocompatibility complex (MHC). Numerous experiments with simple defined immunogens have demonstrated genetic control of immune responsiveness, largely confined to genes within the MHC (Table 4-2).

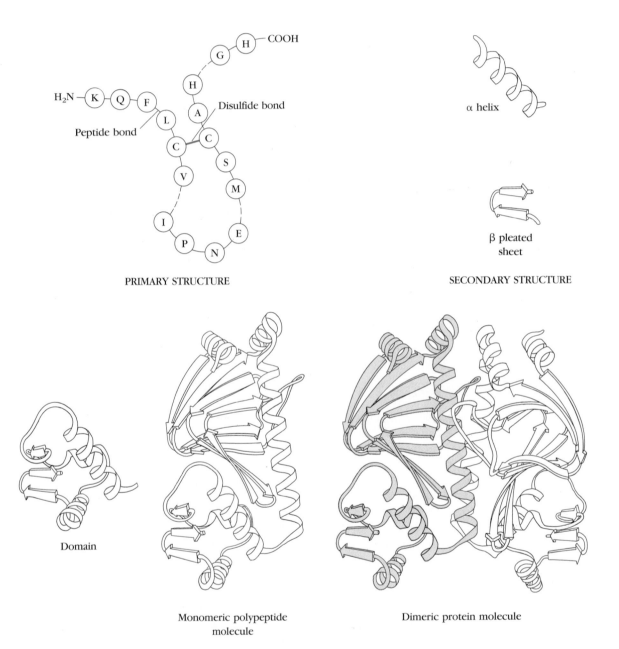

Figure 4-1 The four levels of protein organizational structure. The linear arrangement of amino acids (indicated by single-letter code) and any intrachain disulfide bonds constitute the primary structure. Folding of parts of a polypeptide chain into regular structures (e.g., α helices and β pleated sheets) generates the secondary structure. Tertiary structure refers to the folding of regions between secondary features to give the overall conformation of the molecule or portions of it (domains) with specific functional properties. Quaternary structure results from association of two or more polypeptide chains into a single polymeric protein molecule.

Table 4-2 Effect of MHC haplotype on the immune response to the synthetic copolymers (H,G)-A-L and (T,G)-A-L in mice

MHC haplotype	Representative mouse strains	Antibody response to (H,G)-A-L[*]	Antibody response to (T,G)-A-L[†]
H-2^b	C57	Low	High
H-2^b	C57BL/6	Low	High
H-2^b	C3H.SW	Low	High
H-2^b	I29/J	Low	High
H-2^d	BALB/c	Intermediate	Intermediate
H-2^d	B10.D2	Intermediate	Intermediate
H-2^d	DBA/2	Intermediate	Intermediate
H-2^d	NZB	Intermediate	Intermediate
H-2^k	CBA	High	Low
H-2^k	C3H/HeJ	High	Low
H-2^k	C58J	High	Low
H-2^k	B10.BR	High	Low
H-2^s	B10.S	Low	Low
H-2^s	SJL	Low	Low

[*] Copolymer consists of polylysine backbone with polyalanine side chains to which histidine and glutamic acid residues are attached at the end.

[†] Copolymer consists of polylysine backbone with polyalanine side chains to which tyrosine and glutamic acid residues are attached at the end (see Figure 4-4).

These data indicate that the proteins encoded by the MHC, which function to present processed antigen to T cells, play a central role in determining the degree of immune responsiveness to an antigen. The response of an animal to an antigen also is influenced by the genes encoding B-cell and T-cell receptors and by genes encoding various proteins involved in immune regulatory mechanisms. Genetic variability in all of these genes affects the immunogenicity of a given macromolecule in different animals. These genetic contributions to immunogenicity are discussed more fully in later chapters.

Immunogen Dosage and Route of Administration

For any experimental immunogen there will be some combination of optimal dosage, route of administration, and schedule that will induce a peak immune response in a given animal. An insufficient dose will not stimulate an immune response either because it fails to activate enough lymphocytes or because it induces a nonres-

ponsive state. Conversely, an excessively high dose also can fail to induce a response because it causes lymphocytes to enter a nonresponsive state. In mice the immune response to the purified pneumococcal capsular polysaccharide illustrates the importance of dose. A 0.5-mg dose of antigen fails to induce an immune response in mice, whereas a thousand-fold lower dose of the same antigen (5×10^{-4} mg) induces a humoral antibody response. This phenomenon of "immunologic unresponsiveness," or *tolerance*, is discussed in Chapter 14.

A single dose of most experimental immunogens will not induce a strong response; rather, repeated administration over a period of weeks is required to stimulate a strong immune response. Experimental immunogens generally are administered parenterally—that is, by routes other than the digestive tract. Common administration routes are intravenous, intradermal, subcutaneous, intramuscular, and intraperitoneal. The route of antigen injection determines which immune organs and cell populations will be involved in the response. Antigen administered intravenously is carried first to the spleen, whereas antigen administered subcutaneously moves first to local lymph nodes. Differences in the lymphoid cells populating these organs generate differences in the quality of the subsequent immune response. For each new immunogen a dose-response curve must be established, with variations in dosage, route, and schedule each contributing to peak responsiveness.

Adjuvants

Adjuvants (from Latin *adjuvare*, to help) are substances that, when mixed with an antigen and injected with it, serve to enhance the immunogenicity of that antigen. As seen in Figure 4-2, the antibody response to an influenza vaccine is much higher and longer-lasting when the vaccine is given with an adjuvant than when the vaccine is given alone. Adjuvants are often used to boost the immune response when an antigen has low immunogenicity or when only small amounts of an antigen

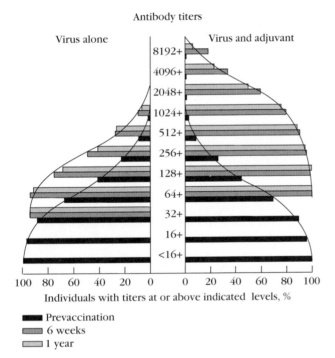

Antibody titers

Virus alone   Virus and adjuvant

Individuals with titers at or above indicated levels, %

- ■ Prevaccination
- ▨ 6 weeks
- ▥ 1 year

Figure 4-2 Effect of incomplete Freund's adjuvant on the immunogenicity of an influenza vaccine. Serum antibody titers to a major influenza antigen were measured before and at two times after immunization in 73 subjects immunized with the influenza vaccine alone and in 101 subjects immunized with the vaccine in adjuvant. The data are graphed as the percentage of individuals with serum antibody titers higher than that indicated by the central scale. The titer is the reciprocal of the last serum dilution to inhibit viral activity; thus, the greater the titer, the higher the antibody level. [Adapted from M. Zanetti, E. Sercarz, and J. Salk, 1987, *Immunol. Today* **8**:23.]

are available, limiting the immunizing dosage. For example, the antibody response in mice following immunization with BSA can be increased by fivefold or more if the BSA is administered with an adjuvant.

Precisely how adjuvants augment the immune response is not entirely known, but several mechanisms appear to be involved (Table 4-3). Some adjuvants serve to prolong the persistence of antigen in the immunized animals. For example, when an antigen is mixed with aluminum potassium sulfate (alum), the salt precipitates the antigen; injection of this alum precipitate results in a slower release of antigen from the injection site, so that the effective time of antigen exposure can be increased from a few days without adjuvant to several weeks with the adjuvant. The increased size of the antigen precipitate may also contribute to the adjuvant action of alum by increasing the likelihood of phagocytosis. Freund's water-in-oil adjuvants also function in this way. Freund's incomplete adjuvant contains antigen in aqueous solution, mineral oil, and an emulsifying agent such as mannide monooleate, which disperses the oil into small droplets surrounding the antigen; the antigen is then released very slowly from the site of injection. Freund's complete adjuvant, which contains heat-killed *Mycobacteria* in the water-in-oil emulsion, is more potent than the incomplete form because a muramyl dipeptide component of the mycobacterial cell wall activates macrophages, increasing production of interleukin 1 and thus augmenting the immune response by activating T_H cells.

Other adjuvants, such as synthetic polyribonucleotides and bacterial lipopolysaccharides, stimulate nonspecific lymphocyte proliferation and thus increase the likelihood of antigen-induced clonal selection of lymphocytes. Some adjuvants stimulate a local, chronic inflammatory response with an increase in phagocytic cells as well as lymphocytes. This cellular infiltration at the site of the adjuvant injection can often result in a dense, macrophage-rich mass of cells called a *granuloma*. Both alum and Freund's complete and incomplete adjuvants cause granuloma formation. The increased numbers of phagocytic cells at the site of the granuloma are thought to facilitate antigen processing and presentation and may also increase production of interleukin 1, thus stimulating activation of T_H cells.

Epitopes

As mentioned in Chapter 1, immune cells do not interact with, or recognize, an entire immunogen molecule; instead, lymphocytes recognize discrete sites on the macromolecule called *epitopes,* or *antigenic determinants.* Epitopes are the immunologically active regions

Table 4-3 Postulated mode of action of some commonly used adjuvants

Adjuvant	Postulated mode of action		
	Prolongs antigen persistence	Induces granuloma formation	Stimulates lymphocytes nonspecifically
Freund's incomplete adjuvant	+	+	−
Freund's complete adjuvant	+	+ +	−
Insoluble aluminum salts (alum)	+	+	−
Mycobacterium tuberculosis	−	+	−
Bordetella pertussis	−	−	+
Bacterial lipopolysaccharide (LPS)	−	−	+
Synthetic polynucleotides (poly IC/poly AU)	−	−	+

of an immunogen that bind to specific membrane receptors for antigen on lymphocytes or to secreted antibodies. Interaction between lymphocytes and a complex antigen may involve several levels of antigen structure. In the case of protein antigens, the structure of an epitope may involve elements of the primary, secondary, tertiary, and even quaternary structure of the protein (see Figure 4-1). In the case of polysaccharide antigens, extensive side-chain branching via glycosidic bonds affects the overall three-dimensional conformation of individual epitopes.

T cells and B cells exhibit fundamental differences in antigen recognition (Table 4-4). B cells recognize soluble antigen when it binds to their membrane-bound antibody receptor. Because B cells bind antigen free in solution, the epitopes they recognize tend to be highly accessible sites on the exposed surface of the immunogen. Such exposed epitopes generally contain hydrophilic amino acids and are often located at bends in the amino acid chain, imparting a greater degree of mobility to these residues. T cells, on the other hand, recognize processed peptides associated with MHC molecules on the surface of antigen-presenting cells and altered self-cells. T cells thus exhibit *MHC-restricted antigen recognition*. The CD4 subpopulation recognizes antigen in association with class II MHC molecules and generally functions as T helper cells whereas the CD8 subpopulation recognizes antigen in association with class I MHC molecules and generally functions as T cytotoxic cells. The CD4 cell is therefore said to be class II restricted and the CD8 cell is said to be class I restricted. Subtle differences in the class I or class II MHC molecules expressed by different individuals influence their ability

to recognize T-cell epitopes. Thus T-cell epitopes cannot be considered apart from their associated MHC molecules.

Determination of the conformation of an epitope is a time-consuming task requiring knowledge of its primary sequence and often of its three-dimensional structure, as well as information on the immune reactivity of each region of that structure. One approach that has been used to identify some T- and B-cell epitopes involves epitope mapping: an immunogenic protein is fragmented into overlapping peptides with proteolytic en-

Table 4-4 Comparison of antigen recognition by T cells and B cells

B cells	T cells
Ig-antigen	Ternary complex: TCR-Ag-MHC
Binds soluble antigen	Unable to bind soluble antigen
No MHC involvement	MHC restricted; recognizes processed antigen displayed by MHC
Antigen: protein, polysaccharide, lipid	Antigen: always protein
Epitope: accessible, often conformational, hydrophilic, mobile	Epitope: internal, denatured linear peptide; hydrophobic; bound by MHC

zymes. The individual peptides are then tested for their ability to bind to an antibody elicited by the native protein or to induce T- or B-cell activation. This approach has been particularly useful in mapping T-cell epitopes since the T cell recognizes short linear peptides complexed with MHC molecules. This method is less effective for determining B-cell epitopes owing to the fact that B-cell-epitopes are often not contiguous amino acid sequences but instead are brought together in the tertiary folded configuration of the protein. These conformational B-cell epitopes cannot be identified by this method.

In a few cases B-cell epitopes have been identified by x-ray crystallographic analysis of antigen-antibody complexes. In this procedure beams of x-rays are passed through a crystal of an antigen-antibody complex. This analysis generates a three-dimensional space-filling model of every atom in the antigen-antibody complex, allowing identification of the epitope and the contact residues of the antibody's binding site. Analysis of the x-ray diffraction patterns is extremely complex and takes years to complete. Consequently only a few antigen-antibody complexes have been analyzed by this method. Needless to say, detailed understanding of epitope structure has not been attained for most immunogens.

Properties of Epitopes Recognized by B cells

Several generalizations have emerged about properties of B-cell epitopes from studies with immunogens in which the conformation of the epitope recognized by B cells has been determined.

The size of a B-cell epitope is determined by the size of the antigen-binding site on the antibody molecules displayed by B cells. The binding of an antibody to an epitope involves weak noncovalent interactions, which operate only over short distances and therefore depend on complementarity between the antibody's binding site and the epitope to maximize these weak interactions. The size of the epitope recognized by a B cell thus is determined by the size, shape, and amino acid residues of the antibody's binding site.

In the 1950s, Elvin A. Kabat designed experiments to determine the size of the B-cell epitope on the glucose polymer dextran. In these experiments, he measured the ability of short glucose oligomers, varying in length from disaccharides to large oligosaccharides, to inhibit the binding of antidextran antibodies to dextran. Kabat reasoned that an oligomer constituting the entire epitope should be able to totally occupy the antibody's antigen-binding site and thus completely inhibit binding of the antibody to the epitope on the immunogen. As he increased the polymer size from trisaccharide to hexasaccharide, the oligomers showed increasing ability to

inhibit the binding of antidextran antibodies to dextran (Figure 4-3). Since heptasaccharides and larger oligosaccharides showed the same inhibitory ability as the hexasaccharide, Kabat predicted that the hexasaccharide best approximated the size of the complete epitope and that additional sugar residues must lie outside the binding site on the antibody molecule. These early studies with small carbohydrate antigens suggested that the antibody's binding site was a cleft of sufficient size to bind 6–7 amino acids or sugar residues (Table 4-5).

In the case of globular protein antigens, the epitope is considerably larger. Determination of the epitope structure on a protein can be achieved only by x-ray crystallographic analysis of antigen-antibody complexes. To date this has only been accomplished for five antigen-antibody complexes: three complexes of antibody with hen egg-white lysozyme and two complexes of antibody with neuraminidase, a glycoprotein on the surface of the influenza virus. In each of these antigen-antibody

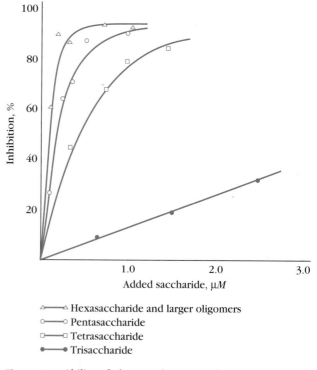

Figure 4-3 Ability of glucose oligomers of various sizes to inhibit the dextran-antidextran reaction. Rabbits were immunized with the glucose polymer dextran, and the antidextran antibodies produced were isolated and incubated with various short oligomers. Binding of the antidextran antibodies to dextran then was determined. Since the greatest inhibition would be expected with oligomers that bound most effectively to the dextran-binding site on the antibody molecules, these data can be used to estimate the size of the dextran epitope recognized by B cells. [Data from E. Kabat, 1974, *J. Am. Chem. Soc.* **76**:3709.]

Table 4-5 Dimensions and molecular weight of B-cell epitopes on some natural and synthetic antigens

Antigen	Determinant*	Size in most extended form (Å)	Molecular weight (Da)
Dextran	Isomaltohexaose	34 × 12 × 7	990
Silk fibroin	Gly [gly$_3$ala$_3$] Tyr	27	632
	Dodecapeptide mixture	44	1000
G^{60}A^{40}, G^{60}A^{30}T^{10}, and G^{42}L^{28}A^{30}	Hexaglutamic acid	36 × 10 × 6	792
Poly-γ-D-Glu	Hexaglutamic acid	36 × 12 × 7	792
Polyalanyl bovine serum albumin	Pentaalanine	25 × 11 × 6.5	373
Polylysine and phosphoryl bovine serum albumin	Pentalysine	27 × 17 × 6.5	659
α-DNP-heptalysine	α-DNP-heptalysine	30 × 17 × 6.5	1080

* Smallest molecule that produces maximal inhibition of antigen-antibody binding.

SOURCE: E. A. Kabat, 1976, *Structural Concepts in Immunology and Immunochemistry*, 2d ed., Holt, Rinehart and Winston. © 1976, 1968 by Holt, Rinehart and Winston; reprinted by permission of Holt, Rinehart and Winston.

complexes the antibody has been shown to make contact with the protein antigen across a large planar face. These studies have revealed that 15–22 amino acids on the surface of the protein antigen make contact with a similar number of residues in the antibody's binding site; the surface area of this large complementary interface is between 650–900 Å^2. For these globular protein antigens, then, the epitope is entirely dependent on the teriary conformation of the native protein.

B-cell epitopes in native proteins generally are hydrophilic amino acids on the protein surface that are topographically accessible to membrane-bound or free antibody. A B-cell epitope must be accessible in order to be able to bind to an antibody. Amino acid sequences that are hidden within the interior of a protein cannot function as B-cell epitopes unless the protein is first denatured. Michael Sela demonstrated the importance of this topographical accessibility in experiments with synthetic branched copolymers in which the accessible amino acids attached to the backbone polypeptide chain were varied. One copolymer, (T,G)-A-L, consisted of a poly-L-lysine backbone with poly D,L-alanine side chains whose N-termini are capped with variable amounts of glutamic acid and/or tyrosine (Figure 4-4). Antibody to (T,G)-A-L reacted largely with the accessible tyrosine and glutamic acid residues at the end of each side chain. Alteration of the synthetic copolymer to A-(T,G)-L, in which poly D,L-alanine residues are in the accessible terminal positions and the glutamic acid and tyrosine residues are in a less accessible position, completely blocked reactivity with the antibody to (T,G)-A-L.

For globular protein antigens, the entire surface of the protein is thought to be potentially antigenic. In general, regions that tend to protrude on the surface of the protein are often recognized as epitopes. Because the residues are accessible, they are often hydrophilic. Of the five crystallized antigen-antibody complexes analyzed to date, the interface between antibody and antigen is highly complementary. The interacting surface between antigen and antibody reveals numerous complementary protrusions and depressions. Contact is made between 15–22 amino acids and has been shown to involve between 75–120 hydrogen bonds as well as ionic and hydrophobic interactions.

B-cell epitopes can contain sequential or nonsequential amino acids. Epitopes may be composed of *sequential* contiguous residues along the polypeptide chain or *nonsequential* residues from segments of the chain brought together by the folded conformation of the protein. Most antibodies elicited by globular protein antigens bind to the protein only when it is in its native conformation. Because denaturation of such antigens usually results in loss of the topographical structure of their epitopes, antibodies to the native protein fail to bind to the denatured protein.

Sperm whale myoglobin is an example of a protein antigen that contains several sequential epitopes. The three-dimensional structure of this protein has been determined by x-ray crystallography. The molecule has an abundance of α-helical regions and five distinct sequential epitopes, each containing six to eight amino acids. Each of these epitopes is on the surface of the molecule

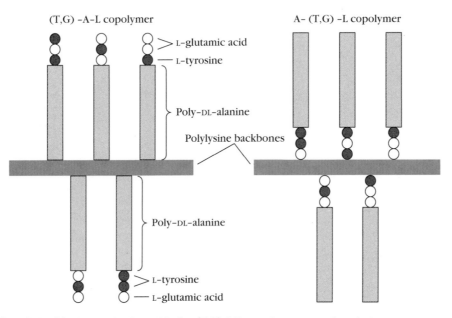

Figure 4-4 Antibodies elicited by immunization with the (T,G)-A-L copolymer react largely with the exposed tyrosine and glutamic acid residues. Anti-(T,G)-A-L antibodies do not react with the A-(T,G)-L copolymer in which the tyrosine and glutamic acid residues are buried. [Adapted from M. Z. Sela, 1969, *Science* **166**:1365.]

at bends between the α-helical regions (Figure 4-5). Recently several additional nonsequential epitopes, or *conformational determinants*, also have been characterized for sperm whale myoglobin. The residues constituting these epitopes are far apart in terms of the primary amino acid sequence but close together in the tertiary structure of the molecule: such epitopes thus

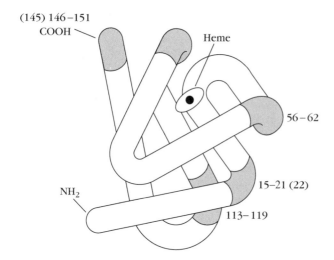

Figure 4-5 Diagram of sperm whale myoglobin showing locations of five sequential B-cell epitopes (light red). [Adapted from M. Z. Atassi and A. L. Kazim, 1978, *Adv. Exp. Med. Biol.* **98**:9.]

are dependent on the native protein conformation for their topographical structure. The epitopes of hen egg-white lysozyme (HEL) and neuraminidase are well-characterized conformational determinants. Figure 4-6 shows the amino acid residues that make up one epitope of HEL and one epitope of neuraminidase. In each case the epitope is composed of nonsequential amino acids, far apart in the primary amino acid sequence, that have been brought together by the tertiary folding of the protein.

Sequential and nonsequential epitopes generally behave differently when a protein is fragmented or reduced. For example, appropriate fragmentation of sperm whale myoglobin can yield five fragments, each retaining one sequential epitope, as demonstrated by the observation that antibody can bind to each fragment. On the other hand, fragmentation of a protein or reduction of its disulfide bonds often destroys any nonsequential epitopes that it contains. For example, HEL has four intrachain disulfide bonds, which determine the final protein conformation. Antibodies to HEL recognize eight different epitopes, most of which are conformational determinants dependent on the overall structure of the protein. If the intrachain disulfide bonds of HEL are reduced with mercaptoethanol, the conformational determinants are lost and antibody to native HEL will not bind to reduced HEL. The inhibition experiment described in Figure 4-7 also demonstrates the importance of these disulfide bonds in determining the structure of HEL epitopes.

(a)

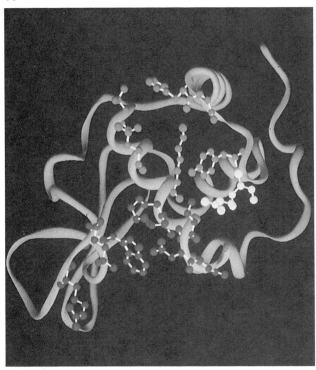

(b)

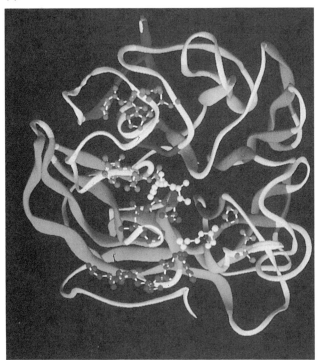

Figure 4-6 Ribbon diagrams of hen egg-white lysozyme (a) and influenza-virus neuraminidase (b) showing the location of one nonsequential epitope (conformational determinant) in each protein. The amino acids that have been shown to contact monoclonal antibody are indicated with shaded balls. [Adapted from W. G. Laver et al 1990, *Cell* **61**:554.]

B-cell epitopes tend to be located in flexible regions of an immunogen and display site mobility. John A. Tainer and his colleagues analyzed the epitopes on a number of protein antigens (myohemerytherin, insulin, cytochrome *c*, myoglobin, and hemoglobin) by comparing the positions of the known B-cell epitopes with the atomic mobility of the same residues. Their analysis revealed that the major antigenic determinants in these proteins generally were located in the most mobile regions. These investigators propose that site mobility of epitopes maximizes complementarity with the antibody's binding site, giving rise to a higher-affinity interaction.

Complex proteins contain multiple overlapping B-cell epitopes. Until recently, it was dogma in immunology that a given globular protein had a small number of epitopes, each confined to a highly accessible region and determined by the overall conformation of the protein. However, it has been shown recently that most of the surface of a globular protein is potentially antigenic. This has been demonstrated by comparing the antigen-binding profiles of different monoclonal antibodies to various globular proteins. For example, when 64 different monoclonal antibodies to bovine serum albumin were compared for their ability to bind to a panel of 10 different mammalian albumins, 25 different overlapping antigen-binding profiles emerged, suggesting that these 64 different antibodies recognized a minimum of 25 different epitopes on bovine serum albumin. Similar findings have emerged for other globular proteins, such as myoglobin and HEL. The surface of a protein, then, must present a large number of potential antigenic sites. The subset of antigenic sites on a given protein that is selected by an individual animal is much smaller than the potential antigenic repertoire, and it varies from species to species and even among individual members of a given species. Within a given animal, certain epitopes are recognized as immunogenic, whereas others are not. Furthermore, some epitopes, referred to as *immunodominant,* induce a more pronounced immune response than other epitopes in a particular animal. It is thought that intrinsic topographical properties of the epitope as well as the animal's regulatory mechanisms influence the immunodominance of particular epitopes.

Properties of Epitopes Recognized by T Cells

Early studies by P. G. H. Gell and Baruj Benacerraf in 1959 suggested that there is a qualitative difference between the T-cell and the B-cell response to protein antigens. Gell and Benacerraf compared the humoral and cell-mediated responses to a series of native and dena-

(a) Hen egg–white lysosome

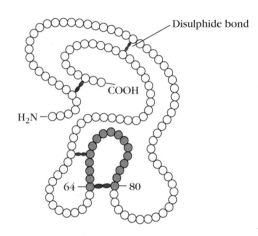

(b) Synthetic loop peptides

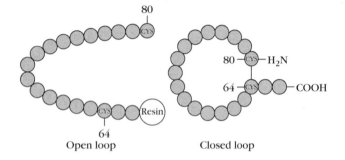

Open loop   Closed loop

(c) Inhibition of reaction between HEL
    loop and anti–loop antiserum

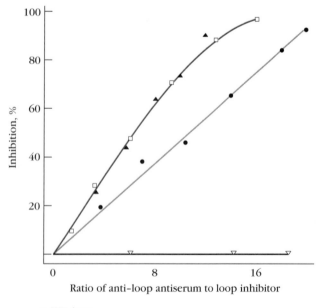

• HEL loop
▲ Natural loop
□ Closed synthetic loop
▽ Open synthetic loop

Figure 4-7 Experimental demonstration that binding of antibody to conformational determinants in hen egg-white lysozyme (HEL) depends on maintenance of the tertiary structure of the epitopes by intrachain disulfide bonds. (a) Diagram of HEL primary structure in which solid balls represent amino acid residues. The loop (red balls) formed by the disulfide bond between the cysteine residues at positions 64 and 80 constitutes one of the conformational determinants in HEL. (b) Synthetic open- and closed-loop peptides showing identity of amino acid residues in the HEL loop epitope. (c) Inhibition of reaction between HEL loop epitope and anti-loop antiserum. Anti-loop antiserum was first incubated with HEL, the natural loop sequence, the synthetic closed-loop peptide, or the synthetic open-loop peptide; the ability of the antiserum to bind the natural loop sequence then was determined. The absence of any inhibition by the open-loop peptide indicates that it does not bind to the anti-loop antiserum. [Adapted from D. Benjamin, J. Berzofsky, I. East et al., 1984, *Annu. Rev. Immunol.* **2**:67.]

tured protein antigens (Table 4-6). They found that if primary immunization was with a native protein, then a secondary antibody response was elicited only with native protein, not with denatured protein. In contrast, the secondary cell-mediated response did not discriminate between native and denatured protein. In other words, a secondary T-cell–mediated response was induced by denatured protein even when the primary immunization had been with native protein. This observation puzzled immunologists until the 1980s, when it became clear that T cells do not recognize soluble native antigen but rather recognize antigen that has been processed and whose peptide fragments are presented in association with MHC. For this reason, destruction of the conformation of a protein by denaturation does not affect its T-cell epitopes.

Oligomeric peptides function as T-cell epitopes. Schlossman synthesized polypeptide polymers containing oligomers of L-lysine residues separated by intervening sequences of D,L-lysine. Only oligomers with a minimum of seven contiguous L-lysines [(L-lysine)7, D-lysine-L-lysine] were capable of stimulating T-cell proliferation. In the case of a complex protein antigen, such as sperm whale myoglobin, I. Berkower and J. Berzofsky found that the smallest peptide that could stimulate a cloned T-cell line specific for sperm whale myoglobin was an 11-aa peptide consisting of residues 136–146. In general, however, many of the peptides of sperm whale myoglobin observed to activate T cells contained on the order of 20 amino acids.

Antigenic peptides recognized by T cells form trimolecular complexes with a T-cell receptor and a MHC molecule. Direct biochemical evidence for an interaction between defined T-cell peptide antigens and class

Table 4-6 Antigen recognition by T and B lymphocytes reveals qualitative differences

Primary immunization	Secondary immunization	Secondary immune response	
		Antibody production	Cell-mediated T_{DTH} response
Native protein	Native protein	+	+
Native protein	Denatured protein	−	+

I and class II MHC molecules has been obtained by several investigators. A class I MHC molecule has been crystallized, revealing a small peptide, presumed to be processed antigen, in the cleft of the molecule (see Figure 9-11d). Although a class II MHC molecule has not yet been crystallized, other experiments suggest that these proteins also bind antigenic peptides. For example, S. Buus and H. M. Grey labeled different antigenic peptides with a radioactive isotope [^{125}I] and demonstrated that the labeled peptides bind to purified class II MHC molecules. In these experiments different peptides were observed to bind to different class II MHC molecules. For example, a peptide of chicken ovalbumin encompassing residues 323–339 was shown to bind to the class II MHC molecule designated IA^d but failed to bind to the class II MHC molecule designated IE^d. As will be discussed later, the binding of a peptide to the MHC also correlated with its ability to activate a T cell.

Antigens recognized by T cells must, therefore, possess two distinct interaction sites: one (the epitope) interacts with the T-cell receptor, and the other, called the *agretope*, interacts with a MHC molecule. Little is understood regarding the nature of the interaction between an agretope and a MHC molecule; the term agretope is not based on clear structural features but simply denotes the functional ability of an antigenic peptide to interact with a MHC molecule. Unlike B-cell epitopes, which can be viewed strictly in terms of their ability to interact with antibody, T-cell epitopes must be viewed in terms of a trimolecular complex involving a T-cell receptor, an antigenic peptide, and a MHC molecule.

The binding of a peptide to the cleft in a MHC molecule does not appear to have the kind of fine specificity exhibited in the interaction between an antibody and its epitope. Instead, a given MHC molecule can selectively bind a variety of different peptides. For example, the class II MHC molecule designated IA^d can bind peptides from ovalbumin (residues 323–339), hemagglutinin (residues 130–142), and lambda repressor (residues 12–26). This broad, but selective interaction suggests that the agretope on these various peptides may share certain structural features, enabling them to bind to the same MHC molecule.

Antigen processing is required to generate peptides that interact specifically with MHC molecules. Experiments suggest that different intracellular processing pathways are involved in the generation of peptides that interact with class I or class II MHC molecules (see Figure 1-9). Endogenous antigens, which are synthesized within a host cell (e.g., viral antigens in a virus-infected cell), appear to be processed into peptides within the cytoplasm and are presented together with class I MHC molecules. Exogenous antigens (e.g., large, soluble protein antigens) are first internalized by antigen-presenting cells and then exposed to proteolytic enzymes within the endosomal-processing system. Within the endosomal pathway, the peptides generated during antigen processing are thought to interact with class II MHC molecules and then to be presented together with these molecules on the membrane of the antigen-presenting cell.

The dependence of T-cell activation on antigen processing has been demonstrated for both class I-restricted T_C cells and class II-restricted T_H cells. K. Ziegler and Emil R. Unanue, for example, observed that T_H-cell activation by bacterial protein antigens was prevented by treating the antigen-presenting cells with paraformaldehyde prior to antigen exposure (Figure 4-8). However, if the antigen-presenting cells were allowed to ingest the antigen and were fixed with paraformaldehyde 1-h later, T_H-cell activation could still occur. In that 1 h time interval, the antigen-presenting cells had converted the antigen into a form able to activate T cells and had displayed it on the membrane. Richard P. Shimonkevitz showed that internalization and processing could be bypassed if antigen-presenting cells were exposed to peptide digests of an antigen instead of the native antigen. In these experiments, antigen-presenting cells were treated with glutaraldehyde and then incubated with native ovalbumin or with ovalbumin that had been subjected to partial enzymatic digestion. The digested ovalbumin was able to interact with the glutaraldehyde-treated antigen-presenting cells, thereby activating ovalbumin-specific T_H cells, whereas the native ovalbumin failed to do so. Similarly, activation of T_C cells can be achieved by treating target cells expressing appropriate

EXPERIMENTAL CONDITIONS   T CELL
                                                                     ACTIVATION

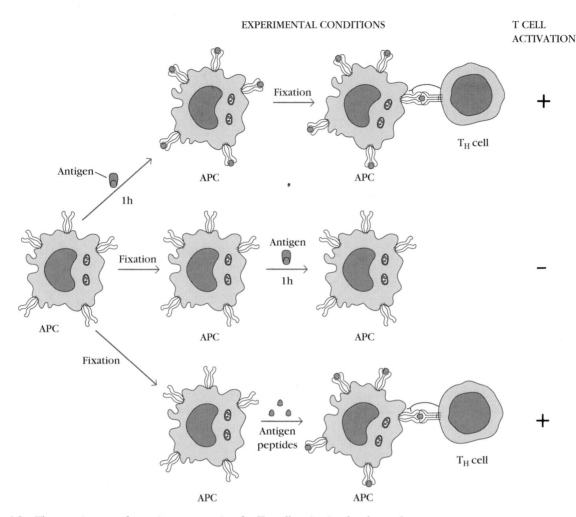

Figure 4-8   The requirement for antigen processing for T_H-cell activation has been shown by fixing antigen-presenting cells (APCs) before antigen exposure or 1 h following antigen exposure. Fixation before antigen exposure (*middle*) completely inhibits the ability of antigen-presenting cells to activate the T_H cells. In contrast, antigen-presenting cells fixed 1 h following antigen exposure (*top*) are able to activate T_H cells. Antigen-presenting cells fixed before antigen exposure but incubated with peptide digests of the protein antigen also are able to activate the T_H cells (*bottom*). T_H-cell activation is determined by measuring a specific T_H-cell response, such as cytokine secretion.

class I MHC molecules with peptide digests, avoiding altogether the requirement for intracellular antigen processing. Taken together, these experiments suggest that antigen processing involves protein digestion with proteolytic enzymes.

Antigens recognized by T cells often contain amphipathic peptides. J. Berzofsky and coworkers have suggested that the primary function of antigen processing may be to unfold an antigen and reveal internal regions that are amphipathic (i.e., possessing both hydrophobic and hydrophilic amino acid sequences). The hydrophobic residues may act as agretopes, interacting with MHC proteins, and the hydrophilic residues may act as epitopes, interacting with T-cell receptors.

To determine whether there might be a correlation between amphipathic peptides and T-cell responsiveness, H. Margalit and her colleagues designed a computer program to analyze peptide sequences within proteins and assigned to each peptide segment an "amphipathic index" based on the amount of amphipathic α helices in it. Comparison of 23 known immunodominant T-cell peptides in various proteins with the amphipathic segments in the same proteins revealed that 18 of the T-cell peptides overlapped with highly amphipathic segments (Table 4-7). This correlation has been used to predict potential T-cell epitopes for synthetic peptide vaccines against a number of diseases, including malaria, influenza, and hepatitis (see Chapter 18). A somewhat similar approach has been used to demonstrate that the known T-cell epitopes in sperm whale myoglobin and hen egg-white lysozyme exhibit minimum protrusion; that is, they tend to be on the "inside" of the protein molecule (Figure 4-9).

Immunodominant T-cell epitopes may be determined in part by the set of MHC cell-surface molecules expressed by an individual (Figures 4-10 and 4-11). The particular set of MHC molecules expressed by an individual determines which antigenic peptides are presented to its T cells. The MHC will therefore play a significant role in determining which T-cell epitopes in a given antigen will be immunodominant in a given individual. A correlation between the ability of a peptide

to bind to an MHC molecule and the T-cell response to that peptide was shown in experiments of S. Buus, A. Sette, and H. M. Grey. They analyzed 14 synthetic peptides, representing overlapping sequences of the entire length of an immunogenic protein. Of these 14 peptides, three were shown to activate T_H cells, and each of these three peptides was also shown to bind to a class II MHC molecule expressed by the same strain of mice (see Figure 4-11).

Another experimental approach for studying the role of the MHC in peptide presentation involves transfection of class II MHC genes into a mouse fibroblast cell line called L cells. Since L cells are not antigen-presenting cells, they do not express their own class II MHC mol-

Table 4-7 Position of known immunodominant T-cell epitopes and amphipathic segments in various protein antigens

Antigen	T-cell epitopes[*]	Amphipathic segments[*]	Amphipathic score[†]
Sperm whale myoglobin	69–78	64–78	14.2
	102–118	99–117	20.1
	132–145	128–145	15.3
Pigeon cytochrome *c*	93–104	92–103	4.3
Influenza hemagglutinin A/PR/8/34 Mt. S.	109–119	97–120	35.3
	130–140	—	—
	302–313	291–314	35.1
Pork insulin	(B)5–16	4–16	5.5
	(A)4–14	1–21	34.0
Chicken lysozyme	46–61	—	—
	74–86	72–86	8.9
	81–96	86–102	13.1
	109–119	—	—
Chicken ovalbumin	323–339	329–346	18.0
Hepatitis B virus pre S	120–132	121–135	8.7
Foot and mouth virus VP1	141–160	148–165	20.3
Beef cytochrome *c*	11–25	9–29	22.7
	66–80	58–78	23.6
Hepatitis B virus major surface antigen	38–52	36–49	7.3
	95–109	—	—
	140–154	—	—
λ Repressor protein CI	12–26	8–25	19.5
Rabies virus-spike glycoprotein precursor	32–44	29–46	20.2

[*] Positions of amino acid residues constituting epitopes and amphipathic segments are shown.

[†] Amphipathic score obtained from computer analysis of peptide segments within the proteins.

SOURCE: Adapted from H. Margalit et al., 1987, *J. Immunol.* **138**:2219.

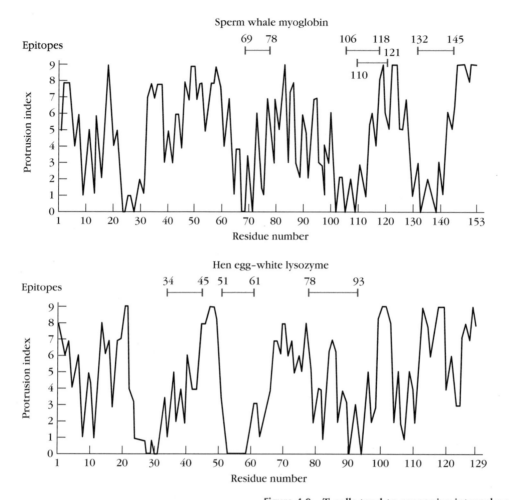

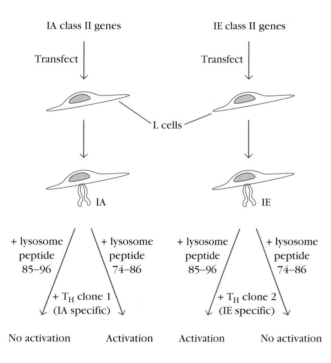

Figure 4-9 T cells tend to recognize internal peptides that are exposed during processing within the antigen-presenting cell. The amino acids of two proteins (sperm whale myoglobin and hen egg-white lysozyme) have been plotted according to their protrusion in the tertiary conformation of the protein. The known T-cell epitopes for each protein are depicted by red bars. Notice that amino acid residues corresponding to the T-cell epitopes are residues with a minimum of protrusion. [From J. Rothbard. et al. 1987, *Modern Trends in Human Leukemia* vol. 7.]

Figure 4-10 Experimental demonstration that MHC molecules exhibit differential interaction with antigenic peptides. In this experiment, the transfected L cells functioned as antigen-presenting cells to two T_H-cell clones, one specific for lysozyme plus class II IA MHC and the other specific for lysozyme plus class II IE MHC. The results indicate that each MHC molecule could present only one of the two lysozyme peptides.

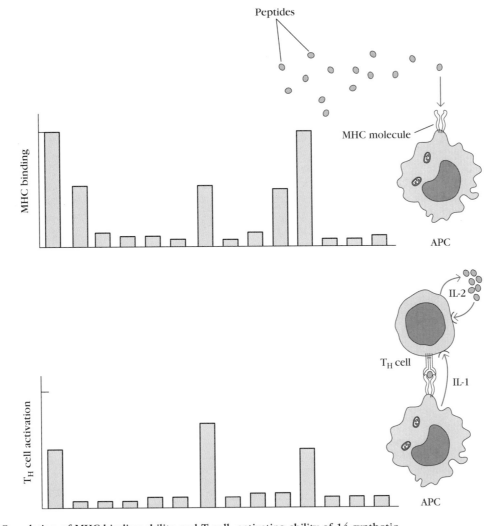

Figure 4-11 Correlation of MHC-binding ability and T-cell–activating ability of 14 synthetic peptides representing overlapping sequences of an immunogenic protein. Of the five peptides that bound to MHC molecules on mouse antigen-presenting cells (*top*), three also stimulated T-cell activation (*bottom*). These data suggest that binding to an MHC protein is necessary, but not sufficient, for a peptide to induce an immune response. [Adapted from H. M. Grey, A. Sette, and S. Buus, 1989, *Sci. Am.* **261**(5):59.]

ecules. However, if a class II gene is transfected under the control of an active promoter, L cells will express the transfected class II gene product. Using this approach, Nilabh Shastri transfected L cells with different class II MHC genes that encoded proteins designated IA and IE; he then tested the ability of the transfected L cells to present various lysozyme peptides to different T_H clones known to be specific for lysozyme plus IA or IE class II MHC. He found that L cells transfected with the IA genes could present lysozyme peptide 74–86 but not peptide 85–96 to the IA-restricted clone; conversely, L cells transfected with the IE genes could present peptide 85–96 but not peptide 74–86 to the T_H-cell clone restricted for IE (see Figure 4-10). In this system, then,

one lysozyme T-cell epitope is immunodominant in the IA-restricted clone and another epitope is immunodominant in the IE-restricted clone, demonstrating that immunodominance is dependent on MHC expression.

Haptens and the Study of Antigenicity

It can be very difficult to study the binding of an individual antibody to a unique epitope on a complex protein. The pioneering work of Karl Landsteiner in the 1920s and 1930s provided a simple, chemically defined system for the study of such binding. In Landsteiner's approach small organic compounds called *haptens* are chemically coupled to larger proteins called *carriers* (Figure 4-12a). When the resulting *hapten-carrier conjugate* is used to immunize animals, it functions as an immunogen, with antibodies being elicited both to the hapten determinant and to unaltered epitopes on the carrier protein; the hapten thus functions as an epitope. Since the chemical conjugation makes it possible for multiple molecules of a single hapten to be coupled to the carrier protein and to be accessible to the immune system, the hapten functions as the immunodominant determinant on a hapten-carrier conjugate. The beauty of the hapten-carrier system is that it provides immunologists with a chemically defined determinant that can be subtly modified by chemical means to determine the effect of various chemical structures on immune specificity.

In the system developed by Landsteiner, hapten alone does not stimulate clonal selection and the ensuing secretion of antibody. That happens only when a hapten is coupled to a protein carrier (Figure 4-12b). Although a hapten behaves as an antigen, in that it can react with antibody, by itself it lacks the property of immunogenicity. It is a hapten's lack of size and valency that prevent it, by itself, from functioning as an immunogen. However, if multiple copies of a hapten are coupled to a large nonimmunogenic homopolymer, the molecule can sometimes behave as an immunogen; the homopolymer provides the requisite size, and the hapten provides the necessary complexity and multivalency.

Landsteiner's studies with haptens demonstrated the fine specificity of the immune system. He immunized rabbits with a hapten-carrier conjugate and then tested the reactivity of the rabbit's immune sera to that hapten

(a)

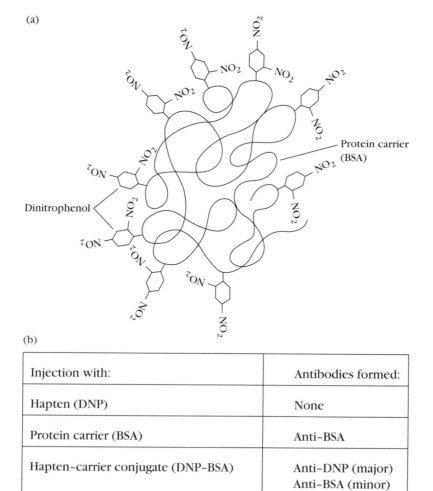

(b)

Injection with:	Antibodies formed:
Hapten (DNP)	None
Protein carrier (BSA)	Anti–BSA
Hapten–carrier conjugate (DNP–BSA)	Anti–DNP (major) Anti–BSA (minor)

Figure 4-12   (a) A hapten-carrier conjugate contains multiple copies of the hapten—a small organic compound such as dinitrophenol (DNP)—chemically linked to a large protein carrier such as bovine serum albumin (BSA). (b) Immunization with DNP alone elicits no anti-DNP antibodies, but immunization with DNP-BSA reveals that the hapten is the immunodominant epitope in a hapten-carrier conjugate.

or to structural modifications of the hapten coupled to a different carrier protein. Thus he could measure, specifically, the reaction of the antihapten antibodies in the immune serum and not that of antibodies to the original carrier epitopes. Landsteiner tested whether an antihapten antibody could bind to other haptens having a slightly different chemical structure. If a reaction occurred, it was referred to as a *cross-reaction*. By observing which hapten modifications prevented or permitted cross-reactions, Landsteiner was able to gain valuable insight into the specificity of the antibody-antigen reaction. Landsteiner found that the overall configuration of the hapten played a major role in determining whether the molecule could react with a given antibody. He produced antisera to aminobenzene and its carboxyl derivatives (*o*-aminobenzoic acid, *m*-aminobenzoic acid, and *p*-aminobenzoic acid). He found that each antiserum was specific for the original immunizing hapten and would not react with any of the isomers. In contrast, if the overall configuration of the

Table 4-8 Reactivity of antisera with various haptens

	Reactivity with			
Antiserum against	Aminobenzene (aniline)	*o*-aminobenzoic acid	*m*-aminobenzoic acid	*p*-aminobenzoic acid
Aminobenzene	+ + +	0	0	0
o-aminobenzoic acid	0	+ + +	0	0
m-aminobenzoic acid	0	0	+ + + +	0
p-aminobenzoic acid	0	0	0	+ + + ±

	Reactivity with			
Antiserum against	Aminobenzene (aniline)	*p*-chloroamino-benzene	*p*-toluidine	*p*-nitroamino-benzene
Aminobenzene	+ + +	+	+ ±	+
p-chloroaminobenzene	± + + ±	+ +	+ +	+ ±
p-toluidine	+ ±	+ +	+ +	+
p-nitroaminobenzene	+	+ +	+ ±	+

KEY: 0 indicates no reactivity; + + + and + + + + indicate strong reactivity; + ±, and + + indicate different degrees of reactivity.

SOURCE: Based on K. Landsteiner, 1962, *The Specificity of Serologic Reactions*. Dover Press. Modified by J. Klein. 1982, *Immunology the Science of Self-Nonself Discrimination*. John Wiley Publishers.

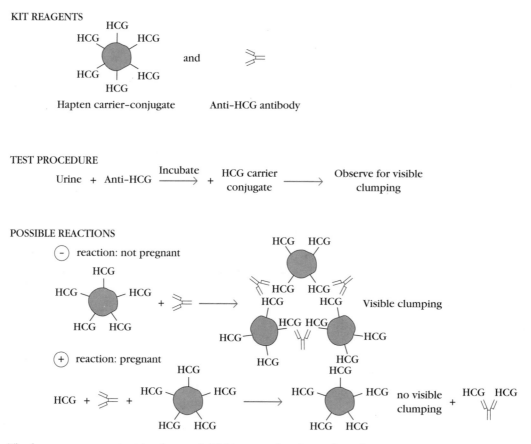

Figure 4-13   The home pregnancy test is a hapten-inhibition test that determines the presence or absence of human chorionic gonadotropin (HCG). If a woman is pregnant, her urine will contain HCG, which will bind to the anti-HCG antibodies in the test kit, thus inhibiting the subsequent binding of the antibody to the HCG-carrier conjugate. Because of this inhibition, no visible clumping occurs if HCG is present.

hapten was kept the same and the hapten was modified in the para position with various nonionic derivatives, then the antisera showed varying degrees of cross-reactivity (Table 4-8). In addition to demonstrating the specificity of the immune system, Landsteiner's work also demonstrated the enormous diversity of epitopes that the immune system is capable of reacting to.

Many biologically important substances, including drugs, peptide hormones, and steroid hormones can function as haptens. By conjugating these haptens to larger protein carriers, it is possible to produce hapten-specific antibody that can then serve to measure the presence of these substances in the body. The home pregnancy test kit, which determines the presence or absence of human chorionic gonadotropin (HCG) in a woman's urine, is a hapten-inhibition assay. If HCG (the hapten) is present in the urine, it inhibits the ability of the kit's anti-HCG antibodies to react with the kit's HCG-carrier conjugate. Since this reaction produces visible clumping, the absence of clumping indicates the presence of HCG, which is a sign of pregnancy (Figure 4-13).

Viral and Bacterial Antigens

The general properties of antigens discussed so far can be illustrated by a closer examination of viral and bacterial antigens. These antigens stimulate the immune response to viral and bacterial infection, thus triggering the body's most effective defense mechanism against infectious disease.

Viral Antigens

Animal viruses consist of nucleic acid (either DNA or RNA) surrounded by a protein coat, called a *capsid,* which is composed of protein subunits called *capsomers.* In simple viruses the capsomers are composed of a single protein; in more complex viruses several capsomer proteins may be present. A capsid with its enclosed nucleic acid is referred to as a *nucleocapsid;* a nucleocapsid may have helical or polyhedral symmetry. Some animal viruses are *naked,* but many have an additional lipoprotein *envelope,* which the virus acquires by modifying the host cell's plasma membrane as it leaves the cell in the process called *budding.* The complete viral particle is called a *virion* (Figure 4-14a). Protein—the principal constituent of animal viruses—is the only component of the capsid and a major component (sometimes in the form of glycoprotein) of the envelope. Proteins are also intimately associated with the viral nucleic acid as internal proteins of the nucleocapsid. Most of these proteins and glycoproteins can be recognized as immunogens by the immune system and will induce a humoral and/or a cell-mediated response.

B cells can recognize a variety of viral proteins and glycoproteins, including components of the envelope and interior components of the nucleocapsid, which may be released from infected host cells prior to complete viral assembly. The subunit structure of the capsid and repeating glycoprotein projections on many enveloped viruses provide the B cell with repeating epitopes. As discussed earlier, immunodominant B-cell epitopes tend to be residues that are accessible, hydrophilic, and mobile; thus surface sequences generated by the tertiary conformation of viral proteins function as the immunodominant B-cell epitopes. During the course of a viral infection, serum levels of antibody to envelope proteins, core proteins, and proteins associated with the viral genome all increase. These antibodies can facilitate virus clearance either by acting as opsonins to enhance phagocytosis or by activating the complement cascade leading to lysis of the enveloped viral particle. These antibodies often play a protective role by binding to viral envelope proteins or glycoproteins and preventing further infection of host cells. The presence of viral-specific antibodies is often used to determine whether an individual has been infected with a particular virus.

Although antibody is produced during a viral infection, in general a cell-mediated immune response is required for protective immunity to a virus. Both T_H and T_C cells can recognize viral proteins. T_H cells are generally class II MHC restricted. These T_H cells recognize viral proteins that have been internalized by the antigen-presenting cell, either by phagocytosis in the case of macrophages or by receptor-mediated endocytosis in the case of the B cells. After processing in the endosomal pathway, antigenic peptides will be displayed, together with class II MHC, on the membrane of these antigen-presenting cells. As mentioned already, the peptides recognized by T_H cells tend to be internal amino acid sequences that have amphipathic properties, enabling them to interact with both a class II MHC molecule and the T-cell receptor. Lymphokines produced by activated T_H cells then serve to activate either B cells or T_C cells.

Many animal viruses are known to replicate within host cells. As viral proteins are produced within the host cell, these endogenously produced proteins may be processed within the cytoplasm and presented together with a class I MHC molecule on the membrane of the infected host cell, inducing a T_C-cell response. The epitopes recognized by T_C cells need not be major, exposed viral components such as the envelope glycoproteins; instead, they often are internal viral proteins produced within the infected host cell. For example, a major influenza antigen recognized by T_C cells is an internal protein called nucleoprotein, which is associated with the viral RNA genome. Activation of T_C cells in response to nucleoprotein peptides appears to play an important role in the elimination of influenza-infected host cells and in recovery from the infection.

Some viruses are capable of substantial variation in the structure of their envelope glycoprotein components. Influenza virus, for example, constantly changes the amino acid sequence of its envelope glycoproteins. Either major amino acid variations (*antigenic shift*) or minor variations (*antigenic drift*) can give rise to new epitopes, allowing the virus to evade the immune system. This antigenic variation is the major cause of repeated influenza outbreaks. This process is discussed more fully in Chapter 19. Rapid changes in an envelope glycoprotein of the human immunodeficiency virus (HIV) of AIDS enable the virus to evade the immune response and thus establish a major obstacle to vaccine development, as will be seen in Chapter 21.

Bacterial Antigens

Bacteria are single-cell organisms, consisting typically of a membrane-bound cytoplasm, containing RNA, DNA, and enzymes, that is surrounded by a cell wall and in some cases enclosed in a capsule. Various processes (flagella, fimbriae, or pili) may protrude from the cell.

(a) Enveloped viral particle

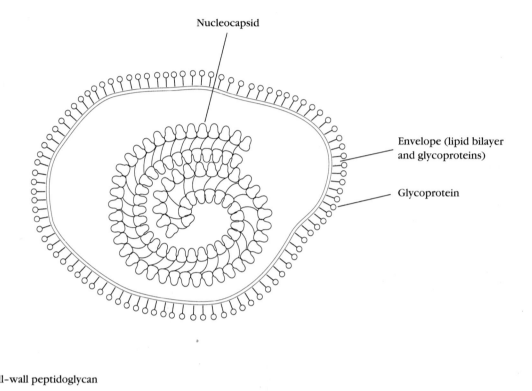

Nucleocapsid

Envelope (lipid bilayer and glycoproteins)

Glycoprotein

(b) Bacterial cell-wall peptidoglycan

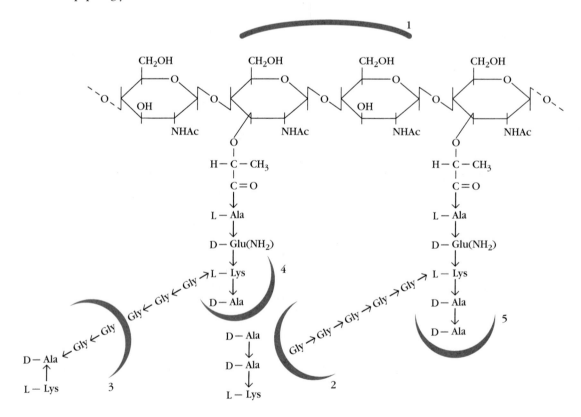

Although a bacterium may secrete soluble products that can serve as immunogens, the major bacterial immunogens are epitopes on surface structures.

The cell wall of so-called *gram-positive* bacteria is composed largely of peptidoglycan, a network of polysaccharides cross-linked by short peptide chains. Intercalated within the gram-positive cell wall are various proteins, polysaccharides, and teichoic acids. Structural differences in these cell-wall components generate unique epitopes, that can be recognized with antibody (Figure 4-14b). The gram-positive *Streptococci*, for example, can be grouped on the basis of antigenic differences in their cell-wall carbohydrate.

Gram-negative bacteria have a thin peptidoglycan layer covered by an outer membrane containing phospholipid, protein, lipopolysaccharide, and lipoprotein. The lipopolysaccharide (LPS) is a major antigenic component of the gram-negative cell wall. The polysaccharide side chains of LPS consist of repeating linear trisaccharides or branched tetra- or pentasaccharides; a chain can include as many as 40 repeat units. The LPS of gram-negative cell walls thus presents the immune system with accessible and multivalent epitopes on the bacterial surface, which are referred to as *O antigens*. Differences in the O-antigen epitope structure of the polysaccharide side chains can induce specific antibodies, which can be used to classify gram-negative bacteria.

The bacterial capsule is a loose polysaccharide or polypeptide layer that lies outside the cell wall. The presence of a capsule is associated with virulence because it interferes with phagocytosis. Most capsules consist of repeating sequences of two or three sugars and have molecular weights as high as 140,000 Da. The accessibility of the capsule, as well as its repeating epitope structure, allows this bacterial component to generate a significant humoral antibody response. In the case of *Pneumococci*, an estimated 4×10^6 antibody molecules can combine with the capsular epitopes expressed on a single bacterial cell. The binding of antibody to capsular epitopes provides another basis for typing bacteria. Differences in capsular polysaccharide sugars and their linkages define more than 80 pneumococcal types.

Figure 4-14 Viral and bacterial antigens. (a) Structure of an enveloped viral particle. The repeating envelope glycoproteins are B-cell epitopes, as are some internal core proteins; both can induce a humoral immune response. Internal proteins that are processed and presented on the membrane of virus-infected cells together with class I MHC molecules induce a cell-mediated response. (b) A portion of the primary structure of the bacterial cell-wall peptidoglycan showing five B-cell epitopes. [From B. Heymer, 1985, in *Immunology of the Bacterial Cell Envelope*, D. E. S. Stewart-Tull and M. Davis, eds., John Wiley and Sons.]

Mitogens

Mitogens are agents that are able to induce cell division in a high percentage of T or B cells. Unlike immunogens which activate only lymphocytes bearing specific receptors, mitogen activation is nonspecific. Mitogens are known as *polyclonal activators* because they activate many clones of T or B cells irrespective of their antigen specificity. A variety of diverse agents function as mitogens. A number of common mitogens are proteins (called *lectins*) that are derived from plants and bind sugars. Lectins recognize different glycoproteins on the surface of various cells, including lymphocytes. Lectin binding to the membrane glycoproteins often leads to agglutination, or clustering, of the cells, which is often followed by cellular activation. Some mitogens preferentially activate B cells, some preferentially activate T cells, and some activate both populations.

Three common mitogens are *concanavalin A*, or *Con A*; *phytohemagglutinin*, or *PHA*; and *pokeweed mitogen*, or *PWM*. *Con A* is a protein derived from jack bean seeds that binds to sugars containing α-D-mannose or α-D-glucose. Con A is a tetramer, with each of the four monomer units containing a carbohydrate binding site. The molecule is therefore able to crosslink glycoproteins on the surface of cells. Con A is a T-cell mitogen. *PHA* is a protein derived from kidney beans that is specific for glycoproteins containing *N*-acetylgalactosamine. Like Con A, it too is a tetramer which is able to crosslink glycoproteins on the surface of cells. PHA also functions as a T-cell mitogen. *PWM* is derived from pokeweed. It binds to di-*N*-acetylchitobiose and is mitogenic for both T and B cells.

Not all mitogens are lectins. The lipopolysaccharide, or *LPS*, component of the gram-negative bacterial cell wall functions as a B-cell mitogen. The mitogenic activity of LPS is due to its lipid A moiety which is thought to interact with the plasma membrane, resulting in a cellular activation signal through, as-yet-unknown mechanisms.

An unusual group of polyclonal activators, known as *superantigens*, are among the most potent T-cell mitogens known. Superantigens were named because of their ability to activate all T cells expressing common sequences in their T-cell receptors, irrespective of their specificity for antigen/MHC. Unlike T-cell epitopes that bind to the cleft of the MHC and are recognized by the T-cell receptor, superantigens appear to recognize residues outside the antigen binding cleft of the MHC and T-cell receptor (Figure 4-15). The superantigen thus binds simultaneously to the T-cell receptor and to the MHC molecule and activates large numbers of T cells. Included among the superantigens are the staphylococcal enterotoxins (SEs) and toxic shock syndrome toxin (TSST1) produced by the gram positive bacterium

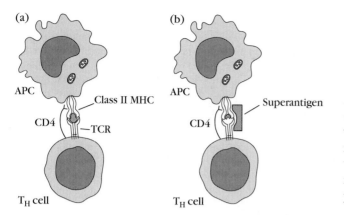

Figure 4-15   (a) Normally T-cell activation occurs after a T cell recognizes both peptide and MHC. (b) Superantigens are thought to bypass the conventional T-cell activation sequence. The superantigen is thought to bind simultaneously to the class II MHC molecule and to the Vβ chain of the TCR. This interaction enables T cells to be activated by MHC molecules bearing peptides for which the T cell is not specific.

Staphylococcal aureus. These toxins appear to activate large numbers of T_H cells by crosslinking the T-cell receptors with any class II MHC molecule expressed on an antigen-presenting cell. Estimates are that one out of every five T cells can be activated by SEs, resulting in the release of abnormally high levels of cytokines. The high levels of cytokines released can lead to shock and death, seen most dramatically in tampon-related toxic shock syndrome caused by the TSST1 superantigen. We will discuss these superantigens more fully in Chapters 11 and 19.

Summary

1.   Immunogenicity is the ability of an antigen to induce an immune response within either the humoral or the cell-mediated branch of the immune system. Antigenicity is the ability of an antigen simply to interact specifically with free antibody and/or with antigen-binding receptors on lymphocytes. B cells and T cells recognize small sites called antigenic determinants, or epitopes, on a complex immunogen.

2.   The foreignness, molecular size, chemical composition and complexity, and degradability of a substance influence its immunogenicity. In addition, several properties of the biological system that an antigen encounters affect its immunogenicity; these include the genotype of the recipient animal, the immunogen dose and route of administration, and the presence or absence of adjuvants.

3.   The size of B-cell epitopes—those epitopes recognized by membrane-bound antibody and free antibody—is determined by the size of antibody's binding site. B-cell epitopes tend to be amino acid sequences within an antigen that are accessible, usually hydrophilic, and mobile. Sequential B-cell epitopes consist of contiguous amino acid residues along the polypeptide chain, whereas nonsequential B-cell epitopes, also called conformational determinants, are formed from noncontiguous segments of the polypeptide chain that are brought into proximity by the three-dimensional folding of a protein.

4.   T-cell epitopes—those epitopes recognized by T-cell receptors—tend to be slightly larger than B-cell epitopes and generally consist of internal amino acid sequences that are hydrophobic or more commonly amphipathic. T-cell epitopes are revealed to the immune system by antigen processing, in which the protein is fragmented into small peptides that interact with class I MHC or class II MHC molecules; the resulting peptide-MHC complexes are then displayed on the surface of altered self-cells or antigen-presenting cells. The immunodominant T-cell epitopes are determined in part by the selective interactions of particular processed peptides with particular MHC molecules.

5.   Haptens are small molecules that can bind to antibodies but cannot by themselves function as immunogens. The study of haptens has allowed immunologists to learn about the structural basis of antibody specificity.

References

BENJAMIN, D., J. BERZOFSKY, I. EAST et al. 1984. The antigenic structure of proteins: a reappraisal. *Annu. Rev. Immunol.* **2**:67.

BERZOFSKY, J. A., K. CEASE, J. CORNETTE et al. 1987. Protein antigenic structures recognized by T cells: potential applications to vaccine design. *Immunol. Rev.* **98**:9.

BERZOFSKY, J., S. BRETT, H. STREICHER, and H. TAKAHASHI. 1988. Antigen processing for presentation to T lymphocytes: function, mechanisms and implications for the T cell repertoire. *Immunol. Rev.* **106**:5.

BUUS, S., A. SETTE, and H. M. GREY. 1987. The interaction between protein-derived immunogenic peptides and Ia. *Immunol. Rev.* **98**:115.

DEMOTZ, S., H. M. GREY, E. APPELLA, and A. SETTE. 1989. Characterization of a naturally processed MHC class II-restricted T cell determinant of hen egg lysozyme. *Nature* **342**:682.

GREY, H. M., A. SETTE, and S. BUUS. 1989. How T cells see antigen. *Sci. Am.* **261**(5):56.

HERMAN, A., J. W. KAPPLER, P. MARRACK, and A. M. PULLEN. 1991. Superantigens: mechanism of T-cell stimulation and role in immune responses. *Annu. Rev. Immunol.* **9**:745.

LAVER, W. G., G. M. AIR, R. G. WEBSTER, and S. J. SMITH-GILL. 1990. Epitopes on protein antigens: misconceptions and realities. *Cell* **61**:553.

ROTHBARD, J. B., and M. L. GEFTER. 1991. Interactions between immunogenic peptides and MHC proteins. *Annu. Rev. Immunol.* **9**:527.

TAINER, J. A., E. GETZOFF, Y. PATERSON, A. OLSON, and R. LERNER. 1985. The atomic mobility component of protein antigenicity. *Annu. Rev. Immunol.* **3**:501.

WERDELIN, O., S. MOURITSEN, B. PETERSEN, A. SETTE, and S. BUUS. 1988. Facts on the fragmentation of antigens in presenting cells, on the association of antigen fragments with MHC molecules in cell-free systems and speculation on the cell biology of antigen processing. *Immunol. Rev.* **106**:181.

Study Questions

1. Indicate whether each of the following statements is true or false. If you think a statement is false, explain why.

   a. Most antigens induce a polyclonal response.

   b. A large protein antigen generally can combine with many different antibody molecules.

   c. A hapten can stimulate antibody formation but cannot combine with antibody molecules.

   d. MHC genes play a major role in determining the degree of immune responsiveness to an antigen.

   e. T-cell epitopes tend to be accessible amino acid residues that can interact with the T-cell receptor.

   f. B-cell epitopes are often nonsequential amino acids brought together by the tertiary conformation of a protein antigen.

   g. Both T_H and T_C cells recognize antigen that has been processed and presented with a MHC molecule.

   h. Each MHC molecule binds a unique peptide.

   i. Internal viral proteins of the nucleocapsid are not likely to be immunogenic because they are not accessible to the immune system.

   j. An influenza hemagglutinin peptide shown to induce potent proliferation of T_H cells in an H-2^k haplotype mouse would be expected to induce potent T_H-cell proliferation in an H-2^d strain as well.

2. Two vaccines are described below. Would you expect either or both of them to activate T_C cells? Explain your answer.

   a. A UV-inactivated ("killed") viral preparation that has retained its antigenic properties but cannot replicate.

   b. An attenuated viral preparation that has low virulence but can still replicate within host cells.

3. You are trying to develop a vaccine to induce cell-mediated immunity to malaria and decide to screen peptides derived from the outer-coat protein of the microorganism that causes malaria for amphipathic properties. What is the rationale for this approach? What other factors must you take into consideration in developing a vaccine by this approach?

4. In the experiment Nilabh Shastri described on page 89, why did he transfect MHC genes into mouse L cells rather than into an antigen-presenting cell such as the macrophage?

5. What are the significant differences between T-cell and B-cell epitopes?

CHAPTER 5

Immunoglobulins: Structure and Function

Immunoglobulins are antibody molecules, the proteins that function both as receptors for antigen on the B-cell membrane and as the secreted products of the plasma cell. These secreted antibodies circulate in the blood and lymph and serve as the effectors of humoral immunity by searching out and neutralizing or eliminating antigens. Like all antibody molecules, immunoglobulins perform two major functions: they bind specifically to an antigen and they participate in a limited number of biological effector functions. This chapter focuses on how the primary, secondary, and tertiary structure of immunoglobulins contributes to both their specificity and their effector functions.

Basic Structure of Immunoglobulins

It has been known since the turn of the century that antibodies—the effector molecules of humoral immunity—reside in the serum. Identification of the serum-protein fraction containing antibodies was accomplished in a classic experiment by A. Tiselius and E. A. Kabat in 1939. They immunized rabbits with a protein antigen, ovalbumin (the albumin of egg whites), and then divided the immunized rabbits' serum into two aliquots. The first serum aliquot was separated by electrophoresis into four fractions: albumin and the alpha (α), beta (β), and gamma (γ) globulins. The second serum aliquot was reacted with antigen, so that antibody bound to the ovalbumin was precipitated and could be removed; then the remaining serum proteins were electrophoresed. A comparison of the electrophoretic profiles of these two serum aliquots revealed that there was a significant drop in the γ-globulin peak in the aliquot that had been subjected to precipitation with antigen (Figure 5-1). Thus the γ-globulin fraction was identified as containing serum antibodies, which were called *immunoglobulins* to distinguish them from any other proteins that might be contained in the γ-globulin fraction.

In the 1950s and 1960s experiments by Rodney Porter and by Gerald Edelman elucidated the basic structure of the immunoglobulin (Ig) molecule. (These experiments were considered of such significance that the two investigators shared a Nobel prize in 1972.) Edelman's and Porter's experimental approaches were quite different. Porter cleaved the Ig molecule with enzymes to obtain fragments, whereas Edelman dissociated the molecule by reducing the interchain disulfide bonds. The results attained by these two approaches complemented each other and allowed the basic structure of the Ig molecule to be elucidated.

Both Porter and Edelman first separated the γ-globulin fraction of serum by ultracentrifugation into a high-molecular-weight fraction with a sedimentation constant of 19S and a low-molecular-weight fraction with a sedimentation constant of 7S. They used the 7S fraction, containing a 150,000-MW γ-globulin designated as immunoglobulin G, or IgG, for their studies. Porter subjected IgG to brief digestion with the enzyme papain and separated the fragments. Although papain has general, nonspecific proteolytic activity and will eventually digest the entire protein, brief treatment cleaves only the most susceptible bonds. Papain digestion of IgG produced two identical fragments (each with a MW of 45,000) called *Fab* fragments because they retained their "antigen-binding" activity and one fragment (MW of 50,000) called the *Fc* fragment because it was found to crystallize during cold storage (Figure 5-2a). A similar experimental approach, but with the enzyme pepsin, was taken by Alfred Nisonoff. Brief pepsin digestion generated a single 100,000-MW fragment composed of two Fab-like fragments and designated $F(ab')_2$. Like the Fab fragments, the $F(ab')_2$ fragment was also able to visibly precipitate antigens. However, with pepsin the Fc fragment was not recovered because it had been digested into multiple fragments.

The chain structure of IgG was first suggested by experiments of Edelman and his colleagues and later confirmed by Porter. Edelman reduced the disulfide bonds of IgG with mercaptoethanol and subjected the denatured protein to starch gel electrophoresis in 8 M urea, which reduces the intrachain as well as the interchain disulfide bonds and allows the molecule to unfold. Two electrophoretic bands were obtained, indicating that the IgG molecule contained more than one protein chain. Porter extended this study by doing a much milder mercaptoethanol reduction, so that only the interchain disulfide bonds were reduced. He then alkylated the exposed sulfhydryl groups with iodoacetamide to prevent random re-formation of the disulfide bonds and added an organic proprionic acid solvent to prevent aggregation. The sample was then chromatographed on a column that separates molecules on the basis of size (Figure 5-2b). This experiment revealed that the 150,000-MW IgG molecule was composed of two polypeptide chains of 50,000 MW, designated as

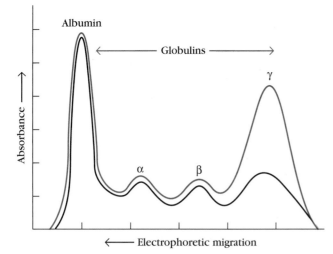

Figure 5-1 Experimental demonstration that antibodies are present in the γ-globulin fraction of serum proteins. After rabbits were immunized with ovalbumin (OVA), their antisera were pooled and electrophoresed, which separates the serum proteins based on electric charge. The red line shows the electrophoretic pattern of untreated antiserum. The black line shows the pattern of antiserum that was first incubated with OVA to remove anti-OVA antibody and then electrophoresed. [Adapted from A. Tiselius and E. A. Kabat, 1939, *J. Exp. Med.* **69**:119.]

(a) Papain digestion of IgG

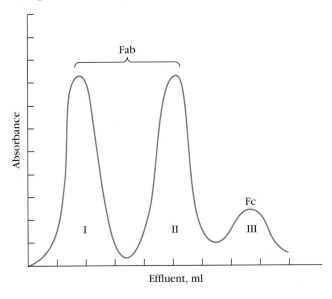

(b) Reduction of IgG interchain disulfide bonds

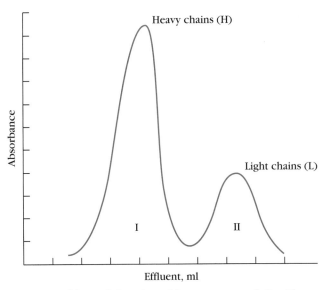

Figure 5-2 (a) Brief digestion of heterogeneous IgG with papain and separation of the digest on a carboxymethylcellulose column revealed three peaks. Peaks I and II contained 45,000-MW Fab fragments and peak III contained the 50,000-MW Fc fragment. Later experiments using homogeneous IgG yielded a single Fab peak, which was the sum of peaks I and II. (b) Separation of the heavy and light chains of IgG was accomplished by mild reduction of the interchain disulfide bonds followed by alkylation with iodoacetamide to prevent re-formation of the disulfide bonds. Gel filtration in organic proprionic acid yielded two peaks. By comparison with known molecular-weight standards, peak I was shown to contain a 50,000-MW heavy chain and peak II was shown to contain a 25,000-MW light chain. [Part (a) adapted from R. R. Porter, 1959, *Biochem. J.* **73**:119; Part (b) adapted from J. B. Fleischman, 1962, *Arch. Biochem. Suppl.* **1**:1974.]

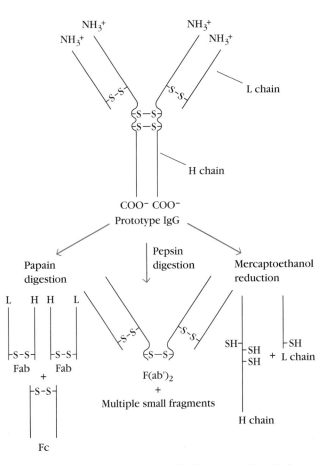

Figure 5-3 Prototype structure of IgG, proposed by Rodney Porter in 1962, showing chain structure and interchain disulfide bonds. The fragments produced by various treatments are also indicated.

heavy (H) *chains*, and two polypeptide chains of 25,000 MW, designated as *light* (L) *chains*.

The remaining puzzle was to determine how the enzyme digestion products—Fab, F(ab')$_2$, and Fc—were related to the heavy-chain and light-chain reduction products. Porter answered this question by using antisera from goats that had been immunized with the Fab fragments and Fc fragments of rabbit IgG. He found that antibody to the Fab fragment could react with both the H and the L chains, whereas antibody to the Fc fragment reacted only with the H chain. These observations led to the conclusion that Fab consists of portions of a heavy and a light chain and that Fc contains only heavy-chain components. Based on these results, Porter proposed a prototype structure for IgG, which has since been confirmed (Figure 5-3). According to this model, the IgG molecule consists of two identical H chains and two identical L chains, which are linked by disulfide bridges. The enzyme papain cleaves just above the interchain disulfide bond linking the heavy chains, whereas the enzyme pepsin cleaves just below this disulfide bond, so that the two proteolytic enzymes generate different digestion products. Mercaptoethanol reduction and alkylation allow separation of the individual heavy and light chains.

Immunoglobulin Sequencing Studies

To understand the molecular nature of immunoglobulins more fully, it was necessary to obtain information about the amino acid sequence of the heavy and the light chains. This proved to be no simple task, and for some time there was no progress. The problem was that sequencing studies require a rather large quantity of a homogeneous protein. Although the basic structure and chemical properties of different antibodies are similar, their antigen-binding specificities, and therefore their exact amino acid sequence, are very different. The γ-globulin fraction consists of a heterogeneous spectrum of antibodies that reflect all the different antigens that have induced an immune response in an animal. Even if immunization is done with a hapten-carrier conjugate, the antibodies formed just to the hapten alone are heterogeneous: They recognize different epitopes of the hapten and have different binding affinities. This heterogeneity of serum immunoglobulin rendered it unsuitable for sequencing studies.

Role of Multiple Myeloma

Sequencing analysis was finally enabled to proceed by the discovery of *multiple myeloma*, a cancer of antibody-producing plasma cells. In a normal individual, plasma cells are end-line cells that secrete specific antibody for a few days and then die. In multiple myeloma plasma cells are no longer end line but divide over and over in an unregulated way without requiring any activation by antigen to induce clonal proliferation. Although such a cancerous plasma cell, called a *myeloma cell*, has been transformed, its protein synthesizing machinery and secretory functions are not altered, and so the cell continues to secrete specific antibody. This antibody is indistinguishable from normal antibody molecules but is referred to as *myeloma protein* to denote its source. In a patient afflicted with multiple myeloma, myeloma protein can account for 95% of the serum immunoglobulins.

In general the antigenic specificity of the myeloma protein in an afflicted individual is unknown; it reflects a prior antigenic commitment of the cancerous plasma cell. A few myeloma proteins have been characterized, however, and shown to bind to known haptens or to known cell-surface determinants of common bacterial pathogens such as phosphorylcholine, the major cell-wall component of pneumococci. In such cases a plasma cell responsive to one of these common bacterial pathogens presumably has become a cancerous myeloma cell, secreting myeloma protein specific for a determinant on a normal pathogen. Most patients with multiple myeloma also secrete large amounts of excess light chains from their myeloma cells. These excess light chains were first discovered in the urine of myeloma patients and were named *Bence-Jones proteins* for their discoverer.

Multiple myeloma also occurs in other animals. In mice it can arise spontaneously, as it does in humans, or can be induced by injecting mineral oil into the peritoneal cavity. The clones of malignant plasma cells that develop are called *plasmacytomas* and are designated MOPCs, denoting the mineral-oil induction of plasmacytoma cells. A large number of mouse MOPC lines secreting different immunoglobulin classes are presently carried by the American type culture collection, a repository of cell lines commonly used in research.

Light-Chain Sequencing

When the amino acid sequences of several Bence-Jones proteins (light chains) were compared, a striking pattern emerged. The amino-terminal half of the chain, consisting of 100–110 amino acids, was found to vary among different Bence-Jones proteins. This region was called the *variable* (*V*) region. The carboxyl-terminal half of the molecule, called the *constant* (*C*) region, had two basic amino acid sequences, which were designated *kappa* (κ) and *lambda* (λ) (Figure 5-4a). In humans 60% of the light chains are kappa, and 40% are lambda. In mice 95% of the light chains are kappa, and only 5% are lambda. A single antibody molecule expresses either κ light chains or λ light chains but never both.

A comparison of the amino acid sequences of λ light chains revealed minor amino acid differences on the basis of which λ light chains are classified into subtypes. In mice there are three subtypes (λ1, λ2, and λ3); in humans there are four subtypes. Single amino acid interchanges at two or three positions are responsible for the subtype differences.

Heavy-Chain Sequencing

For heavy-chain sequencing studies, myeloma proteins were reduced with mercaptoethanol and alkylated, and the heavy chains were separated by gel filtration in a denaturing solvent. When the amino acid sequences of several myeloma protein heavy chains were compared, a pattern similar to that observed with the light chains emerged. The amino-terminal 100–110 amino acids

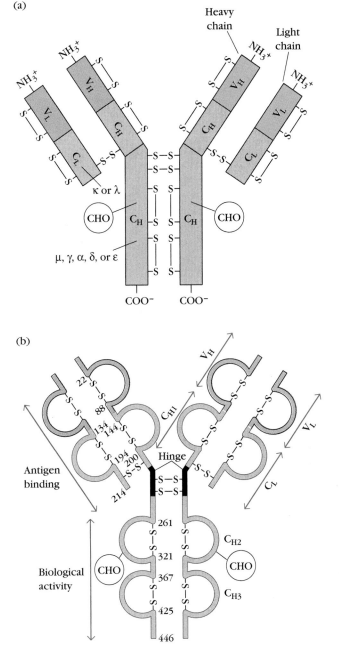

(a)

(b)

Figure 5-4 (a) Sequencing studies revealed that immunoglobulin heavy and light chains each contain an amino-terminal variable (V) region (red) that contains 100–110 amino acids and differs from one antibody to the next. The remainder of the molecule contains a small number of constant (C) regions (gray), designated κ or λ in light chains and μ, γ, α, δ, or ε in heavy chains. (b) Detailed analysis of immunoglobulin sequence data showed that heavy and light chains are organized into domains, each containing about 110 amino acid residues and an intrachain disulfide bond that forms a 60-aa loop. Some heavy chains (γ, δ, and α) also contain a proline-rich hinge region (black). The μ and ε heavy chains lack a hinge region but contain an additional domain in the central portion of the molecule.

Table 5-1 Chain structures of the five immunoglobulin classes in humans

Class	Heavy chain	Light chain	Subclasses	Molecular formula
IgG	γ	κ or λ	$\gamma1$, $\gamma2$, $\gamma3$, $\gamma4$	$\gamma_2\kappa_2$ $\gamma_2\lambda_2$
IgA	α	κ or λ	$\alpha1$, $\alpha2$	$(\alpha_2\kappa_2)_n$ $(\alpha_2\lambda_2)_n$ n = 1, 2, 3, or 4
IgM	μ	κ or λ	None	$(\mu_2\kappa_2)_n$ $(\mu_2\lambda_2)_n$ n = 1 or 5
IgD	δ	κ or λ	None	$\delta_2\kappa_2$ $\delta_2\lambda_2$
IgE	ε	κ or λ	None	$\varepsilon_2\kappa_2$ $\varepsilon_2\lambda_2$

showed great sequence variation from one myeloma heavy chain to the next and was therefore called the variable (V) region. The remaining part of the protein revealed five basic amino acid sequence patterns (μ, γ, α, δ, and ε) corresponding to five different heavy-chain constant (C) regions (see Figure 5-4a). The length of the constant regions was approximately 330 amino acids for α, γ, and δ and 440 amino acids for μ and ε. The heavy chains of a given antibody molecule determine the class of that antibody: IgM, IgG, IgA, IgD, or IgE. Each class can have either κ or λ light chains. A single antibody molecule has two identical heavy chains and two identical light chains (Table 5-1).

Minor differences in the amino acid sequences of the α and of the γ heavy chains led to further classification of the heavy chains into subclasses. In humans there are two subclasses of α heavy chains ($\alpha1$ and $\alpha2$) and four subclasses of γ heavy chains ($\gamma1$, $\gamma2$, $\gamma3$, and $\gamma4$); in mice there are four subclasses of γ heavy chains ($\gamma1$, $\gamma2a$, $\gamma2b$, and $\gamma3$).

Immunoglobulin Fine Structure

The structure of the immunoglobulin molecule is determined by its primary, secondary, tertiary, and quaternary protein structure. The primary amino acid sequence accounts for the variable and constant regions of the heavy and light chains. The secondary structure is formed as the extended polypeptide chain folds back and forth upon itself forming an antiparallel β pleated sheet. The sheet is stabilized by an invariant intrachain

(a)

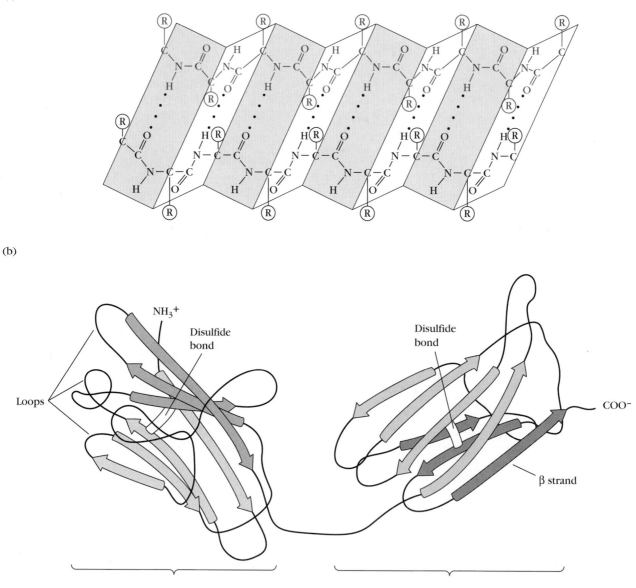

(b)

Figure 5-5 (a) An antiparallel β pleated sheet is shown in which the extended polypeptide chain folds back and forth upon itself. The structure is held together by hydrogen bonds between peptide bonds in neighboring chains. The amino acid side groups (R) are arranged perpendicular to the plane of the sheet. (b) Diagram of immunoglobulin light chain depicting the immunoglobulin-fold structure. Each domain contains two β pleated sheets, which are held together by hydrophobic interactions between them and the conserved disulfide bond. Residues in the amino-terminal loop regions of the variable domains make up the antigen-binding site. Heavy-chain domains have the same characteristic structure. [Part (a) adapted from J. Darnell, H. Lodish, and D. Baltimore, 1990, *Molecular Cell Biology*, Scientific American Books, New York; part (b) adapted from M. Schiffer et al., 1973, *Biochemistry* **12**:4620.]

disulfide bond and by hydrogen bonds that connect the peptide bonds in neighboring chains (Figure 5-5a). The chains are then folded into a tertiary structure of compact globular domains, which are connected to neighboring domains by narrow, more exposed areas. Finally, the globular domains of adjacent heavy and light polypeptide chains interact in the quaternary structure, forming functional domains that enable the molecule to specifically bind antigen and, at the same time, perform a limited number of biological effector functions.

Structure of Immunoglobulin Domains

Careful analysis of the amino acid sequences of immunoglobulin heavy and light chains showed that both chains contain several homologous units of about 110 amino acid residues. Within each unit, termed a *domain*, an intrachain disulfide bond forms a loop of about 60 amino acids. Light chains contain one variable domain (V_L), and one constant domain (C_L); heavy chains contain one variable domain (V_H), and either three or four constant domains (C_H1, C_H2, C_H3, and C_H4), depending on the class (Figure 5-4b).

X-ray crystallographic analysis revealed that immunoglobulin domains were folded into a characteristic compact structure, known as the *immunoglobulin fold*. This structure consists of a "sandwich" of two β pleated sheets, each containing three or four antiparallel β strands of amino acids (Figure 5-5b). The strands are connected by loops of varying lengths. The β strands are characterized by alternating hydrophobic and hydrophilic amino acids whose side chains are arranged perpendicular to the plane of the sheet—the hydrophobic amino acids are oriented toward the interior and the hydrophilic amino acids face outward. The two sheets are stabilized by the hydrophobic interactions between them and by the conserved disulfide bond. An analogy has been made to two pieces of bread, butter between them, and a toothpick holding the slices together. The bread slices represent the two β pleated sheets; the butter represents the hydrophobic interactions between them; and the toothpick represents the intrachain disulfide bond.

Although variable and constant domains have a similar structure, there are subtle differences between them. The V domain is slightly longer than the C domain and contains an extra pair of β strands within the β-sheet structure, as well as an extra loop sequence connecting this pair of β strands. The basic structure of the immunoglobulin fold is uniquely suited to facilitate noncovalent interactions between domains across the faces of the β sheets (Figure 5-6). Interactions occur between identical domains (e.g., C_H2/C_H2, C_H3/C_H3, and C_H4/C_H4), and between nonidentical domains (e.g., V_H/V_L and

C_H1/C_L). The structure of the immunoglobulin fold also allows for variable lengths and sequences of amino acids that form the loops that connect the β strands. As discussed later, the loop sequences of the V_H and V_L domains contain variable amino acids and comprise the antigen-binding site of the molecule.

Variable-Region Domain Structure and Function

Detailed comparisons of the amino acid sequences of the V_L and V_H domains revealed that the sequence variability is concentrated in several *hypervariable regions*. There are three such hypervariable regions in mouse and human heavy and light chains, which constitute 15–20% of the variable domain (Figure 5-7). The remaining 80–85% of the V_L and V_H domains show far less variation; these stretches are referred to as the *framework regions (FRs)*. The hypervariable regions form the *antigen-binding site* of the antibody molecule. Because the antigen-binding site is complementary to the structure of the epitope, the hypervariable regions are also called *complementarity-determining regions (CDRs)*. The framework regions and complementarity-determining regions have distinct locations in the immunoglobulin fold. It is the conserved sequence within the FR that generates the basic β pleated sheet structure of the V_H and V_L domains. The three heavy chain and three light chain CDRs are located on the loops that connect the β strands of the V_H and V_L domains. The three-dimensional structure of the variable domain provides a rigid framework, which is necessary for overall antibody function, and at the same time is able to provide an enormous diversity of antigen-binding sites by varying the length and amino acid residues of the hypervariable loops.

The earliest evidence demonstrating the role of the hypervariable regions in binding antigen was obtained with an experimental technique called *affinity labeling*, which utilizes a synthetic hapten containing groups that can be converted into a chemically reactive state upon ultraviolet activation. The hapten is incubated with its specific antibody in the dark and is then photoactivated, enabling the reactive groups on the hapten to form covalent bonds to neighboring residues in the antibody's binding site. Identification of the amino acids covalently bound to the affinity label has confirmed that hypervariable amino acids within light- and heavy-chain CDRs constitute the antigen-binding site.

Knowledge of the three-dimensional structure of the antibody molecule was necessary to determine precisely how the CDRs are aligned in the antigen-binding site. This has been accomplished by high-resolution x-ray crystallographic analysis of hen egg-white lysozyme

(HEL), the Fab fragment of monoclonal anti-HEL antibody, and the complex between them (Figure 5-8). This analysis revealed that the CDRs of the V_H and V_L domains project outward from the immunoglobulin fold and together make up the antigen-binding site. In this case the antigen-binding site is a rather large, flat region on the surface of the V_H/V_L domain. There is a small cleft into which a glutamine residue of the antigen fits, but most of the interacting residues are located on the surface of

the antigen and the antibody. All of the heavy- and light-chain CDRs in the anti-HEL Fab fragment interact with the antigen; a total of 17 amino acids of the antibody make close contact with 16 residues of the antigen.

A similar crystallographic analysis has also been performed on neuraminidase (the envelope glycoprotein of the influenza virus) and the Fab fragment from a monoclonal antibody to this antigen. As with the anti-HEL Fab, all six CDRs in the neuraminidase Fab fragment interact

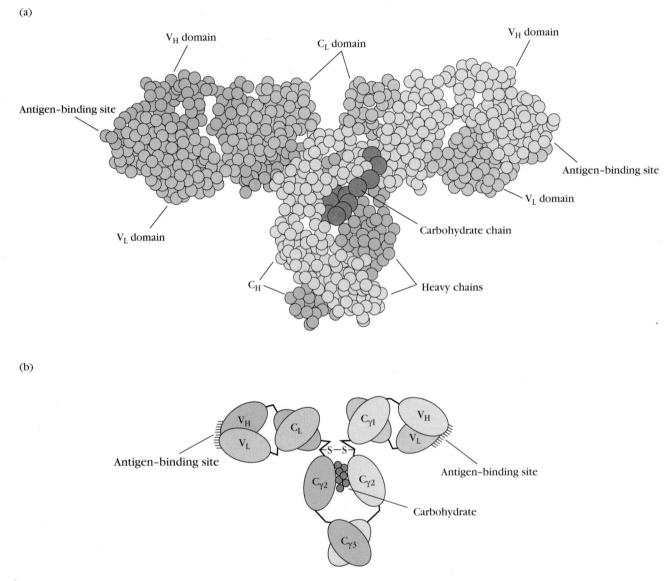

Figure 5-6   (a) Model of IgG molecule, based on x-ray crystallographic analysis, shows associations between domains. Each solid ball represents an amino acid residue. The two light chains are shown in shades of gray, and the two heavy chains are shown in shades of red. (b) A schematic diagram showing the interacting heavy- and light-chain domains. Note that the C_H2/C_H2 domain protrudes due to the presence of carbohydrate in the interior. The protrusion makes this domain more accessible, enabling it to interact with molecules such as certain complement components. [Part (a) from E. W. Silverton, M. A. Navia, and D. R. Davies, 1977, *Proc. Nat. Acad. Sci. USA* **74**:5140.]

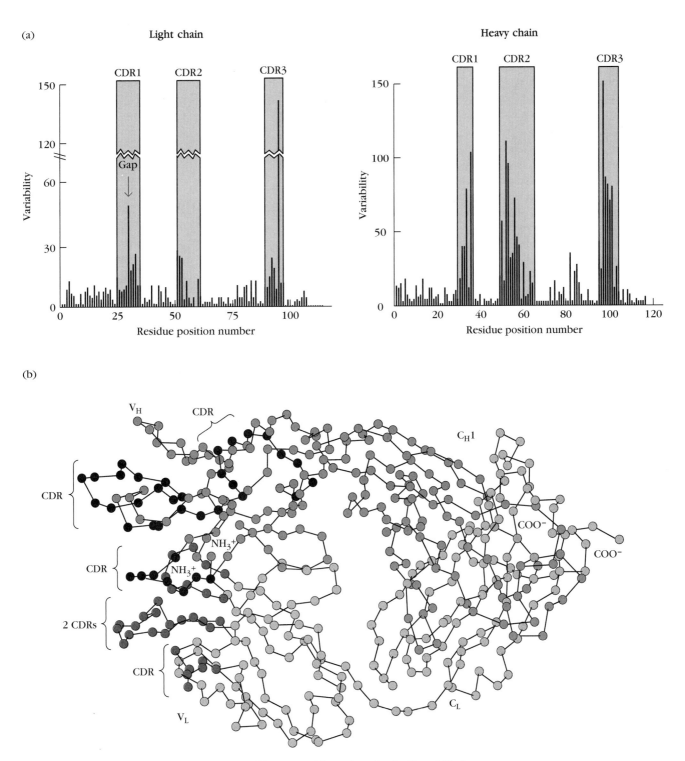

Figure 5-7 (a) Experimental demonstration of hypervariable regions in the V_L and V_H domains of human antibodies. Plots of amino acid variability at each position in antibodies with different specificities revealed three hypervariable regions, also called complementarity-determining regions (CDRs). (b) Model of a Fab fragment in which the α-carbon of each amino acid residue is represented by a ball. The residues making up the light-chain CDRs (black) and heavy-chain CDRs (red) protrude from the molecule and thus are able to contact antigen. [Part (a) from E. A. Kabat, T. T. Wu, and H. Bilofsky, 1977, *Sequence of Immunoglobulin Chains*, U.S. Dept. of Health, Education, and Welfare; part (b) from J. D. Capra and A. B. Edmundson, 1977, *The Antibody Combining Site*, © 1977, vol. 236R(1) Scientific American, Inc.]

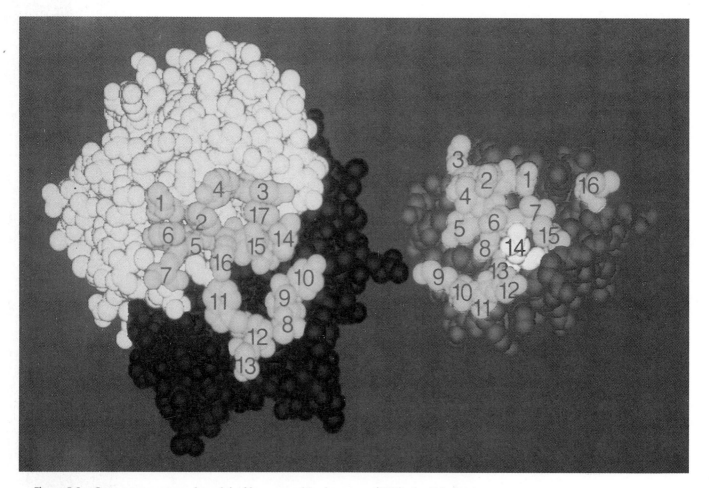

Figure 5-8 Computer-generated model of hen egg-white lysozyme (HEL), the Fab fragment of a monoclonal anti-HEL antibody, and the complex formed between them based on x-ray crystallographic analyses. Unbound HEL and anti-HEL rotated 90° to reveal their interacting surfaces. The amino acid residues that make close contact during binding are numbered. [From A. G. Amit, R. A. Mariuzza, S. E. V. Phillips, and R. J. Poljak, 1986, *Science* **233**:747.]

with the antigen. However, unlike the lysozyme antigen-antibody complex, formation of the neuraminidase antigen-antibody complex is accompanied by a conformational change in both the antigen's epitope and the antibody's antigen-binding site. This conformational change allowed a closer fit between the epitope and the antibody's binding site. As x-ray crystallographic analysis is completed for other antigen-antibody complexes, it will be possible to determine whether this conformational change in the epitope and the antibody's binding site is a common phenomenon.

Constant-Region Domain Structure and Function

The immunoglobulin constant-region domains are associated with various biological functions that are determined by the amino acid sequence of each domain.

C_H1/C_L *Domain*

X-ray crystallographic analysis of immunoglobulins has revealed that the V_H/V_L interaction is quite strong, whereas the C_H1/C_L interaction is weaker, with fewer noncovalent interactions. Until recently the function of the C_H1/C_L domain was thought to be simply to hold the V_H and V_L domains together by virtue of the interchain disulfide bond located in the C_H1/C_L domain (see Figure 5-4b). But recently another important role for the C_H1/C_L domain has emerged. This role of the C_H1/C_L was resolved by first mixing V_H and V_L domains derived from two antibodies having different defined specificities (*a* and *b*). Each V_H and V_L domain was observed to reassociate almost exclusively with its original partner to form V_La/V_Ha and V_Lb/V_Hb complexes (Figure 5-9). In another experiment Fab fragments from antibody *a* and antibody *b* were mildly reduced and denatured to obtain V_HC_H1 and V_LC_L fragments from each antibody. When these longer fragments were mixed, random association occurred, yielding homogeneous complexes containing fragments from either antibody *a* or antibody *b* and heterogeneous complexes containing one *a* and one *b* fragment (Figure 5-9b).

These results suggest that the presence of C_H1 and C_L domains leads to more varied combinations of V_H and V_L domains than would occur if the interaction were driven solely by the V_H and V_L interaction alone. As is discussed in Chapter 8, random rearrangements of the immunoglobulin genes generate unique V_H and V_L sequences for the heavy and light chains expressed by each B lymphocyte. The C_H1/C_L domain increases the likelihood that the unique V_H and V_L sequences expressed in any given B cell will interact to form a unique antigen-binding site and thus contributes to the overall diversity of antibody molecules that can be expressed by an animal. The C_H1/C_L domain also serves to extend the Fab arms, thereby facilitating interaction with antigen and increasing the maximum rotation of the Fab arms.

Hinge Region

The γ, δ, and α heavy chains contain an extended peptide sequence between the C_H1 and C_H2 domains that has no homology with the other domains (see Figure 5-4b). This region, called the *hinge* region, is rich in prolines and is flexible, giving IgG, IgD, and IgA segmental flexibility. As a result, the two Fab arms can assume various angles relative to each other when antigen is bound. This flexibility of the hinge region can be visualized in electron micrographs of antigen-antibody complexes. For example, when a molecule containing two DNP groups reacts with anti-DNP antibody and the complex is captured on a grid, negatively stained, and observed with electron microscopy, large complexes (e.g., dimers, trimers, tetramers) are seen in which the angle between the arms of the Y-shaped antibody molecules varies, reflecting the flexibility of the hinge region (Figure 5-10).

The large number of proline residues in the hinge region confers an extended polypeptide conformation on it, making the hinge region particularly vulnerable to cleavage by proteolytic enzymes; it is this region that is cleaved with papain or pepsin (see Figure 5-3). Although μ and ε chains lack a hinge region, they have an additional 110-aa domain (C_H2/C_H2) that has hingelike features.

Other Constant-Region Domains

In considering the heavy-chain domain functions in the different immunolgobulin classes, the C_H2/C_H2 and C_H3/C_H3 domains of IgA, IgD, and IgG (containing α, δ, and γ heavy chains, respectively) correspond to the C_H3/C_H3 and C_H4/C_H4 domains in IgE and IgM (containing ε and μ heavy chains, respectively). As mentioned already, IgE and IgM lack the hinge region present in the other classes of immunoglobulin. In this region of the molecule, IgE and IgM have an additional immunoglobulin domain, designated C_H2/C_H2. The function of this domain in these classes has not been determined.

X-ray crystallographic analysis has revealed that the C_H2/C_H2 domain of IgA, IgD, and IgG (and the C_H3/C_H3 domain of IgE and IgM) are separated by oligosaccharide side chains; as a result these two globular domains are much more accessible than the other domains to the aqueous environment (see Figure 5-5b). This accessibility accounts for the important biological activity

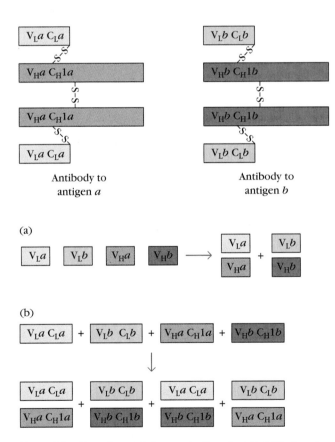

Figure 5-9 Experimental demonstration that C_H1/C_L domain facilitates random association of heavy and light chains. Antibodies with two different specificities (*a* and *b*) were treated to obtain fragments corresponding to the V_L and V_H domains or longer fragments containing the V_HC_H1 and V_LC_L domains. Mixing of the V_H and V_L domains (a) or of the longer VC fragments (b) revealed that the presence of the C_H1 and C_L domains resulted in formation of heterogeneous complexes containing segments from both antibodies.

(a)   (b)

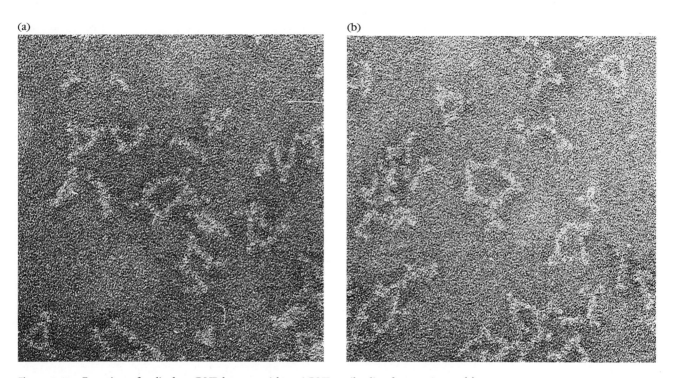

Figure 5-10   Reaction of a divalent DNP hapten with anti-DNP antibodies forms trimers (a) and tetramers (b), as well as other large antigen-antibody complexes. In these electron micrographs of negatively stained preparations, the antibody protein stands out as a light structure against the electron-dense background. Because of the flexibility of the hinge region, the angle between the arms of the antibody molecules varies. [From R. C. Valentine and N. M. Green, 1967, *J. Mol. Biol.* **27**:615.]

of these domains in the activation of complement components by the IgG and IgM classes of antibody molecules.

The carboxyl-terminal domain is designated C_H3/C_H3 in IgA, IgD, and IgG and C_H4/C_H4 in IgE and IgM. The amino acid sequence and the function of this domain differs in membrane-bound antibody on B cells and free antibody secreted by plasma cells. Free antibody has a hydrophilic amino acid sequence of varying lengths at the carboxyl-terminal end. In membrane-bound antibody, this hydrophilic sequence is replaced with three regions: an extracellular hydrophilic "spacer" sequence, a hydrophobic transmembrane sequence, and a cytoplasmic sequence. The transmembrane sequence always contains 26 amino acid residues; the extracellular spacer sequence and cytoplasmic sequence vary in length among immunoglobulin classes.

The carboxyl-terminal domain of a membrane-bound antibody molecule functions to attach the molecule to a B cell and to project the amino-terminal end away from the cell surface, so that it can more easily encounter antigen. In a free antibody molecule, the carboxyl-terminal domain together with the adjacent domain interact with Fc receptors on the surface of various cells. For example, IgG and IgM antibodies bind to Fc receptors on phagocytic cells, mediating opsonization. Some sub-classes of IgG bind to Fc receptors on placental cells and then are transferred across the placenta, allowing maternal IgG antibodies to protect the fetus. Binding of IgE to mast cells and basophils also is mediated by Fc receptors on these cells. As discussed in more detail later, formation of secretory IgA and IgM antibodies involves binding to Fc receptors on mucous membrane epithelial cells. The carboxyl-terminal domains of IgA and IgM also play a role in the polymerization of free IgA and IgM molecules. The presence of cysteine residues in this domain allows disulfide bonds to form between monomeric units, with the result that IgM is secreted by plasma cells as a pentamer and IgA is secreted as a dimer or trimer.

Antigenic Determinants on Immunoglobulins

Since antibodies are glycoproteins, they can themselves function as potent immunogens to induce an antibody response. The antigenic determinants, or epitopes, on immunoglobulin molecules fall into three major categories: *isotypic, allotypic,* and *idiotypic* determinants, which are located in characteristic portions of the molecule (Figure 5-11).

Isotypic Determinants

Isotypes define constant-region determinants that distinguish each heavy-chain class and subclass and each light-chain type and subtype within a species. Each isotype is encoded by a separate constant-region gene, and all members of a species carry the same constant-region genes. Within a species, each normal individual will express all isotypes in their serum. Different species inherit different constant-region genes and therefore express different isotypes. Therefore, when an antibody from one species is injected into another species, the isotypic determinants will be recognized as foreign, inducing an antibody response to the isotypic determinants on the foreign antibody. Anti-isotype antibody is routinely used for research purposes to determine the class or subclass of serum antibody produced during an immune response or to characterize the class of membrane-bound antibody present on B cells.

Allotypic Determinants

Although all members of a species inherit the same set of isotype genes, multiple alleles exist for some of the genes. These alleles encode subtle amino acid differences, called allotypic determinants, that occur in some, but not all, members of a species. In humans allotypes have been characterized for all four IgG subclasses, for one IgA subclass, and for the κ light chain. The γ chain allotypes are referred to as Gm markers. To date, 25 different Gm allotypes have been identified; they are designated by the class and subclass, followed by the allele number [e.g., G1m(1), G2m(23), G3m(11), G4m(4a)]. Of the two IgA subclasses only the IgA2 subclass has allotypes, designated as A2m(1) and A2m(2). The κ light chain has three allotypes, designated κm(1), κm(2), and κm(3). Each of these allotypic determinants represents differences in one to four amino acids that are encoded by different alleles.

Antibody to allotypic determinants can be produced by injecting antibodies from one member of a species into another member of the same species who lacks the allotypic determinant. Antibody to allotypic determinants are sometimes produced by a mother during pregnancy in response to paternal allotypic determinants on the fetal immunoglobulins. Antibodies to allotypic determinants can also arise following a blood transfusion.

Idiotypic Determinants

The unique amino acid sequence of the V_H and V_L domains of a given antibody can function not only as an antigen-binding site but also as an antigenic determinant.

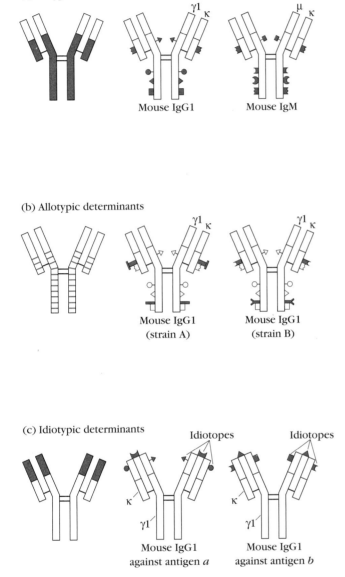

Figure 5-11 Antigenic determinants of immunoglobulins. (a) Isotypic determinants are constant-region determinants that distinguish each Ig class and subclass within a species. (b) Allotypic determinants are subtle amino acid differences encoded by different alleles. Allotypic differences can be detected by comparing the same antibody class among different inbred strains. (c) Idiotypic determinants are generated by the conformation of the amino acid sequences of the heavy- and light-chain variable region specific for each antigen. Each individual determinant is called an idiotope, and the sum of the individual idiotopes is the idiotype. For each type of determinant, the general location of determinants within the antibody molecule is shown (*left*) and two examples are illustrated (*center* and *right*).

The idiotypic determinants are generated by the conformation of the heavy- and light-chain variable regions. Each individual antigenic determinant of the variable region is referred to as an *idiotope* (see Figure 5-11C). In some cases an idiotope may be the actual antigen-binding site, and in some cases an idiotope may comprise variable-region sequences outside of the antigen-binding site. Each antibody will present multiple idiotopes; the sum of the individual idiotopes is called the *idiotype* of the antibody.

Because the antibodies produced by individual B cells derived from the same clone have identical variable-region sequences, they all have the same idiotype. Some idiotypic determinants are shared by antibodies that are not clonally derived. These idiotypic determinants, called public idiotypic determinants, reflect the common usage of the same germ-line variable-region gene by different B cells from the same inbred strain. Anti-idiotype antibody is produced by minimizing isotypic or allotypic differences, so that the idiotypic difference can be recognized. Often a homogeneous antibody such as a myeloma protein or monoclonal antibody is used. Injection of such an antibody into a syngeneic recipient will result in the formation of anti-idiotype antibody to the idiotypic determinants.

One of the earliest experiments demonstrating the presence of idiotypic determinants on antibodies was performed by J. Oudin and M. Michel at the Pasteur Institute in 1963. These researchers injected rabbit anti-*Salmonella* antibody into another rabbit of the same allotype. The rabbit produced antibody that bound to the immunizing antibody but did not bind with other rabbit antibodies from the same donor or with anti-*Salmonella* antibody from other rabbits. Anti-idiotype antibody is produced by animals during the course of an immune response and has been shown to play an important role in regulating the immune response; this phenomenon is discussed in Chapter 11.

Immunoglobulin Isotypes

The various immunoglobulin classes, or isotypes, have been mentioned briefly already. In this section, the structure and effector functions of each isotype are discussed in more detail. Each isotype is distinguished by amino acid sequence differences in the heavy-chain constant region resulting in structural and functional differences between different isotypes. The structures of the five major isotypes are diagrammed in Figure 5-12. The molecular properties and biological activities of the immunoglobulin isotypes are listed in Table 5-2. The effector functions of each isotype results from interactions between its heavy-chain constant regions and other serum proteins or cell membrane receptors.

Immunoglobulin G (IgG)

IgG, the most abundant isotype in serum, constitutes about 80% of the total serum immunoglobulin. The IgG molecule is a monomer consisting of two γ heavy chains and two κ or λ light chains. There are four IgG subclasses in humans, numbered in accordance with their decreasing serum concentrations: IgG1 (9 mg/ml), IgG2 (3 mg/ml), IgG3 (1 mg/ml), and IgG4 (0.5 mg/ml). The four subclasses are encoded by different germ-line C_H genes whose DNA sequences are 90–95% homologous. The structural characteristics that distinguish these subclasses from one another are the size of the hinge region and the number and position of the interchain disulfide bonds between the heavy chains (Figure 5-13). The subtle amino acid differences between subclasses of IgG affect the biological activity of the molecule (see Table 5-2). IgG1, IgG3, and IgG4 readily cross the placenta and play an important role in protecting the developing fetus. Several IgG subclasses are activators of the complement system, although their effectiveness varies. The IgG3 subclass is the most effective complement activator, followed by IgG1; IgG2 is relatively inefficient at complement activation, and IgG4 is not able to activate the complement sequence at all. IgG also functions as an opsonin by binding to Fc receptors on phagocytic cells, but there are subclass differences in this function also. IgG1 and IgG3 bind with a high affinity to Fc receptors. IgG4 has an intermediate affinity, and IgG2 has an extremely low affinity.

Immunoglobulin M (IgM)

IgM accounts for 5–10% of the total serum immunoglobulin, with a serum concentration of about 1 mg/ml. Monomeric IgM is expressed as membrane-bound antibody on B cells. IgM is secreted by plasma cells as a pentamer, in which five monomer units are held together by disulfide bonds linking their carboxyl-terminal domains (see Figure 5-12b). The five monomer subunits are arranged with Fc regions in the center of the pentamer and the 10 antigen-binding sites facing out from the pentamer. Each pentamer contains an additional Fc-linked polypeptide called the *J chain*. The J chain appears to be required for polymerization of the monomers to form pentameric IgM; a single J polypeptide is disulfide-bonded to a carboxyl-terminal cysteine residue of 2 of the 10 H chains.

IgM is the first immunoglobulin class produced in a primary response to an antigen, and it is also the first immunoglobulin class to be synthesized by the neonate. The pentameric structure of the IgM gives the molecule several unique properties. The molecule has increased valency because of its 10 antigen-binding sites. An IgM

(a) IgG

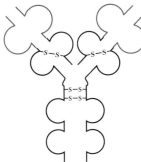

(b) IgM (pentamer)

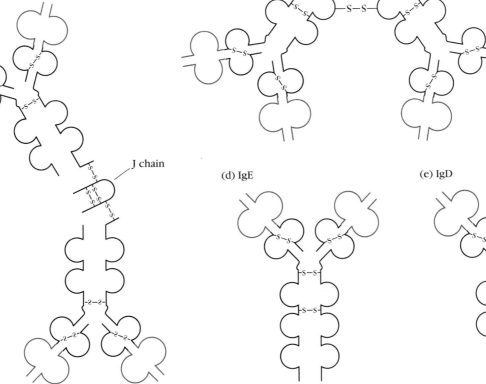

J chain

(c) IgA (dimer)

J chain

(d) IgE

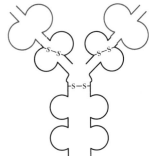

(e) IgD

Figure 5-12 General structures of the five major isotypes of secreted antibody. Variable domains are shown in red and disulfide bonds in black. Note that IgG, IgA, and IgD heavy chains contain four domains and a hinge region, whereas IgM and IgE heavy chains contain five domains but no hinge region. The polymeric forms of IgM and IgA contain a polypeptide, known as the J chain, that is linked by two disulfide bonds to the Fc region in two different monomers. Secreted IgM is always a pentamer; most serum IgA exists as a monomer, although some dimers, trimers, and even tetramers sometimes are present.

molecule can actually bind 10 small hapten molecules, but for larger antigens, steric hindrance limits the binding capacity to only five molecules at a time. The increased valency of pentameric IgM increases its capacity to bind such multidimensional antigens as viral particles and red blood cells (RBCs). For example, when RBCs are incubated with specific antibody, they clump together into large aggregates in a process called *agglutination*. It takes from 100 to 1000 times as many molecules of IgG as of IgM to achieve the same level of agglutination. A similar phenomenon occurs with viral particles—less IgM than IgG is required to neutralize viral infectivity. IgM is also more efficient than IgG at complement activation. Complement activation requires two Fc regions in close proximity, and the pentameric structure of a single molecule of IgM fullfills this requirement.

Because of its large size, IgM does not diffuse well and therefore is found in very low concentrations in the intercellular tissue fluids. The presence of the J chain protein does allow the molecule to bind to receptors on secretory cells where it is transported across epithelial linings to the external secretions that bathe mucosal surfaces. Although IgA is the major isotype found in these secretions, IgM also serves an important accessory role as a secretory immunoglobulin.

Immunoglobulin A (IgA)

Although IgA constitutes only 10–15% of the total immunoglobulin in serum, it is the predominant immunoglobulin class in external secretions such as breast milk, saliva, tears, and mucous of the bronchial, genitourinary, and digestive tracts. In serum, IgA exists primarily as a monomer, although polymeric forms such as dimers, trimers, and even tetramers are sometimes seen. The IgA of external secretions, called *secretory IgA*, is a

Table 5-2 Properties and biological activities* of classes and subclasses of serum immunoglobulins

Property/activity	IgG1	IgG2	IgG3	IgG4	IgA1	IgA2	IgM	IgE	IgD
Molecular weight[†]	150,000	150,000	150,000	150,000	150,000–600,000	150,000–600,000	900,000	190,000	150,000
Heavy-chain component	$\gamma 1$	$\gamma 2$	$\gamma 3$	$\gamma 4$	$\alpha 1$	$\alpha 2$	μ	ε	δ
Normal serum level (mg/ml)	9	3	1	0.5	3.0	0.5	1.5	0.0003	0.03
In vivo serum half-life (days)	23	23	8	23	6	6	5	2.5	3
1st Ab in 1° Response							+		
Activates classical complement pathway	+ +	+	+ +	+/−	−	−	+ +	−	−
Crosses placenta	+	+/−	+	+	−	−	−	−	−
Present on membrane of mature B cells	−	−	−	−	−	−	+	−	+
Binds to macrophage Fc receptors	+ +	+	+ +	+/−	−	−	+	−	−
Present in secretions	−	−	−	−	+ +	+ +	+	−	−
Induces mast-cell degranulation	−	−	−	−	−	−	−	+	−

* Activity levels indicated as follows: + + = high; + = moderate; +/− = minimal; and − = none.

[†] IgG, IgE, and IgD always exist as monomers. IgA can exist as a monomer, dimer, trimer, or tetramer. Membrane-bound IgM is a monomer, but secreted IgM in serum is a pentamer.

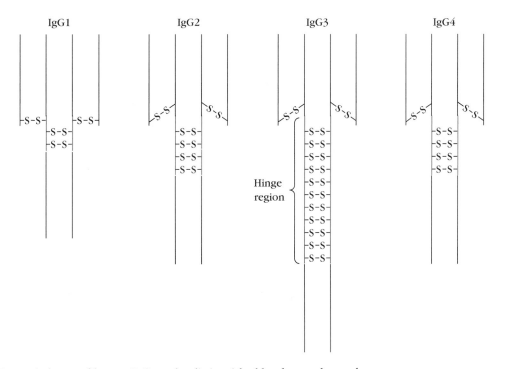

IgG1	IgG2	IgG3	IgG4

Figure 5-13   Four subclasses of human IgG can be distinguished by the number and arrangement of interchain disulfide bonds linking the heavy chains. In the IgG3 subclass, the hinge region (red) is four times as long as the hinge region of the other IgG subclasses and contains 11 interchain disulfide bonds.

dimer or tetramer composed of two or four monomers, a J-chain polypeptide, and a polypeptide chain called *secretory component.* The J-chain polypeptide is identical to that found in pentameric IgM and serves a similar function in facilitating the polymerization of both serum and secretory IgA. The secretory component is a 70,000-MW polypeptide produced by epithelial cells of mucous membranes found in the gastrointestinal and respiratory tracts and in ocular tissue, minor salivary glands, the urinary tract, and the uterus. Surprisingly, more secretory IgA is produced each day than any other immunoglobulin class. The IgA-secreting plasma cells are concentrated along mucous membrane surfaces. Along the jejunum of the small intestines, there are more than 2.5×10^{10} IgA-secreting plasma cells—a number that surpasses the total plasma cells of the bone marrow, lymph, and spleen combined! Each day more than 300 mg of secretory IgA is secreted along the jejunum.

The secretory component is acquired by dimeric IgA as it is transported through the mucosal epithelial cells into their mucous secretions (Figure 5-14). Dimeric IgA binds tightly to a receptor for polymeric immunoglobulin molecules (poly Ig receptor) on the mucous epithelial cells. The receptor-IgA complex is then endocytosed in a membrane vesicle and transported across the cell to the luminal face, where the vesicle fuses with the plasma membrane. The receptor is then

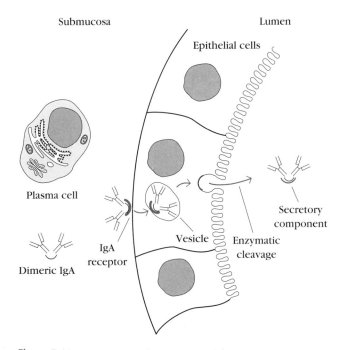

Figure 5-14   Formation of secretory IgA by transport through mucous epithelial cells. Dimeric IgA binds to a specific receptor on the blood-facing surface of an epithelial cell and is internalized by receptor-mediated endocytosis. After transport to the luminal surface, the secretory component remains bound to the dimeric IgA and the secretory IgA is then released.

cleaved enzymatically, and a part of the receptor becomes the secretory component, which is bound to and released together with dimeric IgA into the mucous secretions. The presence of the secretory component appears to protect secretory IgA, rendering it less susceptible to the proteolytic enzymes present in the mucous secretions. Only dimeric IgA can be transported through the mucosal epithelial cells, and it is thought that the receptor actually recognizes the presence of the J chain associated with the dimer. Pentameric IgM can also be transported into mucous secretions by this mechanism, and it is the only other class of immunoglobulin that has an attached J chain.

Secretory IgA serves an important effector function at mucous membrane surfaces. The mucous membrane is the main portal of entry for most pathogenic organisms. Secretory IgA binds to bacterial or viral surface structures and prevents attachment of the pathogen to the mucosal cells. Because attachment is blocked, viral infection and bacterial colonization are inhibited.

Immunoglobulin E (IgE)

The potent biological activity of IgE allowed it to be identified in serum despite its extremely low serum concentration of only 0.3 μg/ml. IgE antibodies mediate the immediate-hypersensitivity reactions that are responsible for the symptoms of hay fever, asthma, hives, and anaphylactic shock. The presence of a serum component responsible for allergic reactions was first demonstrated in 1921 by K. Prausnitz and H. Kustner, who injected serum from an allergic person intradermally into a nonallergic individual. When the appropriate antigen was later injected at the site of injection, a wheal and flare (analogous to hives) developed there. This reaction, called the *P-K reaction*, was the basis for the earliest biological assay for IgE activity.

Actual identification of IgE was accomplished by K. and T. Ishizaka in 1966. They obtained serum from an allergic individual and immunized rabbits with it to prepare anti-isotype antiserum. The rabbit antiserum was then allowed to react with each class of human antibody known at that time (i.e., IgG, IgA, IgM, and IgD). In this way, each of the known anti-isotype antibodies was precipitated and removed from the rabbit anti-serum. What remained was an anti-isotype antibody specific for an unidentified class of antibody. This anti-isotype antibody turned out to completely block the P-K reaction. The new antibody was called IgE (in reference to the E antigen of ragweed pollen, which is a potent inducer of this class of antibody).

IgE binds to Fc receptors on the membranes of blood basophils and tissue mast cells. Cross-linkage of receptor-bound IgE molecules by antigen (allergen) induces

degranulation of basophils and mast cells; as a result, a variety of pharmacologically active mediators present in the granules are released, giving rise to allergic manifestations (Figure 5-15). Localized mast-cell degranulation induced by IgE also may release mediators that facilitate a buildup of various cells necessary for antiparasitic defense (see Chapter 16).

Immunoglobulin D (IgD)

IgD was first discovered when a patient developed a multiple myeloma whose myeloma protein failed to react with anti-isotype antisera against the then-known isotypes: IgA, IgM, and IgG. When rabbits were immunized with this myeloma protein, the resulting antisera identified this same class of antibody at low levels in normal human serum. This new class called IgD has a serum concentration of 30 μg/ml and constitutes about 0.2% of the total immunoglobulin in serum. Its biological function is still not known. IgD, together with IgM, is the major membrane-bound immunoglobulin expressed by mature, immunocompetent B cells, and it is thought to function in the activation of a B cell by an antigen.

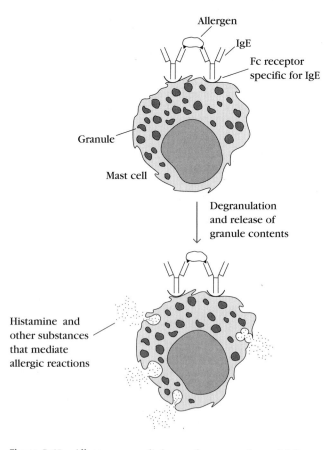

Figure 5-15 Allergen cross-linkage of receptor-bound IgE on mast cells induces degranulation, causing release of substances that mediate allergic manifestations.

The Immunoglobulin Superfamily

The structures of the various immunoglobulin heavy and light chains described earlier share several features, suggesting that they have a common evolutionary ancestry. In particular, all heavy- and light-chain classes have the immunoglobulin-fold domain structure (see Figures 5-4b and 5-5b). The presence of this characteristic structure in all immunoglobulin heavy and light chains suggests that they arose from a common primordial gene encoding a polypeptide of about 110 amino acids.

Gene duplication and later divergence could then have generated the various heavy- and light-chain genes.

In the early 1970s β_2-microglobulin, a small invariant protein associated with class I MHC molecules, was sequenced. Surprisingly, its sequence showed homology to the immunoglobulin heavy- and light-chain constant-region domains, having a length of about 100 amino acids and a conserved intrachain disulfide bond spanning 60 amino acids. Later, x-ray crystallographic analysis revealed that β_2-microglobulin also has the β pleated-sheet structure characteristic of the immunoglobulin fold.

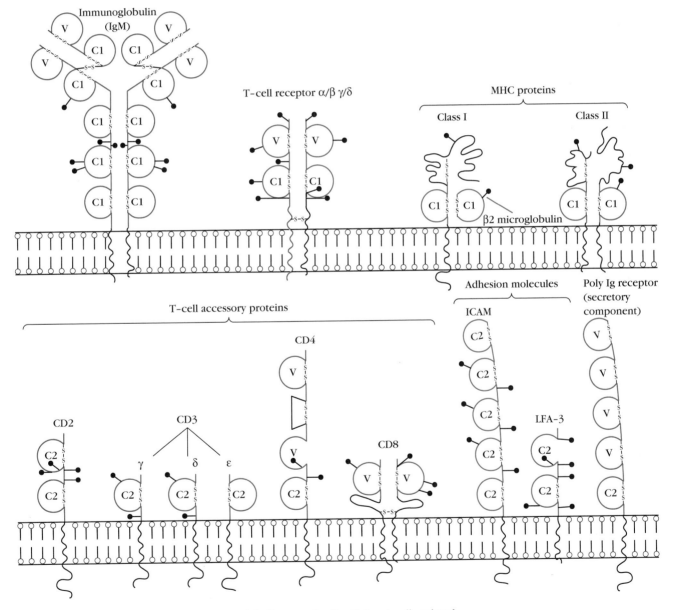

Figure 5-16 Some members of the immunoglobulin superfamily of structurally related glycoproteins, most of which are membrane bound. The loops shown in red represent those portions of the molecule with the characteristic immunoglobulin-fold structure. In all cases the carboxyl-terminal end of the molecule is anchored in the membrane. Many other proteins are members of this family.

Since the discovery of an immunoglobulin-like domain structure in β_2-microglobulin, large numbers of membrane proteins have been shown to possess one or more regions homologous to an immunoglobulin domain. Each of these membrane proteins is classified a member of the *immunolgobulin superfamily*. The term superfamily is used to denote genes derived from a common primordial gene encoding the basic domain structure. These genes have evolved independently and do not share genetic linkage or function. Included in this group of proteins, in addition to the immunoglobulins themselves and β_2-microglobulin, are the following proteins: the T-cell receptor; additional T-cell membrane proteins including the γ, δ, and ε chains of CD3, CD2, CD4 and CD8; class I and class II MHC molecules; the cellular adhesion molecules, LFA-3 and ICAM-1; the poly-Ig receptor for polymeric IgA and IgM; and the platelet derived growth factor (Figure 5-16). Numerous other proteins, some to be discussed in later chapters belong to this group.

Although x-ray crystallographic analysis has not been accomplished for most of the molecules of the immunoglobulin superfamily, the primary amino acid sequence of roughly 110 amino acids, usually with an invariant intrachain disulfide loop spanning 50–70 residues, and the pattern of alternating hydrophilic and hydrophobic amino acids suggests a similar immunoglobulin domain structure with antiparallel sheets of β-pleated strands. Some proteins of the superfamily have V-like domains and some have C-like domains based on their homology to the immunoglobulin V or C domains. Some proteins have a domain that falls between the classical V and C domains. These domains are shorter than the classical immunoglobulin C domain and show equal homology to both V and C domains. These domains are designated C2 domains to distinguish them from the classical immunoglobulin C domains, which are called C1.

Since most of the members of the immunoglobulin superfamily cannot bind antigen, there must be some reason, apart from antigen binding, for so many different membrane proteins to have a similar domain structure with the characteristic immunoglobulin fold. One possibility is that this structure may be particularly suitable to allow interactions between plasma-membrane proteins. It is thought that the basic immunoglobulin fold may facilitate interactions between the faces of β sheets, allowing members of this family of molecules to bind to one another. As discussed earlier, in the immunoglobulins such interactions can occur between homologous domains (e.g., C_H2/C_H2, C_H3/C_H3, and C_H4/C_H4 interactions) and between nonhomologous domains (e.g., V_H/V_L and C_H1/C_L interactions). The observed associations between some members of the immunoglobulin superfamily may depend on interactions between non-homologous immunoglobulin-fold domains. Such associations may allow interactions such as those observed between CD4 and the class II MHC molecule, or CD8 and the class I MHC molecule, or the T-cell receptor and the MHC molecule, or the poly-Ig receptor and polymeric IgA or IgM.

Summary

1.   The basic structure of an antibody molecule consists of two identical light chains and two identical heavy chains, which are disulfide linked. Each heavy and light chain contains a variable sequence in the amino-terminal 110 amino acids and constant sequences in the remainder of each chain.

2.   In any given antibody molecule, the constant region contains one of five basic heavy-chain sequences (μ, γ, δ, α, or ε) and one of two basic light-chain sequences (κ or λ). The constant-region sequences determine the five classes (isotypes) of antibody (IgM, IgG, IgD, IgA, and IgE) and the effector functions of the molecule.

3.   The variable amino acid sequences are not randomly dispersed throughout the variable region but instead are clustered in several hypervariable regions, or complementarity-determining regions (CDRs). These regions form the antigen-binding site of the antibody molecule.

4.   The immunoglobulin molecule consists of a series of interacting domains, each of which is organized in a characteristic structure called the immunoglobulin fold.

5.   Immunoglobulin heavy and light chains are prototype members of a large group of proteins called the immunoglobulin superfamily. All members of this family contain the same basic domain immunoglobulin-fold structure. This basic structure may facilitate homologous and nonhomologous interactions between members of this family.

References

ALZARI, P. M., M. B. LASCOMBE, and R. J. POLJAK. 1988. Three dimensional structure of antibodies. *Annu. Rev. Immunol.* **6**:555.

AMIT, A. G., R. A. MARIUZZA, S. E. PHILLIPS, and R. J. POLJAK. 1986. Three dimensional structure of an antigen-antibody complex at 2.8 Å resolution. *Science* **233**:747.

DAVIES, D. R., E. A. PADLAN, and S. SHERIFF. 1991. Antibody-antigen complexes. *Annu. Rev. Biochem.* **59**:439.

KOSHLAND, M. E. 1985. The coming of age of the J chain. *Annu. Rev. Immunol.* **3**:425.

STANFIELD, R. L., T. M. FIESER, R. LERNER, and I. A. WILSON. 1990. Crystal structures of an antibody to a peptide and its complex with peptide antigen at 2.8 Å. *Science* **248**:712.

UNDERDOWN, B. J., and J. M. SCHIFF. 1986. Immunoglobulin A: strategic defence initiative at the mucosal surface. *Annu. Rev. Immunol.* **4**:389.

WILLIAMS, A. F., and A. N. BARCLAY. 1988. The immunoglobulin superfamily—domains for cell surface recognition. *Annu. Rev. Immunol.* **6**:381.

Study Questions

1. Indicate whether each of the following statements is true or false. If you think a statement is false, explain why.

   a. All myeloma protein molecules derived from a single myeloma clone have the same idiotype and allotype.

   b. A rabbit immunized with human IgG3 will produce antibody that reacts with all subclasses of IgG in humans.

   c. The presence of both IgM and IgD on a single B cell violates one of the tenets of clonal selection—the unispecificity of a given B cell.

   d. All immunoglobulin molecules on the surface of a given B cell have the same idiotype.

   e. All immunoglobulin molecules on the surface of a given B cell have the same isotype.

   f. Folding of the hypervariable regions produces a cleft in which binding of antigen occurs.

   g. All isotypes are normally found in each individual of a species.

   h. The heavy-chain variable region (V_H) is twice as long as the light-chain variable region (V_L).

   i. IgG functions more effectively than IgM in bacterial agglutination.

2. An energetic immunology student has isolated protein X, which he believes is a new isotype of human immunoglobulin.

   a. What structural features would protein X have to have in order to be classified as an immunoglobulin?

   b. You prepare rabbit antisera to whole human IgG, human κ chain, and human γ chain. Assuming protein X is, in fact, a new immunoglobulin isotype, to which of these antisera would it bind? Why?

   c. Devise an experimental procedure for preparing an antiserum that is specific for protein X.

3. IgG, which contains γ heavy chains, developed much more recently during evolution than IgM, which contains μ heavy chains. Describe two advantages and two disadvantages that IgG has in comparison with IgM?

4. a. Draw a diagram of a typical IgG molecule that includes each immunoglobulin domain. Label the following on your diagram: H chains, L chains, interchain disulfide bonds, intrachain disulfide bonds, antigen-binding sites, Fab, Fc, and domains.

   b. How would you have to modify the diagram of IgG to depict an IgA molecule isolated from saliva.

   c. How would you have to modify the diagram of IgG to depict serum IgM.

5. Fill out the table below to indicate the properties of IgG molecules and their various parts. Use ($+$) if positive; ($-$) if negative, and (weakly $+$) if slightly positive.

Property	Whole IgG	H chain	L chain	Fab	F(ab')2	Fc
Binds antigen						
Bivalent antigen binding						
Monovalent antigen binding						
Fixes complement in presence of antigen						
Has V domains						
Has C domains						

6. For each of the following immunization scenarios, state whether the anti-immunoglobulin antibodies would be formed to isotypic, allotypic, or idiotypic determinants:

   a. Anti-DNP antibodies produced in a Balb/c mouse are injected into a C57Bl/6 mouse.

   b. Anti-BGG mab from a Balb/c mouse are injected into another Balb/c mouse.

   c. Anti-BGG antibodies produced in a Balb/c mouse are injected into a rabbit.

   d. Anti-DNP antibodies produced in a Balb/c mouse are injected into an outbred mouse.

   e. Anti-BGG antibodies produced in a Balb/c mouse are injected into the same mouse.

7.   In the table below, write YES of or NO to indicate whether the rabbit antisera listed at the top reacts with the mouse antibody components listed at the left.

	Rabbit antisera to mouse antibody component				
	γ chain	κ chain	IgG Fab fragment	IgG Fc fragment	J chain
Mouse γ chain					
Mouse κ chain					
Mouse IgM whole					
Mouse IgG Fc fragment					

8.   Where are the hypervariable regions located on an antibody molecule and what are their functions?

9.   a.   What are the characteristic structural features of the immunoglobulin fold?
     b.   Many membrane proteins have the basic immunoglobin-fold domain structure. These proteins are classified as members of what family of proteins? How might this structure facilitate the function of these membrane proteins?

10.   A technician wanted to make a rabbit antiserum specific for mouse IgG. She injected a rabbit with purified mouse IgG and obtained an antiserum that reacted strongly with mouse IgG. To her dismay, however, the antiserum also reacted with each of the other mouse isotypes. Explain why she got this result. How could she make the rabbit antiserum specific for mouse IgG?

11.   In the blank after the name of each immunoglobulin class in the column at the left, write the number(s) of the item(s) in the column at the right that are true about that immunoglobulin class. Some of the items in the column at the right may apply to more than one of the immunoglobulin classes; other items may not apply to any of the classes.

IgA _____

IgD _____

IgE _____

IgG _____

IgM _____

1.   Secreted form is a pentamer of the basic H_2L_2 unit
2.   Binds to Fc receptors on mast cells
3.   Multimeric forms have J chain
4.   Present on the surface of mature, unprimed B cells
5.   The most abundant immunoglobulin class in serum
6.   Present in secretions such as saliva, tears, and colostrum
7.   Present on the surface of immature B cells
8.   The first serum antibody made in a primary immune response
9.   Plays an important role in immediate hypersensitivity
10.   Plays an important role in protecting against pathogens that invade through the gut or respiratory mucosa
11.   Multimeric forms present in secretions have secretory piece
12.   Can fix complement by the classical pathway
13.   Can participate in antibody-dependent cell-mediated cytotoxicity (ADCC)

12.   In the table below, indicate whether the antibodies produced would be specific for isotypic, allotypic, or idiotypic determinants:

Immunogen	Animal immunized	Antigenic determinant against which antibodies are produced
IgG from C57Bl/6 mouse	Balb/c mouse	
IgG myeloma protein from C57Bl/6 mouse	C57Bl/6 mouse	
IgG from C57Bl/6 mouse	Rabbit	

Antigen-Antibody Interactions

The antigen-antibody interaction is a bimolecular association similar to an enzyme-substrate interaction but with the important distinction that it does not lead to an irreversible chemical alteration in either the antibody or antigen and therefore is reversible. The interaction between an antibody and an antigen involves various noncovalent interactions between the antigenic determinant, or epitope, of the antigen and the variable-region (V_H/V_L) domain of the antibody molecule, particularly the hypervariable regions, or complementarity-determining regions (CDRs). The exquisite specificity of an antibody for an antigen has led to the development of a variety of immunologic assays. These assays can be used to detect the presence of either antibody or antigen and have played vital roles in diagnosing diseases, monitoring the level of the humoral immune response, and identifying molecules of biological or medical interest. These assays differ in their speed and their sensitivity; some are strictly qualitative, and others are quantitative. In this chapter, the nature of the antibody-antigen interaction is examined, and various immunologic assays that measure this interaction are described.

Strength of Antigen-Antibody Interactions

The noncovalent interactions that form the basis of antigen-antibody binding include hydrogen bonds, ionic bonds, hydrophobic interactions, and van der Waals interactions (Figure 6-1). Because the strength of each of these interactions is weak (compared with that of a covalent bond), a strong antigen-antibody interaction

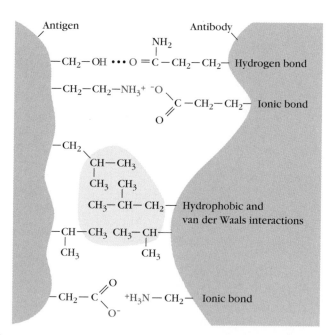

Figure 6-1 The interaction between an antibody and an antigen depends on four types of noncovalent forces: (1) ionic bonds between oppositely charged residues, (2) hydrogen bonds in which a hydrogen atom is shared between two electronegative atoms, (3) hydrophobic interactions in which water forces hydrophobic groups together to maximize hydrogen bonding of water molecules, and (4) van der Waals interactions between the outer electron clouds of two atoms. In an aqueous environment noncovalent interactions are extremely weak and depend upon close structural complementarity between antibody and antigen.

requires a large number of such interactions. Furthermore, each of these noncovalent interactions operates over a very small distance, generally less than 1×10^{-7} mm (1 angstrom, Å); consequently, a strong antigen-antibody interaction depends on a very close fit between the antigen and antibody, which is reflected in the high degree of specificity characteristic of antigen-antibody interactions.

Antibody Affinity

The strength of the sum total of noncovalent interactions between a single antigen-binding site on an antibody and a single epitope is the *affinity* of the antibody for that epitope. Low-affinity antibodies bind antigen weakly and tend to dissociate readily, whereas high-affinity antibodies bind antigen more tightly and remain bound longer. The association between a binding site on an antibody (Ab) with a monovalent antigen (Ag) can be described by the equation

$$Ag + Ab \underset{k_{-1}}{\overset{k_1}{\rightleftharpoons}} Ab - Ag$$

where k_1 is the forward, or association, rate constant and k_{-1} is the reverse, or dissociation, rate constant. The ratio of k_1/k_{-1} is the association constant K, a measure of affinity. It can be calculated from the ratio of the concentration of bound antigen-antibody to the concentrations of unbound antigen and antibody, as follows:

$$K = \frac{k_1}{k_{-1}} = \frac{[Ab - Ag]}{[Ab][Ag]}$$

K values vary for different antibody-antigen complexes and depend upon both k_1, which is expressed in liters/mole/second (L/mol/s) and k_{-1}, which is expressed in 1/second. For small haptens, the forward rate constant can be extremely high; in some cases k_1 values can be as high as 4×10^8 L/mol/s, approaching the theoretical upper limit of diffusion-limited reactions (10^9 L/mol/s). For larger protein antigens, however, k_1 is smaller, with values in the range of 10^5 L/mol/s. The rate at which bound antigen leaves an antibody's binding site (or the dissociation rate constant, k_{-1}) plays a major role in determining the antibody's affinity for an antigen. Table 6-1 illustrates the role of k_{-1} in determining the association constant K for several antibody-antigen interactions. For example, the k_1 for the DNP-L-lysine system is about one-fourth that for the fluorescein system, but its k_{-1} is 200 times greater; consequently, the K for the fluorescein system is about a thousandfold higher than K for the DNP-L-lysine system. Low-affinity antibody-antigen complexes have K values between 10^4 and 10^5 L/mol; high-affinity complexes can have K values as high as 10^{11} L/mol.

Table 6-1 Forward (k_1) and reverse (k_{-1}) rate constants and association constant (K) of three ligand-antibody interactions

Antibody	Ligand	k_1 (L/mol/s)	k_{-1} (s^{-1})	K (L/mol)
Anti-DNP	ε-DNP-L-lysine	8×10^7	1	10^8
Anti-fluorescein	Fluorescein	4×10^8	5×10^{-3}	10^{11}
Anti-bovine serum albumin (BSA)	Dansyl-BSA	3×10^5	2×10^{-3}	1.7×10^8

SOURCE: Adapted from H. N. Eisen, 1990, *Immunology*, 3d ed., Harper and Row Publishers.

The association constant K can be determined by *equilibrium dialysis*. In this procedure a dialysis chamber containing two equal compartments separated by a semipermeable membrane is used. Antibody is placed in one chamber, and in the other chamber is placed a ligand that must be small enough to pass through the semipermeable membrane (Figure 6-2a). Suitable ligands include haptens as well as oligosaccharides and oligopeptides composing the epitope of complex polysaccharide or protein antigens. By radioactively labeling the ligand, it is possible to measure the concentration of a known amount of ligand after equilibrium. At equilibrium part of the labeled ligand will be bound to the antibody, and the unbound ligand will be equally distributed in both compartments. Thus the total concentration of ligand will be greater in the compartment containing antibody (Figure 6-2b). The difference in the ligand concentration in the two compartments represents the concentration of ligand bound to the antibody (i.e., the concentration of Ag-Ab complex). The higher

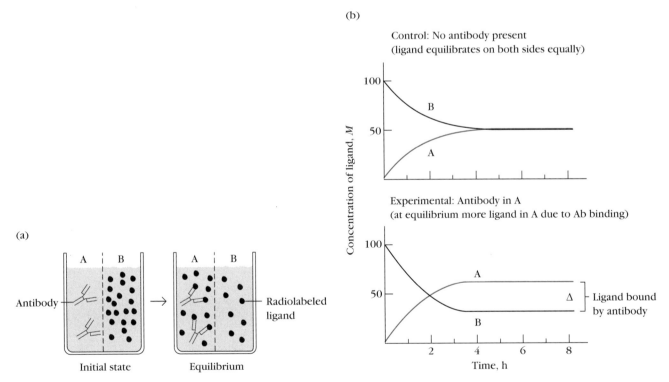

Figure 6-2 Determination of antibody affinity by equilibrium dialysis. (a) The dialysis chamber contains two compartments (A and B) separated by a semipermeable membrane. Antibody is added to one compartment and a radiolabeled ligand to another. At equilibrium the concentration of radioactivity in both compartments is measured. (b) Plot of concentration of ligand in each compartment with time. At equilibrium the difference in the concentration of radioactive ligand in the two compartments represents the amount of ligand bound to antibody.

the affinity of the antibody, the more ligand that is bound.

Since the total concentration of antibody in the equilibrium dialysis chamber is known, the equilibrium equation can be rewritten as

$$K = \frac{[\mathrm{Ab} - \mathrm{Ag}]}{[\mathrm{Ab}][\mathrm{Ag}]} = \frac{r}{(n - r)(c)}$$

where r = the ratio of the concentration of bound ligand to total antibody concentration, c = concentration of free ligand, and n = number of binding sites per antibody molecule. This expression can be rearranged to give the *Scatchard equation*:

$$\frac{r}{c} = Kn - Kr$$

Values for r and c can be obtained by repeating the equilibrium dialysis with the same concentration of antibody but with different concentrations of ligand. If K is a constant, that is, if all the antibodies within the dialysis chamber have the same affinity for the ligand, then a Scatchard plot of r/c versus r will yield a straight line with a slope of $-K$ (Figure 6-3). As the concentration of unbound ligand C increases, r/c approaches 0 and r, therefore, approaches n, the valency. For most antibody preparations, K is not a constant because antibodies (unless they are monoclonal) are heterogeneous and have a range of affinities. A Scatchard plot of heterogeneous antibody yields a curved line whose slope is constantly changing, reflecting the antibody heterogeneity. With this type of Scatchard plot, it is possible to determine the average affinity constant K_o by determining the value of K when half of the antigen-binding sites are filled:

$$K_o = \frac{1}{(2 - 1)c} = \frac{1}{c}$$

Antibody Avidity

The affinity at one binding site does not always reflect the true strength of the antibody-antigen interaction. When complex antigens containing multiple, repeating antigenic determinants are mixed with antibodies containing multiple binding sites, the interaction of antibody with antigen at one site will increase the probability of reaction at a second site. The strength of such interactions between multivalent antibody and antigen is called the *avidity*. The avidity reflects the strength of the interaction between multivalent antibody and antigen and therefore more closely approximates the in-

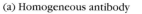
(a) Homogeneous antibody

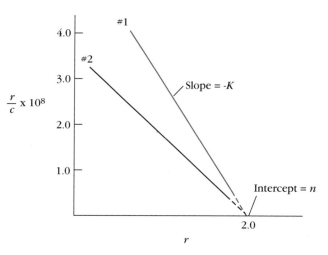

(b) Heterogeneous antibody

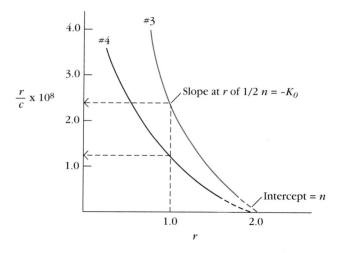

Figure 6-3 If equilibrium dialysis is repeated with the same concentration of antibody but with different concentrations of ligand, then a Scatchard plot can be graphed. In this plot, r = moles bound ligand/mole antibody and c = free ligand. From a Scatchard plot, both the equilibrium constant (K) and the number of binding sites per antibody molecule (n), or its valency, can be obtained. (a) If all antibodies have the same affinity then the Scatchard plot will yield a straight line with slope of $-K$. The Y intercept is the valence of the antibody which is 2 for IgG. In this graph antibody #1 has a higher affinity than antibody #2. (b) If the antibody is heterogeneous then it will have a range of affinities and the Scatchard plot will not give a straight line but instead a line whose slope is constantly changing. The average affinity constant K_0 can be calculated by determining the value of K when one-half of the binding sites are occupied (i.e., when $r = 1$). In this graph antisera #3 has a higher affinity than antisera #4.

teractions seen with biological systems, as in the case of antibody's reaction with determinants on a virus or a bacterial cell. Avidity can compensate for low affinity. For example, secreted pentameric IgM often has a lower affinity than IgG, but because of its high avidity, resulting from its multivalence, it binds effectively to antigen.

Cross-Reactivity

Although the antigen-antibody reaction is highly specific, in some cases antibody elicited by one antigen can cross-react with an unrelated antigen. Such cross-reactions occur if two different antigens share an identical epitope or if antibodies specific for one epitope also bind to an unrelated epitope possessing similar chemical properties. In the latter case the antibody's binding affinity for the cross-reacting epitope is usually less than that for the original epitope.

Cross-reactivity is often observed among polysaccharide antigens that contain similar oligosaccharide residues. The ABO blood-group antigens, for example, are glycoproteins expressed on red blood cells. Subtle differences in the terminal sugar residues distinguish the A and B blood-group antigens. An individual lacking one or both of these antigens will have antibodies to the missing antigen(s). A type O individual thus has anti-A and anti-B antibodies; a type A individual has anti-B; and a type B individual has anti-A. Cross-reactivity is the basis for the presence of these blood-group antibodies, which are induced in an individual not by exposure to red blood cell antigens but by exposure to cross-reacting microbial antigens present on common intestinal bacteria. These cross-reacting microbial antigens induce the formation of antibodies in individuals lacking these antigens. The blood-group antibodies, although elicited by microbial antigens, will cross-react with similar oligosaccharides on red blood cells.

A number of viruses and bacteria possess antigenic determinants identical to or similar to normal host-cell components. In some cases these microbial antigens have been shown to elicit antibody that cross-reacts with the host-cell components, resulting in a tissue-damaging autoimmune reaction. The bacterium *Streptococcus pyogenes* expresses cell-wall proteins called M antigens. Antibodies produced to streptococcal M antigens have been shown to cross-react with several myocardial and skeletal muscle proteins and have been implicated in heart and kidney damage following streptococcal infections. The role of other cross-reacting antigens in the development of autoimmune diseases is discussed in Chapter 17.

Some vaccines also exhibit cross-reactivity. For example, vaccinia virus, which causes cowpox, expresses cross-reacting epitopes with the variola virus, the causative agent of smallpox. This cross-reactivity was the

Table 6-2 Cross-reactivity of three rabbit antialbumin antisera to albumin from various species

Albumin Source	Index of dissimilarity		
	Rabbit antiserum to human albumin	Rabbit antiserum to chimpanzee albumin	Rabbit antiserum to gibbon albumin
Human	1.00	1.09	1.29
Chimpanzee	1.14	1.00	1.40
Gorilla	1.09	1.17	1.31
Orangutang	1.22	1.24	1.29
Siamang	1.30	1.25	1.07
Gibbon	1.28	1.25	1.00
Old World monkeys	2.46	2.22	2.29

* A higher index of dissimilarity indicates less reactivity between specific antibody and an unrelated albumin. The reactivity between each antialbumin antiserum and the albumin used to elicit it is set at 1.00.

SOURCE: V. M. Sarich and A. C. Wilson, 1967, *Science* **158**:1200.

basis of Jenner's method of using vaccinia virus to induce immunity to smallpox, as mentioned in Chapter 1.

Before the development of DNA sequencing, the degree of cross-reactivity between protein antigens of two species was used as an indicator of the evolutionary distance between the species. The basis of this approach is the hypothesis that the evolutionary distance between two species is correlated with the degree of relatedness of their proteins. In one study the relatedness of serum albumins derived from humans, chimpanzees, gorillas, orangutangs, siamangs, gibbons, and six species of Old World monkeys was assessed by this approach. Rabbits were immunized with serum albumin from humans, chimpanzees, and gibbons, and the reactivity of the rabbit antisera was assessed against albumin derived from each of the species. The magnitude of immune cross-reactivity, expressed as an index of dissimilarity, is an indicator of the degree of structural similarity among the albumins and thus of the evolutionary distance between the species. The data in Table 6-2 clearly indicate that the evolutionary distance between humans and Old World monkeys is substantially greater than that between humans and the other species tested.

Table 6-3   Comparative sensitivity of various immunoassays

Assay	Sensitivity,* μg antibody N/ml
Precipitin reaction in fluids	3–20
Precipitin reactions in gels	
Mancini single immunodiffusion	0.2–1.0
Ouchterlony double immunodiffusion	3–20
Immunoelectrophoresis	3–20
Rocket electrophoresis	0.2
Agglutination reactions	
Direct	0.05
Passive agglutination	0.001–0.01
Agglutination inhibition	0.001–0.01
Radioimmunoassay	0.0001–0.001
Enzyme-linked immunosorbent assay (ELISA)	0.0001–0.001
Immunofluorescence	1.0

* The sensitivity depends upon the affinity of the antibody as well as the epitope density and distribution.

SOURCE: Adapted from N. R. Rose, H. Friedman and J. L. Fahey, eds., 1986, *Manual of Clinical Laboratory Immunology*, American Society for Microbiology, Washington, D.C.

Precipitin Reactions

The interaction between an antibody and soluble antigen forms a lattice, which is stabilized by hydrophobic interactions and exhibits few hydrophilic interactions with the solvent, rendering the antigen-antibody complex insoluble. The formation of this lattice depends on the valency of both the antibody and antigen. The antibody must be bivalent; a precipitate will not form with monovalent Fab fragments but can form with $F(ab')_2$ fragments. The antigen must either be bivalent or polyvalent; it must have either two or more copies of the same determinant or different determinants that react with different antibodies present in polyclonal antisera. This requirement for bivalency or polyvalency of protein antigens can be illustrated by precipitin reactions involving myoglobulin. This protein antigen precipitates well with specific polyclonal antisera but fails to precipitate with a specific monoclonal antibody because it contains multiple, distinct antigenic determinants but only a single copy of each determinant. Myoglobin thus can form a cross-linked lattice structure with polyclonal antisera but not with monoclonal antisera. Several common immunologic assays are based on precipitin reactions; the sensitivity of these assays varies considerably, as shown in Table 6-3.

Precipitin Reactions in Fluids

A quantitative precipitin reaction can be performed by placing a constant amount of antibody in a series of tubes and adding increasing amounts of antigen to the tubes. After the precipitate forms, each tube is centrifuged to pellet the precipitate, the supernatant is poured off, and the amount of precipitate is measured. Plotting the amount of precipitate against increasing antigen concentrations yields a precipitin curve. As Figure 6-4 shows, excess of either antibody or antigen interferes with maximal precipitation, which occurs in the so-called *equivalence zone*, when the ratio of antibody to antigen is optimal. As a large multimolecular lattice is formed at equivalence, the complex increases in size and precipitates out of solution. In the region of *antibody excess*, unreacted antibody is found in the supernatant along with small soluble complexes consisting of multiple molecules of antibody bound to a single molecule of antigen. In the region of *antigen excess*, unreacted antigen can be detected and small complexes are again observed, this time consisting of one or two molecules of antigen bound to a single molecule of antibody. Although the quantitative precipitin reaction is seldom used experimentally today, the principles of antigen excess, antibody excess, and equivalence apply to many antigen-antibody reactions.

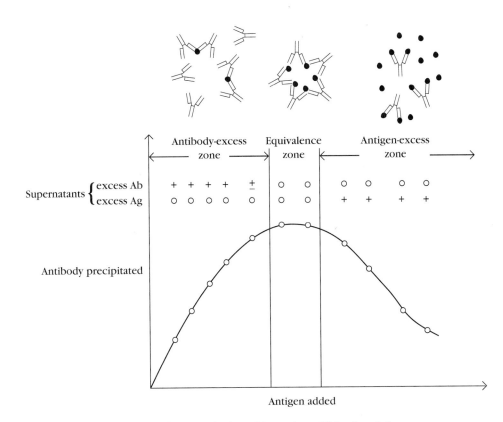

Figure 6-4 A precipitin curve for a system of one antibody and its antigen. This plot of the amount of antibody precipitated versus increasing antigen concentrations (at constant total antibody) reveals three zones: a zone of antibody excess in which precipitation is inhibited and excess antibody can be detected in the supernatant; an equivalence zone of maximal precipitation in which antibody and antigen form large insoluble complexes and neither antibody nor antigen can be detected in the supernatant; and a zone of antigen excess in which precipitation is inhibited and excess antigen can be detected in the supernatant.

The precipitin reaction can also be used as a rapid way to screen for the presence of antibody or antigen. The interfacial, or ring, precipitin test is performed by adding antiserum to a small tube and layering antigen on top. If the antiserum contains antibodies specific for the test antigen, then the antibody and antigen diffuse toward each other and form a visible band of precipitation at the interface within a few minutes (Figure 6-5).

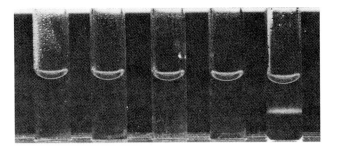

Figure 6-5 The interfacial, or ring, precipitin test is a rapid, qualitative method for determining the presence of antibody or antigen. The antiserum is placed in the bottom of a tube, and then the antigen solution is carefully layered on top. Formation of a visible line of precipitation in the tube at the extreme right indicates a positive reaction. The other four tubes are various controls (e.g., normal serum with antigen and antiserum with buffer). [From J. S. Garvey, N. E. Cremer, and D. H. Sussdorf, 1977, *Methods in Immunology*, 3d ed., W. A. Benjamin Inc., Advanced Book Program.]

Precipitin Reactions in Gels

Immune precipitates can form not only in solution but also in an agar matrix. When antigen and antibody diffuse toward one another in agar or when antibody is incorporated into the agar and antigen diffuses into the antibody-containing matrix, a visible line of precipitation will form (Figure 6-6). As in a precipitin reaction in fluid, visible precipitation occurs in the region of equivalence,

SINGLE IMMUNODIFFUSION

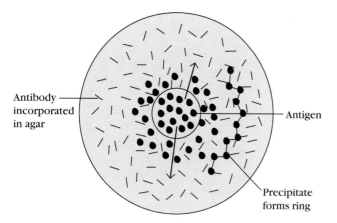

Antibody incorporated into agarose gel

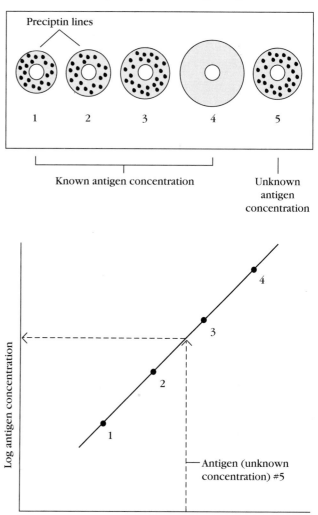

DOUBLE IMMUNODIFFUSION

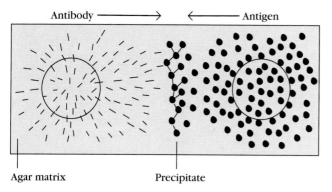

Figure 6-6   Diagrammatic representation of single and double immunodiffusion in a gel. In both cases, large insoluble complexes form in the agar in the zone of equivalence, which are visible as a line of precipitation. As the names imply, only the antigen diffuses in single immunodiffusion, whereas both the antibody and antigen diffuse in double immunodiffusion.

Figure 6-7   The Mancini single radial immunodiffusion technique. Antibody is incorporated into an agar matrix and antigen is added to a well and allowed to diffuse into the agar. At equivalence a precipitin ring will form. The diameter of the ring of precipitation is proportional to the log of the concentration of the antigen. By using known concentrations of antigen wells (1–4) it is possible to obtain a standard curve from which the concentration of an unknown concentration of antigen (well 5) can be determined.

whereas no visible precipitate forms in regions of antibody or antigen excess. These *immunodiffusion* reactions can be used to determine relative concentrations of antibodies or antigens, to compare antigens, or to determine the relative purity of an antigen preparation. Two frequently used immunodiffusion techniques are the single-immunodiffusion (Mancini) method and the double-immunodiffusion (Ouchterlony) method, both are carried out in a semi-solid medium like agar.

Single Immunodiffusion (Mancini Method)

The relative concentrations of an antigen can be determined by a simple quantitative assay in which an antigen sample is placed in a well and allowed to diffuse into agar containing a suitable dilution of an antiserum. As the antigen diffuses into the agar, the region of equivalence is established and a ring of precipitation forms around the well. The diameter of the precipitin ring is

proportional to the concentration of antigen. By comparing the diameter of the precipitin ring with a standard curve (obtained by measuring the precipitin diameters of known concentrations of the antigen), the concentration of the antigen sample can be determined. The Mancini technique is routinely used to quantitate serum levels of IgM, IgG, and IgA by incorporating class-specific anti-isotype antibody into the agar (Figure 6-7). The technique is also applied to determine concentrations of complement components in serum. This method cannot detect antigens present in concentrations below 5–

10 μg/ml; this moderate sensitivity is the major limitation of the Mancini method.

Double Immunodiffusion (Ouchterlony Method)

In the Ouchterlony method both antigen and antibody diffuse radially from wells toward each other, thereby establishing a concentration gradient. As equivalence is reached, a visible line of precipitation forms. This simple technique is an effective qualitative tool for determining the relationship between antigens and for learning how many different antibody-antigen systems are present. The pattern of the precipitin lines that form when two different antigen preparations are placed in adjacent wells indicate whether or not they share epitopes (Figure 6-8). For example, when two antigens share identical epitopes, the antiserum will form a single precipitin line with each antigen that will grow toward each other and fuse to form a pattern called *identity*. If two antigens are unrelated, the antiserum will form independent precipitin lines that cross, a pattern that establishes *nonidentity*. The lines cross because the unrelated antigen and antibody do not precipitate and therefore are free to diffuse past the precipitin line, forming the precipitin line of the unrelated antigen-antibody system. If two antigens share some epitopes but one or the other has a unique epitope, a pattern of *partial identity* is obtained. Antibodies to the common epitope form a line of identity, but antibodies to the unique epitope(s) diffuse past the precipitin line to form a spur, which is a precipitin line formed with the unique epitope(s) of the more complex antigen.

One of the drawbacks of an Ouchterlony double-diffusion assay is that it takes 18–24 h before precipitin lines appear. This limitation can be overcome by using countercurrent electrophoresis. In this method positively charged antibody and negatively charged antigen are added to separate wells in a gel. An electric current is used to drive the immunodiffusion, forming a sharp precipitin line within minutes and with greater sensitivity than in Ouchterlony double diffusion.

Immunoelectrophoresis

Immunoelectrophoresis combines separation by electrophoresis with identification by double immunodiffusion. An antigen mixture is first electrophoresed and

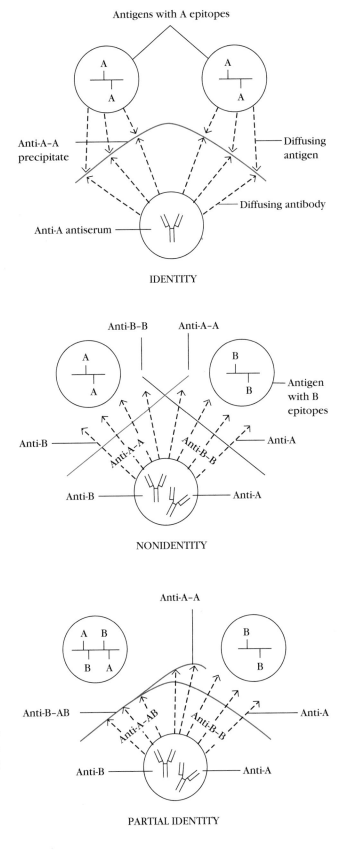

Figure 6-8 Diagram of possible precipitin patterns obtained in double immunodiffusion (Ouchterlony method) of antiserum with different antigen preparations. The pattern of lines (red) indicates whether two antigens have identical epitopes (identity), partially identical epitopes (partial identity), or no epitopes in common (nonidentity).

separated by charge. Troughs are then cut into the agar gel parallel to the direction of the electric field, and antiserum is added to the troughs. The agar gel is then incubated in a humid chamber during which time antigen and antibody diffuse toward each other. The formation of precipitin bands with polyvalent or specific antiserum identifies individual antigen components (Figure 6-9). Immunoelectrophoresis is widely used in clinical laboratories to detect the presence or absence of proteins in the serum. The serum proteins are electrophoresed, and the individual serum components are identified with antisera specific for a given protein or immunoglobulin class. Immunoelectrophoresis can determine whether a patient has an immunodeficiency disease. It can also show if a patient overproduces some serum protein, such as albumin, immunoglobulin, or transferrin. In multiple myeloma the immunoelectrophoretic pattern shows a heavy distorted arc caused by the large amount of myeloma protein, which is monoclonal and therefore uniformly charged.

Immunoelectrophoresis is a strictly qualitative technique that identifies quantitative anomalies only when the departure from normal is striking, as in immunodeficiency and immunoproliferative disorders. *Rocket electrophoresis* overcomes this limitation and makes possible the quantitation of antigen at levels as low as 20 μg/ml. In this technique negatively charged antigen is electrophoresed in a gel containing antibody. The precipitate formed between antigen and antibody has the shape of a rocket, the height of which is proportional

(a)

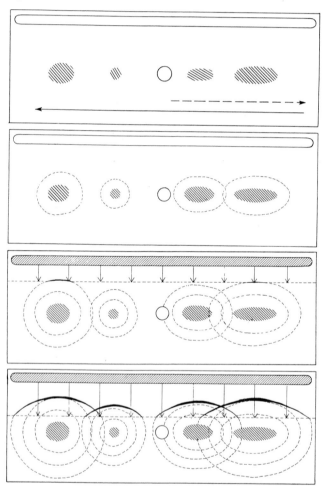

(b)

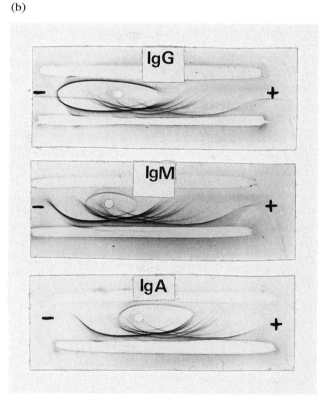

Figure 6-9   Immunoelectrophoresis of an antigen mixture. An antigen preparation is first electrophoresed, which separates the component antigens on the basis of their charge. Antiserum is then added to troughs on either side of the separated antigens and allowed to diffuse; in time, lines of precipitation form where specific antibody and antigen interact. By use of monospecific antiserum, a particular antigen can be identified in a mixture. (b) Comparison of serum from a patient with agammaglobulinemia with normal human serum. The serum samples were electrophoresed and then goat antiserum specific for human serum proteins was placed in the trough between them. The lack of precipitin lines corresponding to IgA, IgM, and IgG in the patient's serum is obvious. [From J. S. Garvey, N. E. Cremer, and D. H. Sussdorf, 1977, *Methods in Immunology*, 3d ed., W. A. Benjamin Inc., Advanced Book Program.]

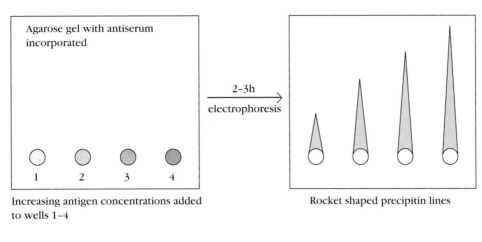

Increasing antigen concentrations added
to wells 1-4

Rocket shaped precipitin lines

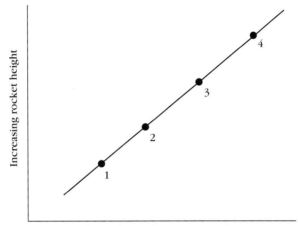

Figure 6-10 In rocket electrophoresis, antigen is electrophoresed in an agarose gel with antiserum incorporated. The height of the rocket-shaped line of precipitation that forms is proportional to the concentration of antigen.

to the concentration of antigen in the well (Figure 6-10). One of the limitations of rocket electrophoresis is the need for the antigen to be negatively charged for electrophoretic movement within the agar matrix. Some proteins, such as immunoglobulins, are not sufficiently charged to be quantitated by this method. Nor is it possible with rocket electrophoresis to quantitate several antigens in a mixture at the same time. A modification of rocket electrophoresis, called *two-dimensional immunoelectrophoresis,* allows one to quantitate several antigens in a complex mixture. In this technique antigen is first separated into components by electrophoresis; the gel is then laid over another agar gel containing antiserum, and electrophoresis is repeated at right angles to the first direction, forming precipitin peaks similar to those obtained with rocket electrophoresis. Measurement of the size of the peaks allows quantitation of a number of proteins in a complex antigen mixture (Figure 6-11).

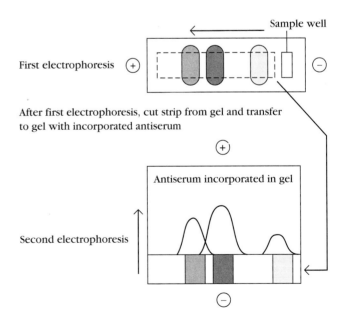

Figure 6-11 Technique of two-dimensional immunoelectrophoresis. With this technique, several antigens in a complex antigen mixture can be quantitated.

Agglutination Reactions

The interaction between antibody and a particulate antigen results in visible clumping called *agglutination*. The agglutination reaction is similar in principal to the precipitation reaction. Just as antibody excess can inhibit the precipitation reaction, an excess of antibody inhibits agglutination reactions; this inhibition, called the *prozone effect*, can be caused by several mechanisms. First, high levels of antibody increase the likelihood that a single antibody will bind to two or more epitopes on a single particulate antigen rather than cross-linking epitopes on two or more particulate antigens. The prozone can also be caused by high concentrations of antibodies that bind to the antigen but do not induce agglutination; these antibodies, called *incomplete antibodies*, are often of the IgG class. At high concentrations of IgG, incomplete antibodies may occupy all of the antigenic sites, thus blocking access by IgM, which is a good agglutinator. The lack of agglutinating activity of an incomplete antibody may be due to restricted flexibility in the hinge region, making it difficult for the antibody to assume the required angle for optimal cross-linking of epitopes on two or more particulate antigens. Alternatively, the density of epitope distribution or the location of some epitopes in deep pockets of a particulate antigen may make it difficult for antibodies, specific for these epitopes, to agglutinate the particulate antigens.

Hemagglutination

Agglutination reactions are routinely performed to type red blood cells (RBCs). Red cells are mixed on a slide with antisera to various RBC membrane antigens. If the antigen is present on the cells, the cells agglutinate on the slide (Table 6-4). By determining which antigens are present or absent it is possible to match blood types for transfusions. At neutral pH red blood cells are surrounded by a negative ion cloud that makes the cells repel one another; this repulsive force is called the zeta potential. Because of its size and pentameric nature, IgM can overcome the zeta potential and cross-link red blood cells, leading to agglutination. Because of its smaller size and bivalency, IgG is less able to overcome the zeta potential. For this reason, IgM is more effective than IgG in agglutinating red blood cells. Antibodies to some RBC antigens (e.g., the Rh antigen) are of the IgG class exclusively. In order to agglutinate Rh$^+$ red blood cells with anti-Rh antibody, the zeta potential must be reduced. This is commonly done by placing the red blood cells in serum albumin, which has a high net negative charge that reduces the effect of the negative ion cloud surrounding the red cells, thus allowing anti-Rh antibody to agglutinate Rh$^+$ cells.

Table 6-4   ABO blood types

Blood type	Antigens or RBCs	Serum antibodies
A	A	Anti-B
B	B	Anti-A
AB	A and B	Neither
O	Neither	Anti-A and anti-B

Bacterial Agglutination

A bacterial infection often elicits the production of serum antibodies specific for surface antigens of the bacterial cells. The presence of such antibodies can be detected by bacterial agglutination reactions. Serum from a patient thought to be infected with a given bacterium is serially diluted in a series of tubes to which the bacteria is added. The last tube showing visible agglutination will reflect the serum antibody titer of the patient. The *agglutination titer* is defined as the reciprocal of the last serum dilution that elicits a positive agglutination reaction. For example, when serial two-fold dilutions of serum are prepared and if the dilution of 1/640 shows agglutination but the dilution of 1/1280 does not, then the agglutination titer of the patient's serum is 640. For some bacteria high-titer serum can be diluted up to 1/50,000 and still show agglutination.

The agglutination titer of an antiserum can be used to diagnose a bacterial infection. For example, in typhoid fever there is a significant rise in the agglutination titer to *Salmonella typhi*. Agglutination reactions also provide a way to type bacteria. For instance, different species of the bacterium *Salmonella* can be distinguished by agglutination reactions with a panel of typing antisera.

Passive Agglutination

The sensitivity and simplicity of agglutination reactions can be extended by coupling soluble antigens to red blood cells and performing *passive agglutination*. In this technique, a soluble antigen is mixed with red blood cells that have been treated with tannic acid or chromium chloride to promote adsorption of protein to the surface of the cells. Serum containing the antibody is serially diluted into microtiter plate wells, and the antigen-coated red blood cells are added to each well;

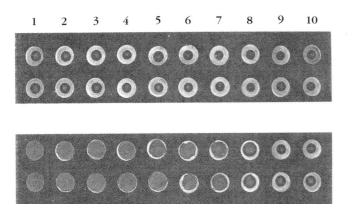

Figure 6-12 Passive hemagglutination test to detect antibodies against BSA-conjugated sheep red blood cells. A constant number of BSA-conjugated red blood cells is placed in each well. Serial dilutions of anti-BSA serum are then added to each well. As seen by the spread pattern, a duplicate reaction in the bottom series indicates positive hemagglutination with an end titer of 64,000 in tube 7, with a slightly positive reaction persisting in tube 8. In the duplicate reaction in the top series, the absence of hemagglution is observed as a solid "button" of settled red blood cells. [From J. S. Garvey, N. E. Cremer, and D. H. Sussdorf, 1977, *Methods in Immunology*, 3d ed., W. A. Benjamin Inc., Advanced Book Program.]

agglutination is assessed by the size of the characteristic spread pattern of agglutinated red blood cells on the bottom of the well (Figure 6-12).

Passive hemagglutination is far more sensitive than precipitin reactions and can detect antibody concentrations as low as 0.001 μg/ml. The sensitivities of precipitation and hemagglutination can be compared by testing an antiserum to hen ovalbumin in a tube-precipitation reaction and in passive hemagglutination with ovalbumin-coated red blood cells. Dilution of the antiserum by 1:5 results in loss of precipitation ability, whereas the antiserum still functions in passive agglutination out to a dilution of 1:10,000. Antigen can also be coupled to particles of latex or the mineral colloid bentonite.

Agglutination Inhibition

A modification of the agglutination assay, called agglutination inhibition, is a highly sensitive assay to detect small quantities of an antigen. One type of pregnancy test uses latex particles coated with human chorionic gonadotropin (HCG) and antibody to HCG (see Figure 4-13). The addition of urine from a pregnant woman, which contains HCG, inhibits agglutination of the latex particles, and so the absence of agglutination indicates pregnancy. Agglutination inhibition can also be used to determine if an individual is using certain types of illegal drugs such as cocaine or heroine. A urine or blood sample containing the suspected drug is first incubated with antibody specific for the drug. Then red blood cells or other particles coated with the drug are added. If the red blood cells are not agglutinated by the antibody, then it suggests that the individual may have been using the illicit drug. One problem with these tests is that some legal drugs have chemical structures similar to those of illicit drugs, and these legal drugs may cross-react with the antibody giving a false positive reaction. Thus a positive reaction must be confirmed by a non-immunologic method.

Agglutination inhibition is also widely used in clinical laboratories to determine if an individual has been exposed to certain types of viruses that cause agglutination of red blood cells. If an individual's serum contains specific antiviral antibodies, then the antibodies will bind to the virus and interfere with hemagglutination by the virus. This technique is commonly used in premarital testing to determine the immune status of women to rubella virus. The reciprocal of the last serum dilution to show inhibition of rubella hemagglutination is the titer of the serum. A titer greater than 10 (1:10 dilution) indicates that a woman is immune to rubella, whereas a titer of less than 10 is indicative of a lack of immunity and the need for immunization with the rubella vaccine.

Radioimmunoassay

Radioimmunoassay (RIA) is a highly sensitive technique that can measure picogram (10^{-12} g) levels of antigen or antibody. The technique was first developed by two endocrinologists, S. A. Berson and Rosalyn Yalow, in 1960 to determine levels of insulin–anti-insulin complexes in diabetics. Although their original attempts to publish a report of this research met with some resistance from immunologists, the technique soon proved its own value for quantitating hormones, serum proteins, drugs, and vitamins. In 1977, some years after Berson's death, the significance of the technique was acknowledged by the award of a Nobel prize to Yalow.

The principle of RIA involves competitive binding of radiolabeled antigen and unlabeled antigen to a high-affinity antibody. The antigen is generally labeled with a gamma-emitting isotope such as ^{125}I. The labeled antigen is mixed with antibody at a concentration that just saturates the antigen-binding sites of the antibody molecule, and then increasing amounts of unlabeled antigen of unknown concentration are added. The antibody does not distinguish labeled from unlabeled antigen, and so the two kinds of antigen compete for available binding sites on the antibody. With increasing concentrations of unlabeled antigen, more labeled antigen will be displaced from the binding sites. By measuring the amount of labeled antigen free in solution, it is possible to determine the concentration of unlabeled antigen.

Several methods have been developed for separating the bound antigen from the free antigen in RIA. One method involves precipitating the antigen-antibody complex with a secondary anti-isotype antiserum. For example, if the Ab-Ag complex contains rabbit IgG antibody, then goat anti-rabbit IgG can precipitate the complex. Another method makes use of the fact that protein A of *Staphylococcus aureus* has high affinity for IgG. If the complex contains an IgG antibody, the complex can be precipitated by mixing with formalin-killed *S. aureus*. After removal of the complex by either of these methods, the amount of free labeled antigen remaining in the supernatant can be quantitated in a gamma counter. A standard curve is then plotted of the percentage of bound labeled antigen versus known concentrations of unlabeled antigen. Once a standard curve had been plotted, unknown concentrations of the unlabeled antigen can be determined from the standard curve.

Various solid-phase RIAs have been developed that make it easier to separate the antigen-antibody complex from the unbound antigen. In some cases the antibody is covalently cross-linked to Sepharose beads. The amount of radiolabeled antigen bound to the beads can be quantitated after the beads have been centrifuged and washed. Alternatively, the antibody can be immobilized on polystyrene or polyvinylchloride and the amount of free labeled antigen in the supernatant can be determined in a gamma counter. In another approach, the antibody is immobilized on the walls of microtiter wells. This procedure is well suited for determining the concentration of a particular antigen in large numbers of samples. For example, a microtiter RIA has been widely used to screen blood for the presence of hepatitis B virus (Figure 6-13). Antibody specific for the surface antigen of the virus (HBsAg) is immobilized on the surface of microtiter wells; [^{125}I]HBsAg and the blood samples are then added to the wells. If a sample is infected, the unlabeled HBsAg will compete with the [^{125}I]HBsAg. A decrease in the radioactivity bound by the solid-phase antibody in the presence of serum indicates that the serum is infected (i.e., contains HBsAg). RIA screening of donor blood has sharply reduced the incidence of hepatitis B infections from blood transfusions.

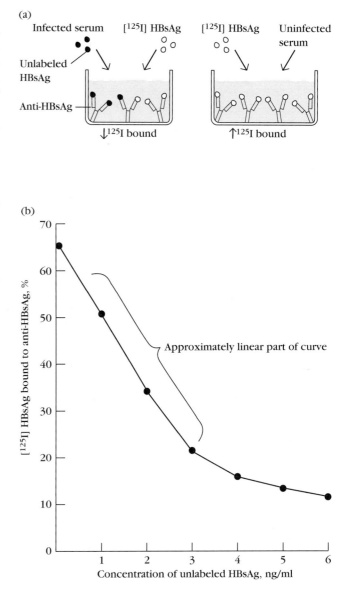

Figure 6-13 A solid-phase radioimmunoassay (RIA) to detect heptitis B virus in blood samples. (a) Microtiter wells are coated with a constant amount of antibody specific for HBsAg, the surface antigen on hepatitis B virions. A serum sample and [^{125}I] HBsAg are then added. After incubation, the supernatant is removed and the amount of radioactivity bound to the antibody is determined. If the sample is infected, the amount of label bound will be less than in controls with uninfected serum. (b) A standard curve is obtained by adding increasing concentrations of unlabeled HBsAg to a fixed quantity of [^{125}I] HBsAg and specific antibody. From the plot of the percentage of labeled antigen bound versus the concentration of unlabeled antigen, the concentration of HBsAg in unknown serum samples can be determined from the linear portion of the curve.

Enzyme-Linked Immunosorbent Assay

Enzyme-linked immunosorbent assay, or ELISA, as it is commonly known, is similar in principle to RIA and has the same sensitivity but depends on an enzyme rather than a radioactive label. An enzyme conjugated to the antibody reacts with a colorless substrate to generate a colored reaction product. A number of enzyme-substrate systems have been employed successfully, including alkaline phosphatase, horseradish peroxidase, and *p*-nitrophenyl phosphatase, each of which generates suitable colored reaction products. These assays approach the sensitivity of RIAs and have the advantage of being safer and less costly. Like a RIA, an ELISA can quantitate either antigen or antibody concentrations. An indirect ELISA, in which antigen is absorbed onto microtiter wells, can detect antibody. Serum or some other sample containing antibody is added to the well and allowed to react with the bound antigen. The wells are then washed, and the presence of antibody bound to the antigen is detected by adding an enzyme-conjugated secondary anti-isotype antibody (Ab_2), which binds to the bound primary antibody. After any free Ab_2 has been washed away, a substrate for the enzyme is added and the colored reaction product is measured by specialized spectro-photometric plate readers, which can measure the absorbance of a 96-well plate in less than one minute.

An indirect ELISA has been the method of choice to detect the presence of serum antibodies against the human immunodeficiency virus (HIV), the causative agent of AIDS. Recombinant envelope and core proteins of HIV are adsorbed as solid-phase antigens to microtiter wells. Individuals infected with HIV will produce serum antibodies to epitopes on the virus. Generally the serum antibodies to HIV can be detected by indirect ELISA within 6 weeks of infection.

Western Blotting

Identification of a specific protein in a complex mixture of proteins, or antibody to a given protein, can be accomplished by a technique known as Western blotting, named for its similarity to Southern blotting, which detects DNA fragments, and Northern blotting, which detects mRNAs. In Western blotting protein is electrophoretically separated on a polyacrylamide slab gel in the presence of SDS. The protein bands are transferred to a nitrocellulose membrane by electrophoresis and the individual protein bands are identified by flooding the nitrocellulose membrane with radiolabeled polyclonal or monoclonal antibody. The antigen-antibody complexes that form are visualized by autoradiography (Figure 6-14). If labeled specific antibody is not available, antigen-antibody complexes can be detected by adding a secondary anti-isotype antibody that is either radiolabeled or enzyme-labeled, and the band is visualized by

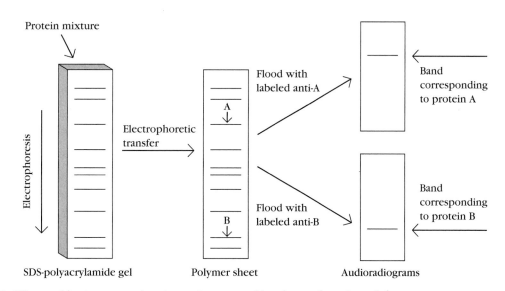

Figure 6-14 In Western blotting a protein mixture is separated by electrophoresis, and the protein bands are transferred by electrophoresis onto a polymer sheet such as nitrocellulose. After flooding the sheet with radiolabeled specific antibodies, the various protein bands can be visualized by autoradiography.

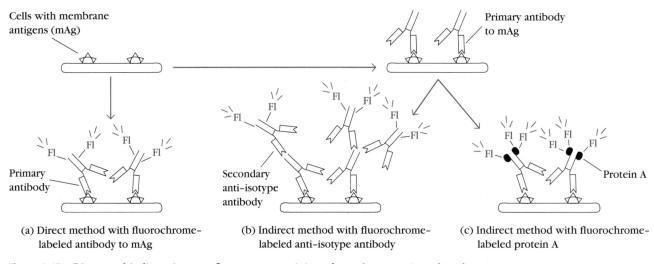

(a) Direct method with fluorochrome-labeled antibody to mAg

(b) Indirect method with fluorochrome-labeled anti-isotype antibody

(c) Indirect method with fluorochrome-labeled protein A

Figure 6-15 Direct and indirect immunofluorescence staining of membrane antigen (mAg). Cells are affixed to a microscope slide. In the direct method (a), cells are stained with anti-mAg antibody that is labeled with a fluorochrome (Fl). In the indirect methods (b and c), cells are first incubated with unlabeled anti-mAg antibody and then stained with a fluorochrome-labeled secondary reagent that binds to the primary antibody. Observation under a fluorescence microscope indicates whether the cells have been stained.

autoradiography or substrate addition. Western blotting can identify either a given protein antigen or specific antibody. For example, Western blotting has been used to identify the envelope and core proteins of HIV and the antibodies to these components in the serum of HIV-infected individuals.

Immunofluorescence

Antibody binding to cells or tissue sections can be visualized by tagging the antibody with a fluorescent dye, or *fluorochrome*. The most commonly used fluorescent dyes are fluorescein and rhodamine. Both dyes can be conjugated to the Fc region of an antibody molecule without affecting the specificity of the antibody. Each of these dyes absorbs light at one wavelength and emits light at a longer wavelength. Fluorescein absorbs blue light (490 nm) and emits an intense yellow-green fluorescence (517 nm); rhodamine absorbs in the yellow-green range (515 nm) and emits a deep red fluorescence (546 nm). The fluorescent emitted light is generally viewed with a fluorescence microscope, which is equipped with a UV light source and excitation filters. By conjugating fluorescein to one antibody and rhodamine to another antibody one can visualize two cell-membrane antigens simultaneously on the same cell.

Fluorescent-antibody staining of cell-membrane molecules or tissue sections can be direct or indirect (Figure

6-15). In direct staining the specific antibody (called the primary antibody) is directly conjugated with fluorescein; in indirect staining the primary antibody is unlabeled and is detected with an additional fluorochrome-labeled reagent. A number of reagents have been developed for indirect staining. The most common is a

Figure 6-16 Separation of fluorochrome-labeled cells with the fluorescence-activated cell sorter (FACS). In the example shown, a mixed cell population is stained with two antibodies, one specific for surface protein A and the other specific for surface protein B. The anti-A antibodies are labeled with fluorescein (Fl) and the anti-B antibodies with rhodamine (Rh). The stained cells are loaded into the sample chamber of the FACS. The cells are expelled, one at a time, from a small vibrating nozzle that generates microdroplets, each containing a single cell. The drops fall past a beam of laser light that excites the fluorochrome; the intensity of the fluorescence emitted by each droplet is monitored by a detector and displayed on an oscilloscope. Those droplets that emit fluorescent light are electrically charged in proportion to their fluorescence; the charged droplets then are separated as they flow past the deflection plates. This mixture of cells contains four subpopulations based on surface proteins A and B: A^+B^-, A^-B^+, A^+B^+, and A^-B^-.

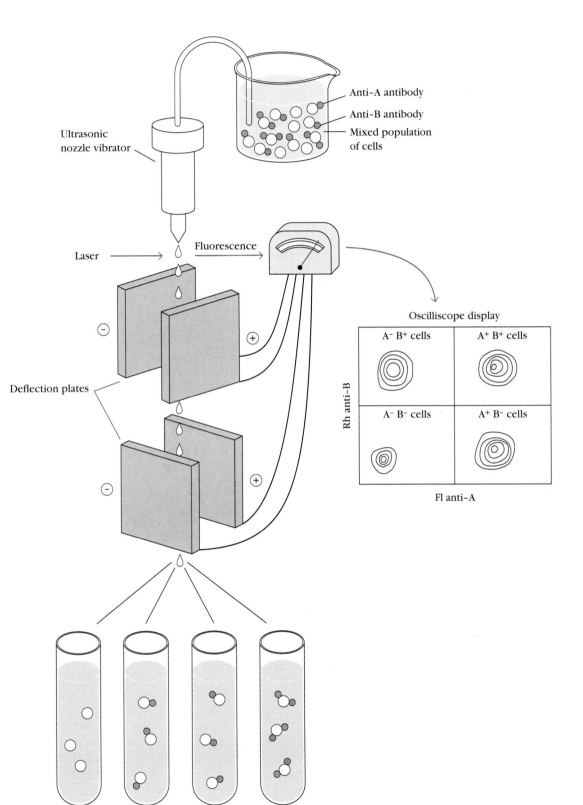

Ultrasonic nozzle vibrator

Anti-A antibody
Anti-B antibody
Mixed population of cells

Laser
Fluorescence

Deflection plates

Oscilliscope display

A⁻ B⁺ cells | A⁺ B⁺ cells
A⁻ B⁻ cells | A⁺ B⁻ cells

Rh anti–B

Fl anti–A

fluorochrome-labeled anti-isotype reagent such as fluo-rescein-labeled goat anti-mouse immunoglobulin. Another reagent is fluorochrome-labeled protein A from *Staphylococcus aureus*; this protein binds with high affinity to the Fc region of IgG antibody molecules. A third approach begins with a biotin-conjugated anti-isotype as the second antibody and then adds fluoro-chrome-conjugated avidin, a protein that binds to the biotin with extremely high affinity. There are two advantages to indirect labeling. One is that the primary antibody does not need to be conjugated with label. Because the supply of primary antibody is often a limiting factor, it is advantageous to avoid loss of antibody in the course of labeling. The second advantage of indirect labeling is that sensitivity is increased because multiple fluorochrome reagents will bind to each primary antibody.

Immunofluorescence has a wide variety of applications. Fluorescent antibodies have been applied to identify a number of subpopulations of lymphocytes, notably the CD4 and CD8 T-cell subpopulations. Fluorescent antibodies can also be used to identify bacterial species, detect antibody-antigen complexes in autoimmune disease, detect complement components in tissues, and localize hormones and other cellular products stained in situ.

Subpopulations of lymphocytes labeled with fluoro-chrome-conjugated antibody can be analyzed and sorted on the basis of the intensity of fluorescent-antibody staining. Labeled cells can be separated in a specialized flow cytometer called a fluorescence-activated cell sorter (FACS), as illustrated in Figure 6-16. The FACS permits separation of fluorescein-stained and rhodamine-stained subpopulations and of high-, medium-, and low-staining cells. Recent advances in flow cytometry make it possible to analyze three fluorochromes on a single stained sample.

Immunoelectron Microscopy

The fine specificity of antibodies has made them powerful tools to identify intracellular tissue components by electron microscopy. In order to visualize the antibody an electron-dense label is either conjugated directly to the Fc portion of the antibody molecule or an indirect labeling technique is employed in which the electro-dense label is conjugated to an anti-immunoglobulin reagent. A number of electron-dense labels have been employed including ferritin and colloidal gold. As the electron dense label absorbs electrons it can be visualized with the electron microscope as small black dots.

In the case of immunogold labeling, different antibodies can be conjugated with different sizes of gold particles, allowing one to indentify several intracellular antigens within a cell by the size of the electron dense gold particle attached to the antibody. These techniques have played an important role in demonstrating that class I and class II MHC molecules may be sequestered along different intracellular processing routes (see Chapter 9).

Summary

1. The antibody-antigen interaction depends on non-covalent interactions including hydrogen bonds, ionic bonds, hydrophobic interactions, and van der Waals interactions. The strength of the antigen-antibody interaction depends on the number of these weak non-covalent interactions between antigen and antibody. The affinity of an antibody for an antigen refers to the strength of these noncovalent interactions between antibody and antigen at a single binding site; the avidity reflects the strength of the interaction of multivalent antibody with multivalent antigen.

2. The interaction of soluble antigen and antibody forms an antigen-antibody complex that has a lattice structure and precipitates out of solution. Precipitin reactions can be performed in liquids or gels. They serve as simple methods for comparing antibodies or antigens, and in some versions can quantitate antibodies or antigens. Electrophoresis can be combined with precipitation in gels in a technique called immunoelectro-phoresis. A variety of immunoelectrophoretic techniques have been developed, including countercurrent electrophoresis, rocket electrophoresis, and two-dimensional electrophoresis.

3. Agglutination reactions occur between antibody and a particulate antigen. In some cases the antigen is a membrane protein on a bacterial cell or red blood cell. In other cases the antigen may be protein attached to a latex particle or adsorbed on the surface of a red blood cell. Agglutination reactions are more sensitive than precipitation reactions and can often detect 100- or 1000-fold lower levels of antigen or antibody than can be detected with a precipitin reaction.

4. Radioimmunoassay utilizes radioactively labeled antigen or antibody and is therefore a highly sensitive technique. Liquid-phase RIA is based on the principle of competition between labeled and unlabeled antigen for a limited amount of antibody. In solid-phase RIA antigen (or antibody) is immobilized on a solid matrix. The main advantage of this technique over liquid-phase RIA is its simplicity of performance and the ease with which the bound antigen-antibody complex can be separated from the unreacted antigen. Both types of RIA can be used to quantitate antibody or antigen.

5. The enzyme-linked immunosorbent assay (ELISA) involves principles similar to those of RIA but depends on an enzyme-substrate reaction that generates a colored reaction product rather than utilizing a radiolabel.

6. In Western blotting, antigen is separated by electrophoresis; then the antigen bands are electrophoretically transferred onto nitrocellulose and identified with labeled antibody.

7. Fluorescent-antibody staining can visualize antigen on cells. Various direct and indirect staining techniques have been developed. The fluorescence-activated cell sorter analyzes and sorts cells labeled with fluorescent antibody.

References

AXELSEN, N. H. 1983. *Handbook of Immunoprecipitation-in-Gel Techniques.* Blackwell Scientific Publications.

EDWARDS, R. 1985. *Immunoassay: An Introduction.* Heinemann Medical Books.

JOHNSTONE, A., and R. THORPE. 1987. *Immunochemistry in Practice,* 2d ed. Blackwell Scientific Publications.

POLAK, J. M., and S. VANNOORDEN. 1987. *An introduction to Immunocytochemistry: Current Techniques and Problems.* Oxford Science Publishers.

WEIR, D. M. 1986. *Handbook of Experimental Immunology,* 4th ed. Vols. I and II. Blackwell Scientific Publications.

JOHNSTONE, A. ed. 1989. *Immunological Techniques.* Current Opinion in Immunology **1**:927.

Study Questions

1. Indicate whether each of the following statements is true of false. If you think a statement is false, explain why.

   a. Indirect immunofluorescence is a more sensitive technique than direct immunofluorescence.

   b. Most antigens induce a polyclonal response.

   c. A papain digest of anti-SRBC antibodies can agglutinate sheep red blood cells (SRBCs).

   d. A pepsin digest of anti-SRBC antibodies can agglutinate SRBCs.

   e. Indirect immunofluorescence can be performed using a Fab fragment as the initial nonlabeled antibody.

   f. For precipitation to occur, both antigen and antibody must be multivalent.

   g. The Ouchterlony technique is a quantitative precipitin technique.

   h. Precipitin tests are generally more sensitive than agglutination tests.

2. Briefly outline the ELISA test for HIV infection indicating which antigen and antibody are used.

3. You have obtained a preparation of purified albumin from normal bovine serum. To determine whether any other serum proteins remain in this preparation of BSA, you decide to use immunoelectrophoresis.

   a. What antigen would you use to prepare the antiserum needed to detect impurities in the BSA preparation?

   b. Assuming that the BSA preparation is pure, draw the immunoelectrophoretic pattern you would expect if the assay was performed with bovine serum in one well, the BSA sample in a second well, and the antiserum you prepared in (a) in the trough between the wells.

4. The labels from four bottles (A, B, C, and D) of hapten-carrier conjugates were accidentally removed. However, it was known that each bottle contained either hapten 1–carrier 1 (H1-C1), hapten 1–carrier 2 (H1-C2), hapten 2–carrier 1 (H2-C1), or hapten 2–carrier 2 (H2-C2). Ouchterlony assays with either anti–H1-C2 or anti–H2-C2 were performed. From the precipitin patterns shown below, determine which conjugate is in each bottle.

Anti–H1-C2
in central well

Anti–H2-C2
in central well

5. The concentration of a hapten can be determined by which of the following assays: (a) ELISA, (b) Ouchterlony method, (c) rocket electrophoresis, and (d) RIA.

6. You perform an Ouchterlony assay in which the central well contains goat antiserum against the F(ab)$_2$ fragment of pooled mouse IgG and the surrounding wells

(a–f) contain six different test antigens. From the resulting precipitin pattern shown below, determine which of the listed test antigens is in each well.

Test antigens	Well number
Fab from an IgG myeloma protein ($\gamma_2\kappa_2$)	
κ light chains	
γ heavy chains	
λ light chains	
F_c from an IgG myeloma protein ($\gamma_2\lambda_2$)	
A mixture of γ heavy chains and κ light chains	

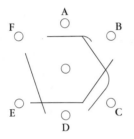

7.   You have a myeloma protein X whose isotype is unknown and several other myeloma proteins of known isotype (i.e., IgG, IgM, and IgA). How could you produce antibodies that could be used to determine the isotype of myeloma protein X? How could you use this anti-isotype antibody to determine the level of that isotype in normal serum?

8.   List an appropriate assay method for each of the following, keeping in mind the sensitivity of the assay and the expected amount of each antigen or antibody.
   a.   IgG in serum
   b.   Insulin in serum
   c.   IgE in serum
   d.   Complement component C3 on glomerular basement membrane
   e.   Anti-A antibodies to blood-group antigen A in serum
   f.   Horsemeat contamination of hamburger
   g.   Syphilis spirochete in a smear from a chancre

9.   You want to develop a sensitive immunoassay for a hormone that occurs in the blood at concentrations around 10^{-7} M. You are offered a choice of three different antisera whose affinities for the hormone have been determined by equilibrium dialysis. The results are shown in the following Scatchard plots:

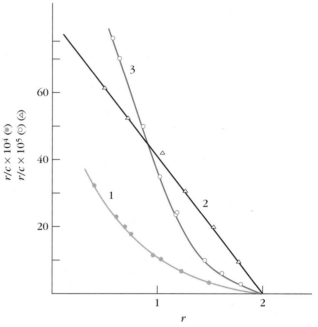

   a.   What is the value of K_0 for each antiserum?
   b.   What is the valence of each of the antibodies?
   c.   Which of the antisera might be a monoclonal antibody?
   d.   Which of the antisera would you use for your assay?

10.   In preparing a demonstration for her immunology class, an instructor purified IgG antibodies to sheep blood cells (SRBCs) and digested some of the antibodies into Fab, Fc, and $F(ab')_2$ fragments. She placed each preparation in a separate tube, labeled the tubes with a water-soluble marker, and left them in an ice bucket. When the instructor returned for her class period, she discovered that the labels had smeared and were unreadable. Determined to salvage the demonstration, she relabeled the tubes 1, 2, 3, and 4 and proceeded. Based on the test results described below, indicate which preparation was contained in each tube and explain why you so identified the contents.

   a.   The preparation in tube 1 agglutinated SRBCs but did not lyse them in the presence of complement.

   b.   The preparation in tube 2 did not agglutinate SRBCs or lyse them in the presence of complement. However, when this preparation was added to SRBCs before the addition of whole anti-SRBC, it prevented agglutination of the cells by the whole anti-SRBC antiserum.

   c.   The preparation in tube 3 agglutinated SRBCs and also lysed the cells in the presence of complement.

   d.   The preparation in tube 4 did not agglutinate or lyse SRBCs and did not inhibit agglutination of SRBCs by whole anti-SRBC antiserum.

CHAPTER

7

Hybridomas and Monoclonal Antibody

The serum antibodies produced in response to an antigen, even a purified one, are heterogeneous because the multiple epitopes on the antigen induce the proliferation and differentiation of a variety of B-cell clones. The polyclonal antibody elicited by an antigen facilitates the localization, phagocytosis, and complement-mediated lysis of that antigen; thus the usual polyclonal immune response has clear advantages in vivo. Unfortunately, the antibody heterogeneity that increases immune protection in vivo often reduces the efficacy of an antiserum for various in vitro uses. Conventional heterogeneous antisera vary from animal to animal and contain undesirable nonspecific or cross-reacting antibodies. Removal of unwanted specificities from a polyclonal antibody preparation is a time-consuming task, involving repeated adsorbtion techniques, which often results in the loss of much of the desired antibody and seldom is very effective in reducing the heterogeneity of an antiserum.

An alternative, simpler approach is to generate pure (monospecific) clones of plasma cells in vitro from which monoclonal antibody with a single antigenic specificity can be obtained (Figure 7-1). For many years this approach was not technically feasible because plasma cells have a short lifespan and cannot be maintained in tissue culture. In 1975, Georges Kohler and Cesar Milstein devised a solution to this technical problem, which was described briefly in Chapter 2. By fusing a normal B cell (plasma cell) with a myeloma cell (a cancerous plasma cell), they were able to generate a hybrid cell, called a hybridoma, that possessed the immortal-growth properties of the myeloma cell but secreted the antibody product of the B cell (see Figure 2-1). The resulting clones of hybridoma cells, which secrete large quantities of monoclonal antibody, can be cultured indefinitely. This basic procedure for producing mono-

clonal antibody is explained in detail in this chapter; several more recent methods for obtaining monoclonal antibody by genetic engineering techniques also are described.

The development of techniques for producing monoclonal antibody gave immunologists (and molecular biologists in general) a powerful and versatile research tool. The significance of the work by Kohler and Milstein was acknowledged when each was awarded a Nobel prize in 1984, along with the eminent theorist Niels Jerne. During the 1980s, monoclonal antibody technology moved out of the research laboratory and now forms the basis for a growing variety of commercial applications, some of which are discussed in this chapter.

Formation and Selection of Hybrid Cells

Since the early 1970s it has been possible to fuse one somatic cell with another to form a hybrid cell called a *heterokaryon*. Fusion can be achieved by incubating a

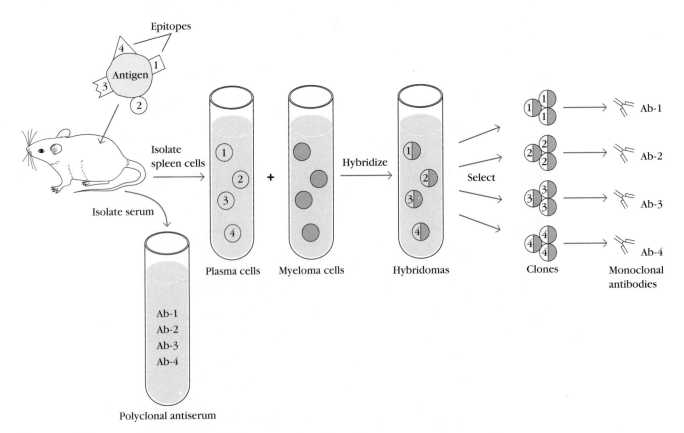

Figure 7-1 The conventional polyclonal antiserum produced in response to a complex antigen contains a mixture of antibodies, each specific for one of the four epitopes shown on the antigen. In constrast, a monoclonal antibody, which is derived from a single plasma cell, is specific for one epitope on a complex antigen. One method for obtaining monoclonal antibody is illustrated.

suspension of two cell types with an inactivated enveloped virus called Sendai virus or with polyethylene glycol, both of which promote the fusion of plasma membranes. In this way the plasma membranes, cytoplasm, and nuclei of two separate cells are brought together into a single hybrid cell.

In the early 1970s L. D. Frye and M. Edidin used heterokaryons to study the fluidity of membrane proteins. In a classic experiment they fused a mouse fibroblast with a human fibroblast, generating a mouse-human heterokaryon, which was then exposed to fluorescein- and rhodamine-tagged antibodies specific for the MHC molecules on human and mouse cells. Immediately after fusion the distribution of labeled antibody revealed that the mouse and human MHC molecules were confined to separate halves of the heterokaryon's plasma membrane. Within a short period of time, however, the fluorescein- and rhodamine-tagged antibodies were seen to diffuse and mix randomly over the surface of the heterokaryon, demonstrating the random diffusion of the mouse and human MHC molecules within the phospholipid bilayer of the heterokaryon's plasma membrane. This experiment was instrumental in the development of the fluid-mosaic model of the cell membrane by J. Singer and G. Nicholson in 1972.

A heterokaryon initially is multinucleated, having two to five separate nuclei (Figure 7-2). In the course of cell division the nuclear membranes disintegrate, and a single large nucleus is formed containing the chromosomes of both parent cells. At this stage the hybrid cell is unstable, and as it continues to divide, it loses a variable number of chromosomes from one or both parent cells until the fused cell stabilizes. Sometimes this random chromosome loss results in loss of a chromosome that is necessary for cell survival, and these hybrids die off. When mouse and human cells are fused, the hybrids eventually lose all of their human chromosomes. The reason for this disparate chromosome loss is not known but presumably is related to the phylogenetic distance between the two species. With selective culture conditions it is possible to select for mouse-human hybrid cells containing one or at most a few human chromosomes. These hybrids have been useful for mapping genes to particular human chromosomes by associating a particular gene function with a particular chromosome.

After fusion the hybrid cells must be separated from unfused parent cells (e.g., A cells and B cells). When Sendai virus or polyethylene glycol is the fusion agent, only a small percentage of the cells actually fuse, and some of the fused cells are homogeneous A-A or B-B cells rather than the desired A-B hybrid. In order to select for the hybrid cells, a selective medium called HAT is employed. HAT selection depends on the fact that mammalian cells can synthesize nucleotides by two different pathways—the de novo and the salvage pathways:

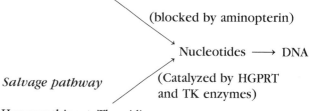

De novo pathway

Phosphoribosyl pyrophosphate + Uridylate

(blocked by aminopterin)

Nucleotides ⟶ DNA

Salvage pathway

(Catalyzed by HGPRT and TK enzymes)

Hypoxanthine + Thymidine

(a)

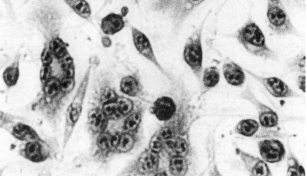

(b)

Figure 7-2 Heterokaryon formation. (a) Unfused cultured mouse cells. (b) Mouse cells fused by treatment with polyethylene glycol. There are two to five nuclei per heterokaryon. [From R. L. Davidson and P. S. Gerald, 1976, *Som. Cell Genet.* **2**:165.]

The de novo pathway, in which a methyl or formyl group is transferred from an activated form of tetrahydrofolate, is blocked by *aminopterin*, a folic acid analog. When the de novo pathway is blocked, cells utilize the salvage pathway, which bypasses the aminopterin block by converting purines and pyrimidines directly into DNA. The enzymes catalyzing the salvage pathway include hypoxanthine-guanine phosphoribosyl transferase (HGPRT) and thymidine kinase (TK). A mutation in either of these two enzymes blocks the salvage pathway. HAT medium contains *a*minopterin to block the de novo pathway and *h*ypoxanthine and *t*hymidine to allow growth via the salvage pathway. When two types of cells, each of which has a mutation in a different enzyme necessary for the salvage pathway, are fused, only the hybrid cells will contain the full complement of the necessary enzymes for growth on HAT medium via the salvage pathway. Culture in HAT medium thus allows only the hybrid cells to grow.

Production of Monoclonal Antibodies

The production of a given monoclonal antibody involves three basic steps: (1) generating B-cell hybridomas by fusing primed B cells and myeloma cells; (2) screening the resulting clones for those which secrete antibody with the desired specificity; and (3) propagating the desired hybridomas.

Generating B-Cell Hybridomas

In their innovative method for producing monoclonal antibodies, Kohler and Milstein applied the techniques of cell fusion and HAT selection of hybrid cells described in the previous section. Their general procedure is outlined in Figure 7-3. The use of myeloma cells that cannot grow in HAT medium (HGPRT⁻ cells) assured that only hybridomas (hybrid myeloma-spleen cells) were selected. The unfused or fused spleen cells did not need

Figure 7-3   The procedure for producing monoclonal antibodies specific for a given antigen developed by G. Kohler and C. Milstein. Spleen cells from an antigen-primed mouse are fused with mouse myeloma cells (HGPRT⁻ and Ab⁻). The spleen cell provides the necessary enzymes for growth on HAT medium, while the myeloma cell provides immortal-growth properties. Unfused myeloma cells or myeloma-myeloma fusions fail to grow due to lack of HGPRT. Unfused spleen cells have limited growth and therefore do not need an enzyme deficiency for elimination with the HAT selection procedure.

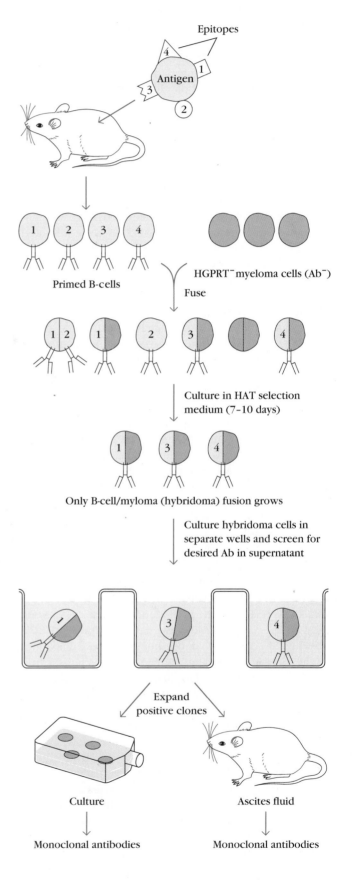

to be selected because they were terminal cells of a differentiation series and were only capable of limited growth in vitro. After 7–10 days of culture in the HAT medium, most of the wells contained dead cells, but a few wells contained small clusters of viable cells, which could be visualized by using an inverted phase contrast microscope. Each cluster represented clonal expansion of a hybridoma (Figure 7-4). After HAT selection, single cells were transferred and cultured in separate wells in an effort to ensure the monoclonality of any secreted antibody. Wells containing single viable clusters were then screened for antibody production; antibody-positive clones were subcultured at low cell densities, again to ensure clonal purity in each microwell. The hybridoma clones obtained by this procedure were isolated, clonally expanded in culture, and shown by Kohler and Milstein to produce monoclonal antibodies, each specific for a single epitope on sheep red blood cells, the original antigen used in their experiments.

The first hybridomas obtained by Kohler and Milstein secreted not only antibody from the splenic B cell but also unwanted antibody from the myeloma cell as well as some hybrid antibody combining heavy or light chains from both original parent cells. To avoid this difficulty, an HGPRT$^-$, Ab$^-$ myeloma cell was chosen as the ideal fusion partner. This fusion partner has the immortal-growth properties of a cancer cell but does not secrete its own antibody gene product. Hybridomas generated with this fusion partner thus secrete only the antibody from the B-cell partner. These hybridomas can be propagated in tissue culture to give rise to large clones secreting homogeneous monoclonal antibody.

Screening for Monoclonal Antibody Specificity

Once pure clones of antibody-secreting hybridomas are obtained, they must be screened for the desired antibody specificity. Although some hybridomas will produce antibody specific for the antigen used for immunization, others will be specific for unwanted antigens. The supernatant of each hybridoma culture contains its secreted antibody and can be assayed for a particular antigen specificity in various ways. Two of the most common screening techniques are ELISA and RIA, both of which are easily adapted to mass screening with 96-well microtiter plates. In both assays, antigen that reacts with the desired antibody is bound to the microtiter wells and washed to remove unbound antigen. Supernatant from each hybridoma well is added to separate wells. After incubation and more washing, an anti-isotype antibody directed against the isotypic determinants on the monoclonal antibody is added. In an ELISA this anti-isotype antibody is conjugated to an enzyme that produces a colored reaction product when the appropriate substrate is added (Figure 7-5). In an RIA the anti-isotype antibody is radiolabeled; bound label can be detected by counting the wells individually in a gamma counter, or the entire plate can be exposed to x-ray film. If the desired monoclonal antibody has specificity for a cell-membrane molecule, immunofluorescent techniques can be used for screening. In this case, target cells with the particular cell-membrane antigen are stained with the monoclonal antibody in microtiter wells and visualized by the addition of a fluorochrome-conjugated anti-isotype antibody (see Figure 6-15). Alternatively, a fluorescence-activated cell sorter can be modified to microsample labeled target cells taken from the microtiter wells.

Zone of lysis

Individual Ab-secreting cells

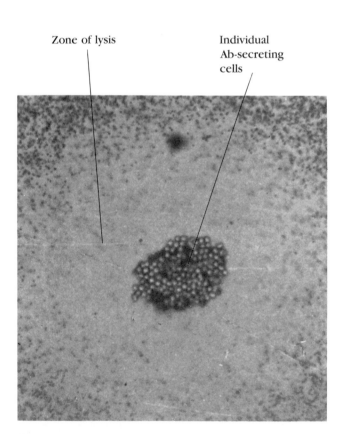

Figure 7-4 Viable hybridoma clone that appeared after culture for 7–10 days in HAT selection medium. The individual cells in the clone are visible. This particular clone secreted monoclonal antibody to sheep red blood cells (SRBCs). When SRBCs and complement were added, the anti-SRBC antibody diffusing out from the secreting cells caused complement-mediated lysis of the red blood cells, producing the visible clear zone. [From C. Milstein, 1980, *Sci. Am.* **243**:67.]

Propagating Hybridomas Secreting Specific Monoclonal Antibodies

Once a hybridoma secreting a monoclonal antibody of the desired specificity has been identified, it should be recloned by limiting dilution to ensure that the culture is truly monoclonal. The cloned hybridoma can then be propagated in one of several ways to produce the desired monoclonal antibody. The hybridoma can be grown in tissue-culture flasks, in which the antibody is secreted into the medium at fairly low concentrations (10–100 μg/ml). The hybridoma also can be propagated in the peritoneal cavity of histocompatible mice, where it secretes the monoclonal antibody into the ascites fluid at much higher concentrations (1–25 mg/ml); the antibody can then be purified from the mouse ascites fluid by chromatography.

To meet the increased demand for monoclonal antibodies, biotechnology companies have been developing various techniques to increase yields. Damon Biotech Company encapsulates hybridomas in alginate gels, which allow nutrients to flow in and waste products and antibodies to flow out. In these capsules, hybridoma cells can achieve much higher densities than in tissue culture; as a result, 100-fold greater yields of antibody production have been attained by this method than with conventional tissue culture. A different approach has been taken by Celltech in England. In this company's method, hybridomas are grown in 1000-liter fermenters, which yield 100 grams of monoclonal antibody in a 2-week period. Further scale-ups to 10,000-liter fermenters are being developed.

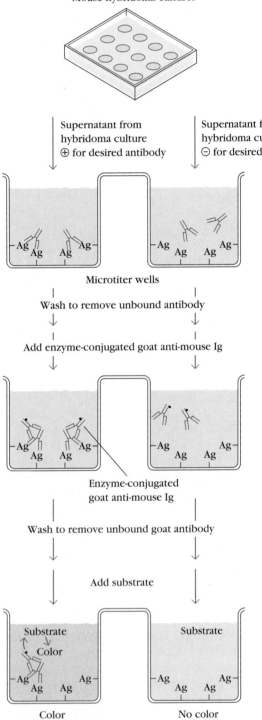

Figure 7-5 ELISA screening of mouse hybridomas for those secreting monoclonal antibody of desired specificity. Microtiter wells are coated with the desired antigen, and supernatant from each hybridoma culture is added to a well. After incubation to allow antibody to bind, the unbound antibody is washed away. An enzyme-conjugated goat anti-mouse antibody is then added. This anti-isotype antibody will bind to the mouse monoclonal antibody. The unbound goat antibody is washed away and a substrate for the conjugated enzyme is added. If the original supernatant contains antibody specific for the antigen, a colored reaction product will be formed on addition of substrate (*left*). The absence of color (*right*) indicates that the tested hybridoma does not secrete the desired antibody.

Producing Human Monoclonal Antibody

The homogeneity and specificity of monoclonal antibodies makes them particularly suitable for in vivo administration in humans for diagnostic or therapeutic purposes. However, a major obstacle to the clinical use of monoclonal antibodies in humans is that they are usually mouse antibodies and therefore are recognized as foreign, inducing an anti-isotype response. For human clinical intervention it is therefore desirable to use human monoclonal antibodies, thus avoiding any anti-isotype response.

The production of human monoclonal antibody has been hampered by a number of technical difficulties. First and foremost is the difficulty of obtaining antigen-primed B cells in humans (equivalent to the mouse spleen cells shown in Figure 7-3). It is possible to obtain B cells primed in response to the antigens in accepted vaccines, but one simply cannot immunize a human volunteer with the range of antigens that can be given to mice or other animals. Immunization in the human system must therefore be done in vitro, which is less effective than in vivo priming of B cells. Such in vitro systems are discussed in Chapter 12.

Another major difficulty in producing human monoclonal antibodies has been finding a suitable fusion partner for the B cell—one that has the three important attributes: immortal growth, susceptibility to HAT selection, and inability to secrete its own antibody. The first human hybridomas were produced by fusing human peripheral blood lymphocytes with human myeloma cells. Unlike mouse myeloma cells, these human myeloma cells did not display immortal growth in culture and instead exhibited a short lifespan in culture. So far, only a few human myeloma cell lines have been adapted to long-term culture, and these cells continue to secrete their own antibodies. In addition, the induction of mutations to allow for HAT selection increased the cells' instability. In an attempt to bypass these limitations of human fusion partners, some researchers have fused human B cells with mouse myeloma cells (Ab⁻, HGPRT⁻). These mouse-human hybrids have proved to be unstable, however, rapidly losing their human chromosomes and thus their antibody genes.

One way to circumvent these limitations of human myeloma cells is to avoid them altogether. Normal human B lymphocytes can be transformed with Epstein-Barr virus (EBV). When lymphocytes are cultured with antigen in the presence of EBV, some of the B cells acquire the immortal-growth properties of a transformed cell while continuing to secrete the desired antibody. By cloning such primed, transformed cells, it is possible to obtain human monoclonal antibody.

Uses for Monoclonal Antibodies

The homogeneity and specificity of monoclonal antibodies makes them the reagents of choice for an exponentially growing market of in vitro and in vivo diagnostic and therapeutic products. As of 1990 monoclonal antibodies had been most widely used in the area of in vitro diagnostics tests. In vivo uses of monoclonal antibodies are just beginning, but analysts predict tremendous growth in the area of in vivo diagnostic tests and immunotherapy with sales expected to reach $6 billion by the mid-1990s (Figure 7-6).

Purification of Proteins

Before the advent of monoclonal antibodies, the purification of minor protein components from a complex mixture of proteins often required numerous chromatographic steps and generally had low yields. However, monoclonal antibody can be made to even a minor protein (X) in a complex mixture, since any hybridoma clones that secrete antibody to proteins other than X are eliminated during the screening phase of monoclonal production. Once monoclonal antibody to a particular protein is available, it can be used to purify that protein.

This approach was used by D. S. Secher and D. C. Burke to obtain highly purified preparations of interferon, which previously had been purified from white blood cells to only a 1% purity level (i.e., 99% of the preparation was contaminating protein). In their work, Secher and Burke produced monoclonal antibody to in-

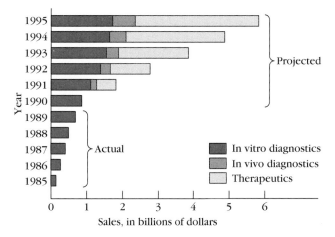

Figure 7-6 Actual and projected sales of monoclonal antibody products used for diagnostic and therapeutic purposes. [Adapted from *Genet. Eng. News*, 1989 (April):5.]

terferon (IFN) using a partially purified preparation to immunize mice. They then attached the anti-IFN monoclonal antibody to beads, thus forming an *immunoadsorbent* column. When they passed a crude IFN preparation through this column, they achieved a 5000-fold increase in interferon purity in a single passage

(Figure 7-7). Large-scale production of interferon is now being performed by a number of biotechnology companies. Interferon is first produced in genetically engineered bacteria, and an anti-IFN immunoadsorbent column is then used to isolate the interferon from the bacterial products and other contaminants.

Identification and Isolation of Lymphocyte Subpopulations and Clones

Monoclonal antibodies can be used to identify and isolate various lymphocyte subpopulations that express characteristic patterns of membrane proteins. Since these proteins reflect the cells' state of differentiation, monoclonal antibodies specific for each of these membrane proteins can be applied to identify the various stages of lymphocyte differentiation. For example, as discussed in previous chapters, T helper cells express CD4 membrane protein and T cytotoxic cells express CD8 membrane protein in both humans and mice. If monoclonal antibodies to CD4 and CD8 are labeled with two different fluorochromes and incubated with a lymphocyte preparation, the T_H cells and T_C cells can then be separated in a fluorescence-activated cell sorter (Figure 7-8); see also Figure 6-6). Alternatively, a given subpopulation can be removed from a preparation by treating the preparation with monoclonal antibody and complement, causing lysis of the cells for which the monoclonal antibody is specific.

Monoclonal antibodies also can be made to cell-membrane proteins that are unique to certain lymphocyte clones. These antibodies, called *clonotypic* monoclonal antibodies, have been useful in the identification of proteins that are unique to a given cell lineage. For example, clonotypic monoclonal antibodies were instrumental in the identification of the T-cell receptor, as is discussed in Chapter 10.

Tumor Detection and Imaging

Monoclonal antibodies can be produced that are specific for certain membrane proteins that are present on tumor cells but are absent (or present at lower levels) on normal cells. The production of these monoclonals is a time-consuming task requiring the screening of large numbers of hybridomas to identify clones secreting antibody specific for tumor-associated antigens. This is illustrated by the work of J. Minna, F. Cuttita, and S. Rosen, who immunized mice with human lung-cancer cells and fused the immunized spleen cells with mouse myeloma cells to generate hybridomas secreting monoclonal antibody to human lung-cancer cells. By screening 20,000 hybridoma clones, they were able to identify 80 clones that

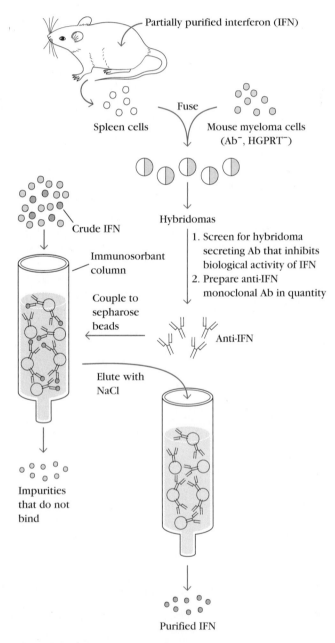

Partially purified interferon (IFN)

Spleen cells

Fuse

Mouse myeloma cells (Ab⁻, HGPRT⁻)

Crude IFN

Hybridomas

1. Screen for hybridoma secreting Ab that inhibits biological activity of IFN
2. Prepare anti-IFN monoclonal Ab in quantity

Immunosorbant column

Couple to sepharose beads

Anti-IFN

Elute with NaCl

Impurities that do not bind

Purified IFN

Figure 7-7   Purification of interferon (IFN) by use of an immunosorbent column. This technique can be used to purify any protein for which a monoclonal antibody is available.

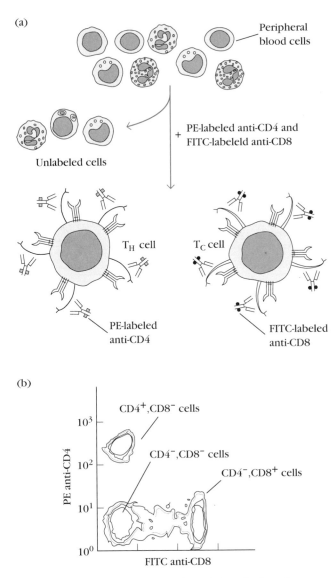

Figure 7-8   Separation of T_H cells and T_C cells from human peripheral blood lymphocytes. (a) Monoclonal antibodies to CD4, which is generally present on T_H cells, and to CD8, which is generally present on T_C cells, are labeled with one of two fluorochromes: phycoerythrin (PE) or fluorescein isothiocyanate (FITC). When the labeled antibodies are incubated with peripheral lymphocytes, the T_H and T_C cells are labeled specifically. (b) Sorting in a FACS reveals three populations of cells, which can be separated.

were specific for various lung-cancer cells and did not react against normal lung cells. One of these monoclonals displayed specificity for small-cell carcinoma of the lung, which accounts for 25% of human lung cancer in the United States. Monoclonal antibodies with such tumor specificity can be used either to detect the spread of tumors or to kill tumor cells.

Certain tumors shed tumor-specific antigen(s) into the blood, and the use of monoclonal antibodies for

detection of such tumors has great potential. For example, in one study monoclonal antibody to a glycolipid antigen shed by colorectal tumors was able to detect this tumor-specific antigen in blood samples from 23 out of 33 patients with advanced colorectal cancer. A monoclonal antibody that detects a shed pancreatic tumor antigen also has been developed. This monoclonal antibody has considerable diagnostic value because the level of this pancreatic tumor antigen in the blood is indicative of the stage of tumor progression. The ability of monoclonal antibody to detect even low levels of this shed tumor antigen may allow early diagnosis of pancreatic cancer, which is not usually diagnosed until an advanced stage.

In another approach, radiolabeled monoclonal antibodies have been used to locate primary or metastatic tumors in patients. For example, monoclonal antibody to breast-cancer cells has been labeled with iodine 131 and introduced into the blood to detect tumor spread to regional lymph nodes. This monoclonal imaging technique can detect breast-cancer metastases that would be undetected by other scanning techniques. Other researchers have labeled monoclonal antibody to breast-cancer cells with the metal gadolinium (Gd), which can be detected by magnetic resonance imaging (MRI) techniques. Following injection of Gd-labeled monoclonal antibody into the blood of breast-cancer patients, pin-head-sized metastases to regional lymph nodes have been visualized.

Although these approaches for detecting and localizing tumors have promise, there are a number of obstacles to widespread use of monoclonal antibodies in tumor detection and imaging. A major problem is that many tumors of a given type, such as breast cancer, do not share common tumor-specific membrane proteins. In one study five monoclonal antibodies to human breast tumors were reacted with breast-cancer biopsy tissue from 45 patients. Most of the biopsy samples reacted with only one of the five antibodies.

Tumor Killing

Monoclonal antibodies can also kill tumor cells, in some cases doing the job directly through complement-mediated lysis. Unconjugated monoclonal antibodies have been used with some success in treating human B-cell lymphomas and T-cell leukemias. In one remarkable study, Ronald Levy and his colleagues successfully treated a 64-year-old man with terminal B-cell lymphoma. At the time of treatment the lymphoma had metastasized to the liver, spleen, bone marrow, and peripheral blood. Because this cancer was of a B cell, the membrane-bound antibody on all the cancerous cells had the same idiotype. These researchers initially fused cancerous B lymphoma cells from the patient with human myeloma cells to obtain a hybridoma secreting the B-lymphoma antibody. This monoclonal antibody bearing the identifying idiotype then served as an antigen to immunize mice, and the mouse spleen cells were fused with mouse myeloma cells. The resulting hybridomas were screened to find one that secreted monoclonal antibody specific for the B-lymphoma idiotype (Figure 7-9). When this mouse monoclonal antibody was injected into the patient, it bound specifically to the B lymphoma cells because these cells expressed that particular idiotype. Since B lymphoma cells are susceptible to complement-mediated lysis, the monoclonal antibody

activated the complement system and lysed the lymphoma cells without harming other cells. After four injections with this anti-idiotype monoclonal antibody, the tumors began to shrink, and as of the last report this patient has been in complete remission.

Although a large number of tumor cells are resistant to complement-mediated lysis, tumor-specific monoclonal antibody can be conjugated to a lethal toxin or a radioisotope to form an *immunotoxin* capable of killing tumor cells. Several toxins lend themselves to this approach, including ricin, *Shigella* toxin, and diphtheria toxin, all of which inhibit protein synthesis and are so potent that a single molecule has been shown to kill a

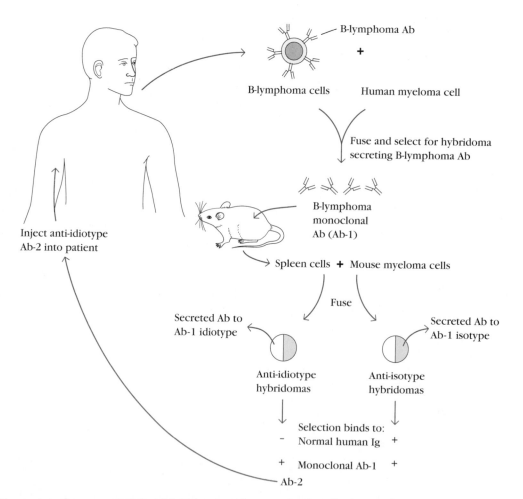

Figure 7-9 Treatment of a man with a B-cell lymphoma with monoclonal antibody specific for idiotypic determinants on the B lymphoma cells. Because all the lymphoma cells are derived from a single transformed B cell, they all express membrane-bound antibody with the same idiotype (i.e., same antigenic specificity). In a two-step procedure, monoclonal antibody against the B-lymphoma idiotype of a patient is produced. When this anti-idiotype antibody (Ab-2) is injected into the patient, it binds to B lymphoma cells, which then are killed by complement-mediated lysis. At least one case in which this approach was successful has been reported.

cell. Each of these toxins consists of two or more functionally distinct polypeptide components, one the toxin itself and the other a ligand that binds to receptors on cell surfaces; without the binding polypeptide the toxin can not get into cells and therefore is harmless. An immunotoxin is prepared by replacing the binding polypeptide with a monoclonal antibody having specificity for a particular tumor cell (Figure 7-10a). In theory, the attached monoclonal antibody will target the toxin specifically to tumor cells, where it will cause cell death by inhibiting protein synthesis (Figure 7-10b). The high toxicity of the toxin is important, since very few molecules of an immunotoxin will actually make contact with the tumor mass. A number of in vitro studies with toxin-conjugated monoclonal antibodies have demonstrated their ability to kill tumor cells without killing normal healthy cells.

Diagnostic Reagents

There are currently over 100 different monoclonal antibody products for detecting pregnancy; diagnosing infectious protozoan, bacterial, and viral pathogens; monitoring therapeutic drug levels; detecting heart damage; matching histocompatibility antigens; detecting diabetes; and detecting tumor cells. Many of these test kits utilize strips of paper impregnated with an appropriate monoclonal antibody. These diagnostic products are highly specific and relatively inexpensive to produce, and many biotechnology companies have entered the field. Monoclonal antibody–based products for detecting diabetes, colorectal cancer, and pregnancy are expected to generate $521 million in sales by 1992. Similar market success has been predicted for monoclonal antibody tests for therapeutic drug monitoring and for drug abuse testing.

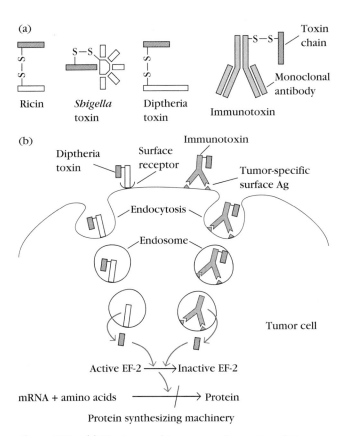

Figure 7-10   (a) Toxins used to prepare immunotoxins include ricin, *Shigella* toxin and diphtheria toxin. Each toxin contains an inhibitor chain and a binding component. To make an immunotoxin, the binding component of the toxin is replaced with a monoclonal antibody. (b) Diphtheria toxin binds to a cell-membrane receptor (*left*) and a diphtheria-immunotoxin binds to a tumor-associated antigen (*right*). In either case the toxin is internalized in an endosome. The toxic chain is then released into the cytoplasm, where it inhibits protein synthesis by catalyzing the inactivation of elongation factor 2 (EF-2).

Engineering Monoclonal Antibodies

When monoclonal antibodies are used as immunotoxins for tumor killing they must generally be given in high concentrations to bind sufficient amounts of antibody to the tumor. However, because these are mouse monoclonal antibodies they are recognized as foreign and evoke an antibody response against the isotypic and idiotypic determinants of the mouse antibody. This results in the formation of complexes of mouse and human antibodies. The buildup of these complexes in organs such as the kidney can cause serious and, in some cases, life-threatening allergic reactions. These undesirable reactions place limitations on the use of mouse monoclonal antibodies for tumor detection and killing in humans. Clearly, one way to overcome at least some of these complications is to use human monoclonal antibodies. However, as discussed previously, the development of human monoclonal antibodies has been hampered by considerable technical difficulties. Because of the problems in producing human monoclonal antibodies and the complications resulting from in vivo use of mouse monoclonal antibodies, researchers have begun engineering monoclonal antibody using recombinant DNA technology.

Chimeric Monoclonal Antibodies

One approach to engineer an antibody is to clone recombinant DNA containing the promoter, leader, and variable-region sequences from a mouse antibody gene and the constant-region exons from a human antibody gene (Figure 7-11). The antibody encoded by such a recombinant gene is a mouse-human chimera. Its antigenic specificity, which is determined by the variable region, is derived from the mouse DNA; its isotype, which is determined by the constant region, is derived from the human DNA (Figure 7-12a). Because their constant regions are encoded by human genes, these chimeras have fewer mouse antigenic determinants and are far less immunogenic when administered to humans.

Because the mouse variable region in the chimeric antibodies can also induce an antibody response in humans, chimeric antibodies containing only mouse CDRs have been developed. In this novel approach, the CDRs of a mouse antibody are grafted together with human framework regions (FRs) to construct a variable region retaining the human β-strand framework with only the hypervariable loops of mouse origin (Figure 7-12b). Since the hypervariable loops comprise the antigen-binding site, it is sometimes possible for these engineered antibodies to retain their antigen-binding specificity. So far, three different antibodies have been engineered by this approach and have been shown to retain the antigen-binding specificity of the original mouse monoclonal antibody. These antibodies are less

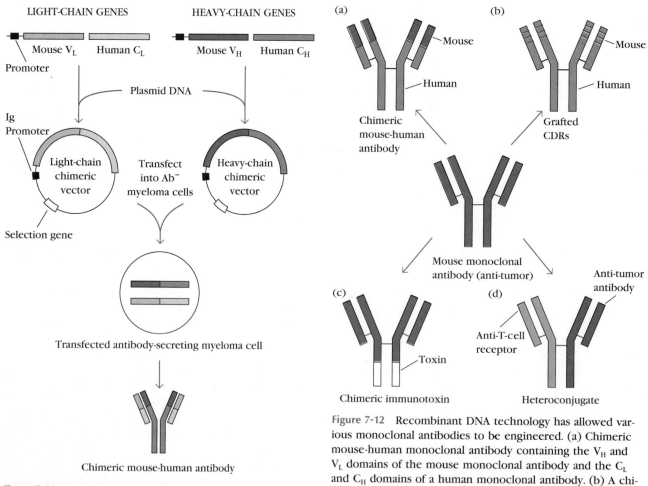

Figure 7-11 Production of chimeric mouse-human monoclonal antibodies. Chimeric mouse-human heavy- and light-chain λ expression vectors are produced. These vectors are transfected into myeloma cells that are Ab⁻. Culture in ampicillin medium selects for transfected myeloma cells, which secrete the chimeric antibody. [Adapted from M. Verhoeyen and L. Reichmann, 1988, *BioEssays* **8**:74.]

Figure 7-12 Recombinant DNA technology has allowed various monoclonal antibodies to be engineered. (a) Chimeric mouse-human monoclonal antibody containing the V_H and V_L domains of the mouse monoclonal antibody and the C_L and C_H domains of a human monoclonal antibody. (b) A chimeric monoclonal antibody containing only the CDRs of a mouse monoclonal antibody grafted within the framework regions of a human monoclonal antibody. (c) A chimeric monoclonal antibody in which the terminal Fc domain is replaced by a toxin. (d) A heteroconjugate in which one-half of the molecule is specific for a tumor antigen and the other half is specific for the CD3/T-cell receptor complex.

immunogenic in humans than the mouse-human chimeric antibodies containing the entire mouse variable region.

The chimera approach also can be used to engineer an antibody with a constant region possessing a given biological effector function. For example, the $\gamma 1$ constant region in humans is very effective at mediating complement lysis. By engineering antitumor antibodies with a $\gamma 1$ constant region, it is hoped that complement-mediated destruction of tumor cells can be enhanced. Another approach has been to replace the terminal constant-region domain with a toxin (Figure 7-12c). These antibodies serve as immunotoxins, and because they lack the terminal domain of the Fc, they are not able to bind to cells bearing Fc receptors.

Monoclonal Antibody Heteroconjugates

Heteroconjugates are hybrids of two different antibody molecules (Figure 7-12d). Various heteroconjugates have been designed in which one half of the antibody has specificity for a tumor and the other half has specificity for a surface molecule on an immune effector cell, such as a NK cell, an activated macrophage, or a CTL. The heteroconjugate thus serves to crosslink the immune effector cell to the tumor. Some heteroconjugates have been designed to activate the immune effector cell when it is crosslinked to the tumor cell. For example, the T-cell receptor is always expressed as a complex with an associated membrane molecule, CD3 which is involved in signal transduction. Heteroconjugates consisting of anti-CD3 and an antitumor monoclonal antibody have been shown to crosslink CTLs to tumor cells. Not only does the heteroconjugate crosslink the CTL to the tumor cell, but it also appears to activate the CTL so that it begins to mediate tumor-cell destruction.

Generation of Monoclonal Antibodies from Immunoglobulin-Gene Libraries

Recently a new technology has been developed for generating monoclonal antibodies without hybridomas or even immunization. In this approach, the polymerase chain reaction is used to amplify the DNA encoding antibody heavy-chain and light-chain Fab fragments from hybridoma cells or plasma cells (see Figure 2-8). Separate heavy- and light-chain libraries are constructed in bacteriophage λ. Each heavy- and light-chain construct contains an EcoRI restriction site, downstream for the heavy chain and upstream for the light chain. By cleaving with EcoRI and joining the heavy and light chains, numerous random heavy-light combinations are obtained (Figure 7-13). This procedure generates an enormous diversity of antibody combinations; clones containing these random combinations can be rapidly screened for those secreting antibody to a particular antigen. For example, in one study a million clones were screened in just 2 days, with over 100 being identified that produced antibody specific for the desired antigen. The technique has the potential of producing an enormous repertoire of antibody specificities without the limitations of antigen priming and hybridoma technology that currently complicate the production of monoclonal antibodies.

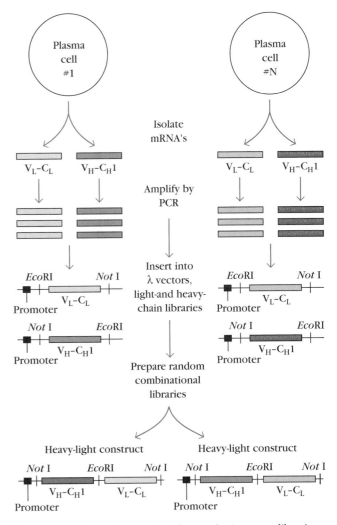

Figure 7-13 General procedure for producing gene libraries encoding Fab fragments. In this procedure isolated heavy- and light-chain genes are amplified by the polymerase chain reaction (PCR). Random combinations of heavy- and light-chain genes generate an enormous number of heavy-light constructs encoding Fab fragments. [Adapted from W. D. Huse et al., 1989, Science 246:1275.]

Catalytic Monoclonal Antibodies (Abzymes)

The binding of an antibody to its antigen is similar in many ways to the binding of an enzyme to its substrate. In both cases the binding involves weak, noncovalent interactions and exhibits high specificity and often high affinity. What distinguishes an antibody-antigen interaction from an enzyme-substrate interaction is that the antibody does not alter the antigen, whereas the enzyme catalyzes a chemical change in its substrate. The enzyme uses its binding energy to stabilize the transition state of the substrate, thus reducing the activation energy for chemical modification of the substrate.

Because of the similarities between antigen-antibody interactions and enzyme-substrate interactions, R. A. Lerner and his colleagues wondered whether some antibodies might behave like enzymes and catalyze chemical reactions. To investigate this possibility, they produced a hapten-carrier complex in which the hapten structurally resembled the transition state of an ester undergoing hydrolysis (Figure 7-14). Using this conjugate, they generated antihapten monoclonal antibodies. When these monoclonal antibodies were incubated with the ester substrate, some of them accelerated hydrolysis by about 1000-fold; that is, they acted like the enzyme that normally catalyzes the substrate's hydrolysis. The catalytic activity of these antibodies was highly specific, as they hydrolyzed only esters whose transition-state structure closely resembled that of the hapten in the immunizing conjugate.

Catalytic monoclonal antibodies have been generated that catalyze ester hydrolysis and carbonate hydrolysis. These antibodies have been called *abzymes* in reference to their dual role as antibody and enzyme.

The development of immunoglobulin-gene libraries was pioneered by Lerner to produce an enormous antibody repertoire without the requirement of antigen priming, so that large numbers of antibodies could be screened for their catalytic activity. As more and more abzymes are generated by this method, it may be possible to produce a battery of abzymes that cut peptide bonds at specific amino acid residues, much as restriction enzymes cut DNA at specific sites. Such enzymes would be invaluable tools in facilitating structural and functional analysis of proteins. Additionally, it may be possible to generate abzymes with the ability to dissolve blood clots or to cleave viral glycoproteins at specific sites, thus blocking viral infectivity. Abzymes are likely to represent a major technological advance that will impact on various branches of science in the coming years.

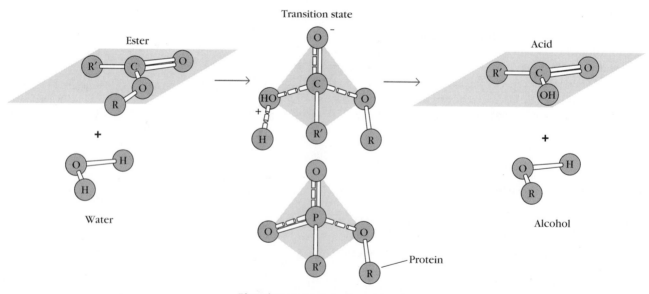

Figure 7-14 Because of its tetrahedral shape and partial negative charge, a phosphonate ester (PE) is an analog of the unstable transition state of an ester undergoing hydrolysis. Anti-PE monoclonal antibodies have been obtained by immunizing mice with a PE-carrier conjugate. Some of these anti-PE antibodies catalyze ester hydrolysis, presumably by binding to and stabilizing the transition state. [Adapted from R. A. Lerner and A. Tramontano, 1988, *Sci. Am.* **258**:58.]

T-Cell Hybridomas

The hybridomas discussed so far are produced by fusion of primed B cells with cancerous plasma cells; these B-cell hybridomas secrete monoclonal antibody. T-cell hybridomas can be produced by fusing primed T cells with cancerous T cells (called thymoma cells) in a similar procedure. T-cell hybridomas do not secrete antibody, but rather possess other immunologic functions (e.g., secretion of lymphokines and expression of T-cell receptors with specificity for antigen-MHC). Antigen-specific T helper, suppressor, and cytotoxic hybridomas have all been cloned and have facilitated the identification of various T-cell–specific molecules. For example, an ovalbumin-specific, class II MHC–restricted T-cell hybridoma was used to identify the T-cell receptor for antigen (see Chapter 10). This particular T-cell hybridoma was produced by fusing a T_H cell specific for ovalbumin with a T-cell thymoma. The resulting hybridoma, which displayed the antigenic specificity and MHC restriction of the parent T_H cell, could be assayed for T_H function by its capacity to secrete interleukin 2 in response to ovalbumin on an appropriate antigen-presenting cell. Because T-cell hybridomas grow as tumors, large cell numbers can be attained within a short period of time; this property has facilitated the biochemical isolation and purification of various T-cell products, including several T-cell lymphokines.

Summary

1. With the technique of cell fusion and HAT-medium selection, primed splenic lymphocytes can be fused with mouse myeloma cells (HGPRT$^-$, Ab$^-$). These hybrid cells, called B-cell hybridomas, continue to secrete the specific antibody of the primed B cell but possess the immortal-growth properties of the myeloma cell.

2. Unlike polyclonal antibodies, a monoclonal antibody is a homogeneous preparation specific for a single epitope on a complex antigen.

3. Monoclonal antibodies have been used to purify antigens, to detect cellular subpopulations, and to detect and kill specific tumor cells. In addition, monoclonal antibodies are presently used in over 100 diagnostic tests.

4. Recombinant DNA technology has been used to engineer chimeric monoclonal antibodies consisting of the mouse variable regions and human constant regions. These chimeras do not elicit an anti-isotype response when injected into humans.

5. Monoclonal Fab fragments have been produced by random combination of heavy- and light-chain gene libraries constructed in bacteriophage λ. This procedure allows the production of monoclonal antibodies without antigen priming or hybridoma technology.

6. Several catalytic monoclonal antibodies, or abzymes, have been identified. Future screening of large numbers of monoclonal antibodies generated from immunoglobulin-gene libraries may identify other abzymes with useful catalytic functions.

7. T-cell hybridomas, produced by fusion of primed T cells with T-cell thymomas, have been useful in isolating and purifying various cytokines secreted by T cells.

References

DE YOUNG, G. 1986. Monoclonal antibodies: promises fulfilled. *High Technology* (Feb.):32.

HUSE, W. D., L. SASTRY, S. A. IVERSON, A.S. KING et. al. 1989. Generation of a large combinatorial library of the immunoglobulin repertoire in phage lambda. *Science* **246**:1275.

JUNG, G., and H. J. MULLER EBERHARD, 1988. An in vitro model for tumor immunotherapy with antibody heteroconjugates. *Immunol. Today* **9**:257.

KOHLER, G., and C. MILSTEIN. 1975. Continuous cultures of fused cells secreting antibody of predefined specificity. *Nature* **256**:495.

LERNER, R. A., and S. J. BENKOVIC. 1988. Principles of antibody catalysis. *BioEssays* **9**:107.

LIU, A. Y., R. R. ROBINSON, K. E. HELLSTROM, E. D. MURRAY JR. et al. 1987. Chimeric mouse-human IgG1 antibody that can mediate lysis of cancer cells. *Proc. Natl. Acad. Sci. USA* **84**:3439.

MARX, J. 1982. Monoclonal antibodies in cancer. *Science* **216**:283.

MILSTEIN, C. 1980. Monoclonal antibodies. *Sci. Am.* **243**:66.

MORRISON, S. L., and V. T. OI. 1989. Genetically engineered antibody molecules. *Adv. Immunol.* **44**:65.

OLSNES, O., K. SANDVIG, O. W. PETERSEN, and B. VAN DEURS. 1989. Immunotoxins-entry into cells and mechanisms of action. *Immunol. Today* **10**:291.

REICHMAN, L., M. CLARK, H. WALDMANN, and G. WINTER. 1988. Reshaping human antibodies for therapy. *Nature* **332**:323.

VERHOEYEN, M., and L. RIECHMANN. 1988. Engineering of antibodies. *BioEssays* **8**:74.

Study Questions

1. Indicate whether each of the following statements is true or false. If you think a statement is false, explain why.

    a. An HGPRT$^-$ myeloma cell requires hypoxanthine for growth.

    b. When a heterokaryon initially is formed, it is multinucleated.

    c. Chromosome loss from heterokaryons occurs randomly.

    d. Hypoxanthine is added to HAT medium to prevent cell growth by the salvage pathway.

    e. An HGPRT$^+$ revertant myeloma cell would be a good fusion partner for production of B-cell hybridomas because it would not be able to grow in HAT medium.

2. The myeloma cells used in the production of B-cell hybridomas have three properties that make them suitable fusion partners. List these properties and explain why they are necessary for the production of hybridomas that secrete B-cell antibodies.

3. What would be the consequences if you omitted aminopterin from the HAT medium used to select hybridomas in the standard procedure for producing monoclonal antibodies.

4. In order to treat a patient with terminal B-cell lymphoma, Levy and his coworkers produced two hybridomas. One hybridoma was obtained by fusing B lymphoma cells from the patient with human myeloma cells; the other was obtained by fusing primed mouse spleen cells with mouse myeloma cells.

    a. What is the purpose in producing these two hybridomas and what was the desired monoclonal antibody secreted by each?

    b. Outline a screening assay for identifying hybridomas that produce the desired monoclonal antibody. What kind of control should be included in the screening assay?

5. You immunize a mouse with human interleukin 2 (IL-2) and purify the antibodies against IL-2 from its serum. List three ways in which these antibodies differ from a monoclonal antibody specific for IL-2.

6. Polyclonal antibodies usually precipitate soluble protein antigens, whereas monoclonal antibodies to the same protein antigens often fail to do so. What might account for this difference?

7. Although monoclonal antibodies are by definition reactive with a single antigenic determinant, they sometimes react with more than one antigen. Explain this finding.

8. You have produced a monoclonal antibody that binds to a particular protein antigen, as determined by a solid-phase ELISA. Even though this antibody has a high affinity for the antigen, why might it fail to react in (a) an immunodiffusion assay, (b) a Western-blot assay, and (c) a tube precipitation assay.

9. You produced a monoclonal antibody to HIV and suspect that it has been stolen by a colleague and is now being marketed by a biotechnology company. You want to prove that the company's product is the same as the monoclonal antibody that you isolated.

    a. Describe quick and inexpensive immunologic tests that you could perform to determine if the two antibodies might be identical.

    b. Assuming these initial tests suggest that the two antibodies are identical, what more expensive and time-consuming procedures could you use to demonstrate unequivocally whether or not the two antibodies are the same?

10. You fuse spleen cells with myeloma-cell preparations differing in their immunoglobulin heavy-chain (HC) and light-chain (LC) genotype. Predict how many different types of antibody would be produced by hybridomas formed from myeloma fusion partners having the following genotypes: (a) HC$^+$, LC$^+$ (b) HC$^-$, LC$^+$; and (c) HC$^-$, LC$^-$. In each case, diagram the chain structure of the various antibodies, indicating whether the chains originate from the spleen (s) or myeloma (m) fusion partner.

11. An immunotoxin is prepared by conjugating a monoclonal antibody specific for a tumor antigen with diphtheria toxin. If the antibody part of the immunotoxin is degraded in vivo and the toxin is not, will normal cells be killed?

CHAPTER

8

Organization and Expression of Immunoglobulin Genes

One of the most remarkable features of the vertebrate immune system is its ability to respond to an apparently limitless array of foreign antigens. As immunoglobulin-sequence data accumulated, virtually every antibody molecule studied was found to contain a unique amino acid sequence in its variable region but only one of a limited number of invariant sequences in its constant region. An understanding of the genetic basis of such tremendous variation, and at the same time constancy within a single protein molecule, came from studies showing that in germ-line DNA, multiple gene segments encode a single immunoglobulin heavy or light chain. These gene segments are carried in the germ cells but cannot be transcribed and translated into heavy and light chains until they are arranged into functional genes. During B-cell differentiation in the bone marrow, these gene segments are randomly shuffled by a dynamic genetic system capable of generating more than 10^8 specificities. This process is carefully regulated: B-cell differentiation from an immature pre-B cell to a mature cell involves an ordered progression of immunoglobulin-gene rearrangements. By the end of this process a mature, immunocompetent B cell will contain a single, functional variable-region DNA sequence for its heavy chain, and a single, functional variable-region DNA sequence for its light chain, so that the individual B cell is antigenically committed to a specific epitope. After antigenic stimulation, further rearrangement of constant-region gene segments can generate changes in the isotype expressed and consequently changes in the associated biological effector functions without changing the specificity of the immunoglobulin molecule (Table 8-1).

This chapter describes the detailed organization of the immunoglobulin genes, the process of gene rearrangement, and the role of differential RNA processing of the primary transcript in the expression of immunoglobulin genes. The relationship of gene rearrangements to various stages in B-cell differentiation also is explored. Finally, the various mechanisms by which the dynamic immunoglobulin genetic system generates more than 10^8 different antibody specificities are discussed.

Development of a Genetic Model Compatible with Immunoglobulin Structure

The results of the immunoglobulin-sequencing studies discussed in Chapter 5 revealed a number of features of immunoglobulin structure that were difficult to reconcile with classic genetic models. Any viable model of the immunoglobulin genes has to account for (a) the vast diversity of antibody specificities, (b) the presence of a variable region at the amino-terminal end and of a

Table 8-1 Sequence of B-lymphocyte maturation and antigen-induced differentiation

	Stem cell	Pre-B cell	Immature B cell
Site of maturation	Bone marrow	Bone marrow	Bone marrow
Immunoglobulin expressed	None	Cytoplasmic μ heavy chain	Membrane IgM (κ or λ light chain)
Isotype switching	—	—	—
Role of antigen	—	—	—

	Mature B cell	Activated B cell	Plasma cell
Site of maturation	Periphery	Periphery	Periphery
Immunoglobulin expressed	Membrane IgM + IgD	Membrane Ig low level secreted Ig	Low level membrane Ig; high level secreted Ig
Isotype switching	—	+	+
Role of antigen	—	+	+

constant region at the carboxyl-terminal end of heavy and light chains, and (c) the existence of isotypes with the same antigenic specificity, which result from the association of a given variable region with different heavy-chain constant regions.

Problems Faced by Classical Genetic Models

It has been estimated that the mammalian immune system can generate more than 10^8 different antibody specificities, allowing an animal to respond to a vast number of potential antigens. Since antibodies are proteins and proteins are encoded by genes, it follows that this tremendous diversity in antibody structure must arise from a genetic system capable of generating tremendous diversity. For several decades immunologists sought to imagine a genetic mechanism that might generate such diversity. There emerged two very different sets of theories to explain the observed variability in antibody specificity at the gene level. The *germ-line* theories maintained that the genome contains a large repertoire of immunoglobulin genes sufficient to generate more than 10^8 different antibody specificities; thus no special genetic mechanisms were invoked to account for antibody diversity in these theories. In contrast, the *somatic-variation* theories maintained that the genome contains a relatively small number of immunoglobulin genes from which a large number of antibody specificities are generated in the somatic cells by mutational or recombinational mechanisms.

As the amino acid sequences of more and more immunoglobulins were determined, it became clear that there was a need not only for a mechanism for generating antibody diversity but also for some means of maintaining constancy. In other words, whether diversity was generated by germline or somatic mechanisms, a paradox remained: how could stability be maintained in the constant (C) region while some kind of diversifying mechanism generated the variable (V) region? Germline proponents found it difficult to account for an evolutionary mechanism that could generate diversity in the variable part of each gene while preserving the constant region unchanged. Somatic-variation proponents found it difficult to conceive of a mechanism that could diversify the variable region of a single gene in the somatic cells by mutation or recombination without allowing a single alteration in the amino acid sequence encoded by the constant region.

The third structural feature of immunoglobulins requiring an explanation was first recognized when amino acid sequencing of a human myeloma protein called Til revealed that identical variable-region sequences were associated with both γ and μ heavy-chain constant regions. A similar phenomenon was observed in rabbits by C. Todd, who found that a particular allotypic marker in the heavy-chain variable region could be associated with α, γ, and μ heavy-chain constant regions. Considerable additional evidence has confirmed that a single variable-region sequence, defining a particular antigenic specificity, can be associated with multiple heavy-chain constant-region sequences; in other words, different classes, or isotypes, of antibody (e.g., IgG, IgM) can be expressed having identical variable-region sequences.

Dryer and Bennett Genetic Model

In an attempt to develop a genetic model consistent with these findings about the structure of immunoglobulins, W. Dryer and J. Bennett suggested, in their classic theoretical paper of 1965, that two separate genes encode a single immunoglobulin heavy or light chain, one gene encoding the V region and one gene encoding the C region. They suggested that these two genes must somehow come together at the DNA level to form a continuous message that can be transcribed and translated to yield a single heavy or light protein chain. Moreover, they proposed that hundreds or thousands of V-region genes were carried in the germ line, whereas only single copies of C-region class and subclass genes need exist. The strength of this type of recombinational model (which combined elements of the germ-line and somatic-variation theories) was that it allowed for the great diversity of antibody specificities in the variable region while conserving invariant constant-region sequences to provide necessary biological effector functions. It suggested a way for a single V gene to join with various C-region genes and also for the association of innumerable V-region genes with a single C gene.

If Dryer and Bennett were correct and two genes did encode a single immunoglobulin heavy and light chain, the first question to be addressed was whether joining took place at the DNA, RNA, or protein level. Dryer and Bennett proposed that V-C joining occurred at the DNA level. Certainly, joining at the protein level was an unlikely prospect, since classical peptide-bond formation was never observed between two protein chains after translation. Evidence that joining was in fact not at the protein level came from experiments in which plasma cells were briefly incubated and pulse-labeled with radioactive amino acids. The immunoglobulin heavy and light chains were then isolated, and the location of the radioactive amino acids in the newly synthesized chains was determined. The results showed that the maximal radioactivity was at the carboxyl-terminal end of each chain, proving that complete heavy and light chains are translated without interruption from the amino terminus of the V region to the carboxyl terminus of the C region. If V-C joining had taken place during translation, the incorporated radioactivity should have shown two peaks: one at the carboxyl-terminal end of the C region and one at the carboxyl-terminal end of the V region. This was not the case, thus ruling out joining at the protein level. There remained the question of whether joining was accomplished at the RNA or DNA level.

At first, support for the Dryer and Bennett hypothesis was indirect. The model could account for those immunoglobulins in which a single V region was combined with various C regions. By postulating a single constant-region gene for each immunoglobulin class and subclass, the model also could account for the conservation of necessary biological effector functions while allowing for evolutionary diversification of variable-region genes. Early studies of DNA hybridization kinetics using a radioactive constant-region DNA probe indicated that the probe hybridized with only one or two genes, confirming the model's prediction that only one or two copies of each constant-region class and subclass gene existed. Yet the evidence in support of the Dryer and Bennett model continued to be indirect, and there was stubborn resistance to their hypothesis in the scientific community. The suggestion that two genes coded a single polypeptide contradicted the existing one gene–one polypeptide principle and was without precedent in any system in cell or molecular biology.

As so often is the case in science, theoretical and intellectual understanding of immunoglobulin-gene organization progressed ahead of the available methodology. Although the Dryer and Bennett model provided a theoretical framework for reconciling the dilemma between immunoglobulin-sequence data and gene organization, actual validation of their hypothesis had to wait for several major technological advances in the field of molecular biology. These advances, described in Chapter 2, included mRNA isolation and purification, restriction-endonuclease cleavage of DNA, nucleic acid hybridization by Southern or Northern blotting, DNA cloning, DNA sequencing, and gene transfer by transfection or transgenic techniques. In time, the Dryer and Bennett hypothesis was proved to be essentially correct. Indeed, far more complex genetic mechanisms have been shown to be involved than could ever have been imagined at the time that Dryer and Bennett published their paper.

Early Verification of the Dryer and Bennett Hypothesis

In 1976 S. Tonegawa and N. Hozumi provided the first direct evidence that separate genes encode the V and C regions and are rearranged in the course of B-cell differentiation. Their experimental approach was to cleave DNA from embryonic cells and from adult myeloma cells into fragments with various restriction endonucleases. These fragments were then separated by size by means of agarose gel electrophoresis and analyzed for their ability to hybridize with a radiolabeled κ-chain mRNA probe. The results showed that two separate restriction fragments from the embryonic DNA hybridized with the mRNA, whereas only a single restriction fragment of the myeloma DNA hybridized with the probe (Figure 8-1). The interpretation of these results by Tonegawa and Hozumi was that during differentiation of lymphocytes from the embryonic state to the fully differentiated plasma-cell stage (represented in their system by myeloma cells), there is a rearrangement of the V and C genes. In the embryo the V and C genes are separated by a large distance containing a restriction endonuclease site, but in the differentiated myeloma cells the V and C genes occupy a single restriction fragment, showing that during differentiation the DNA is

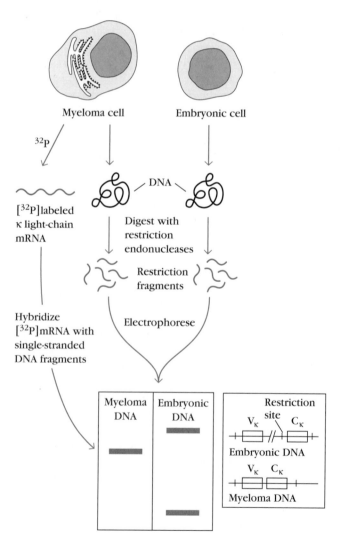

rearranged in such a way as to bring the V and C chains closer together.

Later experiments used an approach similar to that taken by Tonegawa and Hozumi but used the newly developed technique of Southern blotting. The restriction DNA fragments no longer needed to be eluted from the gel slices and instead were transferred by blotting onto nitrocellulose. The arrangement of the kappa, lambda, and heavy-chain genes of non-B cell lineage cells (including embryonic cells and liver cells) was compared to the arrangement of B-cell lineage cells (represented by the myeloma cell) by Southern blot analysis with their respective radiolabeled mRNA probes. In each case the variable- and constant-region genes of the embryonic DNA were shown to be separated by a large distance containing a restriction enzyme site and therefore the respective radiolabeled mRNA probes hybridized with two bands: one band containing the variable-region sequence and one band containing the constant region sequence. In the fully differentiated plasma cell stage (represented by the myeloma cell), the variable- and constant-region genes had rearranged and were now together on a single restriction DNA fragment and therefore the radiolabeled mRNA probe hybridized with a single band. These results demonstrated that the Dryer and Bennett two-gene model—one gene encoding the variable region and one gene encoding the constant region—applied to both heavy- and light-chain genes.

Multigene Organization of Immunoglobulin Genes

As cloning and sequencing of the light- and heavy-chain DNA was accomplished, even greater complexity was revealed than had been predicted by Dryer and Bennett. The κ and λ light chains and the heavy chains are en-

Figure 8-1 Experimental demonstration that the genes encoding κ light chains are rearranged during B-cell development. DNA isolated from embryonic cells and from myeloma cells, which are equivalent to differentiated plasma cells, was digested with restriction endonucleases and separated by size by agarose gel electrophoresis. The electrophoretic gel was then cut into slices and the DNA fragments were eluted from the slice, denatured into single-stranded DNA, and analyzed by hybridization with a [^{32}P] labeled mRNA encoding κ light chains. The mRNA probe hybridized with two bands from the embryonic DNA but with only a single band from the myeloma DNA. This finding indicates that in embryonic cells the κ exons (presumably V and C exons) are separated by a long stretch of DNA containing a restriction-enzyme cleavage site, whereas in myeloma cells the κ exons are closer together and are not separated by a restriction-enzyme cleavage site (inset). [Adapted from N. Hozumi and S. Tonegawa, 1976, *Proc. Natl. Acad. Sci. USA* **73**:3628.]

Table 8-2 Chromosomal locations of immunoglobulin genes in human and mouse

	Chromosome	
Gene	Human	Mouse
λ Light chain	22	16
κ Light chain	2	6
Heavy chain	14	12

coded by separate multigene families situated on different chromosomes (Table 8-2). Each of these multigene families contains a series of coding sequences, called *gene segments*. The κ and λ light-chain families contain L, V, J, and C gene segments; the heavy-chain family contains L, V, D, J, and C gene segments. Functional immunoglobulin genes are generated during B-cell maturation by a process, to be described later, whereby the gene segments are rearranged and brought together. The rearranged VJ gene segments encode the variable region of the light chains; the rearranged VDJ gene segments encode the variable region of the heavy chain. The C gene segments encode the constant regions of the light or heavy chains. The L gene segment encodes a short leader peptide that guides the heavy or light chain through the endoplasmic reticulum but is cleaved before assembly of the finished immunoglobulin molecule; thus amino acids corresponding to L gene segments do not appear in light and heavy chains.

λ-Chain Multigene Family

The first evidence that the light-chain variable region was actually encoded by two gene segments was provided when Tonegawa cloned the germ-line gene encoding the variable region of mouse λ light chain and determined the complete nucleotide sequence. When the nucleotide sequence was compared with the known amino acid sequence of the λ-chain variable region, an unusual discrepancy was observed. Although the first 97 amino acids of the λ-chain variable region corresponded to the nucleotide codon sequence, the remaining 13 carboxyl-terminal amino acids of the protein's variable region did not correspond to the sequential nucleotide sequence. It turned out that a separate, 39-bp gene segment, called J for joining, encoded the remaining 13 amino acids of the λ-chain variable region. Thus a functional λ variable-region gene contains two coding segments—a 5' V segment and a 3' J segment—which are separated in unrearranged germ-line DNA.

(a) λ-chain DNA

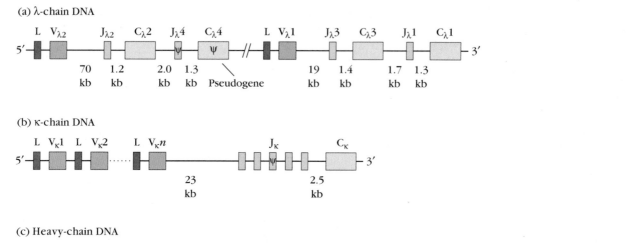

(b) κ-chain DNA

(c) Heavy-chain DNA

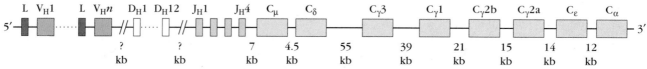

Figure 8-2   Germ-line organization of (a) λ light-chain, (b) κ light-chain, and (c) heavy-chain gene segments in the mouse. The λ and κ light chains are encoded by L, V, J, and C gene segments. The heavy chain is encoded by L, V, D, J, and C gene segments. The V and J gene segments of the light chain and the V, D, and J gene segments of the heavy chain are separated in the germ-line DNA. Boxes with symbol ψ indicate nonfunctional pseudogenes.

The λ multigene family in the mouse contains two V_λ gene segments, four J_λ gene segments, and four C_λ gene segments (Figure 8-2a). The $J_\lambda 4$ and $C_\lambda 4$ gene segments are defective genes, called pseudogenes, which are indicated with the psi symbol (ψ). The V_λ and J_λ gene segments encode the variable region of the λ light chain; the C_λ gene segments encode the constant regions of the three λ-chain subtypes (λ_1, λ_2, and λ_3).

κ-Chain Multigene Family

The κ-chain multigene family in the mouse contains approximately 300 V_κ gene segments, each with an adjacent leader sequence a short distance upstream (i.e., on the 5′ side). There are five J_κ gene segments (one of which is a nonfunctional pseudogene) and a single C_κ gene segment (Figure 8-2b). As in the λ multigene family, the V_κ and J_κ gene segments encode the variable region of the κ light chain, and the C_κ gene segment encodes the constant region. Since there is only one C_κ gene segment, there are no subclasses of κ light chains. Comparison of Figure 8-2a and b shows that the arrangement of the gene segments is quite different in the κ and λ gene families.

Heavy-Chain Multigene Family

The organization of the mouse immunoglobulin heavy-chain genes is similar to but more complex than that of the κ and λ light-chain genes (Figure 8-2c). An additional gene segment encodes part of the heavy-chain variable region. The existence of this gene segment was first proposed by Leroy Hood and his colleagues, who compared the heavy-chain variable-region amino acid sequence with the V_H and J_H nucleotide sequences. The V_H gene segment was found to encode amino acids 1 to 101 and the J_H gene segment was found to encode amino acids 107 to 123; however, neither of these gene segments carried the information to encode amino acids 102 to 106. When the nucleotide sequence was determined for rearranged myeloma DNA and compared with the germ-line DNA sequence, an additional nucleotide sequence was observed between the V_H and J_H gene segments. This nucleotide sequence corresponded to amino acids 102 to 106 of the heavy chain. Hood proposed that a third germ-line gene segment must join with the V_H and J_H gene segments to encode the entire variable region of the heavy chain. Because this gene segment encoded amino acids within the third complementarity-determining region (CDR3), it was designated

D, for diversity, in reference to its contribution to the generation of antibody diversity. Tonegawa and his colleagues located the D gene segments within mouse germ-line DNA with a cDNA D-region probe, which hybridized with a stretch of DNA lying between the V_H and J_H gene segments.

The heavy-chain multigene family on chromosome 12 in the mouse has an estimated 300–1000 V_H gene segments, located an as-yet-unknown distance upstream to a cluster of about 12 D_H gene segments. As with the light-chain genes, each V_H gene segment has a leader sequence a short distance upstream from it. Downstream from the D_H gene segments are four J_H gene segments, followed by a series of C_H gene segments. Each C_H gene segment encodes the constant region of an immunoglobulin heavy-chain isotype. The C_H gene segments are organized into a series of coding exons and noncoding introns. Each exon encodes a separate domain of the heavy-chain constant region (see Figure 5-6b).

The conservation of important biological effector functions of the antibody molecule is maintained by the limited number of heavy-chain constant-region genes. In the mouse the C_H gene segments are arranged sequentially in the following order: C_μ-C_δ-$C_\gamma 3$-$C_\gamma 1$-$C_\gamma 2b$-$C_\gamma 2a$-C_ε-C_α. This sequential arrangement is no accident; it is generally related to the developmental appearance of the immunoglobulin classes in the course of an immune response. During B-cell differentiation there are notable changes in the class of immunoglobulin expressed, while the specificity remains the same. The changes are accomplished by DNA rearrangements mediating class switching, which will be discussed in a later section.

Variable-Region Gene Rearrangements

The previous sections have shown that the assembly of functional chains encoding immunoglobulin light and heavy chains involves recombinational events at the DNA level. Variable-region gene rearrangements occur in an ordered sequence during B-cell maturation in the bone marrow. The heavy-chain variable-region genes rearrange first, then the light-chain variable-region genes. At the end of this process, each B cell contains a single, functional variable-region DNA sequence for its heavy chain and a single, functional variable-region DNA sequence for its light chain. In other words, this process leads to generation of mature, immunocompetent B cells each of which is antigenically committed to a single epitope and expresses membrane-bound antibody on its surface. As is discussed in the next section, rearrangement of heavy-chain constant-region genes occurs later, generating changes in the immunoglobulin class expressed by a B cell without changing its antigenic specificity. Although variable-region gene rearrangements occur in an ordered sequence, they are random events that result in the random determination of B-cell specificity. The order, mechanism, and consequences of these rearrangements are described in this section.

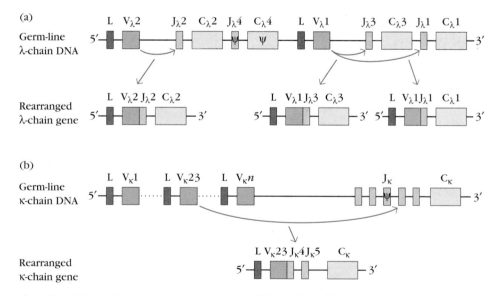

Figure 8-3 Examples of variable-region gene rearrangements in λ light-chain (a) and κ light-chain (b) germ-line DNA. Lambda light chain rearrangement can join $V_\lambda 2$ with $J_\lambda 2$ or it can join $V_\lambda 1$ with either $J_\lambda 1$ or $J_\lambda 3$. Kappa light chain gene rearrangements can join any one of the V_κ gene segments with any one of the four functional J_κ segments. In this case $V_\kappa 23$ has joined J 4.

V-J Rearrangements in Light-Chain DNA

Expression of both λ and κ light chains requires rearrangement of the variable-region V and J gene segments. In the case of the λ light chain, DNA rearrangement can join the $V_\lambda 1$ gene segment with either the $J_\lambda 1$ or $J_\lambda 3$ gene segments, or the $V_\lambda 2$ gene segment can be joined with the $J_\lambda 2$ gene segment. In the case of the κ light chain, any one of the estimated 300 V_κ gene segments can be joined with any one of the four functional J_κ gene segments. Rearranged κ and λ light-chain genes consist of a short leader (L) gene segment, followed by an intervening noncoding DNA sequence (intron), followed by the joined VJ gene segment, followed again by an intron and finally by the C gene segment (Figure 8-3). Upstream from the leader gene segment is a promoter sequence. The rearranged light-chain sequence is transcribed by RNA polymerase from the L segment through the C gene segment, generating a light-chain primary RNA transcript (Figure 8-4). The introns in the primary transcript are removed by RNA-processing enzymes, and the resulting light-chain messenger RNA then exits from the nucleus. The light-chain mRNA binds to polyribosomes and is translated into the light-chain protein. The leader sequence at the amino terminus pulls the growing polypeptide chain into the lumen of the rough endoplasmic reticulum and is then cleaved and is therefore absent from the finished light-chain protein product.

V-D-J Rearrangements in Heavy-Chain DNA

Generation of a functional immunoglobulin heavy-chain gene requires two separate rearrangement events within the variable region. As illustrated in Figure 8-5, a D_H gene segment first joins to a J_H segment; the resulting $D_H J_H$ segment then moves next to and joins a V_H segment to generate a $V_H D_H J_H$ unit that encodes the entire variable region. In heavy-chain DNA, variable-region rearrangement produces a rearranged gene consisting of the following sequences starting from the 5' end: a short L segment, an intron, a joined VDJ segment, another intron, and a series of C gene segments. As with the

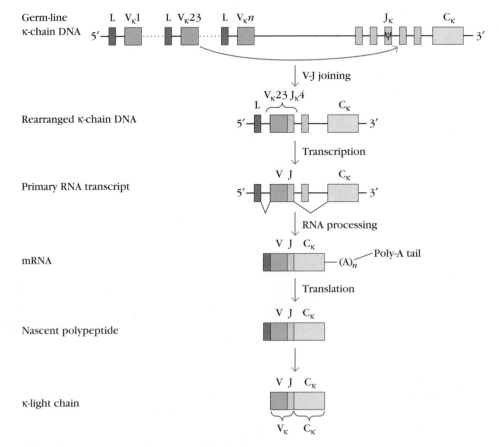

Figure 8-4   Kappa light chain-gene rearrangements and RNA processing events required to generate the finished kappa light-chain protein product. In this case $V_\kappa 23$ has joined $J_\kappa 4$.

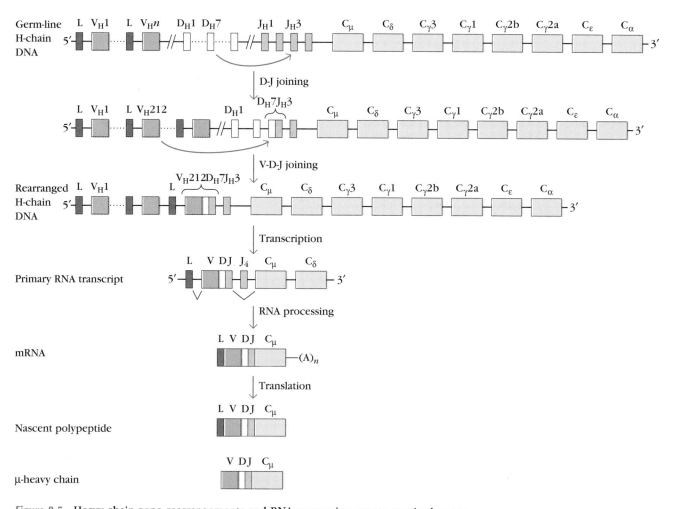

Figure 8-5 Heavy-chain gene rearrangements and RNA processing events required to generate the finished μ heavy-chain protein product. Two DNA rearrangements are necessary to generate a functional H chain gene: a D_H to J_H rearrangement and a V_H to D_H-J_H rearrangement. In this illustration V_H212 has joined with D_H7 and J_H3. Expression of functional heavy-chain genes, although generally similar to expression of light-chain genes, involves differential RNA processing, which generates several different heavy-chain products.

light-chain genes, a promoter sequence is located a short distance upstream from each heavy-chain leader sequence.

Once heavy-chain gene rearrangement is accomplished, RNA polymerase can bind to the promoter sequence and transcribe the entire heavy-chain gene, including the introns. Initially, both C_μ and C_δ gene segments are transcribed. RNA-processing enzymes remove the introns and process the primary transcript to generate mRNA, encoding either C_μ or C_δ. These two mRNAs then are translated, and the leader peptide of the resulting nascent polypeptide is cleaved, generating finished μ and δ chains. Since two different heavy-chain mRNAs are produced following heavy-chain variable-region gene rearrangement, a mature, immunocompetent B cell expresses both IgM and IgD with identical antigenic specificity on its surface.

Mechanism of Variable-Region DNA Rearrangements

Considerable research has been directed toward elucidating the mechanism by which variable-region gene rearrangements occur during maturation of B cells. The details of this process and the means by which it is regulated are discussed in this section.

Recombination Signal Sequences Direct Rearrangements

Discovery of two closely related conserved sequences in variable-region germ-line DNA paved the way toward fuller understanding of the mechanism of gene rearrangements. DNA sequencing studies revealed the presence of unique DNA recombination signal sequences (RSS's) flanking each other germ-line V, D, and J gene segments, which function as signals for the recombination events. Each RSS contains a conserved palindromic heptamer sequence and a conserved AT-rich nonamer sequence (Figure 8-6a). The heptamer and nonamer sequences on the 3' side of kappa and lambda light-chain V exons show inverted complementarity to the heptamer and nonamer sequences on the 5' side of the J exons. Similar conserved complementary DNA sequences were observed flanking the heavy-chain V, D, and J gene segments. Nonamer and heptamer sequences were found on both sides of the D gene segment, on the 3' side of the V gene segment and on the 5' side of the J gene segment.

The nonamer and heptamer sequences are separated by a sequence referred to as a *spacer*. The spacers have an unusual property: although the base sequence of the spacers varied, the length was conserved at either 12 base pairs or 23 base pairs. Leroy Hood observed that these lengths correspond respectively to one or two turns of the DNA helix. The V_κ signal sequence was found to have a 12-bp spacer, and the J_κ signal sequence was found to have a 23-bp spacer. In λ light-chain DNA, the V_λ signal sequence has a 23-bp spacer and the J_λ signal sequence has a 12-bp spacer. In the heavy-chain

DNA, a 23-bp spacer occurs in the recognition signal sequences of the V_H and J_H gene segments and a 12-bp spacer occurs in the recognition signals on either side of the D_H gene segment (Figure 8-6b). Signal sequences having a 12-bp spacer can only join with sequences having a 23-bp spacer (the so-called 12/23 joining rule). This 12/23 joining rule ensures that a V_L segment only joins to a J_L segment and not to another V_L segment; the rule likewise ensures that V_H, D_H, and J_H segments join in proper order and that segments of the same type do not join each other.

Recombination Activating Genes (RAG-1 and RAG-2) Mediate Joining

A number of events must occur for proper V(D)J joining: the recognition of the recombination signal sequences, followed by endonucleolytic cleavage of the RSS, and then ligation to rejoin the cleaved DNA. The genes involved in the recombination machinery are still in an early stage of research identification. Two genes that have been shown to act synergistically to mediate V(D)J joining are the *recombination activating genes*, RAG-1 and RAG-2. These genes were recently identified by David Schatz, Majorie Oettinger, and David Baltimore.

The RAG-1 gene was identified by designing a retro-

(a) Nucleotide sequence of recognition signals

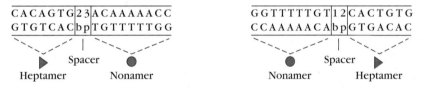

(b) Location of recognition signals in germ-line immunoglobulin DNA

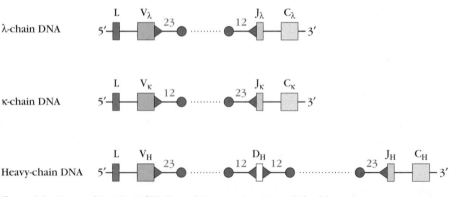

Figure 8-6 Recombination of V, D, and J exons is accomplished by unique conserved recognition sequences which are located 3' to the V exons, 5' and 3' to the D_H exon and 5' to the J exons. (a) The recognition sequences consist of a palindromic heptamer, CACAGTG sequence and an AT-rich nonamer sequence. The heptamer and nonamer recognition sequences are separated by nonconserved spacers of 12 or 23 base pairs. (b) The locations of the recognition signals within λ-chain, κ-chain, and heavy-chain germ-line DNA are shown. The joining process always joins a gene segment with a 12-bp spacer to one with a 23-bp spacer, assuring that the proper V-J and V-D-J joinings occur.

viral construct containing germline V_κ and J_κ genes with their adjacent RSS's together with a gene that conferred resistance to the drug mycophenolic acid. The researchers then transfected a variety of cells with this construct. Those cells that could rearrange the V_κ and J_κ gene segments acquired resistance to the mycophenolic acid. By using this system they demonstrated that only pre-B cells and pre-T cells were able to rearrange the V_κ and J_κ gene segments. (As will be discussed in Chapter 10, the pre-T cell employs the same RSS's to rearrange the genes for its TCR which is why it also proved to be positive in this assay.) Mature B and T cells did not possess the ability to rearrange the retroviral construct, indicating that the recombinase activity is limited to an early stage in B or T cell maturation.

Having established that the retroviral construct could be rearranged in pre-B cells, the research team then set out to isolate the recombination genes from the pre-B cell. First fibroblasts were transfected with the retroviral construct and then the fibroblasts were transfected with genomic DNA from the pre-B cell. In this way a gene was identified which mediated recombination of the retroviral construct and it was named the recombination activating gene, RAG-1. RAG-1 was shown to be present in both pre-B cells, pre-T cells, and in the central nervous system. The expression of RAG-1 in the central nervous system is intriguing and may suggest that similar recombination events may take place within the central nervous system.

It soon became apparent that RAG-1 was not the whole story. When RAG-1 cDNA was transfected into the fibroblasts, it was no more efficient at mediating recombination than the genomic DNA. It had been expected that the purified cDNA would have a 100–1000 fold increase in recombination efficiency compared to genomic DNA. The puzzle was finally solved by comparing the sequence of the cDNA and genomic clones. RAG-1 was shown to be encoded by a single 6.6 kb exon. The 18 kb genomic clone contained an additional 12 kb sequence of unknown function. To determine whether an additional gene was encoded in this 12 kb sequence of genomic DNA they transfected the fibroblasts with the cDNA RAG-1 gene alone, with the genomic DNA alone or with a mixture of both cDNA and genomic DNA. They found that co-transfection with both RAG-1 cDNA and the genomic DNA resulted in a 100-fold increase in the frequency of recombination compared to either DNA alone. A second closely linked gene, designated RAG-2 was identified. Cotransfection with both RAG-1 and RAG-2 resulted in over a 1000-fold increase in recombination in their fibroblast model system. It has not yet been determined whether RAG-1 and RAG-2 play a direct role as part of the recombination machinery or whether they play a regulatory role leading to the expression of other, as yet unidentified enzymes, involved in recombination.

Joining of Gene Segments

The conservation throughout evolution of the complementary nonamer and heptamer sequences as well as the intervening 12- or 23-base-pair spacers reflects the role of the recognition signals in the process of V_L-J_L and V_H-D_H-J_H joining. Several models have been proposed for the joining process, and the exact mechanism is still somewhat speculative. Figure 8-7 depicts two types of V_κ-J_κ joining—deletional and inversional—depending on the $5' \rightarrow 3'$ orientation of the V_κ segment. In both inversional and deletional joining, the DNA loops around, bringing a V_κ and J_κ signal sequence into proximity. It is believed that all or part of the double-stranded signal

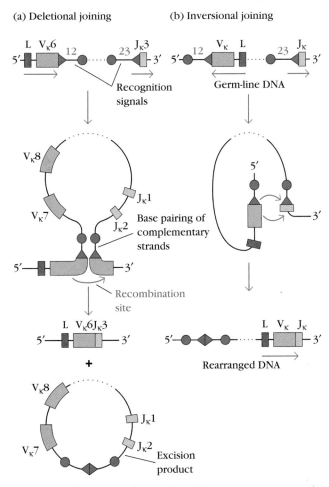

Figure 8-7 Hypothetical model for V-J joining in κ-chain germ-like DNA. Joining occurs by a deletional mechanism (a) when the V_κ and J_κ to be joined have the same transcriptional orientation (small red arrows) and by an inversional mechanism (b) when they have the opposite orientation. Recognition signals adjacent to V and J segments specify the sites at which joining can occur. In deletional joinings, the excised DNA is lost from the cell. In inversional joinings, all of the DNA is conserved.

sequence unwinds and that one strand from the V_κ signal associates by hydrogen-bonded base pairing with the complementary strand in the J_κ signal. When the transcriptional orientation of the two segments are in the same directions, an intermediary stem-loop structure is formed (Figure 8-7a). A recombinase enzyme is postulated to recognize the stem-loop structure, excise it, and join the V_κ and J_κ segments. The joining process will result in the loss of the entire stem structure containing the intervening DNA gene segments. This process contributes to the *commitment* of the B cell to an antibody specificity. There continue to be V genes 5′ of the rearrangement, and in some B-cell lines additional rearrangements have indeed been observed, but this is not thought to be the general situation. When the transcriptional orientation of V_κ and J_κ are in opposite directions, looping of DNA involves an inversion that orients the two segments in the same 5′ → 3′ direction; in such inversional joining, the intervening DNA is conserved, as shown in Figure 8-7b. Joining of variable-region gene segments in λ light-chain genes and in heavy-chain genes is also thought to occur by deletional or inversional mechanisms.

Productive and Nonproductive Joining

V-D-J rearrangements do not take place at a precise site relative to the recognition signal sequences. Instead, there is a certain flexibility in the joining. This flexibility allows for greater generation of antibody diversity by contributing to the hypervariability of the antigen-combining site. (This will be covered in more detail later in the chapter). In-phase joining maintains a correct reading frame for translation of the resulting VJ or VDJ unit into a polypeptide (Figure 8-8); this is called a *productive* rearrangement. If the gene segments are joined out of phase (for example, if joining introduces one or two nucleotides instead of three nucleotides), then the triplet reading frame is not preserved and frequent stop codons will be generated; this is called a *nonproductive* rearrangement. Most evidence suggests that nonproductive rearrangements occur with a high frequency. If one allele rearranges nonproductively, the cell can go on to rearrange the other allele and may generate a productive rearrangement. A productive heavy-chain V-D-J rearrangement must take place before a light-chain V-J rearrangement can occur. The κ light chain is

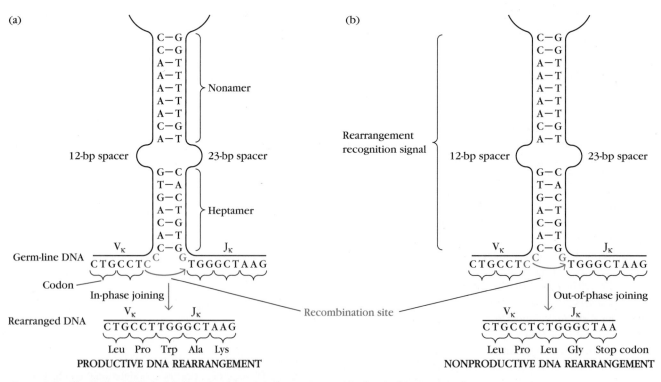

Figure 8-8 Flexibility of V_κ-J_κ joinings. In-phase joining generates productively rearranged DNA, which can be translated into protein. Out-of-phase joining leads to nonproductively rearranged DNA, which contains stop codons and is not translated into protein. Although this flexibility generates considerable diversity in variable-region DNA, it also results in many nonproductive joinings.

thought to rearrange after the heavy chain. If κ rearrangement is nonproductive for both alleles, the λ-chain genes will rearrange. If both light-chain arrangements are nonproductive, the B cell presumably ceases to mature.

Allelic Exclusion

B cells, like all somatic cells, are diploid and contain both maternal and paternal chromosomes. Even though a B cell is diploid, it expresses the rearranged heavy-chain genes from only one chromosome and the rearranged light-chain genes from only one chromosome. This process, called *allelic exclusion*, ensures that functional B cells never contain more than one $V_H D_H J_H$ and one $V_L J_L$ unit (Figure 8-9). This is, of course, essential for the antigenic specificity of the B cell, because the expression of both alleles would render the B cell multispecific. This suggests that once there has been a productive variable-region rearrangement in the heavy- and light-chain, genes, the enzymatic machinery responsible for rearrangements must be turned off, so that the heavy- and light-chain genes on the other chromosome are not expressed.

G. D. Yancopoulos and F. W. Alt have proposed a model to account for allelic exclusion (Figure 8-10). They suggest that once a productive rearrangement is attained, its encoded protein is expressed and the presence of this protein acts as a signal to prevent further gene rearrangement. According to their model, the presence of μ heavy chains signals the maturing B cell to turn off rearrangement of the other heavy-chain allele and to turn on rearrangement of the κ light-chain genes. If a productive κ rearrangement occurs, κ light chains are produced and then pair with μ heavy chains to form a complete antibody molecule. The presence of this antibody then turns off further light-chain rearrangement. If κ rearrangement is nonproductive for both alleles, rearrangement of the λ-chain genes begins. If neither λ allele rearranges productively, the B cell presumably ceases to mature and soon dies out.

Two studies with transgenic mice have supported the hypothesis that the protein products encoded by rearranged heavy- and light-chain genes regulate rearrangement of the remaining alleles. In one study, transgenic mice (see Chapter 2) were prepared carrying a rearranged μ heavy-chain transgene. The μ transgene product was expressed by a large percentage of the B cells, and rearrangement of the endogenous immunoglobulin heavy-chain genes was blocked. Similarly, cells from a transgenic mouse carrying a rearranged κ light-chain gene did not rearrange the endogenous κ-chain genes if the κ transgene was expressed and was associated with a heavy chain to form complete immunoglobulin.

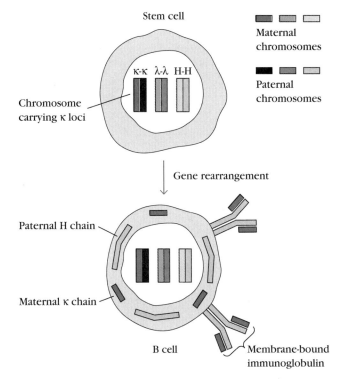

Figure 8-9 Because of allelic exclusion, which is unique to B lymphocytes, the immunoglobulin heavy- and light-chain genes of only one parental chromosome are expressed per cell. This process ensures that a single B lymphocyte will be specific for a given epitope.

These studies suggest that expression of the heavy- and light-chain proteins may indeed prevent gene rearrangements of the remaining alleles and thus account for allelic exclusion.

Rearrangements Bring Promoter into Proximity of Enhancer

Each V_H and V_L gene segment has a promoter located just upstream from the leader sequence (Figure 8-11a). The promoter is a relatively short sequence of DNA extending about 200 bp upstream from the transcription initiation site. Like other promoters, the immunoglobulin promoters contain a highly conserved AT-rich sequence, called the TATA box, to which RNA polymerase II binds. After binding to the TATA box the RNA polymerase starts transcribing the DNA from the initiation site, located about 25–35 bases downstream of the TATA box.

In unrearranged germ-line DNA, the rate of transcription of V_H and V_L coding regions is almost negligible. Following V-D-J and V-J rearrangement the rate of transcription increases. The increase is due to the effects of

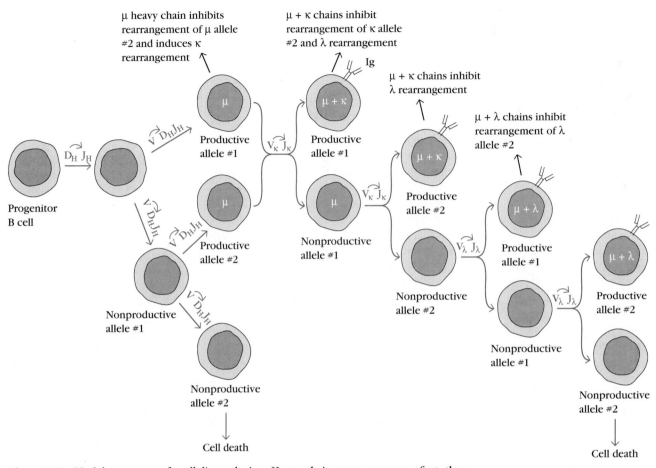

Figure 8-10 Model to account for allelic exclusion. Heavy-chain genes rearrange first, then κ light-chain genes, and finally λ light-chain genes. Once a productive heavy-chain gene rearrangement occurs, the μ protein product prevents rearrangement of the other heavy-chain allele and initiates light-chain gene rearrangement. Once a complete immunoglobulin is formed, further light-chain gene rearrangement ceases. If a nonproductive rearrangement occurs for one allele, then the cell attempts rearrangement of the other allele. [Adapted from G. D. Yancopoulos and F. W. Alt, 1986, *Annu. Rev. Immunol.* 4:339.]

an enhancer region. Enhancers are *cis*-acting DNA sequences that activate transcription from the promoter sequence. The mechanism by which enhancers activate transcription is still not known; it is thought that DNA-binding factors bound to the enhancer may alter chromatin structure in the vicinity, thereby facilitating the formation of a stable transcription-initiation complex at the promoter site. One heavy-chain enhancer is located within the intron between the last J gene segment and the switch site (see next section) for the first C gene (C_μ) (see Figure 8-11a). The location of this heavy-chain enhancer allows it to continue to function after class-switching events. Recently another heavy-chain enhancer has been detected 3′ of the C_α gene segment. One kappa light-chain enhancer is located between the J_κ segments and the C_κ segment, and another enhancer

is located 3′ of the C_κ gene segment. The recently discovered enhancers of the lambda light chain are 3′ of $C_\lambda 4$ and 3′ of $C_\lambda 1$.

Variable-region gene rearrangement brings the promoter within 2 kb of the enhancer so that the enhancer can influence transcription. As a result, the rate of transcription of a rearranged $V_L J_L$ or $V_H D_H J_H$ unit is as much as 10^4 times the rate of transcription of unrearranged V_L or V_H segments. The importance of the enhancer region in the transcription of immunoglobulin genes has been demonstrated experimentally. In one such study, B cells transfected with rearranged heavy-chain genes from which the enhancer had been deleted did not transcribe the genes. In contrast, B cells transfected with similar genes that contained the enhancer transcribed the transfected genes at a high rate.

DNA-Binding Proteins Regulate Immunoglobulin-Gene Expression

The activity of the immunoglobulin promoter and enhancer sequences are regulated by DNA-binding proteins, some of which are found in many cell types and some of which are mostly restricted to cells of the lymphoid lineage. Evidence suggesting that lymphoid cells have lineage-restricted transcription factors was first demonstrated by experiments in which rearranged light-chain or heavy-chain DNA was introduced into the germ-line DNA of mouse embryos to yield transgenic mice carrying the rearranged genes in all their somatic cells. Even though all the cells in the transgenic mice contained the rearranged genes, these genes were expressed only in cells of the spleen, and not in cells of

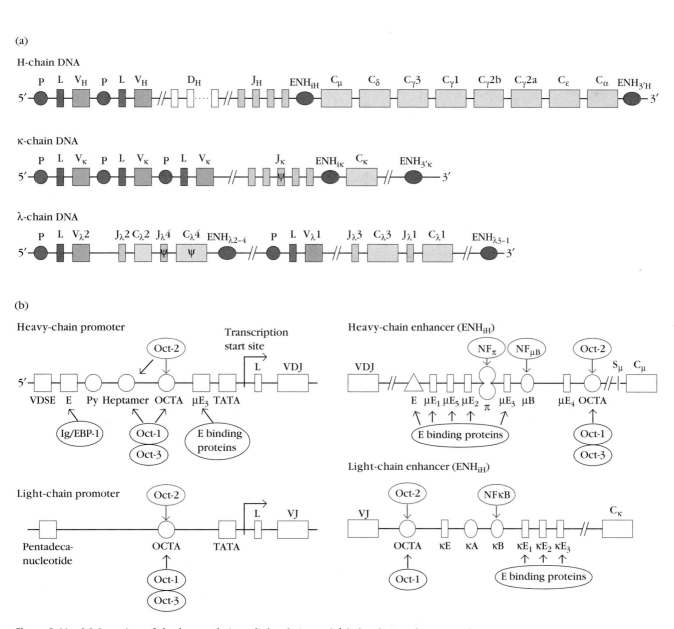

Figure 8-11   (a) Location of the heavy-chain, κ light-chain, and λ light-chain enhancer and promoter sequences in germ-line DNA. DNA rearrangement of the heavy chain and κ light chain moves the promoter closer to the enhancer enabling the enhancer to activate transcription from the promoter. (b) DNA-binding proteins bind to conserved sequences in the promoter and enhancer regions and regulate transcription. Lineage-specific DNA-binding factors are shown in color above the promoter or enhancer region while DNA-binding factors that are found in many other types of cells are shown below.

the testis, liver, kidney, heart, muscle, brain, or thyroid gland. This finding suggests that B cells produce lineage-specific transcription factors that limit the transcription of the immunoglobulin genes to B-lineage cells.

The immunoglobulin promoter contains a number of conserved sequences (or motifs) that are recognized by DNA-binding proteins (Figure 8-11b). These include a heptamer motif, an octamer motif (OCTA), a pyrimidine-rich motif (Py), two enhancer motifs (μE3 and E), the TATA box, and a motif responsive to IL-5 plus antigen (VDSE). Different combinations of DNA-binding proteins bind to these motifs and act together to regulate gene transcription. Most of these conserved sequences and their associated DNA-binding proteins are found in a wide variety of cells. However, the OCTA motif and one of its associated DNA-binding proteins called Oct-2 has a limited distribution and is found only in B cells and a few other cell lineages. The OCTA sequence acquired its name because it originally was thought to contain eight conserved bases. However, later it was shown to be a decamer sequence containing nine conserved bases and one variable base but its name has not been changed to reflect its true nature. The OCTA sequence is regulated by B-lineage specific DNA-binding factors. Evidence for this came from engineering the OCTA sequence upstream of a TATA sequence on a β-globulin gene promoter. When the engineered β-globulin gene is transfected into B-cell lines and into fibroblast cells, the transfected B cells express 20-fold higher levels of the β-globulin gene than the transfected fibroblasts. A B-cell lineage-specific OCTA-binding protein called Oct-2 is expressed by B cells when D_H-J_H joining occurs. The Oct-2 DNA-binding protein is a member of the POU domain family of DNA-binding proteins. The POU family is defined by the presence of a 60-aa domain, the homeodomain, and a 75-aa POU domain. Both the homeodomain and POU domain are required for Oct-2 binding to the OCTA motif. The positive regulatory role of Oct-2 on the immunoglobulin promoter can be seen by transfecting the immunoglobulin gene and its promoter into a fibroblast cell line. The construct is inactive in these transfected cells unless the cell is also transfected with an Oct-2 expression vector.

The immunoglobulin enhancer regions are also regulated by lineage-specific factors (see Figure 8-11b). The heavy-chain enhancer contains three sequences (π, μB, and OCTA), thought to bind lineage-specific transcription factors as well as a number of sequences (E motifs) that bind factors that are not specific to B cells. The enhancer OCTA sequence is the same as the OCTA sequence in the immunoglobulin promoter; thus Oct-2 binds to both the promoter and to the heavy-chain enhancer. The π and μB DNA-binding proteins have not yet been cloned. The E-motif binding proteins include a group of transcription factors, characterized by two

13 aa amphipathic α helices separated by a loop of variable length (helix-loop-helix, HLH, proteins). Members of this group of transcription factors form homodimers or heterodimers that interact with E motifs within the enhancer sequence. The κ light-chain enhancer also contains an OCTA sequence, various E motifs, and a lineage-specific sequence called κB that binds a protein called NF-κB. The κB sequence is also present in several other genes, including the IL-2 gene. NF-κB is found in the cytoplasm in an inactive form bound to an inhibitor. Upon B-cell activation, protein kinase C phosphorylates the inhibitor, releasing the NF-κB that enters the nucleus and binds to the κ enhancer (Figure 8-12). NF-κB can be induced in other cells, including activated T cells, but in such cells its appearance is only transient.

DNA Rearrangements Mediating Class Switching

Following antigenic stimulation of a B-cell, the heavy-chain DNA can undergo a further rearrangement in which the $V_H D_H J_H$ unit can combine with any C_H gene segment. The exact mechanism of this process, called *class switching*, is unclear, but evidence suggests that short DNA flanking sequences (termed *switch sites*) located 2–3 kb upstream from each C_H segment (except C_δ) are involved. These switch sites are rather large but are composed of multiple copies of short repeated sequences. It is proposed that a series of class-specific recombinase proteins may bind to these switch sites and thereby facilitate DNA recombination. The choice of the particular immunoglobulin class to be expressed might then depend on the specificity of the recombinase protein expressed.

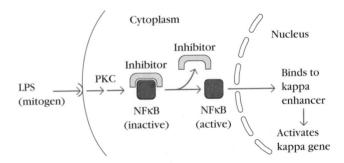

Figure 8-12 Nuclear factor-κB (NF-κB) is found in the cytoplasm in an inactive form bound to an inhibitor. After the B cell is activated by antigen or a mitogen (LPS), protein kinase C phosphorylates the inhibitor, releasing NF-κB, which enters the nucleus and binds to the κB sequence on the enhancer.

Various lymphokines secreted by activated T_H cells have been shown to induce B cells to class-switch to a particular isotype. Interleukin 4 (IL-4), for example, induces class switching from C_μ to $C_\gamma 1$ or C_ε. K. Yoshida, H. Sakano, and colleagues have demonstrated that IL-4 induces class switching in a successive manner: first from C_μ to $C_\gamma 1$ and then from $C_\gamma 1$ to C_ε (Figure 8-13). They were able to demonstrate this by identifying the circular DNA containing the intervening DNA sequences that are excision products produced during class switching. The class switch from C_μ to $C_\gamma 1$ was shown to generate a circular excision product containing C_μ together with the 5′ end of the $\gamma 1$ switch site ($S_\gamma 1$) and the 3′ end of the μ switch site (S_μ). The switch from $C_\gamma 1$ to C_ε was shown to generate two circular excision products containing $C_\gamma 1$ together with portions of the switch sites. The role of lymphokines in immunoglobulin class switching is discussed more fully in Chapter 12.

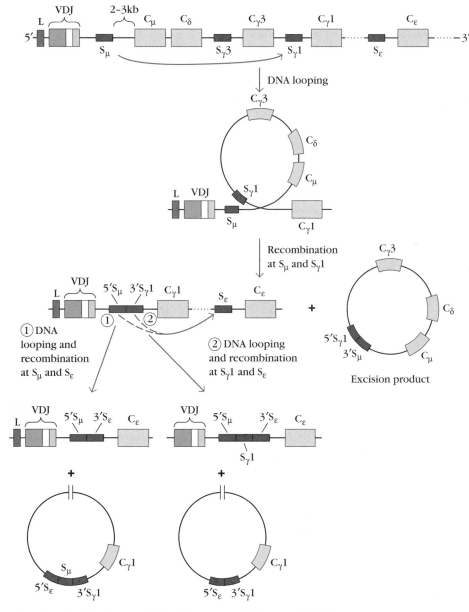

Figure 8-13 Proposed mechanism for class switching in rearranged immunoglobulin heavy-chain genes induced by interleukin 4. Switch sites are located upstream from each C_H segment except C_δ. Identification of the indicated circular excision products containing portions of the switch sites suggested that IL-4 induces sequential class switching from C_μ to $C_\gamma 1$ to C_ε.

Expression of Immunoglobulin Genes

As in the expression of other genes, post-transcriptional processing of immunoglobulin primary transcripts is required to produce functional mRNAs (see Figure 8-4). The first step in this RNA processing, which occurs while transcription is proceeding, is addition of a 7-methylguanosine residue to the 5′ end of the primary transcript. This forms the 5′ cap structure, which plays a role in translation of mRNA on the polyribosomes. Once transcription is completed, the primary RNA transcript is cleaved some 15–30 nucleotides downstream of a highly conserved AAUAAA sequence (called the *polyadenylation signal*). An enzyme called poly-A polymerase recognizes the signal sequence and adds sequential adenylate residues derived from ATP to the 3′ end of the primary transcript, forming a poly-A tail of about 250 residues.

Following capping and polyadenylation, the introns of a primary transcript are excised and their flanking exons are connected by a process called RNA splicing. Short, moderately conserved splice sequences, or splice sites, which are located at the intron-exon boundaries of a primary transcript, signal the positions at which splicing occurs. After heavy-chain and light-chain DNA rearrangement is completed, the DNA continues to contain intervening DNA sequences. These intervening sequences include noncoding introns and J gene segments not lost during V-D-J rearrangement. In addition the heavy-chain C gene segments are organized as a series of coding exons and noncoding introns. Each exon of the C_H gene segment corresponds to a domain or hinge region of the heavy polypeptide chain. Processing of the primary transcript in the nucleus removes each of these intervening sequences to yield the final mRNA product. The mRNA is then exported from the nucleus and goes to polyribosomes for translation into the complete H or L chain.

Differential RNA Processing of Primary Transcripts

In some cases, processing of an immunoglobulin primary transcript can lead to production of different mRNAs. Such differential RNA processing of heavy-chain transcripts explains the production of secreted or membrane-bound forms of a particular immunoglobulin and the simultaneous expression of IgM and IgD.

Expression of Membrane-Bound or Secreted Immunoglobulin

As discussed in Chapter 5, a particular immunoglobulin can exist in a membrane-bound form or in a secreted form. The two forms differ in the amino acid sequence

of the heavy-chain carboxyl-terminal domains (C_H3/C_H3 in IgA, IgD, and IgG and C_H4/C_H4 in IgE and IgM). The secreted form has a hydrophilic sequence of about 20 amino acids in the carboxyl-terminal domain: this is replaced in the membrane-bound form with a sequence of about 40 amino acids containing a hydrophilic segment, a hydrophobic transmembrane segment, and a short hydrophilic cytoplasmic segment at the carboxyl terminus (Figure 8-14a). For some time the existence of these two forms seemed inconsistent with the structure of germ-line heavy-chain DNA, which had been shown to contain a single C_H gene segment corresponding to each class and subclass (see Figure 8-2c).

The explanation of this apparent paradox came from DNA sequencing of the C_μ gene segment, which consists of four exons ($C_\mu1$, $C_\mu2$, $C_\mu3$, and $C_\mu4$) corresponding to the four domains of the IgM molecule. The $C_\mu4$ exon contains a nucleotide sequence at its 3′ end that encodes the hydrophilic sequence in the C_H4 domain of secreted IgM. Two additional exons called M1 and M2 are located just 1.8 kb downstream from the 3′ end of the $C_\mu4$ exon. The M1 exon encodes the transmembrane segment, and M2 encodes the cytoplasmic segment of the C_H4 domain in membrane-bound IgM. Later DNA sequencing revealed that all the C_H gene segments have two additional downstream M1 and M2 exons encoding the transmembrane and cytoplasmic segments.

The primary transcript produced by transcription of a rearranged μ heavy-chain gene contains two polyadenylation signal sequences, or poly-A sites. Site 1 is located at the 3′ end of the $C_\mu4$ exon and site 2 at the 3′ end of the M2 exon. If cleavage of the primary transcript and addition of the poly-A tail occurs at site 1, the M1 and M2 exons are lost. Excision of the introns and splicing of the remaining exons then produces mRNA encoding the secreted form of the μ heavy chain. (Figure 8-14b). If cleavage and polyadenylation of the primary transcript occur instead at site 2, then a different pattern of splicing occurs. The sequence of the $C_\mu4$ exon contains a splice signal toward its 3′ end. Splicing en-

Figure 8-14 Expression of secreted and membrane forms of the μ heavy chain by alternative RNA processing. (a) Amino acid sequence of the carboxyl-terminal end of secreted and membrane μ heavy chains. Residues are indicated by the single-letter code. Hydrophilic residues are shaded red, and hydrophobic residues are shaded gray. Charged amino acids are indicated with a + or − . The rest of the sequence is identical in both forms. (b) Structure of a rearranged heavy-chain gene showing the C_μ exons and poly-A sites. Polyadenylation of the primary transcript at either site 1 or site 2 produces two RNA transcripts. Subsequent splicing (indicated by V-shaped lines) generates mRNAs encoding secreted or membrane μ chains.

(a)

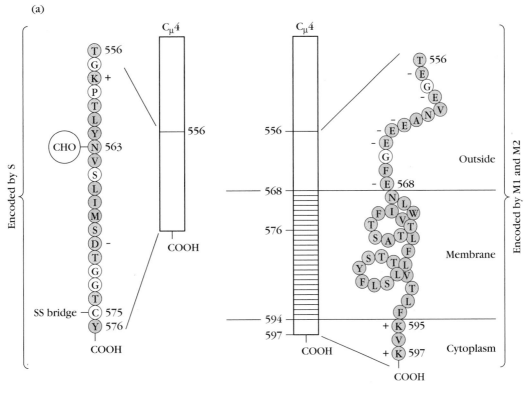

Secreted μ

Membrane μ

(b)

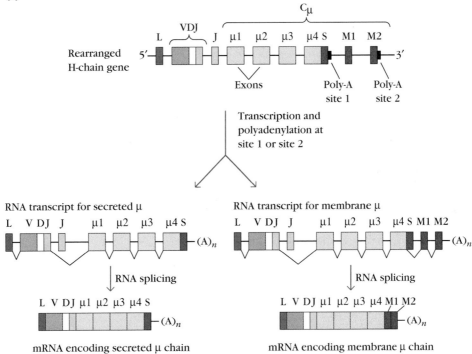

zymes, however, recognize this splice signal only if another splice signal lies downstream, as it does when the M1 and M2 exons are present. In this case, splicing removes the 3′ end of the $C_\mu 4$ exon that encodes the hydrophilic sequence of the secreted form and joins the remainder of the $C_\mu 4$ exon with the M1 and M2 exons, producing mRNA for the membrane form of the μ heavy chain.

Production of the secreted or membrane form of an immunoglobulin thus depends on differential processing of a common primary transcript. As noted previously, mature B cells produce only membrane-bound antibody, whereas differentiated plasma cells produce secreted antibodies. Presumably some mechanism exists in unprimed B cells and in plasma cells that directs RNA processing preferentially toward the production of mRNA, encoding either the membrane form or secreted form of an immunoglobulin.

Simultaneous Expression of IgM and IgD

The phenomenon of differential RNA processing also explains the simultaneous expression of membrane-bound IgM and IgD by mature B cells. As mentioned already, transcription of rearranged heavy-chain genes in mature B cells produces primary transcripts containing both the C_μ and C_δ gene segments. One explanation for this is that the close proximity of C_μ and C_δ, which are only about 5 kb apart, and the lack of a switch site between them permits the entire $VDJC_\mu C_\delta$ region to be transcribed into a long primary RNA transcript, about 15 kb long, which contains four poly-A sites (Figure 8-15a). Sites 1 and 2 are associated with C_μ, as described in the previous section; sites 3 and 4 are located at similar places in the C_δ gene segment. If the transcript is cleaved and polyadenylated at site 1 or 2 after the C_μ exons, then the mRNA will encode the membrane or secreted

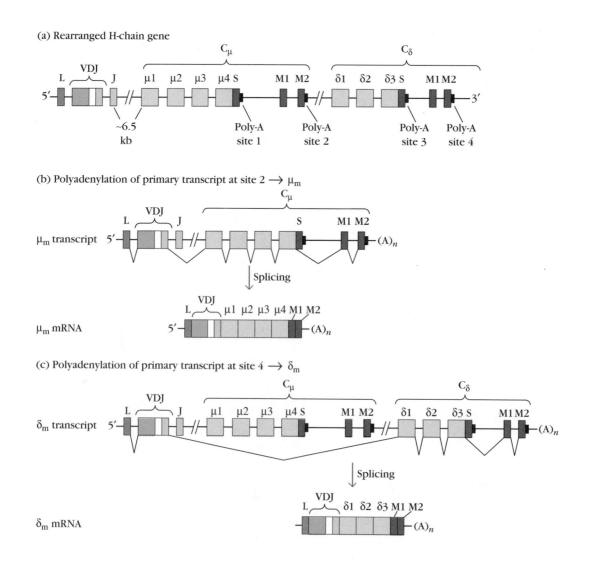

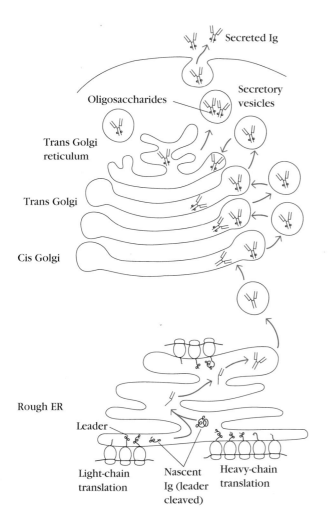

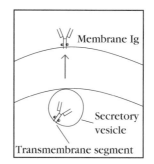

Figure 8-16 Synthesis, assembly, and secretion of the immunoglobulin molecule. The heavy and light chains are synthesized upon separate polyribosomes (polysomes). The assembly of the chains to form the disulfide-linked and glycosylated immunoglobulin molecule occurs as the chains pass through the cisternae of the endoplasmic reticulum into the Golgi apparatus and then into secretory vesicles. The main figure depicts assembly of a secreted antibody. The inset depicts a membrane-bound antibody, which contains the carboxyl-terminal transmembrane segment. This form becomes anchored in the membrane of secretory vesicles and then is inserted into the cell membrane when the vesicle fuses with the membrane.

forms of the μ heavy chain (Figure 8-15b); if polyadenylation is instead further downstream at sites 3 or 4 after the C_δ exons, then RNA splicing will remove the intervening C_μ exons and produce mRNA for the membrane or secreted forms of the δ heavy chain (Figure 8-15c). Since the mature B cell expresses both IgM and IgD on its membrane, processing by both pathways must occur simultaneously.

Figure 8-15 Expression of μ_m and δ_m heavy chains by alternative RNA processing. (a) Structure of rearranged heavy-chain gene showing C_μ and C_δ exons and poly-A sites. (b) Structure of μ_m transcript and μ_m mRNA resulting from polyadenylation at site 2 and splicing. (c) Structure of δ_m transcript and δ_m mRNA resulting from polyadenylation at site 4 and splicing. Both processing pathways can proceed in a given B cell.

Synthesis, Assembly, and Secretion of Immunoglobulins

Immunoglobulin heavy- and light-chain mRNAs are translated on separate polyribosomes of the rough endoplasmic reticulum (RER). Newly synthesized chains contain an amino-terminal leader sequence, which serves to guide the chains into the lumen of the RER where it is then cleaved off. The assembly of light (L) and heavy (H) chains into the disulfide-linked and glycosylated immunoglobulin molecule occurs as the chains pass through the cisternae of the RER into the Golgi apparatus and then into secretory vesicles, which fuse with the plasma membrane (Figure 8-16). The order of chain assembly varies among the immunoglobulin classes. In the case of IgM, the H and L chains assemble within the RER to form half-molecules, and then two half-molecules assemble to form the complete molecule. In the case of IgG, two H chains assemble, then an H_2L intermediate is assembled, and finally the complete H_2L_2 molecule is formed. Interchain disulfide bonds are formed, and the polypeptides are glycosylated as they move from the endoplasmic reticulum into the Golgi apparatus. If the molecule contains the transmembrane sequence of the membrane form, it becomes anchored in the membrane of a secretory vesicle and is inserted into the plasma membrane as the vesicle fuses with the plasma membrane. If the molecule contains the hydrophilic sequence of secreted immunoglobulins, it is transported as a free molecule in a secretory vesicle and is released from the cell when the vesicle fuses with the plasma membrane.

Correlation of B-Cell Differentiation with Gene Rearrangements and Alternative RNA Processing

The discussion in Chapters 1 and 3 indicated that formation of antibody-secreting plasma cells occurs in two phases: an initial antigen-independent phase followed by an antigen-dependent phase (see Figure 1-13). In the antigen-independent phase, lymphoid stem cells in the bone marrow differentiate first into progenitor B cells and then into mature, immunocompetent B cells. Rearrangement of the immunoglobulin V_H and V_L gene segments occurs during this first phase. A mature B cell thus leaves the bone marrow expressing membrane-bound immunoglobulins (IgM and IgD) with a single antigenic specificity. Mature B cells circulate in the blood and lymph and are carried to the secondary lymphoid organs (most notably the spleen and lymph nodes). If a B cell interacts with the antigen for which its membrane-bound IgM and IgD is specific, it undergoes clonal expansion and differentiation, generating a population of plasma cells and B memory cells. This antigen-dependent phase depends on the participation of antigen-presenting cells (e.g., macrophages) and activated T_H cells (see Figure 1-13).

Once the immunoglobulin-gene rearrangements described earlier in this chapter had been elucidated, various researchers tried to correlate these molecular events with the different stages in B-cell differentiation. Such studies, however, require large populations of homogeneous B cells at different stages of differentiation. As described in Chapter 2, primary cell cultures of lymphocytes have a limited lifespan and are heterogeneous; thus they are unsuitable for this type of study. One approach to obtaining large numbers of homogeneous cells is to produce hybridomas by fusing normal B cells with myeloma cells (see Figure 2-1). Such hybridomas retain the gene rearrangements of the B-cell fusion partner but exhibit the immortal-growth properties of the myeloma cell. Chapter 7 described fusion of plasma cells with myeloma cells to produce hybridomas that secrete

monoclonal antibody. However, B cells at other stages of differentiation can also be used to produce hybridomas expressing the immunoglobulin characteristic of that stage. For example, if fetal liver cells are fused with myeloma cells, some of the resulting hybridomas represent the pre-B cell stage during which the μ heavy chain is expressed in the cytoplasm but there is no detectable membrane immunoglobulin.

Tumor-cell lines representing a given differentiation stage have also proved useful for analyzing the stages of B-cell differentiation. There are currently more than 1000 human lymphoid cell lines representing various stages of B- or T-cell differentiation (see Table 2-2). Although some investigators have pointed out that these are aberrant cells, such cell lines have nonetheless made it possible to detect immunoglobulin-gene rearrangements or membrane markers that were later shown to occur in normal cells. Cell lines also make it possible to express cloned DNA by serving as hosts for transfection. Transfection of rearranged or nonrearranged immunoglobulin genes into various lymphoid or nonlymphoid cell lines has shed light on the mechanisms involved in immunoglobulin-gene regulation.

Antigen-Independent Phase

Figure 8-17 outlines the immunoglobulin-gene rearrangements and changes in RNA processing that occur at various stages of B-cell differentiation. The earliest distinctive B-lineage cell—the *progenitor B cell*—expresses a lineage-specific cell-surface marker called B220. At this stage, the heavy-chain D_H-J_H rearrangement occurs. However, since progenitor B cells lack any functional immunoglobulin genes, they do not synthesize any heavy or light chains. During the next stage the V_H-D_H-J_H rearrangement occurs, resulting in pre-B cells. Allelic

Figure 8-17 Sequence of events in antigen-independent and antigen-dependent phases of B-cell diffferentiation. The earliest B-lineage cells to apppear—progenitor B cells—express a B-cell surface marker (B220) but no immunoglobulin chains. Sequential gene rearrangements and changes in RNA processing of heavy-chain transcripts leads to formation of mature B cells, which coexpress membrane-bound IgM and IgD. Interaction of a mature B cell with antigen and T_H-cell derived lymphokines results in activation, clonal selection, and proliferation, generating plasma cells and memory B cells. Activated B cells and memory B cells (red) can undergo class switching, allowing expression of different isotypes. A given plasma cell secretes only one isotype. Some memory cells express the membrane form of a single isotype, whereas others express two isotypes.

exclusion, which was described earlier, operates at this stage, so that either the maternal or paternal allele, but never both, is rearranged. If a productive rearrangement occurs, the resulting heavy-chain gene is transcribed into a primary transcript containing $V_H D_H J_H C_\mu C_\delta$. Differential RNA processing of this primary transcript produces mRNA that encodes the membrane form of the μ heavy chain (see Figures 8-14 and 8-15). Pre-B cells thus express cytoplasmic μ heavy chains, as well as the B220 surface marker.

The light-chain V_L-J_L rearrangement occurs next, generating the *immature B cell*. As illustrated in Figure 8-10, this rearrangement begins with the κ gene segments; if it is productive, the cell stops light-chain rearrangement. If rearrangement of both κ alleles is nonproductive, the λ light-chain gene segments undergo rearrangement. Completion of the light-chain rearrangement commits the cell to a particular antigenic specificity determined by the cell's heavy-chain VDJ sequence and light-chain VJ sequence. Immature B cells synthesize κ or λ light chains; differential processing of the heavy-chain primary transcript leads to synthesis of the membrane form of the μ heavy chain. Assembly of

the light and heavy chains results in expression of monomeric IgM on the surface of Immature B cells. Further differentiation of the immature B cell leads to the coexpression of IgD and IgM on the membrane, which characterizes *mature B cells*. This progression presumably involves some change in RNA processing of the heavy-chain primary transcript to permit production of two mRNAs, one encoding the membrane form of the μ chain and the other encoding the membrane form of the δ chain.

Antigen-Dependent Phase

Up to this point, B-cell differentiation is an antigen-independent process. The subsequent steps, however, involve antigen-driven clonal selection of mature B cells, leading to development of *plasma cells* and *B memory cells*. B memory cells can undergo class switching, resulting in expression of a new isotype on the membrane (i.e., IgG, IgA or IgE). Some B memory cells express a single isotype, whereas others express two isotypes (IgM + IgG, IgM + IgA, or IgM + IgE). It is not known

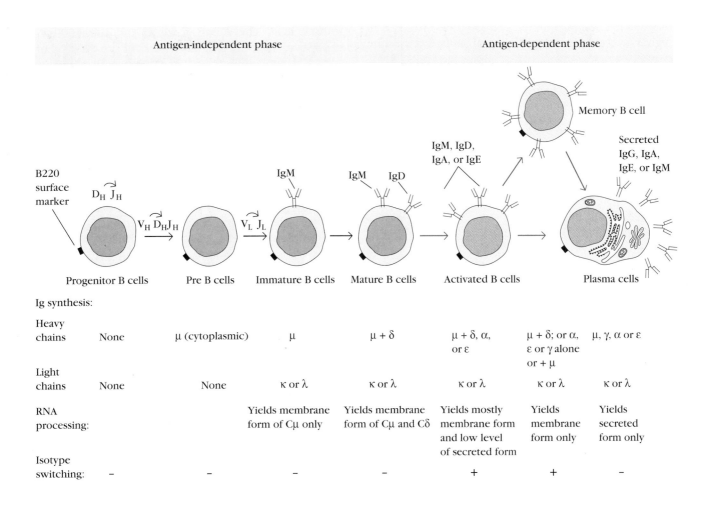

	Antigen-independent phase			Antigen-dependent phase		
	Progenitor B cells	Pre B cells	Immature B cells	Mature B cells	Activated B cells	Memory B cell	Plasma cells

Ig synthesis:							
Heavy chains	None	μ (cytoplasmic)	μ	$\mu + \delta$	$\mu + \delta$, α, or ε	$\mu + \delta$; or α, ε or γ alone or + μ	μ, γ, α or ε
Light chains	None	None	κ or λ	κ or λ	κ or λ	κ or λ	κ or λ
RNA processing:		Yields membrane form of Cμ only	Yields membrane form of Cμ and Cδ	Yields mostly membrane form and low level of secreted form	Yields membrane form only	Yields secreted form only	
Isotype switching:	–	–	–	–	+	+	–

how a B memory cell can express both IgM and another isotype whose constant-region gene is 50–100 kb away. It is possible that the μ-chain mRNA is long-lived, so that μ heavy chains continue to be expressed after class switching to another isotype. It is also possible that molecular mechanisms other than class switching may be responsible for coexpression of IgM with IgG, IgA, or IgE. For example, some very long primary transcripts containing $V_H D_H J_H$ and multiple C_H gene segments have been detected in B memory cells. Differential processing of such long transcripts might generate different isotypes within a given memory cell; this would be analogous to the coexpression of IgM and IgD in a mature B cell. At a later stage, class switching by the mechanism described earlier (see Figure 8-12) would lead to irreversible deletion of intervening C_H segments and the sequential appearance of the various isotypes in the order they appear in the DNA.

Plasma cells generally lack detectable membrane-bound immunoglobulin and instead synthesize high levels of secreted antibody. Differentiation of mature B cells into plasma cells must involve a change in RNA processing so that the secreted form of the heavy chain rather than the membrane form is synthesized. In addition, the rate of transcription of heavy- and light-chain genes increases significantly in plasma cells. Several authors have suggested that the increased transcription by plasma cells might be explained by their synthesis of higher levels of immunoglobulin enhancer factors compared with less-differentiated B-lineage cells. Some mechanism also must coordinate the increase in transcription of heavy-chain and light-chain genes, even though these genes are on different chromosomes.

Generation of Antibody Diversity

As the organization of the immunoglobulin genes was deciphered, the sources of the vast diversity in the variable region began to come clear. The germ-line theory, mentioned earlier, argued that the entire variable-region repertoire is encoded in the germ line of the organism and is transmitted from parent to offspring via the germ cells (egg and sperm). The somatic-variation theory, held that the germ line contains a limited number of variable genes, which are diversified in the somatic cells by either mutational or recombinational events during development of the immune system. As the cloning and sequencing of the immunoglobulin genes was completed, both models were partially vindicated. The sources of antibody diversity in the mouse and the number of different specificities generated cumulatively by these mechanisms are summarized in Table 8-3. The total number of possible combinations is conservatively estimated

at 10^8, the commonly quoted figure for the number of different antibody specificities that can be generated by the mammalian immune system.

Multiple Germ-Line V, D, and J Gene Segments

DNA hybridization studies have demonstrated that mouse germ-line DNA contains about 300 V_κ gene segments and 300–1000 V_H gene segments but only two V_λ gene segments. The existence of multiple J_L, D_H, and J_H segments expands the germ-line contribution to diversity. In the mouse, there appear to be 4 functional J_H, 4 functional J_κ, 3 functional J_λ, and an estimated 12 D_H gene segments. Although the numbers of germ-line genes are far fewer than predicted by early proponents of the germ-line model, it is still obvious that multiple germ-line, V, D, and J genes do contribute to diversity of the antigen-binding sites in antibodies.

Combinatorial V-J and V-D-J Joining and Chain Association

Further diversification of the germ-line genes is of course generated combinatorially during rearrangement in the somatic cells. The ability of any of the 300–1000 V_H gene segments to combine with any of the 12 D_H gene segments and any of the 4 J_H gene segments allows an enormous amount of diversity to be generated ($300 \times 12 \times 4 = 1.4 \times 10^4$ possible combinations). Similarly 300 V_κ gene segments randomly combining with 4 J_κ gene segments has the potential of generating 1.2×10^3 diverse combinations. With only 2 V_λ and 3 J_λ gene segments the combinatorial diversity of the λ light chain is much less.

Because the specificity of an antibody's antigen-binding site is determined by the variable regions in both its heavy and light chains, additional diversity is generated by the combinatorial association of heavy and light chains. Assuming that any one of the 1.4×10^4 possible heavy-chain genes and any one of the possible 1.2×10^3 κ light-chain genes can occur randomly in the same cell, then the total possible combinations containing κ light chains and heavy chains is 1.7×10^7.

Junctional Flexibility

The enormous diversity generated by means of V, D, and J combinations is further augmented by flexibility in the joining process. Although this flexibility can lead to many nonproductive rearrangements (see Figure 8-8), it also increases antibody diversity by generating several productive combinations encoding alternative amino acids at each joining site (Figure 8-18a). These joining sites have been shown to fall within the third hypervariable region (CDR3) in immunoglobulin heavy-chain and κ light-chain genes. Since hypervariable regions make up a significant portion of the antigen-binding site on the antibody molecule, it is obvious that an amino acid change generated by joining flexibility can have major impact in generating antibody diversity. On the average, joining flexibility generates three different amino acids at each junction (V_L-J_L, D_H-J_H, and V_H-D_H-J_H) and therefore the heavy-chain diversity is increased by a factor of nine and the light-chain diversity is increased by a factor of three. Junctional flexibility thus increases the total possible combinations in heavy-chain genes to 1.3×10^5 ($1.4 \times 10^4 \times 3 \times 3$) and in κ light-chain genes to 3.6×10^3 ($1.2 \times 10^3 \times 3$).

N-Region Nucleotide Addition

The V-D and D-J joining boundaries in immunoglobulin heavy chains have been shown to contain short amino acid sequences that are not encoded by the V, D, or J gene segments. These amino acids are encoded by nu-cleotides that are randomly added during joining by the mechanism shown in Figure 8-18b; nucleotide addition is catalyzed by a terminal deoxynucleotidyl transferase. Thus a complete heavy-chain variable region is encoded by a $V_H N D_H N J_H$ unit. The additional heavy-chain diversity generated by N-region nucleotide addition is quite large because the N regions appear to consist of wholly random sequences. Since this diversity occurs at joining sites, it is localized in the CDR3 of heavy-chain genes.

Somatic Mutation

All the antibody diversity discussed so far stems from mechanisms that operate during formation of specific variable regions by gene rearrangement. The implicit assumption throughout this chapter has been that once a functional variable-region gene unit is formed, it is not altered. This assumption turns out to be false, and additional antibody diversity is generated in rearranged variable-region gene units by a process called *somatic mutation*. As a result of somatic mutation, individual nucleotides in VJ or VDJ units are replaced with alternative bases, thus potentially altering the specificity of the encoded immunoglobulins.

Table 8-3 Cumulative generation of antibody diversity in the mouse

Mechanism of diversity	Possible combinations		
		Light chains	
	Heavy chain	κ	λ
Multiple germ-line gene segments:			
V	300	300	2
D	12	0	0
J	4	4	3
Combinatorial V-J and V-D-J joining	$300 \times 12 \times 4 = 1.4 \times 10^4$	$300 \times 4 = 1.2 \times 10^3$	$2 \times 3 = 6$
Junctional flexibility*	$9 \times 1.4 \times 10^4 = 1.3 \times 10^5$	$3 \times 1.2 \times 10^3 = 3.6 \times 10^3$	$3 \times 6 = 18$
N-region nucleotide addition[†]	+	−	−
Somatic mutation[†]	+	+	+
Combinatorial association of heavy and light chains	$>1.3 \times 10^5 \times (>3.6 \times 10^3 + >18) = \gg 4.7 \times 10^8$		

* On average three different productive rearrangements can occur at each junction.

[†] A + indicates mechanism makes significant contribution to diversity but to an unknown extent. A − indicates mechanism does not operate.

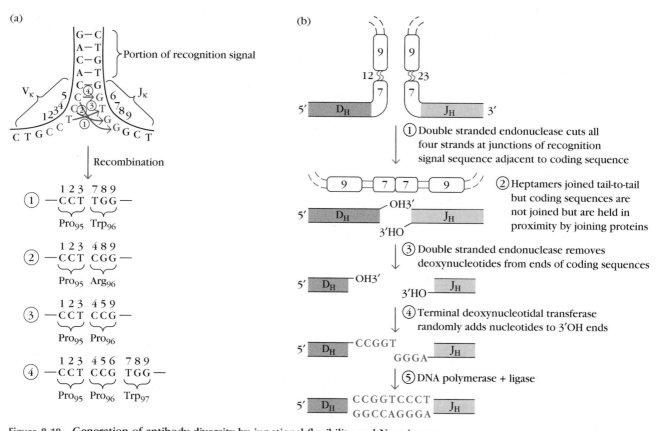

Figure 8-18 Generation of antibody diversity by junctional flexibility and N-region nucleotide addition. (a) Flexibility in joining has been shown to generate four different sequences at the V-J junction in κ light chains. The nucleotides in the junction region are numbered for convenience; the positions of the amino acids in the finished κ chains are indicated by subscripts. Note that recombination (4) adds an amino acid residue to the sequence. Similar flexibility occurs during joining of variable-region gene segments in λ light-chain and heavy-chain genes. (b) Random addition of nucleotides occurs during D-J and V-D-J joinings in heavy-chain genes. This process has not been demonstrated in light-chain genes.

Comparisons of germ-line variable-region DNA sequences with the DNA sequences expressed by somatic cells has demonstrated somatic mutation in both light- and heavy-chain genes. In one such study, L. E. Hood and his colleagues investigated the antibody response in mice to the hapten phosphorylcholine. This particular antigen-antibody system was chosen because a single V_H gene segment, T-15, was utilized by all the antibodies produced to phosphorylcholine. Hood cloned the T-15 germ-line DNA and sequenced it to determine the germ-line prototype sequence. He then sequenced the heavy-chain variable region in 19 phosphorylcholine-specific myeloma proteins and compared these with the germ-line V_H prototype sequence (Figure 8-19). Of the 19 expressed sequences, 10 were identical with the prototype sequence; the other 9 differed from the prototype by from one to eight amino acid substitutions. Of additional interest was the observation that all nine heavy-chain, variable-region variants were present in the

IgG or IgA myeloma proteins; none were present in IgM. This finding suggests a possible association of somatic mutation with class switching or, at least, that the additional cell divisions a cell undergoes in the process of class switching may increase the likelihood of somatic mutation occurring. Furthermore, the estimated rate of somatic mutation in B cells is quite high, being 10^{-3} mutations per base pair per cell division. This rate is 10^6 times higher than the spontaneous mutation rate in other genes, again suggesting that for some reason B cells are predisposed to somatic mutation.

The numbers of mutations generated by the process of somatic mutation has been shown to increase in the secondary and tertiary antibody responses to an antigen. Claudia Berek and Cesar Milstein were able to sequence the mRNA encoding antibodies produced in response to a primary, secondary or tertiary immunization with a hapten-carrier conjugate. The hapten that they chose was 2-phenyl-5-oxazolone (phOx) coupled to a protein

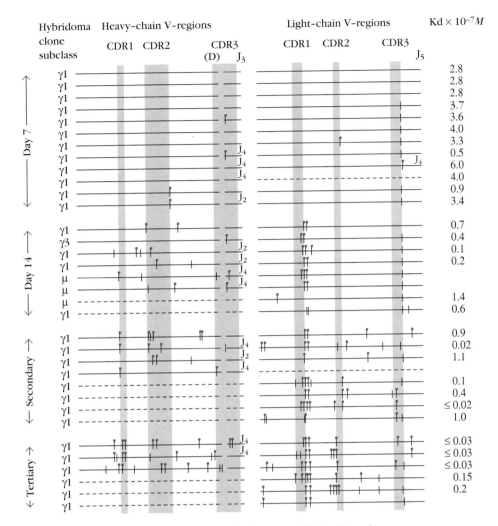

Figure 8-19 Diagram comparing the mRNA sequences of the heavy and light chains from hybridomas specific for the ph-Ox hapten. The solid lines represent the germline V_H Ox-1 and V_K Ox-1 sequences. Dashed lines represent sequences derived from other germline genes. Vertical lines show the position of mutations and the red circles indicate that the mutation encodes a different amino acid from the germline codon sequence. In hybridomas derived following secondary and tertiary immunizations there is an increase in the number of mutations as well as an increase in the overall affinity of the antibody as indicated by a decrease in the dissociation constant (Kd) obtained by equilibrium dialysis. Note that most of the mutations are clustered within CDR1 and CDR2 of both heavy and light chains. [Adapted from C. Berek and C. Milstein. 1987. *Immunol. Rev.* **96**:23.]

carrier. They chose this hapten because it had previously been shown to induce production of a majority of antibodies encoded by a single germline V_H and V_K gene segment. Berek and Milstein immunized mice with the phOx-carrier conjugate and then used the mice spleen cells to prepare hybridomas secreting monoclonal antibodies specific for the phOx hapten. The mRNA sequence for the H chain and κ light chain of each hybridoma was then determined (see Figure 8-19). They found that of 12 hybridomas obtained from mice seven days after a primary immunization, all used the V_H Ox-1 gene and all but one use the V_K Ox-1 gene. Only a

few hybridomas showed mutations from the germline sequence. By day 14 after primary immunization, analysis of eight hybridomas revealed that six continued to use the germline V_H Ox-1 gene and all continued to use the V_K Ox-1 gene. Now, however, a majority of the hybridomas showed mutations from the germline sequence. Hybridomas analyzed from the secondary and tertiary responses showed a larger percentage utilizing germline V_H genes other than the V_H Ox-1 gene. In those hybridoma clones that utilized the V_H Ox-1 and V_K Ox-1 gene segments there were progressively more mutations from the germline sequence as the response progressed following secondary and tertiary immunizations. Most of the mutations were clustered in CDR1 and CDR2 hypervariable regions. And, what was most interesting, was that the overall affinity of the antibodies progressively increased from the primary to the secondary and tertiary response. Although the process of somatic mutation is random, and can therefore generate antibodies of lower affinity as well as higher, the ability of an antigen to drive clonal expansion will selectively increase the proliferation of B cells that have higher-affinity membrane-bound antibody on their surface.

Summary

1. Immunoglobulin κ light chains, λ light chains, and heavy chains are encoded by three separate multigene families located on different chromosomes. In germ-line DNA, each multigene family contains numerous gene segments. The variable-region gene segments are designated V and J in light-chain DNA and V, D, and J, in heavy-chain DNA. Multiple constant-region (C) gene segments also are present.

2. Functional light-chain and heavy-chain genes are generated by random rearrangement of the variable-region gene segments in germ-line DNA. Conserved DNA sequences, termed recognition signal sequences, flank each V, D, and J gene segment and direct the joining of segments. Each recognition signal contains a conserved hepatamer sequence, a conserved nonamer sequence, and either a 12-bp or 23-bp spacer; the length, but not the nucleotide sequence, of these spacers is conserved. During rearrangement, gene segments flanked by a 12-bp spacer join only to segments flanked by a 23-bp spacer. This 12/23 joining rule assures proper V_L-J_L or V_H-D_H-J_H joining.

3. Immunoglobulin-gene rearrangements occur in sequential order, with heavy-chain rearrangements occurring first followed by light-chain rearrangements. These rearrangements are carefully regulated so that the immunoglobulin DNA of only one parental chromosome is rearranged to form a functional light-chain or heavy-chain gene. This allelic exclusion is necessary to assure that a mature B cell expresses immunoglobulin with a single antigenic specificity.

4. Differential RNA processing of the immunoglobulin heavy-chain primary transcript can generate either membrane-bound or secreted antibody. Differential processing is also responsible for expression of IgM alone by immature B cells and the coexpression of IgM and IgD by mature B cells.

5. After antigenic stimulation of mature B cells, additional rearrangement of their heavy-chain gene segments

can occur. Such class switching results in expression of different classes of antibody (IgG, IgA, and IgE) with the same antigenic specificity.

6. Differentiation of progenitor B cells into mature B cells has been correlated with variable-region gene rearrangements. This antigen-independent phase of B-cell differentiation occurs in the bone marrow. During the antigen-dependent phase of differentiation, antigenically primed B cells undergo class switching and changes in RNA processing. This phase leads to formation of B memory cells that express different membrane isotypes and plasma cells that secrete various isotypes.

7. The various mechanisms contributing to antibody diversity can generate, at a minimum, about 10^8 possible combinations. Major sources of antibody diversity are the random joining of multiple V, J, and D germ-line gene segments and the random association of a given heavy-chain and light-chain in a particular cell. Other mechanisms that augment antibody diversity by a significant but unknown extent are variability in the nucleotide sequences at the joints between gene segments and somatic mutation following antigenic stimulation.

References

AKIRA, S., K. OKAZAKI, and H. SAKANO. 1987. Two pairs of recombination signals are sufficient to cause immunoglobulin V-(D)-J joining. *Science* **238**:1134.

CALAME, K. 1985. Mechanisms that regulate immunoglobulin gene expression. *Annu. Rev. Immunol.* **3**:159.

CALAME, K., and S. EATON. 1988. Transcriptional controlling elements in the immunoglobulin and T cell receptor loci. *Adv. Immunol.* **43**:235.

CHUN, J. J. M., D. G. SCHATZ, M. A. OETTINGER, R. JEANISCH, and D. BALTIMORE. 1991. The recombination activating gene-1 (RAG-1) transcript is present in the murine central nervous system. *Cell* **64**:189.

HONJO, T., F. W. ALT, and T. H. RABBITS, eds. 1989. *Immunoglobulin Genes.* Academic Press.

HOZUMI, N., and S. TONEGAWA. 1976. Evidence for somatic rearrangement of immunoglobulin genes coding for variable and constant regions. *Proc. Natl. Acad. Sci. USA* **73**:3628

OETTINGER, M. A., D. G. SCHATZ, C. GORKA, and D. BALTIMORE. 1990. RAG-1 and RAG-2, adjacent genes that synergistically activate V(D)J recombination. *Science* **248**:1517.

BEREK, C., and C. MILSTEIN. 1987. Mutation drift and repertoire shift in the maturation of the immune respose. *Immunol. Rev.* **96**:23.

SEN, R., and D. BALTIMORE. 1989. Factors regulating immunoglobulin-gene transcription. In *Immunoglobulin Genes.* Academic Press.

STAUDT, L. M., and M. J. LENARDO. 1991. Immunoglobulin gene transcription. *Annu. Rev. Immunol.* 9:373.

TONEGAWA, S. 1983. Somatic generation of antibody diversity. *Nature* **302**:575.

WALL, R., and M, KUEHL. 1983. Biosynthesis and regulation of immunoglobulin. *Annu. Rev. Immunol.* **1**:393.

YANCOPOULOS, G. D., and F. W. ALT. 1986. Regulation of the assembly and expression of variable region genes. *Annu. Rev. Immunol.* **4**:339.

Study Questions

1. Indicate whether each of the following statements is true of false. If you think a statement is false, explain why.

   a. V_λ gene segments sometimes join to C_κ gene segments.

   b. Immunoglobulin class switching usually is mediated by DNA rearrangements.

   c. Separate exons encode the transmembrane portion of the membrane immunoglobulins.

   d. Although each B cell carries two alleles encoding the immunoglobulin heavy and light chains, only one allele is expressed.

   e. Primary transcripts are processed into functional mRNA by removal of introns, capping, and polyadenylation.

   f. The primary transcript is an RNA copy of the DNA and includes both introns and exons.

2. Draw a schematic diagram illustrating each of the following forms of immunoglobulin heavy-chain DNA, RNA, or protein in the mouse:

   a. The DNA arrangement in a liver cell.

   b. The DNA arrangement in a mature B cell.

   c. The primary RNA transcript in a mature B cell.

   d. The mRNA in a mature B cell.

   e. The protein product observed on the membrane of a mature B cell.

   f. The DNA arrangement in a plasma cell secreting IgE.

3. Explain why a V_H cannot join directly with a J_H in heavy-chain gene rearrangement?

4. Ignoring junctional diversity and somatic mutation, how many different antibody molecules potentially could be generated from germ-line DNA containing 500 V_L and 4 J_L gene segments and 300 V_H, 15 D_H, and 4 J_H gene segments?

5. Multiple choice (more than one answer may be correct each):

   1. Recombination of the immunoglobin gene segments serves to:

   a) promote Ig diversification
   b) assemble a complete Ig coding sequence
   c) allow changes in coding information during development
   d) a and b
   e) a, b, and c

   2. Somatic mutation accounts for:
   a) allelic exclusion
   b) class switching from IgM to IgG
   c) affinity maturation
   d) all of the above
   e) none of the above

   3. Somatic hypermutation is most active during:
   a) differentiation of pre-B cells into mature B cells
   b) differentiation of pre-T cells into mature T cells
   c) generation of memory B cells
   d) antibody secretion by the plasma cell

   4. Kappa and lambda light chain genes:
   a) are located on the same chromosome
   b) associate with only one type of heavy chain
   c) can be expressed by the same B cell
   d) all of the above
   e) none of the above

   5. Combinatorial diversity of immunoglobins involves:
   a) mRNA splicing
   b) DNA rearrangement
   c) recombination signal sequences
   d) 12/23 joining rule
   e) switch sites

6. You have a fluorescein-labeled antibody to the μ heavy chain and a rhodamine-labeled antibody to the δ heavy chain. Describe the fluorescent antibody staining pattern of the B-cell maturational stages assuming that you can visualize both membrane and cytoplasmic staining: (a) progenitor B cell; (b) pre-B cell; (c) immature B cell; (d) mature B cell; and (e) plasma cell.

7. What mechanisms generate the three hypervariable regions (complementarity-determining regions) of immunoglobulin heavy and light chains? Why is the third hypervariable region of the light and heavy chain more variable than the other two hypervariable regions?

8. You have been given a cloned myeloma cell line that secretes IgG with the molecular formula $\gamma_2\lambda_2$. Both the heavy- and light-chain genes in this cell line are derived from allele 1. In the table on the next page, indicate the form(s) in which each of the genes would occur in this cell line using the following symbols: G = germ-line configuration; R = productively rearranged gene; NP = nonproductively rearranged configuration. State the reason for the form(s) you indicate in each case.

	Configurations		
Gene	Possible	Not possible	Reason
Heavy chain, allele 1			
Heavy chain, allele 2			
κ chain, allele 1			
κ chain, allele 2			
λ chain, allele 1			
λ chain, allele 2			

Event	YES	NO
IgM to IgD		
IgM to IgA		
IgE to IgG		
IgA to IgG		
IgM to IgG		

9. You have a B-cell lymphoma which has made non-productive rearrangements for both heavy-chain alleles. What is the arrangement of its κ light-chain DNA? Why?

10. Describe one advantage and one disadvantage of the random addition and deletion of nucleotides at the V-D-J junctions during rearrangement of immunoglobulin gene segments.

11. Indicate whether the following class-switching events can occur by marking an X in the column marked YES or NO.

12. DNA was isolated from three sources: liver cells, pre-B lymphoma cells, and IgM-secreting myeloma cells. Each sample (designated A, B, or C) was digested separately with *Bam*HI and *Eco*RI, and the digested samples were analyzed by Southern blotting. The *Bam*HI digests were hybridized to a radiolabeled $C_\mu 1$ probe (blot #1), and the *Eco*RI digests were hybridized to a radiolabeled C_κ probe (blot #2). Based on the restriction maps and the Southern blots below, show which DNA sample was isolated from which source in the following table:

Source	*Sample*
Liver cells	_____
Pre-B lymphoma cells	_____
IgM-secreting myeloma cells	_____

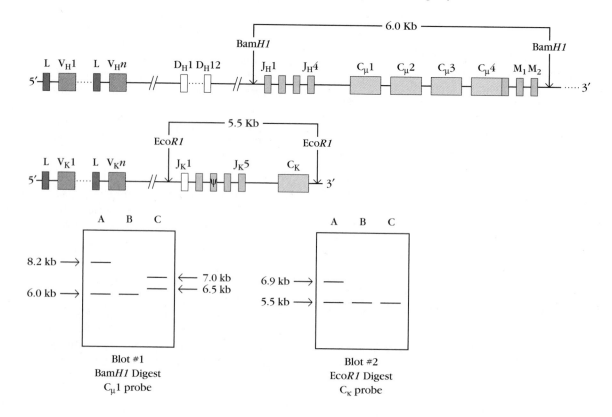

9

Major Histocompatibility Complex

Every mammalian species studied to date possesses a tightly linked cluster of genes—the major histocompatibility complex (MHC)—whose products are associated with intercellular recognition and with self/nonself discrimination. The MHC complex is a region of multiple loci that play major roles in determining whether transplanted tissue will be accepted as self (histocompatible) or rejected as foreign (histoincompatible).

The MHC plays a central role in the development of both humoral and cell-mediated immune responses. As discussed in previous chapters, the

T-cell requirement for MHC-restricted antigen recognition confers upon these molecules a critical role in antigen recognition by T cells. As antigen-presenting structures, the individual differences in MHC molecules expressed by an individual will influence the repertoire of antigens to which the T_H cells and T_C cells can respond. The MHC thus influences the response of an individual to antigens of infectious organisms and has been implicated in the susceptibility to disease and to the development of autoimmunity. This chapter will examine the organization and inheritance of MHC genes and the structure and function of the MHC molecules which play such a central role in the immune response.

General Organization and Inheritance of the MHC

The concept that the rejection of foreign tissue is the result of an immune response to cell-surface molecules (now called histocompatibility antigens) came from the work of R. A. Gorer and G. D. Snell in the mid-1930s. Gorer was using inbred strains of mice to identify blood-group antigens. In the course of these studies, he identified four groups of genes, designated I through IV, that encoded blood-cell antigens. Later work by Gorer and Snell established that the group II antigens were involved in the rejection of transplanted tumors and other tissue. Snell called these genes "histocompatibility genes"; their designation as histocompatibility-2 (H-2) genes was in reference to Gorer's group II blood-group antigens. The significant contribution of this early work of Snell was highlighted when he was awarded a Nobel prize in 1980.

Location of MHC Loci

The major histocompatibility complex is a collection of 40–50 genes arrayed within a long continuous stretch of DNA on chromosome 6 in humans and on chromosome 17 in mice. The MHC is referred to as the *HLA complex* in humans and as the *H-2 complex* in mice. Although the organization of genes is somewhat different in the human HLA and the mouse H-2 complex, certain features are common to both. In both cases the MHC genes are organized into regions encoding three classes of molecules: class I, class II, and class III. The class I genes encode glycoproteins expressed on the surface of nearly all nucleated cells, where they present peptide antigens of altered self-cells necessary for the activation of T_C cells. The class II genes encode glycoproteins expressed primarily on antigen-presenting cells (macrophages, dendritic cells, and B cells), where they present processed antigenic peptides to T_H cells (see

Figure 1-13). The class III genes encode somewhat different products that are also associated with the immune process. These include a number of soluble serum proteins (including components of the complement system), steroid 21-hydroxylase enzymes, and tumor necrosis factors.

Class I MHC molecules are encoded by the K and D regions in mice and by the A, B, and C regions in humans (Figure 9-1). Additional regions, designated Qa and Tla, also encode class I molecules in mice and are closely linked to the H-2 complex. Class II molecules are encoded by the I region in mice and by the D region in humans. The terminology is somewhat confusing, since the D region in mice encodes class I MHC molecules, whereas the D region in humans encodes class II MHC molecules! It is a relief that the class III molecules are encoded by regions with descriptive designations of S (for soluble protein) in the mouse and C4, C2, Bf (designating some of the individual complement proteins encoded here) in humans.

MHC Haplotypes

As discussed in more detail later, the loci constituting the MHC are highly *polymorphic;* that is, many alternate forms of the gene, or *alleles*, exist at each locus. The MHC loci are closely linked, having a recombination frequency of only 0.5%. For this reason, an individual inherits the alleles encoded by these closely linked loci as two sets, one from each parent. Each set of alleles is referred to as the *haplotype*. An individual inherits one haplotype from the mother and one haplotype from the father. In an outbred population the offspring are generally heterozygous at many loci and will express both maternal and paternal MHC alleles. The alleles are therefore codominantly expressed, that is both maternal and paternal gene products are expressed in the same cells. In inbred mice, however, each H-2 locus is homozygous because the maternal and paternal haplotypes are identical, and all offspring express identical haplotypes.

Certain inbred mice strains have been designated as prototype strains, and the haplotype expressed by these strains is designated by an arbitrary superscript (e.g., H-2^a, H-2^b, H-2^d, H-2^k). The arbitrary designation simply is a way of referring to the set of inherited alleles within a strain without having to refer to each allele individually (Table 9-1). If another inbred strain has inherited the same set of alleles as the prototype strain, its MHC haplotype is the same as the prototype strain, as illustrated in Figure 9-2a. For example, the CBA, C3H and AKR strains all have the same MHC haplotype (H-2^k). The three strains differ, however, in genes outside the H-2 complex. If two inbred strains of mice having different MHC haplotypes are bred, the F_1 generation inherits

Mouse H-2 complex

Complex	H-2							Tla	
MHC class	I	II		III			I	I	I
Region	K	IA	IE	S			D	Qa	Tla
Gene products	H-2K	IA αβ	IE αβ•	Complement proteins	Tumor necrosis factor TNF-α	TNF-β	H-2D	H-2L	Qa	Tla, Qa

Human HLA complex

Complex	HLA							
MHC class	II			III		I		
Region	DP	DQ	DR	C4, C2, BF		B	C	A
Gene products	DP αβ	DQ αβ	DR αβ	Complement proteins	Tumor necrosis factor TNF-α	TNF-β	HLA-B	HLA-C	HLA-A

Figure 9-1 Simplified organization of the major histocompatibility complex (MHC) in the mouse and human. The MHC is referred to as the H-2 complex in mice and as the HLA coding class I (red) class II (light red), and class III (gray) gene products.• IEβ gene is actually located in the IA region.

Table 9-1 H-2 haplotypes of some mouse strains

Prototype strain	Other strains with the same haplotype	Haplotype	MHC regions				
			K	A	E	S	D
CBA	AKR, C3H, B10.BR, C57BR	k	k	k	k	k	k
DBA/2	BALB/c, NZB, SEA, YBR	d	d	d	d	d	d
C57BL/10 (B10)	C57BL/6, C57L, C3H.SW, LP, 129	b	b	b	b	b	b
A	A/He, A/Sn, A/Wy, B10.A	a	k	k	k	d	d
A.SW	B10.S, SJL,	s	s	s	s	s	s
A.TL		t1	s	k	k	k	d
DBA/1	STOLI, B10.Q, BDP	q	q	q	q	q	q

haplotypes from both parental strains and therefore expresses both parental alleles at each MHC locus. For example, if strain C57BL/6 (H-2^b) is crossed with strain CBA (H-2^k), then the F$_1$ inherits both parental sets of alleles and is said to be H-2$^{b/k}$ (Figure 9-2b). Because such an F$_1$ expresses the MHC proteins of both parental strains on its cells, it is histocompatible with both strains and able to accept grafts from either parental strain.

As noted above, in an outbred population, each animal is generally heterozygous at each locus. Furthermore, both the maternal and paternal alleles at each MHC locus are expressed (this differs from expression of the immunoglobulin genes, which exhibit allelic exclusion, so that only one allele is expressed). The F$_1$ offspring of two heterozygous parents inherits one set of MHC alleles (i.e., one haplotype) from the father and one set from the mother (Figure 9-2c). Such an F$_1$ expresses only half of the paternal and half of the maternal class I MHC molecules on its nucleated cells. If this F$_1$ is grafted with tissue from either parent, it will recognize the foreign MHC molecules on the parental graft and reject the graft. Because the MHC loci are closely linked and are inher-

(a) Hypothetical allelic composition of mouse MHC haplotypes

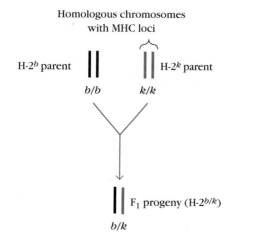

Strain	Haplotype	K	A_β	A_α	E_β	E_α	D	L
				Alleles				
CBA	k	3	22	54	11	97	13	80
C3H	k	3	22	54	11	97	13	80
C57BL/10	b	12	74	3	18	20	5	65

(b) Mating of inbred mouse strains with different MHC haplotypes

(c) Mating of outbred mouse strains with different MHC haplotypes

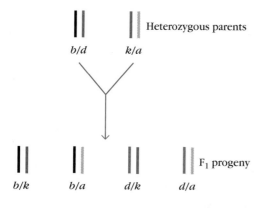

Figure 9-2 (a) Illustration of MHC haplotype designation. Strain CBA inherits a particular allele, indicated by a hypothetical number, at each MHC locus. The complete set of alleles is arbitrarily designated as the H-2^k haplotype. Any inbred strain (e.g., C3H) that has the same set of MHC alleles is designated as an H-2^k strain. Strains with a different set of MHC alleles (e.g., C57BL/10) are given a different haplotype designation. (b) and (c) Because the MHC loci are closely linked and inherited as a set, the MHC haplotype of F$_1$ progeny from mating of inbred and outbred strains can be predicted easily.

ited as a haplotype, there is a one in four chance in outbred populations that siblings will inherit the same paternal and maternal haplotypes and therefore be histocompatible (unless, of course, the father and mother share a haplotype in common).

The inheritance and expression of class II MHC molecules is complicated by the fact that class II MHC molecules contain two different polypeptide chains (α and β), which are encoded by different loci in the IA and IE subregions of the H-2 complex (see Figure 9-1). The F$_1$ offspring obtained from crossing two inbred mouse strains express not only the parental class II molecules but also heterologous hybrid molecules containing one parent's α chain and the other parent's β chain. For example, an H-2^k haplotype mouse expresses IA^k and IE^k class II molecules (i.e., IA$\alpha^k\beta^k$ and IE$\alpha^k\beta^k$); similarly an H-2^b haplotype mouse expresses IA^b and IE^b molecules (i.e., IA$\alpha^b\beta^b$ and IE$\alpha^b\beta^b$). The F$_1$ offspring obtained from crossing these two mice will express a variety of class II MHC molecules distinct from either parent. These class II MHC molecules are formed by the association of the α and β chains encoded by each parental allele. The class II MHC molecules expressed by the F$_1$ would include the four homologous parental proteins (IA$\alpha^b\beta^b$, IA$\alpha^k\beta^k$, IE$\alpha^b\beta^b$, IE$\alpha^k\beta^k$) and heterologous hybrid proteins (IA$\alpha^b\beta^k$, IA$\alpha^k\beta^b$, IE$\alpha^k\beta^b$, IE$\alpha^k\beta^k$). The number of different class II gene products expressed per cell may actually approach 10–20 because, in addition to the association of maternal and paternal α and β chains, more than one functional β gene is found within the IA and IE loci. As discussed previously, MHC proteins function in the presentation of processed antigen to T cells. The heterozygosity generated by expression of both MHC alleles and by production of heterologous class II MHC molecules presumably increases the number of different antigenic peptides that can be presented and thus is advantageous to the organism.

Congenic MHC Mouse Strains

Detailed analysis of the H-2 complex in mice was made possible by the development of congenic mouse strains. Two strains are *congenic* if they are genetically identical except at a single genetic locus or region. Any phenotypic differences that can be detected between congenic strains are related to the genetic region that distinguishes the strains. Congenic strains that are identical to each other except at the major histocompatibility complex can be produced by a series of crosses, backcrosses, and selections. Figure 9-3 outlines the steps by which the H-2 complex of homozygous strain B can be introduced into the background genes of homozygous strain A to generate a congenic strain, denoted A.B.

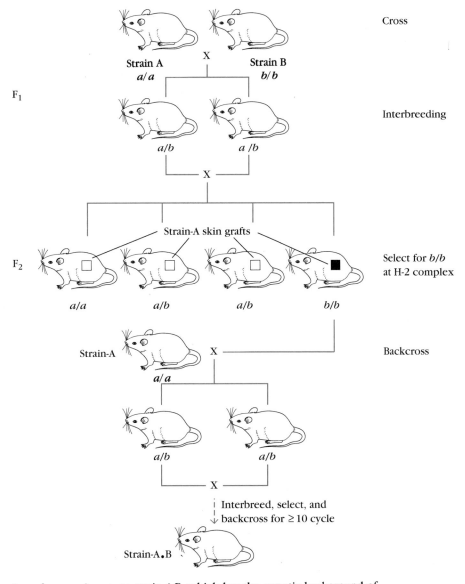

Figure 9-3 Production of congenic mouse strain A.B, which has the genetic background of parental strain A but the H-2 complex of strain B. Crossing inbred strain A (H-2^a) with strain B (H-2^b) generates F_1 progeny that are heterozygous (a/b) at all H-2 loci. The F_1 progeny are interbred to produce an F_2 generation, which includes a/a, a/b, and b/b individuals. The F_2 progeny homozygous for the B-strain H-2 complex are selected by their ability to reject a skin graft from strain A; any progeny that accept an A-strain graft are eliminated from future breeding. The selected b/b homozygous mice are then back-crossed to strain A; the resulting progeny are again interbred and their offspring are again selected for b/b homozygosity at the H-2 complex. This process of backcrossing to strain A, intercrossing, and selection for rejection of an A-strain graft is repeated for at least 12 generations. In this way A-strain homozygosity is restored at all loci except the H-2 locus, which is homozygous for the B strain.

The congenic strain will be genetically identical to strain A except for the MHC locus or loci contributed by strain B.

During production of congenic mouse strains, a crossover event sometimes occurs within the H-2 complex, yielding a recombinant strain that differs from the parental strains or the congenic strain at one or a few loci within the H-2 complex. Figure 9-4 illustrates several recombinant congenic strains that were obtained during production of a B10.A congenic strain. Such recombinant strains have been extremely useful in analyzing the MHC because they permit comparisons of functional differences between strains that differ in only a few genes within the MHC.

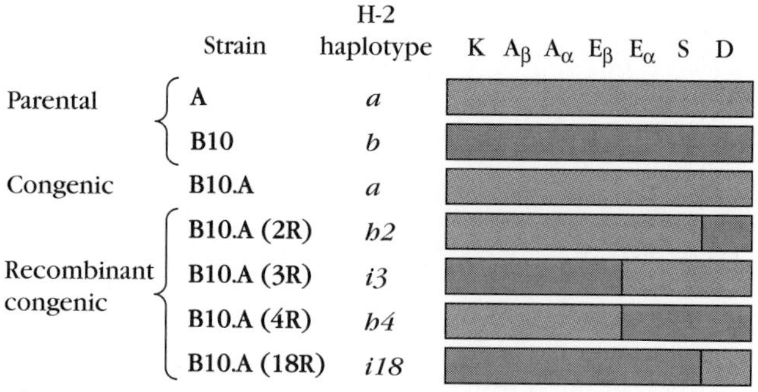

Figure 9-4 Examples of recombinant congenic mouse strains generated during production of the congenic B10.A strain from parental strain B10 (H-2^b) and parental strain A (H-2^a). Crossover events within the H-2 complex produce recombinant strains, which have *a*-haplotype alleles (red) at some H-2 loci and *b*-haplotype alleles (gray) at other loci.

Mapping the MHC

Once congenic and recombinant congenic mouse strains were available, mapping of the position and function of the individual genes within the H-2 complex became possible. In these studies, both serologic and functional assays were used to assess the gene products encoded by the MHC genes. More recently, cloning of both mouse and human MHC genes has permitted restriction-enzyme mapping of the MHC.

Serologic Mapping

When cells from one inbred strain are injected into a genetically different inbred strain, antibodies are elicited against the unique epitopes of the foreign MHC molecules. These antibodies can define different groups of MHC antigenic specificities. The epitopes that are unique to a given haplotype are *private specificities*, whereas epitopes shared by more than one haplotype are *public specificities*. Antisera specific for different public or private MHC antigenic specificities have been used to identify different MHC gene products and to determine whether or not they are encoded by separate loci. It was on the basis of early serologic results that the *K* and *D* loci of the mouse H-2 complex were first identified. Serologic studies eventually led to the identification of K, D, L, IA, and IE gene products and their mapping within the H-2 complex.

Functional Mapping

A functional map of the mouse H-2 complex was developed by use of various assays based on the immunologic function of class I, II, and III MHC molecules. A few examples of these functional assays are described here; others are discussed in later chapters.

Class I Functional Assays

When an animal is immunized with *allogeneic* cells (i.e., cells from a genetically distinct individual of the same species), it generates cytotoxic T lymphocytes (CTLs) specific for the MHC molecules on the allogeneic cells. The functional activity of the specific CTLs induced by the allogeneic cells can be assayed by *cell-mediated lympholysis* (CML). In the CML assay splenic lymphocytes from an immunized animal are incubated in vitro with the same allogeneic cells used for immunization except that the cells are labeled intracellularly with radioactive ^{51}Cr. As the immune CTLs attack the radiolabeled allogeneic cells, ^{51}Cr is released from the cells into the medium (Figure 9-5a). The amount of ^{51}Cr released into the culture medium is proportional to the level of cell-mediated cytotoxicity. CML assays performed with congenic recombinant mouse strains differing in various regions within the MHC have shown that a difference in either the K or the D region significantly affects CTL-mediated killing of allogeneic cells, indicating that this activity maps to the class I regions.

The CML assay also can be used to measure CTL-mediated killing of virus-infected cells. In this case, an animal is infected with a virus and the cytotoxic activity of its lymphocytes is assessed with syngeneic cells that have been infected with the same virus and intracellularly labeled with ^{51}Cr (Figure 9-5b). The immune CTLs were found to kill virally infected cells only if the class I MHC K or D regions of the target cell were the same as the CTL cell's, indicating that this activity maps to the class I region of the MHC.

Class II Functional Assays

The earliest function associated with the MHC class II region—its ability to influence immune responsiveness to various antigens—was discovered quite unexpectedly by B. Benacerraf in 1963. He had been trying to produce homogeneous antibody by immunizing guinea pigs with simple synthetic immunogens containing a limited number of epitopes, such as DNP–poly-L-lysine (DNP-PLL). Much to his surprise, injection with DNP-PLL induced a good antibody response in some animals (designated as *responders*) but no antibody response in other animals (designated as *nonresponders*). Similar results were obtained for other simple synthetic polypeptides, such as a glutamic acid–alanine copolymer and a glutamic acid–tyrosine copolymer. The genetic control over responsiveness or nonresponsiveness was shown to be inherited in a simple Mendelian fashion (Table 9-2). When responder guinea pigs were mated with nonresponder guinea pigs, all the F_1 offspring were responders; backcrossing of the F_1 to the nonresponder parent yielded 50% nonresponders and 50% responders, suggesting that a single dominant genetic region controlled immune responsiveness. These studies were extended by Hugh McDevitt, who injected different inbred strains of mice. These studies revealed that the class II MHC region controlled immune responsiveness to simple synthetic peptide antigens. The results of additional studies with congenic recombinant strains differing in various regions within the MHC showed that the genetic control of immune responsiveness to these simple synthetic-peptide antigens mapped to a subregion between K and S. McDevitt designated this subregion as the Ir region, for immune responsiveness (Table 9-2). This region is now known to comprise the IA and IE subregions encoding the class II MHC molecules. Since these early studies with synthetic amino acid polymers, the immune response to a wide variety of antigens, both synthetic and naturally occurring, has been shown to be under the control of I-region genes in both IA and IE subregions. It was not until the late 1970s and early 1980s

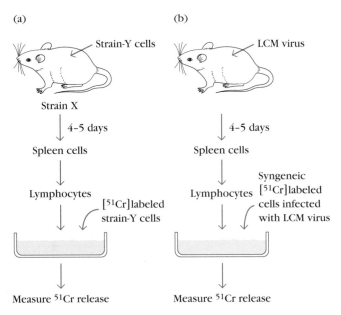

Figure 9-5 The in vitro cell-mediated lympholysis (CML) assay can measure the activity of cytotoxic T lymphocytes (CTLs) against allogeneic cells (a) or virus-infected cells (b). In both cases the release of ^{51}Cr into the supernatant indicates the presence of CTLs that can lyse the target cells.

Table 9-2 Demonstration of Mendelian inheritance of immune responsiveness to synthetic peptide antigens

	Immune response*				
Synthetic antigen	Strain 2	Strain 13	2 × 13 (F_1)	F_1 × 2	F_1 × 13
DNP–poly-L-Lys	+	−	+ (100%)	+ (100%)	+ (50%) − (50%)
Glu-Ala copolymer	+	−	+ (100%)	+ (100%)	+ (50%) − (50%)
Glu-Tyr copolymer	−	+	+ (100%)	+ (50%) − (50%)	+ (100%)

* Determined by production (+) or no production (−) of specific serum antibody following immunization with antigen. In crosses, the values in parentheses indicate the percentage of animals showing a + or − response.

that the role of the I region in governing immune responsiveness began to be unraveled with the discovery of the central role of the class II MHC molecules as antigen-presenting molecules for T_H activation.

Class II MHC molecules also play a role in T-cell proliferation in response to antigens on allogeneic cells. For example, when lymphocytes from two different inbred strains are cultured together, the cells begin to proliferate in response to the antigenic differences on the allogeneic lymphocytes. The intensity of this *mixed lymphocyte reaction (MLR)* can be quantified by adding [³H] thymidine to the culture medium. As the cells proliferate, the radioactive thymidine is incorporated into the DNA of the daughter cells. The amount of radioactivity in the DNA can be measured by harvesting the cells, lysing them, and measuring the amount of radioactive thymidine incorporated into the DNA, which is directly proportional to the level of cell proliferation. When allogeneic lymphocytes are mixed together, both populations of lymphocytes proliferate. This type of reaction is called a *two-way MLR*. To measure the proliferative response of only one population of lymphocytes a *one-way MLR* is performed; in this assay the proliferative response of one lymphocyte population is inhibited by treatment with x-rays to induce chromosomal damage or with mitomycin C to inhibit spindle formation. In the one-way MLR the untreated cells are referred to as *responders* and the treated cells, which can no longer proliferate, are called *stimulators* (Figure 9-6). By performing one-way MLRs between different congenic recombinant strains of lymphocytes, it was possible to determine which region of the MHC induced the strongest MLR reaction. The experiments revealed that an MHC difference between responder and stimulator cells in the I region resulted in the most intense proliferative response (Figure 9-7). As is discussed later, the MLR measures proliferation of the T helper cell; indeed the critical role of class II MHC proteins in T_H-cell activation was first revealed by means of this assay.

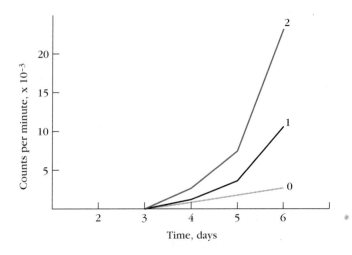

Figure 9-6   One-way mixed-lymphocyte reaction (MLR). This assay measures the proliferation of lymphocytes from one strain (responder cells) in response to allogeneic cells that have been x-irradiated or treated with mitomycin C to prevent proliferation (stimulator cells). The amount of [³H] thymidine incorporated into the DNA is directly proportional to the level of proliferation.

Figure 9-7   The amount of [³H] thymidine uptake in a one-way MLR in which the stimulator and responder cells have no class II MHC differences (curve 0), have one class II MHC difference (curve 1), or have two class II MHC differences (curve 2). These results demonstrate that lymphocyte proliferation in response to allogeneic cells depends on differences in class II MHC molecules.

Molecular Mapping

The availability of congenic and recombinant congenic mouse strains as well as the functional and serological mapping of the mouse MHC led to rapid progress in mapping the mouse MHC genes. Molecular dissection of the MHC began in the early 1980s with the isolation of cDNA clones encoding class I, class II, or class III MHC molecules. In each case, mRNA encoding a particular MHC molecule was isolated and converted with reverse transcriptase into cDNA, which was then cloned (see Figure 2-4). Meanwhile, large fragments of chromosomal DNA from the BALB/c mouse strain were cloned in cosmid vectors (see Figure 2-5). These genomic DNA cosmid clones were then screened with a cDNA probe to identify the clones containing MHC genes.

The position of the individual MHC genes could then be determined by restriction-enzyme mapping. Each cosmid clone shown to hybridize with a cDNA probe was digested by several restriction endonucleases so that an ordered DNA map could be constructed (see Figure 2-3). The distal ends of the mapped region were subcloned, converted into single-stranded DNA, and used as probes to identify another set of overlapping cosmid clones. Each of these clones was again mapped by restriction-enzyme mapping and again the 5′ and 3′ ends were subcloned to serve as new probes that could recognize still more overlapping cosmid clones, thus extending the map in both the 5′ and 3′ directions (Figure 9-8). This technique, called *chromosome walking*, has made it possible to map large sequences of the mouse and human MHC complex.

Restriction-enzyme mapping of the HLA complex in humans has revealed 40–50 genes within a 3500-kb span of DNA. It is interesting to note that this span is approximately the size of the entire *E. coli* genome of 5000 genes. Each MHC gene therefore spans about 100 times as much DNA as a single *E. coli* gene; this greater length may reflect the inclusion of more complex regulatory sequences in mammalian genes than in the genes of a less complex organism such as *E. coli*. Mapping has been important in confirming or correcting the original maps derived from functional or serologic analysis. Molecular mapping has revealed a number of additional genes that map to class I, class II, or class III regions within the MHC (Figure 9-9). In some cases, the genes are defective and represent pseudogenes. In other cases, genes that had been identified by functional or serologic assays were not revealed by restriction-enzyme mapping. For example, early functional and serologic mapping had identified a subregion called IJ, but cloning of the MHC showed that the I region does not include an IJ subregion, so that other explanations must account for the functions attributed to IJ.

Molecular mapping of the MHC has revealed additional genes, many of whose functions are only beginning to be unraveled. In humans, the class I region has been shown to contain at least three additional loci, designated as E, F, and G, as well as the previously described A, B, and C loci. A large number of class I-like genes have also been identified outside of the MHC and telomeric to the HLA-A gene. A number of these nonclassical class I genes are pseudogenes and do not encode a protein product but others encode class I-like products of yet unknown function. These genes are thought to be analogous to the Qa and Tla genes that are adjacent to the mouse H-2 complex.

Molecular mapping of the class II MHC has revealed additional β chain genes, which have been identified in both mouse and human class II regions. In the human DR region, for example, there are two or three functional β chain genes. Each of these β chain genes can be expressed together with the α chain gene, thereby increasing the number of antigen-presenting molecules on a single cell. In humans, the class II region has also been shown to contain additional class II-like sequences designated DZ, DO, DX, and DV. Some of these sequences are pseudogenes and others encode protein products of unknown function. Genes encoding molecules, which are thought to function as peptide transporters, also map within the class II region. These molecules are thought to transport peptides from the cytoplasm into the endoplasmic reticulum, enabling the peptide to interact with newly synthesized class I MHC molecules.

The class III region of the MHC in humans and in mice contains a heterogeneous collection of genes encoding several components of the complement system: (C2, factor B, and C4), the microsomal cytochrome P-450 steroid 21-hydrolase, two heat shock proteins (hsp70-1 and hsp70-2), and two cytokines (TNFα and TNFβ). It is not known why this heterogeneous group of genes maps in the middle of the MHC, but there is speculation that at least some of the relationship of the MHC to certain diseases may be due to gene products of the class III region. A number of abnormalities of the complement system have been linked to autoimmune diseases: The cytokines (TNFα and TNFβ) have been shown to induce increased expression of the class I and class II MHC molecules which may contribute to some diseases. The heat shock proteins are an unusual group of highly conserved proteins that are released by cells in response to various stresses including heat shock (for which they were named), nutrient deprivation, oxygen radicals, and viral infection. Some of these proteins are thought to bind incompletely- or aberrantly-folded proteins and may be involved in the intracellular trafficking of proteins for proper antigen presentation; during heat

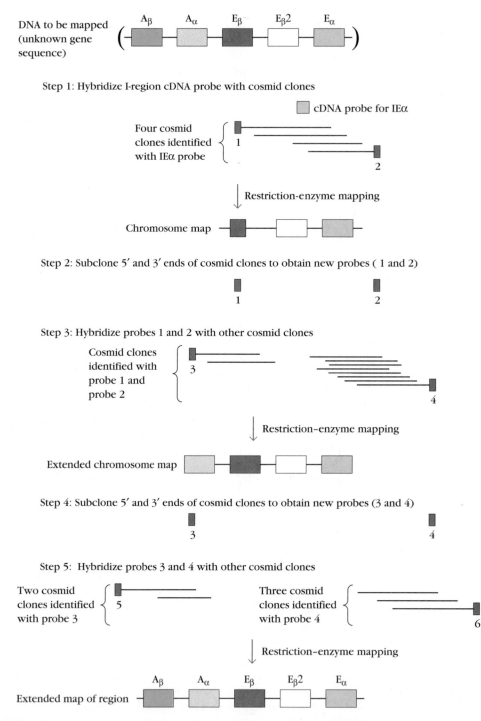

Figure 9-8　Mapping of I region of mouse H-2 complex by the technique of chromosome walking. Initially, an mRNA encoding an I-region gene product is converted into labeled cDNA with reverse transcriptase, and a series of large chromosomal fragments are cloned in cosmid vectors. The cDNA is used to probe the cosmid clones to identify those containing the I-region gene. Each identified clone is mapped by restriction-enzyme mapping and ordered relative to each other. The most distal 5′ and 3′ ends of the cosmid clones (numbered black boxes) are then subcloned and used as probes to identify still more cosmid clones. By repeating this process over and over, the map can be extended in both directions.

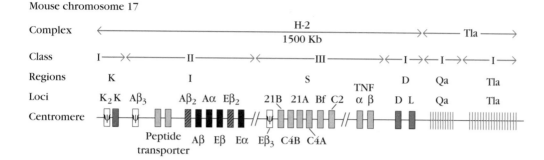

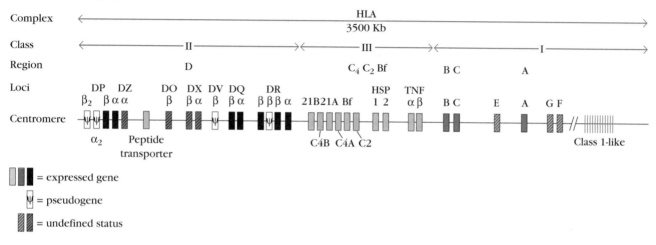

Figure 9-9 Organization of the mouse and human MHC loci reveals additional complexity. Class I genes are depicted by red, class II genes by black, and class III genes by light gray. Molecular mapping has revealed a number of additional genes. Included among these genes are three new human class I genes (HLA-E, F, and G), the peptide transporter genes located within the class II region of both the mouse and human and the heat shock protein (HSP 1 & 2) located within the class III region of humans. Several class II MHC loci contain multiple α and β genes, which vary among different alleles. Some of the newly identified genes (indicated by an open box) are pseudogenes and may be important sources of DNA involved in gene conversion. Other genes (indicated by a light red and dark gray boxes) have an as yet undefined status.

shock these proteins associate with ribonucleoproteins in the nucleus. There is speculation that the heat shock proteins may be linked to certain autoimmune diseases; this will be discussed in Chapter 16.

Class I MHC Molecules and Genes

Class I MHC molecules contain a large α chain associated noncovalently with a much smaller β_2-microglobulin molecule (Figure 9-10). The α chain is encoded by genes within the A, B, and C regions of the human HLA complex and within the K and D/L regions of the mouse H-2 complex (see Figure 9-9). In the mouse, the genes in the Qa and Tla regions, which are downstream from the

H-2 complex and closely linked to it, also encode class I MHC molecules. These genes, however, are less polymorphic than the classic class I MHC genes and show different patterns of expression. For example, the Tla gene products are expressed only in thymocytes, activated T cells, and some thymic leukemia cells, whereas the class I MHC gene products are expressed in nearly all nucleated cells. In addition, a number of Qa gene products are expressed as secreted proteins, whereas class I MHC molecules are only expressed on membranes. Also, many of the genes in the Qa and Tla regions appear to be pseudogenes having no identified protein product.

Class I MHC molecules function to present processed antigenic peptides produced in altered self-cells to T_C cells. The class I molecules are found on the membranes

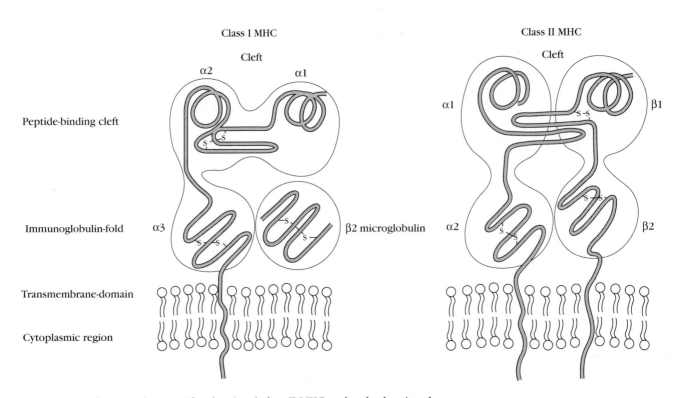

Figure 9-10 Schematic diagram of a class I and class II MHC molecule showing the external domains, the transmembrane segment and the cytoplasmic region. The peptide binding cleft is formed by the membrane distal α1 and α2 domains of the class I MHC and by the α1 and β1 domains of the class II MHC. The membrane proximal domains of both class I and class II molecules are organized with the basic immunoglobulin-fold and therefore these molecules are classified as members of the immunoglobulin superfamily.

of all nucleated cells with the exception of sperm and the trophoblast, however, the level of class I expression varies considerably among different cell types. The highest levels of class I molecules are expressed by lymphocytes where they constitute approximately 1% of the total plasma-membrane proteins, or some 5×10^5 molecules per cell. Fibroblasts, muscle cells, liver hepatocytes, and neural cells express very low levels of class I MHC molecules. The low level of class I MHC expressed by the liver hepatocytes may reduce the likelihood of graft recognition by cytotoxic T lymphocytes of the recipient and is thought to contribute to the considerable success with liver transplants.

Isolation of Class I Molecules

The isolation of class I MHC molecules is difficult because they are membrane bound and have a relatively low level of expression, accounting for at most only 1% of the membrane proteins. Their isolation from the mem-

brane of lymphoid cell lines was ultimately achieved by two methods. In one method lymphoid cells are treated with Nonidet P-40 detergent, which extracts the class I molecule intact but renders it insoluble in aqueous

Figure 9-11 Structure of class I MHC molecules. (a) Schematic diagram showing various regions of the molecule. The α_3 domain and β_2-microglobulin have the immunoglobulin-fold structure (light red). (b) Representation of the human class I HLA-A2 molecule determined by x-ray crystallographic analysis. The β strands are depicted as thick arrows (light red) and the α helices as helical ribbons (dark red). Disulfide bonds are represented as two interconnected spheres. (c) Representation of the α_1 and α_2 domains as viewed from the top of a class I MHC molecule showing the cleft consisting of a base of antiparallel β strands and sides of α helices. (d) Computer representation of a crystallized class I MHC molecule showing a peptide, which had cocrystallized with the molecule, bound in the cleft. [Part (d) from P. J. Bjorkman, M. A. Saper, B. Samraoui et al. 1987. *Nature* **329**:506.]

(a)

Class I MHC α-chain

α_2

α_1

H_2N

α_3

β_2-microglobulin

S—S
S—S

S
S
S
S

Exterior

Cell
Membrane

Interior

Transmembrane
segment

Cytoplasmic tail

COOH

(b)

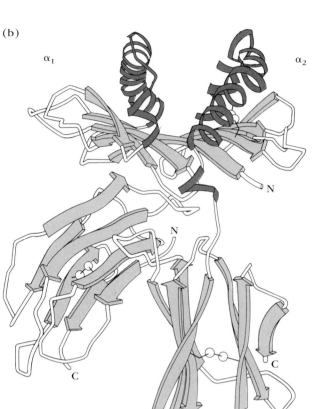

α_1

α_2

N

N

β_2-microglobulin

C

C

α_3

(c)

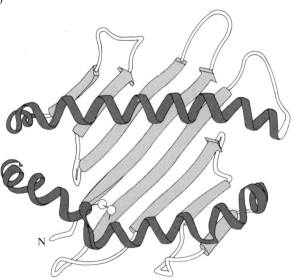

N

(d)

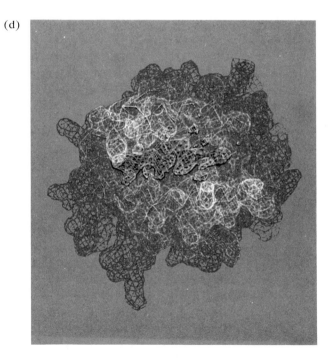

solutions. In the other method cells are treated with the enzyme papain, which cleaves the exposed hydrophilic, soluble portion of the molecule from its hydrophobic, insoluble transmembrane tail. The cleaved portion is then concentrated by passage through an affinity column of lectin bound to Sepharose beads. Glycoproteins, including class I MHC molecules, are bound by lectin and can be eluted from a Sepharose column by free sugar. The class I molecules in this enriched preparation can be immunoprecipitated with specific antibody.

Structure of Class I Molecules

As noted already, each class I MHC molecule consists of a heavy chain—the α chain—associated noncovalently with a light chain, which is β_2-microglobulin. The α chain is a polymorphic transmembrane glycoprotein of about 45 kilodaltons (kD) encoded by class I MHC loci. The β_2-microglobulin is an invariant protein of about 12 kD encoded by genes on a separate chromosome. Association with β_2-microglobulin is required for expression of class I molecules on cell membranes. The α chain is anchored in the plasma membrane by its hydrophobic transmembrane segment and hydrophilic cytoplasmic tail.

Peptide mapping and amino acid sequencing have revealed that the α chain of class I MHC molecules is organized into three external domains each containing approximately 90 amino acids (α_1, α_2, and α_3), a transmembrane domain of about 40 amino acids, and a cytoplasmic anchor segment of 30 amino acids (Figure 9-11a). In size and organization β_2-microglobulin is similar to the external domains. Comparison of sequence data has shown that considerable homology exists between the α_3 domain, β_2-microglobulin, and the constant-region domains in immunoglobulins. The enzyme papain cleaves the α chain just 13 residues proximal to its transmembrane domain, releasing the extracellular portion of the molecule consisting of α_1, α_2, α_3, and β_2-microglobulin. Purification and crystallization of the extracellular portion revealed two pairs of interacting domains: a membrane-distal pair made up of the α_1 and α_2 domains and a membrane-proximal pair comprised of the α_3 domain and β_2-microglobulin.

The α_1 and α_2 domains interact to form a platform of eight antiparallel β strands spanned by two long α-helical regions. The structure forms a deep groove, or cleft, approximately 25 Å × 10 Å × 11 Å, with the long α helices as sides and the β strands of the β sheet as a bottom (Figure 9-11b). This groove is on the top surface of the molecule and is thought to be the peptide-binding site of the class I MHC molecule, having a sufficient size to bind a peptide of 10–20 amino acids. The great surprise

in the x-ray crystallographic analysis of the class I molecule was the finding of a small peptide in the cleft that had cocrystallized with the molecule. It is speculated that this peptide may, in fact, be processed antigen bound to the α_1 and α_2 domains in this deep groove.

The α_3 domain and β_2-microglobulin are organized into two β pleated sheets each formed by antiparallel β strands of amino acids (Figure 9-11c). As described in Chapter 5, this structure, known as the immunoglobulin fold, is characteristic of immunoglobulin domains (see Figure 5-6a). Because of this structural similarity, which is not surprising given the considerable sequence homology with the immunoglobulin constant regions, class I MHC molecules and β_2-microglobulin are classified as members of the immunoglobulin superfamily. The α_3 domain appears to be highly conserved among class I MHC molecules and contains a sequence that is recognized by the CD8 T cell membrane molecule. β_2-microglobulin interacts extensively with the α_3 domain and also interacts with amino acids of the α_1 and α_2 domains. The interaction of β_2-microglobulin appears to be necessary for the proper conformation of the class I MHC molecule. Peptide binding to the groove in the α_1/α_2 domain appears to enable the α_3 domain to interact with β_2-microglobulin, allowing the molecule to assume its proper conformation. Without β_2-microglobulin the class I molecule will not be expressed on the membrane. The Daudi tumor cell line is unable to synthesize β_2-microglobulin. These cells transcribe class I genes and translate the mRNA into protein but are unable to express the class I molecule on the membrane. If the Daudi cells are transfected with a functional gene for β_2-microglobulin they will begin to express the class I molecule on the membrane.

Structure of Class I Genes

A number of class I MHC genes have been cloned and sequenced. Comparison of the amino acid sequence of the protein product with the DNA sequence has revealed that separate exons encode each domain (Figure 9-12a). The mouse *K, D, L, Qa,* and *Tla* genes and human *A, B,* and *C* genes all have a 5′ leader exon encoding a short signal peptide followed by five or six exons encoding the α chain of the class I molecule. The signal peptide serves to facilitate insertion of the α chain into the endoplasmic reticulum and is later removed following translation by proteolytic enzymes in the endoplasmic reticulum. The next three exons encode the extracellular α_1, α_2, and α_3 domains. The next downstream exon encodes the transmembrane region; finally a 3′-terminal exon or two exons encode the cytoplasmic domains.

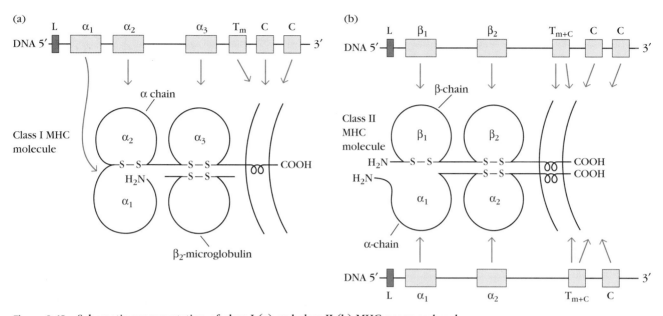

Figure 9-12 Schematic representation of class I (a) and class II (b) MHC genes and molecules showing the correspondence between exons (red) and the domains in the gene product. Each exon, with the exception of the leader (L) exon, encodes a separate domain of the MHC molecule. T_m = transmembrane; C = cytoplasmic.

Class II MHC Molecules and Genes

Class II MHC molecules contain two different polypeptide chains, designated α and β. Both chains are encoded by genes within the D region of the human HLA complex and within the I region of the mouse H-2 complex (see Figure 9-9). The mouse I region is divided into two subregions—IA and IE, and the human D region is divided into at least three subregions—DP, DQ, and DR. Each of these subregions contains at least one α and one β gene, encoding the α and β chains of a class II MHC molecule. In addition both the mouse and the human class II regions contain some additional genes for which no protein product has been identified (see Figure 9-9). These genes include; SXα, SXβ, DZα, DOβ, DXα, DXβ, and DRβ2 in humans and Aβ_2 and Eβ_2 in mice.

Unlike class I MHC molecules, class II molecules are expressed only by certain immune-system cells, notably macrophages, dendritic cells, thymic epithelial cells, B cells, and in humans activated T cells. Class II MHC proteins function to present processed antigenic peptides to T_H cells.

Structure of Class II Molecules

The same methods described earlier for isolating class I MHC molecules have been used to isolate class II molecules.

Class II MHC molecules are similar to the Class I molecules in that they also are membrane-bound glycoproteins containing external domains, a transmembrane segment, and a cytoplasmic anchor segment. In mice there are two isotypic forms of class II molecules (IA and IE), and in humans there are three (DP, DQ, and DR). Amino acid sequencing comparisons of the mouse and human class II molecules suggests that there are structural and functional similarities between the IA and DQ molecules and between IE and DR; there does not appear to be a mouse equivalent for the human DP molecule. A class II MHC molecule contains a 33-kD α chain and a 28-kD β chain, which associate by noncovalent interactions. An additional, invariant chain, called Ii, is transiently associated with the heterodimer during transport to the plasma membrane.

Each chain in a class II molecule contains two external

domains: α_1 and α_2 domains and β_1 and β_2 domains (Figure 9-11b). The membrane-proximal α_2 and β_2 domains, like the membrane-proximal α_3 domain of class I MHC molecules, bear sequence homology to the immunoglobulin-fold domain structure; for this reason, class II MHC molecules also are classified in the immunoglobulin superfamily. The membrane-distal domain of a class II molecule is composed of the α_1 and β_1 domains, which are thought to form an antigen-binding cleft for processed antigen. The three-dimensional structure of the α_1 and β_1 domains awaits further clarification by x-ray crystallographic analysis.

Structure of Class II Genes

Like class I MHC genes, the class II genes are organized into a series of exons and introns mirroring the domain structure of the α and β chains (Figure 9-10b). Both the α and the β genes encoding mouse and human class II MHC molecules have a leader exon, an α_1 or β_1 exon, an α_2 or β_2 exon, a transmembrane exon, and one or more cytoplasmic exons.

Class III MHC Molecules

As noted earlier, several structurally and functionally diverse proteins are encoded within the third region of the MHC. These class III molecules include several complement components (C2, C4A, C4B, and factor B), two steroid 21-hydroxylase enzymes (21-OHA and 21-OHB), and tumor necrosis factors α and β (TNF-α and TNF-β). The location of the genes encoding these proteins within the MHC is shown in Figure 9-1.

Unlike class I and class II MHC molecules, the class III molecules are not membrane proteins and have no role in antigen presentation. It is not known why the class III genes are situated within the MHC complex. There is speculation that the observed genetic association of some MHC alleles with certain diseases may in some cases reflect regulatory disorders of the class III region. For example, ankylosing spondylitis is strongly associated with an allele of the *B* locus of the HLA complex (the *HLA-B27* allele). This disease is characterized by destruction of cartilage, and it has been suggested that because of the close linkage of the *TNF-α* and *TNF-β* genes with the *HLA-B* locus, these cytokines may be involved in cartilage destruction. Systemic lupus erythematosus is another disease which is associated with certain alleles of the MHC. This disease is characterized by autoantibody production, deposition of immune complexes, and complement-mediated damage; it is possible that regulatory defects in the expression of class III complement components may contribute to the severity of this disease.

Probing MHC Structure and Function

Additional information about the structure and function of various MHC molecules has been obtained from studies with hybrid and mutated MHC genes and from transfection experiments.

Exon Shuffling and Site-Directed Mutagenesis

Hybrid class I and class II MHC genes can be constructed by shuffling of homologous exons using genetic engineering techniques. Since each exon encodes a separate protein domain, these hybrid genes can be used to produce MHC molecules containing domains from genetically distinct individuals. Figure 9-13 illustrates the production of MHC genes containing alleles from two different haplotypes. By means of such hybrid MHC genes, researchers have been able to assess the role of the membrane-distal α_1/α_2 and α_1/β_1 domains in class I and class II molecules, respectively, in antigen presentation and in antigen recognition by T cells. These experiments have revealed that both the α_1 and the α_2 domains are required for class I MHC–restricted recognition by CD8$^+$ cells and that both the α_1 and the β_1 domain are required for class II MHC-restricted recognition by CD4$^+$ cells.

In another experimental approach, chemical or oligonucleotide-directed mutagenesis is used to induce single amino acid substitutions in the various external domains of class I and class II MHC molecules. The effect of these mutations on antigen presentation and activation of specific T-cell clones can then be studied. Experiments with mutated class I MHC molecules, for example, have confirmed the importance of both the α_1 and the α_2 domains in T_C-cell recognition, suggesting that the T-cell receptor interacts with residues in both domains. In some studies a single amino acid substitution in just one of the domains has been shown to inhibit antigen recognition by T_C cells.

Transfection of MHC Genes

Another way to study the function of a specific MHC gene is to transfect it into cells that do not express that particular MHC gene. In this way it is possible to study antigen presentation by a single MHC gene product, eliminating the complicating effect of other MHC gene products. For example, the L cell is not an antigen-presenting cell and therefore does not express any class II MHC molecules. For this reason, L cells transfected with a class II MHC gene express only the class II molecule encoded by the transfected gene. Transfection studies with specific IA and IE genes have shown that

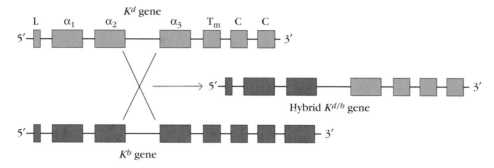

Figure 9-13 Hybrid class I and class II MHC genes can be constructed by exon shuffling. In this example, mouse H-2 *K* genes with the *b* (black) or *d* (red) haplotype were shuffled to produce a hybrid *K* gene containing some *b*-haplotype exons and some *d*-haplotype exons.

different haplotypes differ in their ability to present particular peptides to T_H cells.

The same general approach can be used to study class I MHC function. Since the mouse L cell is a fibroblast cell line derived from a H-2^k haplotype mouse, it contains the K^k, D^k, and L^k class I alleles and expresses the gene products of these alleles on its membrane. By transfecting class I MHC genes of a different haplotype into L cells, it is possible to assess antigen presentation to T_C cells by comparing the transfected L cells with untransfected L-cell controls. If, for example, some L cells are transfected with the K^b gene and other L cells are transfected with the D^b gene, any difference in the ability of K^b and D^b molecules to present particular peptides to T_C cells can be detected.

In transfection experiments, a selection gene (e.g., thymidine kinase) is transfected in addition to the MHC gene. If the MHC gene is present in excess, most L cells that take up the selection gene also will take up the MHC gene. When the cells are cultured in the appropriate selection medium, only transfected cells will be able to grow. Transfection of MHC genes can be combined with exon shuffling or site-directed mutagenesis in a powerful experimental approach for studying the effect of various alterations in MHC molecules on T-cell activation.

Regulation of MHC Expression

Complex mechanisms must regulate the expression of class I and class II MHC molecules, but not much is known about these mechanisms. As noted already, class I MHC molecules are expressed by nearly all nucleated cells, but the level of their expression is very different among different types of cells; the reason for this dif-

ferential expression is not at all clear. As for class II MHC molecules, regulatory mechanisms must limit their expression to antigen-presenting cells. And even among the antigen-presenting cells, class II MHC expression is regulated by the stage of differentiation of the cell. For example, class II MHC molecules cannot be detected on pre-B cells but are expressed on the membrane of mature B cells. Similarly, macrophages have been observed to increase their expression of class II MHC molecules after they have been activated. Both class I and class II MHC genes are flanked by 5′ regulatory gene sequences which bind sequence-specific DNA-binding proteins. Several regulatory sequences have been identified for class I and class II genes, but presently the nuclear binding proteins that regulate these sequences are poorly understood.

A number of cytokines have been shown to affect class I and class II expression. Interferons (IFNs) α, β, and γ and tumor necrosis factor (TNF) have each been shown to increase expression of class I MHC molecules on cells. IFNγ appears to induce the formation of a specific nuclear binding protein that binds to a regulatory sequence flanking the class I MHC genes. Binding of this nuclear binding protein to the regulatory sequence appears to upregulate transcription of the class I MHC gene. IFNγ also has been shown to increase the level of class II MHC expression. In some cases high concentrations of IFNγ has been shown to induce class II expression on a variety of cells including skin keratinocytes, intestinal epithelial cells, vascular endothelium, and pancreatic β cells. The regulation of MHC expression by other lymphokines is limited only to certain cells. For example, IL-4 appears to increase expression of class II MHC molecules only on resting B cells. MHC expression has also been shown to be downregulated by certain agents: corticosteroids and prostaglandins have been shown to downregulate class II MHC expression; and certain viruses, including adenovirus, have been shown to downregulate class I MHC expression.

A number of diseases have been associated with increased or decreased expression of class I or class II MHC molecules. For example, certain malignant tumor cells have been shown to completely lack class I MHC molecules. Since T_C cells recognize antigen in association with class I molecules, their absence on a malignant tumor may contribute to its ability to escape immune destruction. The finding that interferons induce increased expression of class I MHC molecules on cells has led to clinical trials with interferon in cancer patients in an effort to restore class I MHC expression on malignant tumors (see Chapter 23). Conversely, in some autoimmune diseases there appears to be inappropriate expression of class II MHC molecules by nonantigen-presenting cells; this inappropriate class II expression may facilitate the presentation of self-antigens to T_H cells, thus activating an autoimmune response. In animal models of autoimmune disease, it has been possible to reverse the development of autoimmunity by injecting the animal with monoclonal antibodies specific for class II MHC molecules (see Chapter 17). A family of genetic diseases, called *bare lymphocyte syndrome*, involves impaired expression of class I and/or class II MHC molecules on cells. In some cases the absence of class I or class II MHC molecules in these syndromes may be due to a defect in the promoter region of the MHC genes, preventing binding of transcriptional activating factors. Children born with this disease appear to have a severely reduced immune response and suffer from recurrent bacterial and viral infections resulting in death generally by five years of age (see Chapter 20).

MHC and Immune Responsiveness

As discussed earlier, immune responsiveness to exogenous antigens, as measured by the production of serum antibodies, is under the control of class II MHC genes. Two explanations have been proposed to account for the variability in immune responsiveness observed among different haplotypes (see Table 9-3). According to the *determinant-selection* model, different class II MHC molecules differ in their ability to bind processed antigen. The alternative *holes-in-the-repertoire* model suggests that T cells bearing receptors that recognize foreign antigens closely resembling self-antigens may be eliminated during thymic processing. Since the T-cell response to an antigen involves a trimolecular complex of the T cell's receptor, an antigenic peptide, and a MHC molecule, both models may be correct. That is, the absence of a MHC molecule that can bind and present a given peptide *or* the absence of T-cell receptors that

can recognize a given peptide–MHC molecule complex could result in the absence of immune responsiveness and so account for the observed relationship between MHC haplotype and immune responsiveness.

Determinant-Selection Model

The determinant-selection model assumes that the structure of a particular MHC molecule determines the strength of its association with any given antigen. Animals that respond, for example, to antigen A must express at least one class II MHC molecule whose structure facilitates interaction with antigen A, whereas animals that do not respond must express class II MHC molecules that do not interact effectively with antigen A. According to this model, the MHC polymorphism within a species will generate different patterns of responsiveness and nonresponsiveness to different antigens.

If this model is correct, then class II molecules from responder and nonresponder strains should show differential binding of antigen. Table 9-4 presents data on the binding of various radiolabeled peptides to class II IA and IE molecules with the H-2^d or H-2^k haplotype. Each of the listed peptides binds significantly to only one of the class II molecules. Furthermore, as predicted, the haplotype of the class II molecule showing the highest-affinity binding for a particular peptide generally is the same as the haplotype of responder strains for that peptide.

In other experiments the nonresponder status of some strains has been linked to the deletion of a class II MHC gene. For example, H-2^b and H-2^s haplotype mice have undergone deletion of the E_α gene and therefore do not express class II IE. These strains are nonresponders to a synthetic Glu-Lys-Phe peptide and to pigeon cytochrome c. When an E_α gene is introduced into a fertilized egg in these nonresponding strains, the resulting transgenic mice express the class II IE molecule and are now able to respond to both the synthetic Glu-Lys-Phe peptide and to pigeon cytochrome c.

Holes-in-the-Repertoire Model

The influence of the MHC on immune responsiveness can also be caused by an absence of functional T cells capable of recognizing a given antigen–MHC molecule complex. A good example is documented in the peptide-binding data presented in Table 9-4. The λ repressor peptide (residues 12–26) binds best in vitro to IE^d, yet the MHC restriction for this peptide is known to be associated not with IE^d but instead with the IA^d and IE^k. The suggested explanation is that T cells recognizing

Table 9-3 Effect of H-2 haplotype on immune responsiveness of mice to the synthetic copolymer antigens (H,G)-A-L and (T,G)-A-L

Mouse strain	H-2 alleles					(H,G)-A-L Response[*]	(T,G)-A-L Response[*]
	K	IA	IE	S	D		
A	*k*	*k*	*k*	*d*	*d*	High	Low
A.TL	*s*	*k*	*k*	*k*	*d*	High	Low
B10.A (4R)	*k*	*k*	*b*	*b*	*b*	High	Low
B10	*b*	*b*	*b*	*b*	*b*	Low	High
B10.STA62	*w*27	*b*	*w*27	*w*27	*w*27	Low	High
A.SW	*s*	*s*	*s*	*s*	*s*	Low	Low

[*] Indicated by production of specific serum antibodies.

Table 9-4 Differential binding of peptides to mouse class II MHC molecules and correlation with MHC restriction

Labeled peptide[*]	MHC restriction of responders[†]	Percentage of labeled peptide bound to[‡]			
		IA^d	IE^d	IA^k	IE^k
Ovalbumin (323–339)	IA^d	**11.8**	0.1	0.2	0.1
Influenza hemagglutinin (130–142)	IA^d	**18.9**	0.6	7.1	0.3
Hen egg-white lysozyme (46–61)	IA^k	0.0	0.0	**35.2**	0.5
Hen egg-white lysozyme (74–86)	IA^k	2.0	2.3	**2.9**	1.7
Hen egg-white lysozyme (81–96)	IE^k	0.4	0.2	0.7	**1.1**
Myoglobin (132–153)	IE^d	0.8	**6.3**	0.5	0.7
Pigeon cytochrome *c* (88–104)	IE^k	0.6	1.2	1.7	**8.7**
λ repressor (12–26)[§]	$IA^d + IE^k$	1.6	**8.9**	0.3	2.3

[*] Amino acid residues included in each peptide are indicated by the numbers in parentheses.

[†] Refers to class II molecule (IA or IE) and haplotype associated with a good response to the indicated peptides as determined by studies such as that shown in Table 9-3.

[‡] Binding determined by equilibrium dialysis. Bold-faced values indicate binding was significantly greater ($p < 0.05$) than to the other three class II molecules tested.

[§] The λ repressor is an exception to the rule that high binding correlates with the MHC restriction of high-responder strains. In this case, the T_H cell specific for the λ peptide plus IE^d has been deleted; this is an example of the hole-in-the-repertoire mechanism.

SOURCE: Adapted from S. Buus et al., 1987, Science **235**:1353.

this λ repressor peptide in association with IE^d may have been eliminated during thymic processing leaving a hole in the T-cell repertoire.

An absence of functional T cells capable of recognizing a given antigen–MHC complex has been observed in several experimental systems. For example, the synthetic peptide poly Glu-Tyr induces an immune response in DBA/2 mice but not in BALB/c mice, although both strains have the H-2^d haplotype and the antigen-presenting cells of both strains are capable of presenting this peptide. T cells from the responder strain were shown to respond to poly Glu-Tyr on antigen-presenting cells from both responder and nonresponder strains, whereas T cells from the nonresponder strain did not respond to this peptide whether it was presented by responder or nonresponder antigen-presenting cells. These results suggest that the T cells specific for poly Glu-Tyr have been functionally inactivated or clonally deleted in the nonresponder strain. A number of elegant studies with transgenic mice designed to evaluate the role of self-tolerance in influencing the T-cell repertoire are described in later chapters.

Polymorphism of Class I and Class II MHC Molecules

The loci that encode class I and class II MHC molecules are the most polymorphic known in higher vertebrates. That is, within a given species, there is an extraordinarily large number of different alleles at each locus. Analysis of human HLA class I molecules has so far revealed 23 A alleles, 49 B alleles, and 8 C alleles. In mice the polymorphism is equally staggering, with more than 55 alleles now identified at the K locus and 60 alleles identified at the D locus. The current estimate of actual polymorphism in both the human and the mouse MHC, suggested by serologic and functional analysis, is more than 100 alleles for each locus. This enormous polymorphism results in a tremendous diversity of MHC proteins within a species. Given 100 different alleles for each gene within the mouse MHC, the theoretical MHC diversity possible for the species is

$$100(K) \times 100(A_\alpha) \times 100(A_\beta) \times$$
$$100(E_\alpha) \times 100(E_\beta) \times 100(D) = 10^{12}!!$$

In humans the theoretical diversity is even larger, because humans have more class I and class II genes. However, because these genes are tightly linked and are inherited as a haplotype, the actual diversity within a species is less than the theoretical estimate. Still, this enormous polymorphism creates a major obstacle when it comes to matching MHC molecules for successful organ transplants.

A comparison of the amino acid sequences of several allelic MHC molecules encoded at a single locus reveals a sequence divergence of between 5 and 10%. This degree of variation is unusually high. Indeed, the sequence divergence among alleles of the MHC *within a species* is as great as the divergence observed for the genes encoding a single enzyme (e.g., lactate dehydrogenase) *across species lines*. What is also unusual is that the sequence variation among MHC molecules is not randomly distributed along the entire polypeptide chain but instead is clustered in short stretches, largely within the α_1 and α_2 domains of class I molecules and within the α_1 and β_1 domains of class II molecules (Figure 9-14). The clustered distribution of the sequence variation is thought to arise through *gene conversion*, a process whereby short donor DNA sequences base-pair with partially homologous DNA sequences in a recipient gene; excision repair or replication then inserts the donor sequence into the recipient DNA. By this process gene conversion transfers information unidirectionally from a donor DNA sequence to a partially homologous recipient DNA sequence. The molecular mechanism of gene conversion has not yet been defined, but conversion has been shown to occur in yeasts, trypanosomes, and human fetal globulin genes in addition to the class I and class II MHC genes. The large number of unexpressed pseudogenes in the MHC, such as the class I–like genes of the mouse *Tla* locus or the human *DX*, *DO*, and *DZ* loci, may serve as a pool of related gene sequences from which short, nearly homologous gene sequences can be transferred to functional class I or class II genes (see Figure 9-9).

Recent work has begun to establish the location of these polymorphic residues within the membrane-distal domains of class I and class II molecules, and analysis is under way to determine whether these polymorphic differences correlate with functional differences among various class I or class II molecules. Experiments have shown that class II MHC molecules bind specifically to various peptides (see Table 9-4), and the binding site has been located in the membrane-distal α_1/β_1 domain, the very regions that display localized polymorphism within class II molecules. A number of researchers have suggested that differences in these polymorphic amino acids in the class II MHC molecules expressed on antigen-presenting cells, might influence the cells' ability to recognize a given peptide. The polymorphic amino acids of class I MHC molecules also are clustered in the membrane-distal α_1/α_2 domain. Now that high-resolution crystallographic analysis of human class I HLA-A2 has been completed, it is possible to locate the polymorphic residues within the structure of the α_1 and α_2 domains. P. J. Bjorkman determined the location of the polymorphic class I residues by comparing their primary position to crystallization analysis of the HLA-A2 molecule. Of 17 amino acid residues previously shown to display significant polymorphism, 15 turn out to be in the groove thought to be the class I binding site for processed antigen (see Figure 9-11c, d). The location of so many polymorphic amino acids within the putative binding site for processed antigen is postulated to influence the ability of a given class I MHC molecule to interact with a given processed antigen.

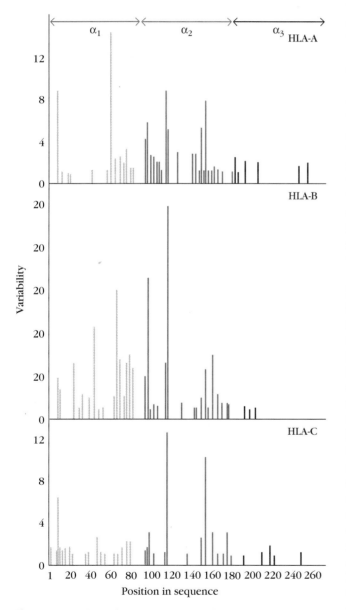

Figure 9-14 Plots of the variability in the amino acid sequence of allelic class I MHC molecules in humans versus residue position demonstrate that the variable residues are clustered in the α_1 and α_2 domains. [Adapted from D. A. Lawlor et al., 1990, *Annu. Rev. Immunol.* **8**:23.]

Role of the MHC in Susceptibility to Infectious Diseases

As mentioned earlier, certain diseases have been shown to be associated with particular MHC alleles. Included among these diseases are a large number of autoimmune diseases, susceptibility to certain viral pathogens, disorders of the complement system, certain neurologic disorders, and some types of allergies. In most MHC-associated diseases, however, a number of other genes, outside the MHC, as well as external environmental factors also appear to play a role; therefore, it has been difficult to unravel these associations. The relation of the MHC to autoimmune diseases is discussed in Chapter 17, and the discussion here is limited to the relationship of the MHC to diseases caused by pathogenic organisms.

A number of hypotheses have been suggested to account for the role of the MHC in disease. Susceptibility to a given pathogen may reflect the role of particular MHC alleles in responsiveness or nonresponsiveness to the pathogen. Variations in antigen presentation by different MHC alleles may determine the effectiveness of the immune response to a given pathogen. If major epitopes on a given pathogen mimic certain self–MHC molecule complexes, it is possible that an animal may lack functional T cells for that pathogen. Various MHC alleles may also provide binding sites for specific viruses, bacteria, or their products.

Some recent evidence suggests that a reduction in MHC polymorphism within a species may predispose that species to disease. Cheetahs, for example, have been shown to be far more susceptible to viral disease than other big cats. Because the present cheetah population arose from a limited breeding stock, the species suffers from a loss of MHC diversity. The increased susceptibility of cheetahs to various viral diseases may result from a reduction in the number of different MHC molecules available to the species as a whole and a corresponding limitation on the range of processed antigens with which these MHC molecules can interact. Thus the high level of MHC polymorphism that has been observed in various species may be advantageous by providing a broad range of antigen-presenting MHC molecules. Because of this extreme polymorphism, some individuals within a species probably will not be able to develop an immune response to any given pathogen and therefore will be susceptible to infection by it. On the other hand, and perhaps of more importance, MHC polymorphism ensures that at least some members of a species will be able to respond to any one of a very large number of potential pathogens. In this way, MHC diversity appears to protect a species from a wide range of infectious diseases.

In a few cases the presence or absence of certain MHC alleles has been associated with specific diseases.

In chickens, for example, susceptibility to the virus causing Marek's disease has been linked to inheritance of certain MHC alleles. Chickens expressing the *B19* MHC allele are susceptible to the virus, whereas birds expressing the *B21* allele are not susceptible. An interesting link between the MHC and disease susceptibility in humans came from a study of Dutch immigrants to South America. In 1845 a group of Dutch immigrants consisting of 367 individuals from 50 families emigrated from Europe to South America. Within two weeks of their arrival an epidemic of typhoid fever killed 50% of the immigrants, and six years later an epidemic of yellow fever killed another 20% of the population. Thereafter the annual mortality rate was relatively low, and the survivors remained and intermarried. Recently the MHC polymorphism of the "selected" descendants of the survivors was analyzed and compared with that of a similar number of Dutch families living in the Netherlands. The descendants in South America exhibited significant relative decreases in some HLA alleles, such as *B7*, and significant increases in other alleles, such as *B13*, *Bw38*, and *Bw50*. It is hypothesized that these descendants may carry MHC alleles that enable them to respond more effectively to pathogens endemic to their South American environment.

MHC and Antigen Presentation

Both class I and class II MHC molecules on the membranes of self-cells can associate with processed antigen and present that antigen to various T-cell subpopulations. As discussed in Chapter 1, class I MHC molecules bind peptides derived from endogenous antigen synthesized within altered self-cells (e.g., virus-infected cells), whereas class II MHC molecules bind peptides derived from exogenous antigen that has been internalized by antigen-presenting cells (e.g., macrophages, B cells, dendritic cells).

Preferential Binding of Peptides by MHC Molecules

As described earlier in this chapter, x-ray crystallographic analysis of a class I MHC molecule revealed a peptide-binding cleft in which processed antigen peptides are thought to lie, contacting amino acid residues lining the floor and the sides of the cleft (see Figure 9-10). Although a class II MHC molecule has not yet been crystallized, a similar peptide-binding cleft has been proposed. Differences in the amino acid sequence in this region of class I and class II MHC molecules pre-

sumably determine which peptides can be presented. The observed clustering of polymorphic amino acids within this groove enables allelic MHC molecules to interact with different peptides.

The binding of a peptide to the cleft in an MHC molecule does not have the kind of fine specificity characteristic of the binding of an antibody with its epitope. Instead a given MHC molecule can selectively bind a variety of different peptides. For example, as shown in Table 9-4, the IA^d class II MHC molecule binds strongly to specific peptides from ovalbumin and hemagglutinin, binds weakly to peptides from hen egg-white lysozyme and λ repressor, and does not bind to several other tested peptides. This broad, but selective, interaction between the agretope and the MHC suggests that structural features common to a variety of antigenic peptides may enable them to bind to the same MHC molecule. Nevertheless, since each individual MHC molecule selectively binds only some peptides and not others, the repertoire of MHC alleles inherited by an individual will determine which peptides can be presented to the T cells.

Assembly and Transport of MHC Molecules

Like other proteins, MHC molecules are synthesized on polysomes in the rough endoplasmic reticulum (RER). Class I MHC molecules appear to bind antigenic peptides within the RER, whereas class II MHC molecules do not.

Recent experiments suggest that the binding of a peptide to a class I MHC α chain may induce a conformational change in the molecule, enabling it to associate with β_2-microglobulin and then be transported to the cell membrane (Figure 9-15a). Evidence for the role of peptide in the assembly and transport of class I molecules came from the discovery of a mutant cell line called RMA-S. This particular cell line expresses about 5% of the normal levels of class I MHC molecules on its membrane. These cells synthesize both class I MHC molecules and β_2-microglobulin, but both remain intracellular instead of appearing on the membrane. A clue to the mutation in the RMA-S cell line was the discovery by Alain Townsend and his colleagues that "feeding" these cells predigested peptides restored their level of membrane class I MHC to normal. This led them to speculate that perhaps a defect in antigen processing or peptide transport might account for decreased expression of a class I MHC molecule on cell membranes. They suggested that peptide might be required to stabilize the interaction between a class I MHC molecule and β_2-microglobulin. Recently, peptide-transport proteins have been discovered that serve to transport peptides from the cytoplasm into the

(a)

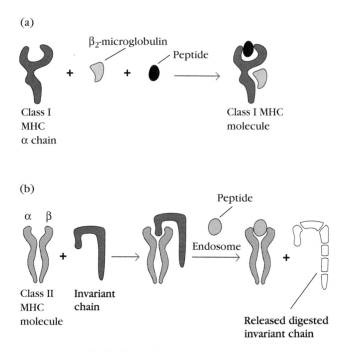

Figure 9-15   (a) Binding of an antigenic peptide to a class I MHC α chain within the endoplasmic reticulum is thought to stabilize association of the α chain with β_2-microglobulin. (b) Within the endoplasmic reticulum, the noncovalently associated α and β chains of a class II MHC molecule bind an invariant (Ii) chain. As long as the Ii chain occupies the peptide-binding site, the class II MHC molecule cannot bind peptide.

Segregation of Class I and Class II MHC Molecules within Antigen-Processing Pathways

Some of the first evidence suggesting that class I and class II MHC molecules present antigen that has been processed along different routes was obtained by studying two clones of T_C cells specific for influenza virus. One cytotoxic clone was a usual $CD8^+$, class I–restricted T cell, but the other was unusual in that it was $CD4^+$ and therefore class II restricted. As discussed in Chapter 3, the association between functional T-cell populations and MHC restriction is not absolute. There are increasing reports of T cells that cross functional lines ($CD8^+$ T_H clones that are class I restricted and $CD4^+$ T_C clones that are class II restricted). Influenza is one antigen that has been shown to induce both $CD8^+$ T_C cells which are class I restricted and $CD4^+$ T_C cells that are class II restricted. L. A. Morrison and T. J. Braciale analyzed two such cytotoxic T-cell clones, one specific for the influenza hemagglutinin molecule together with class I and the other specific for hemagglutinin and class II.

By comparing the ability of target cells treated in various ways to induce these two CTL clones, Morrison and Braciale sought to determine whether antigen is processed along different pathways for association with class I or class II MHC molecules. In one set of experiments, target cells that expressed both class I and class II MHC molecules were incubated with infectious influenza virus or with UV-inactivated influenza virus. (The UV-inactivated virus retained its antigenic properties but was no longer capable of replicating within the target cells.) The target cells were then incubated with the class I–restricted or class II–restricted CTLs and subsequent lysis of the target cells was determined. Their results, presented in Table 9-5, show that the class II–restricted CTLs responded to target cells treated with infectious or noninfectious influenza virions, whereas the class I–restricted CTLs responded to target cells treated with infectious virions but not to target cells treated with noninfectious virions. Similarly, target cells that had been treated with infectious influenza virions in the presence of emitine, which inhibits viral protein synthesis, stimulated the class II–restricted CTLs but not the class I–restricted CTLs. Just the opposite results were obtained with target cells that had been treated with infectious virions in the presence of chloroquine, an inhibitor of phagolysosome formation in the phagocytic pathway.

These results support the distinction made in Chapter 1 between exogenous and endogenous antigens and the preferential association of exogenous antigens with class II MHC molecules and of endogenous antigens with class I MHC molecules. In other words, the mode of

endoplasmic reticulum where they can interact with class I MHC molecules. It has been suggested that the defect in the RMA-S cell line may be in these transporter proteins. Interestingly, the genes for these transporter proteins map to the class II MHC region.

Since antigen-presenting cells express both class I and class II MHC molecules, some mechanism must exist for preventing class II molecules from binding to the same set of antigenic peptides as the class I molecules. Recent studies have shown that when a class II MHC molecule is synthesized within the RER, it associates with another protein called the invariant (Ii) chain. This protein interacts with the peptide-binding cleft of the class II molecule, preventing any endogenously derived peptides from binding to the cleft while the class II molecule is within the endoplasmic reticulum (Figure 9-15b). In addition to its role in preventing peptide binding to class II MHC molecules, the I chain also appears to be involved in the routing of class II MHC molecules to lysosomes, where exogenous antigen is processed. After loss of the I chain, the class II molecules bind antigenic peptides and move to the cell membrane.

antigen entry into cells and its subsequent processing within either the endosomal-processing pathway (exogenous antigens) or the cytoplasm (endogenous antigens) determines whether antigen associates with class I or class II MHC molecules. In the Morrison and Braciale experiments, association of viral antigen with class II MHC molecules did not require viral replication or protein synthesis. On the other hand, association of viral antigen with class I MHC molecules required replication of the influenza virus and viral protein synthesis within the target cells. These findings suggest that there are separate routes by which endogenous and exogenous antigens are processed and presented with class I and class II MHC molecules, respectively.

Recent evidence suggests that routing of class I and class II MHC molecules to separate intracellular compartments dictates whether they interact with cytosolic peptides of biosynthetic origin or with peptides derived from exogenous antigens degraded in the endosomal-processing pathway (Figure 9-16). The class I MHC molecules are thought to bind peptides within the endoplasmic reticulum. These peptides are thought to be

Table 9-5 Effect of antigen presentation on activation of class I and class II MHC–restricted CTLs

Treatment of target cells*	CTL activity	
	Class I restricted	Class II restricted
Infectious virus	+	+
UV-inactivated virus (noninfectious)	−	+
Infectious virus + emitine	−	+
Infectious virus + chloroquine	+	−
Hemagglutinin protein	−	+
Hemagglutinin gene	+	−
Synthetic hemagglutinin peptides	+	+

* Target cells, which expressed both class I and class II MHC proteins, were treated with the indicated preparations of influenza virus. Emetine inhibits viral protein synthesis, and chloroquine inhibits the endosomal-processing pathway. The influenza hemagglutin (HA) gene was introduced into target cells as part of a recombinant vaccinia virus vector that contained the HA gene but no HA polypeptide.

† Determined by lysis (+) or no lysis (−) of the target cells.

SOURCE: Adapted from Braciale, T. J., L. A. Morrison, M. T. Sweetser, J. Sambrook et al., 1987, *Immunol. Rev.* **98**:95.

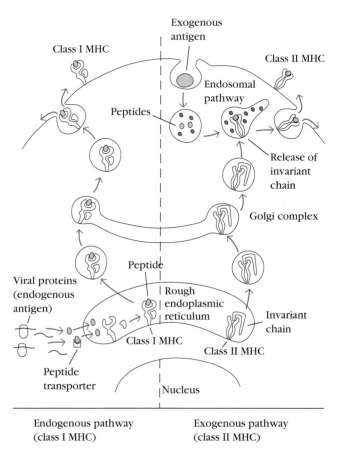

Endogenous pathway (class I MHC)   Exogenous pathway (class II MHC)

Figure 9-16 Model of separate antigen-presenting pathways for endogenous and exogenous antigens. Routing of class I and class II MHC molecules to separate intracellular compartments may determine the type of antigenic peptide that each class of MHC molecule binds. Class I MHC molecules are thought to interact with peptides that have been carried into the rough endoplamsic reticulum by transporter proteins. Upon peptide binding, the interaction between a class I MHC α chain and β_2-microgobulin is thought to be stabilized, and the complex is routed through the Golgi to the plasma membrane. The presence of the invariant (Ii) chain is thought to prevent peptide binding to class II MHC molecules within the endoplasmic reticulum and to facilitate their routing to the cell compartment where exogenous antigen is processed. Late in the endosomal-processing pathway. Vesicles containing class II MHC molecules and the Ii chain, fuse with lysosomes. Enzymes within the lysosomes degrade the Ii chain, enabling the class II MHC molecules to bind peptides.

synthesized within the cytoplasm of the cell and are thought to be transported across the ER membrane by peptide transporters. Once in the ER, the peptide is thought to bind to the class I MHC, inducing a conformational change in the molecule enabling it to associate with β_2-microglobulin. The peptide/class I MHC molecule is then routed through the Golgi to the cell membrane. Endogenously synthesized peptide does not bind to class II MHC within the ER because of the presence of the invariant chain. Exogeneous antigen that has entered the cell through endocytosis or phagocytosis will enter the endosomal pathway where it is degraded by proteolytic enzymes. The class II molecules, together with associated invariant chains are thought to be routed from the ER to enter the endosomal pathway at a late point in structures related to lysosomes. Here within the lysosomes, proteolytic enzymes are thought to degrade the invariant chain, exposing the binding cleft of the class II molecule to the peptides contained within the lysosome. The lysosomes containing peptide-bound class II MHC molecules then fuse with the plasma membrane.

Summary

1. The major histocompatibility complex (MHC) is a tightly linked group of genes that encode proteins associated with intercellular recognition and antigen presentation to T lymphocytes. The MHC, called the H-2 complex in mice and the HLA complex in humans, is organized into regions encoding class I, class II, and class III molecules. Class I molecules are encoded by the K and D regions in mice and the A, B, and C regions in humans. Class II molecules are encoded by the I region in mice and the D regions in humans. Class III molecules are encoded by the S region in mice and the C4,C2,BF region in humans. Many alleles exist for each class I and class II MHC gene; the entire set of alleles present on each chromosome in a given animal is its haplotype.

2. Class I MHC molecules consist of a large glycoprotein α chain, encoded by the class I MHC genes, and a much smaller molecule of β_2-microglobulin, encoded by a gene outside of the MHC. The α chain contains three external domains (α_1, α_2, and α_3), a hydrophobic transmembrane segment, and a cytoplasmic tail. The latter two domains anchor the α chain to the cell membrane, and the α_1 and α_2 domains interact to form a cleft that is thought to bind antigenic peptides. The class I MHC genes are organized as a series of exons and introns, with each exon encoding a separate domain of the α chain.

3. Class II MHC molecules are heterodimers composed of two noncovalently associated glycoproteins, the α and β chain, which are encoded by separate class II genes. Each chain contains two external domains, a transmembrane segment, and a cytoplasmic tail. The class II MHC genes are organized as a series of exons and introns, with each exon encoding a separate domain of the α or β chain.

4. Because portions of both class I and class II MHC molecules exhibit the immunoglobulin-fold structure, these molecules are considered members of the immunoglobulin superfamily. In addition to a similarity in structure, both class I and class II MHC molecules function to present antigen to T cells. Class I molecules, which are present on nearly all nucleated cells, present processed endogenous antigen to CD8[+] cells. Class II molecules, which are expressed on a limited number of antigen-presenting cells (macrophages, dendritic cells, B cells), present processed exogenous antigen to CD4[+] cells. The preferential association of class I molecules with endogenous antigen and class II molecules with exogenous antigen appears to involve segregated antigen-presenting pathways.

5. Studies with hybrid and mutated MHC genes have demonstrated that the two membrane-distal domains in both class I and class II MHC molecules are required for antigen presentation. Studies with congenic and recombinant congenic mouse strains and with L cells transfected with MHC genes have shown that the MHC haplotype influences immune responsiveness and the ability to present antigen.

6. The variation in amino acid sequence (i.e., the polymorphism) that characterizes class I and class II MHC molecules is found primarily in the membrane-distal domains. In class I MHC molecules, the polymorphic residues have been shown to be localized largely in the groove thought to be the antigenic peptide-binding site.

References

ACCOLLA, R. S., C. AUFFRAY, D. S. SINGER, and J. GUARDIOLA. 1991. The molecular biology of MHC genes. *Immunol. Today* **12**:97.

AJITKUMAR, P., S. S. GEIER, K. V. KESARI, F. BORRIELLO et al. 1988. Evidence that multiple residues on both the α-helices of the class I MHC molecules are simultaneously recognized by the T cell receptor. *Cell* **54**:47.

BENOIST, C. and D. MATHIS. 1990. Regulation of major histocompatibility complex class II genes: X, Y, and other letters of the alphabet. *Annu. Rev. Immunol.* **8**:681.

BJORKMAN, P. J., M. A. SAPER, B. SAMRAOUI, W. S. BENNET et al. 1987. Structure of the human class I histocompatibility antigens. *Nature* **329**:506.

BJORKMAN, P. J., and P. PARHAM. 1990. Structure, function and diversity of class I major histocompatibility complex molecules. *Annu. Rev. Biochem.* **59**:253.

KAPPES, D. and J. L. STROMINGER. 1988. Human class II major histocompatibility complex genes and proteins. *Annu. Rev. Biochem.* **57**:991.

KLEIN, J. 1986. *Natural History of the Major Histocompatibility Complex.* John Wiley and Sons.

KOLLER, B. H., D. E. GERAGHTY, R. DEMARS, L. DUVICK et al. 1989. Chromosomal organization of the human major histocompatibility complex class I gene family. *J. Exp. Med.* **169**:469.

LAWLOR, D. A., et al. 1990. Evolution of class I MHC genes and proteins: from natural selection to thymic selection. *Annu. Rev. Immunol.* **8**:23.

PETERS, P. J., J. J. NEEFJES, V. OORSCHOT, H. L. PLOEGH, and H. J. GEUZE. 1991. Segregation of MHC class II molecules from MHC class I molecules in the golgi complex for transport to lysosomal compartments. *Nature* **349**:669.

ROCHE, P. A., and P. CRESSWELL.1990. Invariant chain association with HLA-DR molecules inhibits immunogenic peptide binding. *Nature* **345**:615.

SCHAEFFER, E. B., et al. 1989. Relative contribution of determinant selection and holes in the repertoire to T cell responses. *Proc. Natl. Acad. Sci. USA* **86**:4649.

SPIES, T., M. BRESNAHAN, S. BAHRAM, D. ARNOLD, G. BLANCK et al. 1990. A gene in the human major histocompatibility complex class II region controlling the class I antigen presentation pathway. *Nature* **348**:744.

TOWNSEND, A., et al. 1989. Association of class I major histocompatibility heavy and light chains induced by viral peptides. *Nature* **340**:443–448.

Study Questions

1. Indicate whether each of the following statements is true or false. If you think a statement is false, explain why.

   a. A monoclonal antibody specific for β_2-microglobulin can be used to detect both class I MHC K and D molecules on the surface of cells.

   b. Antigen-presenting cells express both class I and class II MHC molecules on their membrane.

2. You wish to produce a syngeneic and a congenic mouse strain. Indicate which of the following statements applies to production of syngeneic (S), congenic (C), or both (S and C) mice.

   a. Requires the greatest number of generations. _____
   b. Requires backcrosses. _____
   c. Yields mice that are genetically identical. _____
   d. Requires selection for homozygosity. _____
   e. Requires sibling crosses. _____
   f. Can be started with outbred mice. _____
   g. Yields progeny that are genetically identical to the parent except for a single genetic region. _____

3. You have generated a congenic A.B strain mouse that has been selected for the MHC.

   a. What is the genetic background of this mouse?
   b. What is the haplotype of the MHC of this mouse?
   c. To produce this congenic strain, the F_1 progeny are always backcrossed to which strain?
   d. Why was backcrossing to the parent performed?
   e. Why was inbreeding performed?
   f. Why was selection necessary and what kind of selection was performed?

4. You cross a C57Bl/6 ($H\text{-}2^b$) mouse with a CBA ($H\text{-}2^k$) mouse. What MHC molecules will the F_1 progeny express on its liver cells and on its macrophages?

5. To carry out studies on the structure and function of the class I MHC molecule K^b and the class II MHC molecule IA^b, you decide to transfect the genes encoding these proteins into a mouse fibroblast cell line (L cell) derived from the C3H strain ($H\text{-}2^k$). In the following table, indicate which of the listed MHC molecules will ($+$) or will not ($-$) be expressed on the membrane of the transfected L cells.

Transfected gene	MHC molecules expressed on the membrane of the transfected L cells					
	D^k	D^b	K^k	K^b	IA^k	IA^b
None						
K^b						
A_α^b						
A_β^b						
A_α^b and A_β^b						

6. a. The E_β locus in the IE region of the MHC is deleted in the SJL mouse strain (H-2^s). List the MHC molecules that would be expressed on the membrane of macrophages from this strain.

b. If the class II IE genes (E_α and E_β) from a H-2^k strain are transfected into SJL macrophages, what additional MHC molecules would be expressed on the transfected macrophages?

7. Draw diagrams illustrating the general structure, including the domains, of class I MHC molecules, class II MHC molecules, and membrane-bound antibody on B cells; include molecules that are associated with these proteins. Label each chain and the domains within it, the antigen-binding regions, and regions that have the immunoglobulin-fold structure.

8. Where are the polymorphic amino acid residues located in MHC molecules? What is the significance of this location? How is MHC polymorphism thought to be generated?

9. As a student in an immunology laboratory class, you have been given spleen cells from a mouse immunized with the LCM virus. You determine the antigen-specific functional activity of these cells with two different assays. In assay 1, the spleen cells are incubated with macrophages that have been briefly exposed to the LCM virus; the production of interleukin 2 (IL-2) is a positive response. In assay 2, the spleen cells are incubated with LCM-infected target cells; lysis of the target cells represents a positive response in this assay. The results of the assays using macrophages and target cells of different haplotypes are presented in the table below. Note that the experiment has been set up in a way to exclude alloreactive responses.

a. Which cell populations are detected in each of the two assays?

b. From the results of this experiment, which MHC molecules are required, in addition to the LCM virus, for specific reactivity of the spleen cells in each of the two assays?

c. Which additional experiments would you need to do to unambiguously confirm the MHC molecules required for antigen-specific reactivity of the spleen cells?

d. Which of the mouse strains listed in the table could have been the source of the immunized spleen cells tested in the functional assays? Give your reasons.

For use with Question 9.

| Mouse strain used as source of macrophages and target cells | MHC haplotype of macrophages and virus-infected target cells | | | | Response of spleen cells | |
	K	A	E	D	IL-2 production in response to LCM-pulsed macrophages (assay 1)	Lysis of LCM-infected cells (assay 2)
C3H	k	k	k	k	+	−
BALB/c	d	d	d	d	−	+
(BALB/c × B10.A)F$_1$	d/k	d/k	d/k	d/d	+	+
A.TL	s	k	k	d	+	+
B10.A (3R)	b	b	b	d	−	+
B10.A (4R)	k	k	—	b	+	−

10. A T_C-cell clone recognizes a particular measles virus peptide when it is presented by the MHC molecule D^b. Another MHC molecule is identical to D^b in the antigen-binding groove but differs from D^b at several other amino acids in the α_1 and α_2 domains. Could the second MHC molecule present the measles virus peptide to this T_C clone? Briefly explain your answer.

11. How can you determine if two different inbred mouse strains have identical MHC regions.

12. Red blood cells are not nucleated and do not express any MHC molecules. Why is this property fortuitous for blood transfusions?

T-Cell Receptor

Although the antigen-specific nature of T-cell responses clearly implies that they possess an antigen-specific and clonally restricted receptor, the nature of the T-cell receptor for antigen was unknown as recently as the early 1980s. Experimental results within the field were contradictory and difficult to conceptualize within a single model because the T-cell receptor differs from the B-cell antigen-binding receptor in two important ways. First, the T cell does not secrete its receptor as the B cell does, so that any assessment of receptor structure and specificity had to rely on complex cellular assays. Second, the T-cell receptor (TCR) is specific, not for antigen alone, but for antigen in association with one of the molecules of the major histocompatibility complex. This property prevents purification of the T-cell receptor by antigen-binding techniques and adds complexity to any experimental system designed to investigate the receptor. In 1982, the authors of a workshop report titled "T-Cell Receptors; Through a Glass Darkly," summarized the workshop by stating, "At present we approach the T-cell receptor as the blind men in the fable approached the elephant. Even with our eyes wide open, we do not know if one person's helper T cell is in any way related to another's, nor whether molecules isolated from different T cells are encoded by the same or independent genes."

Within two short years of this workshop, new investigative tools—notably monoclonal antibodies and nucleic acid probes—were used to isolate T-cell receptors and their genes for the first time. The T-cell receptor was identified as a heterodimer composed of either alpha and beta or gamma and delta chains. Surprisingly, the genomic organization and the mode of generation of diversity for each chain were found to be similar to that of the B-cell receptor's immunoglobulin chains. Two important differences that distinguish the T-cell receptor from immunoglobulin were also discovered. First, was the restricted ability of the T-cell receptor to recognize antigen only as a complex with self-MHC molecules. Second, was the finding that the T-cell receptor, unlike immunoglobulin, is associated on the membrane with accessory molecules (CD3 and CD4 or CD8), which may function to transduce signals or augment MHC restriction. The knowledge that emerged in the 1980s about the structure, specificity, and function of T-cell receptors has provided a framework for greater understanding of cell-mediated immunity and of the similarities and differences between B cells and T cells.

Isolation of T-Cell Receptors and Their Genes

In the 1970s and early 1980s investigators learned much about T-cell function but were thwarted in their attempts to identify and isolate its antigen-binding receptor. Several properties, unique to the T-cell receptor, hampered its identification.

Functional Assays for the T-Cell Receptor

Because the T cell does not secrete its receptor, complex cellular assays are required to assess TCR structure, specificity, and function. The general practice is to challenge T cells with antigen and then measure various functions indicative of T-cell activation. For example, activation of T helper (T_H) cells can be assayed by proliferation of the T_H cells, by secretion of various cytokines, or by the ability of activated T_H cells to activate B cells and T

cytotoxic (T_C) cells. Activation of T_C cells can be assayed by lysis of target cells or by secretion of cytokines such as interferon gamma (IFN-γ). The requirement for complex cellular assays to assess receptor structure or specificity made it difficult to tell whether an agent that specifically stimulated or blocked the T-cell's response did so by having a direct effect on the TCR or by acting indirectly at some other level to enhance or block the cellular function being assessed.

Properties of the T-Cell Receptor Revealed in Early Studies

Even before the T-cell receptor was isolated, researchers had demonstrated several properties related to its general structure and interaction with antigen. Several experiments that revealed these properties are described here.

T-Cell Receptor Is Not Immunoglobulin

In early studies to determine whether the T-cell receptor is similar in structure to antibody, T cells were incubated with fluorescent antibodies directed against either immunoglobulin heavy-chain constant-region determinants or light-chain constant-region determinants (i.e., isotypic determinants; see Figure 5-11). In both cases, the T cells failed to stain with the anti-isotype antibodies, thus indicating that the T-cell receptor does not share the immunoglobulin heavy- and light-chain constant regions. However, when T cells were incubated with fluorescent anti-idiotype antibodies (i.e., antibodies directed against the antigen-binding site on an antibody), a low percentage of T cells stained, indicating that the T cells expressed a cross-reacting idiotype and suggesting that the T-cell receptor has a variable region with at least some structural features in common with immunoglobulins.

Various theories were proposed to account for these fluorescent-antibody results. Some investigators suggested that T cells might express the same variable-region gene segments as antibodies but might have a heavy-chain constant region with a new isotype, an "IgT." But why, then, did T cells not stain with anti-light-chain antibody? Was the TCR light chain of a different class as well? Others suggested that perhaps T cells expressed a known isotype for heavy and light chains but that the receptor was so deeply buried in the membrane that only its variable regions were accessible. It was hard to imagine, however, how the hydrophilic domains of an antibody molecule could be buried in the plasma membrane of a T cell.

The debate as to whether the T-cell receptor is encoded by the immunoglobulin genes was settled by a number of experiments published between 1980 and 1983 by M. Kronenberg, Leroy Hood, and their colleagues. By using a variety of cDNA probes specific for immunoglobulin variable-region gene sequences, these researchers analyzed the organization of the immunoglobulin genes in a variety of T-cell clones. These experiments demonstrated that there were no complete rearrangements of the immunoglobulin genes in T cells. The T cell's antigen-binding receptor could therefore not be immunoglobulin. Its nature remained a mystery.

The T-Cell Receptor Is MHC Restricted

For a number of years it was recognized that one could generate T_C cells specific for hapten-conjugated target cells. Mice could be primed with syngeneic target cells that had been chemically modified with the hapten TNP. The T_C cells from these immunized mice could then be shown to kill the TNP target cells in vitro. Yet these same T_C cells failed to bind free hapten (TNP) or hapten conjugated to a protein carrier TNP-BSA. Why did the T cytotoxic cell not bind the soluble antigen? The answer came when it was shown that T cells recognized antigen only when it was in association with class I or class II molecules of the MHC.

Since the T-cell receptor does not bind soluble antigen, its specificity cannot be assessed by simple antigen-binding assays similar to those used to determine an antibody's specificity. Much more complex assay systems had to be devised. In a classic experiment R. Zinkernagel and P. Doherty showed in 1974 that T_C cells only recognize antigen associated with class I self-MHC molecules on the surface of a cell. In this assay, mice were immunized with a virus and several days later the spleen cells, which included T_C cells specific for the virus, were added to virus-infected target cells of different MHC haplotypes. The results showed that the T_C cells could only kill virally infected target cells bearing a syngeneic class I MHC haplotype. In other words, the T cytotoxic cell could bind the viral antigen only when it is presented in the proper context of a class I self-MHC molecule (Figure 10-1). Other experiments performed during this same time period by D. Katz and B. Benaceraff and by E. M. Shevach and A. Rosenthal demonstrated that T_H cells also display MHC restriction, recognizing antigen only in the context of class II self-MHC molecules.

Early Models for the T-Cell Receptor

In an attempt to explain the MHC restriction of the T-cell receptor, two models were proposed. The *dual-receptor model* envisioned a T cell as having two separate receptors, one for antigen and one for class I or class II MHC molecules. The *altered-self model* proposed that there is a single receptor capable of recog-

nizing foreign antigen complexed to a self-MHC molecule. Unlike the dual-receptor model, in which antigen and MHC are recognized separately, the altered-self model predicts that a single receptor recognizes the alteration in a MHC molecule induced by its association with foreign antigen.

The debate between proponents of these two models was waged for a number of years, until an elegant experiment by J. Kappler and P. Marrack provided a means to test each model. Two different T cells with specificities for different antigen-class II MHC complexes were used for the experiment: one T cell was a T-cell hybridoma specific for ovalbumin (OVA) in the context of class II MHC molecules with the H-2^k haplotype, the other T cell was a normal T cell reactive to keyhole limpet hemocyanin (KLH) in the context of the H-2^f

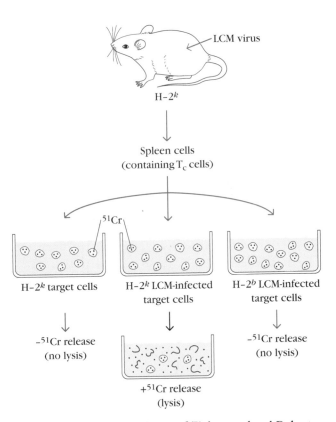

Figure 10-1 Classic experiment of Zinkernagel and Doherty demonstrating that antigen recognition by T cells exhibits MHC restriction. H-2^k mice were primed with the lymphocytic choriomeningitis (LCM) virus to induce cytotoxic T lymphocytes (CTLs) specific for the virus. Spleen cells from this LCM-primed mouse were then added to target cells of different H-2 haplotypes that were intracellularly labeled with [^{51}Cr] (dots) and either infected or not with the LCM virus. CTL-mediated killing of the target cells, as measured by the release of [^{51}Cr] into the culture supernatant, occurred only if the target cells were infected and had the same MHC haplotype as the CTLs.

class II MHC molecule. The experimentors fused these two cells to produce a T-cell hybridoma expressing the receptors of both fusion partners (Figure 10-2). If the dual-receptor model were correct, then the hybrid cells should express separate receptors for each antigen and separate receptors for each class II MHC molecule; therefore, the hybrid cells should respond to both antigens presented by either H-2^k or H-2^f antigen-presenting cells. In fact, Kappler and Marrack found

that the hybrid cells continued to respond only to OVA presented by H-2^k cells and to KLH presented by H-2^f cells. In other words, the original specificity for antigen and MHC haplotype appeared to segregate together in the membrane of these hybrid cells. This finding provided early support for the altered-self model.

Isolation of T-Cell Receptors with Monoclonal Antibodies

Identification and isolation of the T-cell receptor finally was accomplished by producing large numbers of monoclonal antibodies to various T-cell clones and then screening those monoclonal antibodies to find one that was clone specific, or *clonotypic*. This approach was based on the assumption that since the T-cell receptor is specific for both antigen and a MHC molecule, there should be significant structural differences in the receptor from clone to clone. Identification of the T-cell receptor using this approach was first accomplished by J. P. Allison in 1982, closely followed by E. Reinherz and S. Schlossman and by J. Kappler and P. Marrack.

The experimental approach of Kappler and Marrack illustrates how clonotypic monoclonal antibody can be used to identify and isolate the T-cell receptor. They had characterized a T$_H$-cell clone (hybridoma) that was specific for OVA and the H-2^d haplotype. This particular clone responded to OVA on an H-2^d antigen-presenting cell (APC) by secreting interleukin 2 (IL-2), which could be assayed in the culture supernatant. Kappler and Marrack set out to produce various monoclonal antibodies to membrane proteins of this antigen-specific T-cell clone, hoping to find a clonotypic monoclonal antibody that reacted only with the antigen-specific clone and not with other, related T-cell clones. After immunizing mice with the T-cell clone, they fused the spleen cells from the immunized mice with Ab$^-$, HGPRT$^-$ myeloma cells to make various hybridomas secreting monoclonal antibodies to epitopes on the T$_H$ cells. They screened the wells for a monoclonal antibody that blocked IL-2 secretion by the immunizing T$_H$ clone in response to OVA on class II^d antigen-presenting cells. They reasoned that such a monoclonal antibody would be specific for the T-cell receptor if it was clonotypic and specifically inhibited the response of the immunizing clone to its antigen-class II molecule. Kappler and Marrack were, indeed, successful in identifying such a clonotypic monoclonal antibody, as the data in Table 10-1 show. Once having obtained a specific anti-TCR antibody, they used this antibody preparation to precipitate the T-cell receptor from a solubilized membrane extract of the original T$_H$ clone. The clonotypic antibody precipitated a disulfide-linked glycoprotein that contained a 40-kD α chain and a 43-kD β chain.

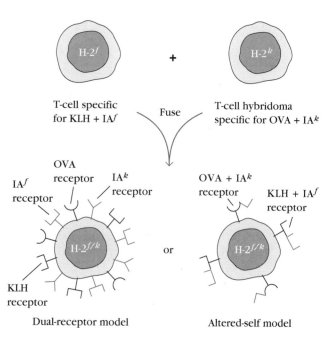

Response of fused cells				
		Expected response		
Antigen	MHC on APCs	Dual-receptor model	Altered-self model	Actual response
OVA	IA^k	+	+	+
OVA	IA^f	+	−	−
KLH	IA^k	+	−	−
KLH	IA^f	+	+	+

Figure 10-2 Fusion of T cells with two different specificities allowed the dual-receptor (DR) and altered-self (AS) models of T-cell recognition to be tested. One fusion partner was specific for ovalbumin (OVA) + the class II MHC molecule IA^k on antigen-presenting cells (APCs), and the other was specific for keyhole limpet hemocyanin (KLH) + IA^f. Comparison of the expected responses of the fused cells, assuming the dual-receptor or altered-self model to be correct, with the actual responses supports the altered-self model. [Based on J. Kappler et al., 1981 *J. Exp. Med.* **153**:1198.]

Table 10-1 Inhibition of IL-2 secretion by T cells specific for OVA on H-2^d APCs with clonotypic monoclonal antibodies

Antigen	APC haplotype	Clonotypic antibody	IL-2 secretion by T cells (units/ml)
OVA	H-2^d	–	2000
OVA	H-2^d	+	5
—	H-2^d	–	5
OVA	H-2^k	–	5

By taking a similar approach, Allison isolated a similar $\alpha\beta$ heterodimer from the T-cell membrane. He carried the characterization of the T-cell receptor one step further by showing that some antisera bound to $\alpha\beta$ heterodimers from all T-cell clones, whereas other antisera was clone specific. This finding suggested that the TCR α and β chains, like the immunoglobulin heavy and light chains, each have a constant and variable amino acid sequence. Later, a second TCR heterodimer consisting of δ and γ chains was also identified. The great majority of T cells (more than 95%) express the $\alpha\beta$ heterodimer; the remaining 2–5% of T cells express the $\gamma\delta$ heterodimer.

Identifying and Cloning the TCR Genes

In order to identify and isolate the TCR genes, S. M. Hedrick and M. M. Davis sought to isolate mRNA encoding the α and β chains from a T$_H$-cell clone. This was no easy task. Because the T cell does not secrete its antigen receptor, the receptor mRNA does not represent a sizable fraction of the mRNA, as it does, for example, in the plasma cell, where immunoglobulin is a major secreted cell product and mRNAs encoding the heavy and light chains are relatively easy to purify. The successful scheme of Hedrick and Davis for isolating TCR genes depended on a number of well-thought-out assumptions, which proved to be correct.

Hedrick and Davis reasoned that the mRNA encoding the T-cell receptor must, like the mRNAs encoding other integral membrane proteins, be bound to polyribosomes rather than to free cytoplasmic ribosomes. They therefore isolated the membrane-bound polyribosomal mRNA from a T$_H$-cell clone and used reverse transcriptase to synthesize [^{32}P] labeled cDNA probes (Figure 10-3). Because only 3% of lymphocyte mRNA is in the membrane-bound polyribosomal fraction, this step eliminated the

97% of the mRNA that did not encode any integral membrane protein.

Hedrick and Davis next used a technique called DNA subtractive hybridization to remove all the [^{32}P] cDNA that was not unique to T cells from their preparation. Their rationale for this step was that since T cells and B cells are derived from a common progenitor cell, they should express many genes in common. Earlier measurements by Davis had shown that 98% of the genes expressed in lymphocytes are common to B cells and T cells. Hedrick and Davis sought to enrich for the 2% of the expressed genes that are unique to T cells, which should include the genes encoding the T-cell antigen receptor. Therefore, by hybridizing B-cell mRNA with their T$_H$-cell [^{32}P] cDNA, they were able to remove, or substract, all the cDNA that was common to B cells and T cells. The unhybridized [^{32}P] cDNA remaining after this step presumably represented the expressed polyribosomal mRNA that was unique to the T$_H$-cell clone, including the mRNA encoding its T-cell receptor.

Cloning of the unhybridized [^{32}P] cDNA generated 10 different cDNA clones. To determine which of these T-cell–specific cDNA clones might represent the T-cell receptor, Hedrick and Davis used these clones as probes to look for genes on the genomic DNA that rearranged in mature T cells. This approach was based on the assumption that since the $\alpha\beta$ heterodimer appeared to have constant and variable regions, its genes should undergo DNA rearrangements like those observed in B cells. The two investigators isolated genomic DNA from T cells, B cells, liver cells, and macrophages, cleaved it with restriction endonucleases, and subjected each DNA sample to Southern-blot analysis (see Figure 2-7) using the 10 [^{32}P] cDNA probes to identify unique T-cell genomic DNA sequences. They looked for bands that showed DNA rearrangement in T cells but not in liver cells, B cells, or macrophages. One [^{32}P] cDNA probe showed the same Southern-blot patterns for DNA isolated from liver cells, B cells, and macrophages but six different patterns for the DNA from six different mature T-cell lines (Figure 10-3). These patterns presumably represented rearranged TCR genes. Such results would be expected if rearranged TCR genes occur only in mature T cells. The observation that all six T-cell lines showed different Southern-blot patterns is consistent with the differences in TCR specificity to be expected in each cell line.

The cDNA clone identified by the Southern-blot analysis shown in Figure 10-3 has all the hallmarks of a putative TCR gene: It represents a gene sequence that rearranges, is expressed as a membrane-bound protein, and is expressed only in T cells. This cDNA clone was found to encode the β chain of the T-cell receptor. Later, cDNA clones were identified encoding the α chain, the γ chain, and finally the δ chain.

Organization and Rearrangement of Germ-Line TCR Genes

Once cDNA clones encoding the α, β, γ, and δ chains of the T-cell receptor were available, they were used as probes to isolate the corresponding genes in germ-line DNA. Nucleotide sequencing of germ-line TCR genes soon revealed a remarkable similarity to the multigene organization of the immunoglobulin genes.

TCR Multigene Families

Germ-line DNA contains four multigene families each encoding one of the TCR chains. As in the case of immunoglobulin genes, functional TCR genes are produced by gene rearrangements involving V and J segments in the α-chain and γ-chain families and V, D, and J segments in the β-chain and δ-chain families. In the mouse the α-, β-, and γ-chain gene segments are located on chromosomes 14, 6, and 13, respectively. The δ-chain gene segments are located on chromosome 14 between the V_α and J_α segments. This location of the δ-chain gene family is significant: A productive rearrangement of the α-chain gene segments deletes C_δ, so that the αβ TCR receptor cannot be coexpressed with the γδ receptor in a given T cell.

Mouse germ-line DNA contains 75–100 V_α and 50 J_α gene segments and a single C_α segment. The δ-chain gene family contains about 10 V gene segments, which are largely distinct from the V_α gene segments, although some sharing of V segments has been observed in rearranged α- and δ-chain genes. Two D_δ and two J_δ gene segments and one C_δ segment also have been identified. The β-chain gene family has approximately 30 V gene

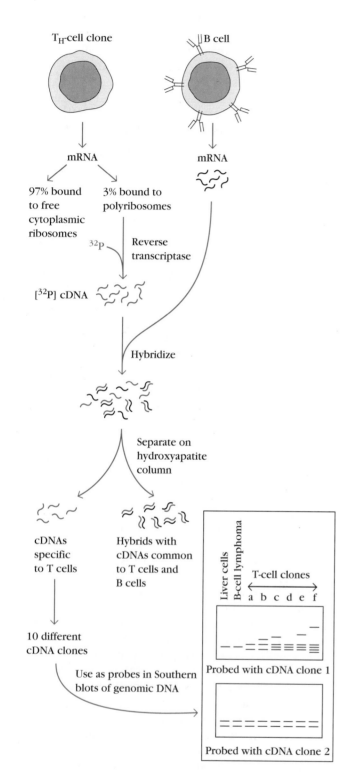

Figure 10-3 Production and identification of a cDNA clone encoding the T-cell receptor. The flow chart outlines the procedure used by S. Hedrick and M. Davis to obtain [32P] cDNA clones corresponding to T-cell–specific mRNAs. The technique of DNA subtractive hybridization enabled them to isolate [32P] cDNA unique to the T-cell. (*Inset*) The labeled cDNA clones were used as probes in Southern-blot analyses of genomic DNA from liver cells, B-lymphoma cells, and six different T_H-cell clones (a–f). Probing with cDNA clone 1 produced a distinct blot pattern for each T-cell clone, whereas probing with cDNA clone 2 did not. Assuming that the liver cells and B cells contained unrearranged germ-line DNA and that each of the T-cell clones contained different rearranged TCR genes, the results using cDNA clone 1 as probe identified the T-cell receptor. The other cDNA clone 2 identified another T-cell membrane molecule encoded by DNA that does not undergo rearrangement. [Based on S. Hedrick et al., 1984, *Nature* **308**:153.]

segments and two repeats of D, J, and C segments, each repeat consisting of one D_β, six J_β and one C_β. The γ-chain gene family consists of seven V exons and three different functional J-C repeats. The organization of the gene segments within each multigene family is shown in Figure 10-4.

Variable-Region Gene Rearrangements

The mechanisms by which TCR germ-like DNA is rearranged to form functional receptor genes appear to be similar to the mechanisms used in immunoglobulin-gene rearrangements. For example, conserved heptamer and nonamer recognition signals sequences (RSS), containing either 12- or 23-bp spacer sequences, have been identified flanking each V, D, and J gene segment in TCR germ-line DNA. The recognition signals in T cells have the same heptamer and nonamer sequences as those in B cells (see Figure 8-6). All of the TCR-gene rearrangements follow the 12/23 joining rule observed for the immunoglobulin genes. A recombinase enzyme recognizes the heptamer and nanomer recognition signals and catalyzes V-J and V-D-J joining by the same deletional or inversional mechanisms that occur in the immunoglobulin genes (see Figure 8-8). Circular excision products thought to be generated by looping-out and deletion in TCR rearrangement have been shown to be present in thymocytes. Like the pre-B cell, the pre-T cell has also been shown to express the recombination activating genes, RAG-1 and RAG-2. These genes are either a part of the recombination machinery for both cell types or else they play a role in regulating the recombination machinery.

A number of experiments have suggested that T cells utilize the same recombinase enzyme system as B cells in V-(D)-J joining. In one experiment G. D. Yancopoulos transfected unrearranged TCR β-chain genes into B-lineage precursor cells having active recombinase activity. He found that the recombinase enzyme of the B cells could rearrange the transfected TCR β-chain genes. Another experimental system that has shed light on the mechanisms of V-(D)-J joining in T- and B-cell lineages is a mutant mouse strain designated CB17-*scid*. This strain lacks functional T and B cells and therefore manifests severe combined immunodeficiency disease (SCID). These mice have been maintained in a sterile germ-free environment, and their immune defect has been extensively analyzed. Both the T cells and B cells of these mutant mice show abnormal gene rearrangements such that the J gene segment is deleted during the D-J rearrangement of both the immunoglobulin genes and TCR genes. This finding lends support to the notion that the same recombinase enzyme may be involved in V-D-J rearrangements in B cells and in T cells and that a defect in this recombinase system may give rise to the immune deficiency in *scid* mice. The fact that the immunoglobulin genes are not normally rearranged in T cells and that TCR genes are not rearranged in B

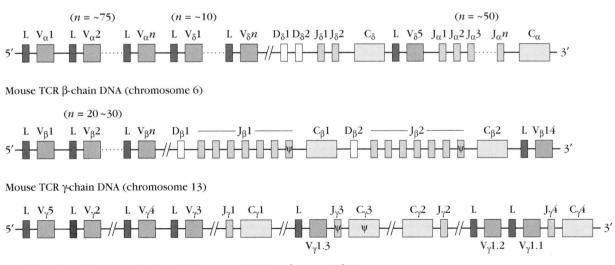

Figure 10-4 Germ-line organization of the mouse TCR α-, β-, γ-, and δ-chain gene segments. The estimated numbers of the variable-region V, D, and J gene segments are listed in Table 10-1. Each C gene segment is composed of a series of exons and introns, which are not shown. [Adapted from D. Raulet, 1989, *Annu. Rev. Immunol.* **7**:175.]

cells suggests that there must be mechanisms that regulate the recombinase enzyme system in each cell lineage. Presumably, differences in chromatin configuration of the immunoglobulin genes and TCR genes within B- and T-cell lineages account for the preferential rearrangement of immunoglobulin genes in B cells and TCR genes in T cells.

As with the immunoglobulin genes, rearrangement of the T cell receptor genes also exhibits allelic exclusion. Once a productive rearrangement occurs for one allele, the rearrangement of the other allele is inhibited. The phenomenon of allelic exclusion can be demonstrated by transgenic mice into which the rearranged genes for the $\alpha\beta$ TCR have been introduced. Expression of the rearranged TCR gene inhibits gene rearrangements of the endogeneous TCR genes.

Generation of Diversity in T-Cell Receptor

Although the T-cell receptors are encoded by far fewer V-gene exons than the immunoglobulin molecules, a number of features contribute to generating even greater diversity in the TCR. Table 10-2 compares the cumulative diversity of antibodies and T-cell receptors. As in immunoglobulin diversity, *combinatorial joining* of V-J and V-D-J gene segments generates a large number of random gene combinations for the $\alpha\beta$ or $\gamma\delta$ chains (Figure 10-5). For example, 75 V_α gene segments and 50 J_α gene segments can generate 3.75×10^3 possible combinations. Similarly, 25 V_β gene segments, 2 D_β gene segments, and 12 J_β gene segments can give 6×10^2 possible combinations. Although there are far fewer TCR

Table 10-2   Comparison of possible diversity in mouse immunoglobulin and TCR genes

| Mechanism of diversity | Possible combinations[*] | | | | | |
| | Immunoglobulins | | $\alpha\beta$ TCR | | $\gamma\delta$ TCR | |
	H chain	κ chain	α chain	β chain	γ chain	δ chain
Multiple germ-line gene segments						
V	300	300	75	25	7	10
D	12	0	0	2	0	2
J	4	4	50	12	2	2
Combinatorial V-J and V-D-J joining	$300 \times 12 \times 4$ $= 1.4 \times 10^4$	300×4 $= 1.2 \times 10^3$	75×50 $= 3.75 \times 10^3$	$25 \times 2 \times 12$ $= 6 \times 10^2$	7×2 $= 14$	$10 \times 2 \times 2$ $= 40$
Alternative joining of D gene segments	−	−	−	+ (some)	−	+ (often)
Junctional flexibility	+	+	+	+	+	+
N-region nucleotide addition[†]	+	−	+	+	+	+
Somatic mutation	+	+	−	−	−	−
Total estimated diversity[‡]	$\sim 10^{11}$		$\sim 10^{15}$		$\sim 10^{18}$	

[*] A (+) means that indicated mechanism makes a significant contribution to diversity but exactly how much is unknown. A (−) means that the indicated mechanism does not operate.

[†] There are theoretically 5461 permutations possible at each junction due to N-region nucleotide addition. The total possibilities for immunoglobulin V_H-D_H-J_H joining $= 3.0 \times 10^7$ and for TCR joinings are as follows: V-J $= 5.5 \times 10^3$, V-D-J $= 3.0 \times 10^7$, and V-D-D-J $= 1.6 \times 10^{11}$.

[‡] Total estimated diversity includes contribution from combinatorial association of chains.

Source: Adapted from M. Davis and P. J. Borkman, 1988, Nature **334**:397.

GENERATION OF DIVERSITY

(a) T-CELL RECEPTOR

(b) IMMUNOGLOBULIN

Random joining VDJ VJ

V DJ

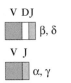 β, δ

V J

α, γ

V DJ

H

V J

L

Junctional diversity

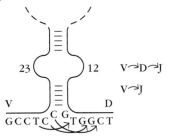

23   12   V⤳D⤳J

V⤳J

V   D

$\overline{\text{GCCTC}}$ $^{C}_{}$ $^{G}_{}$ $\overline{\text{TGGCT}}$

23   12   V⤳D⤳J

V⤳J

$\overline{\text{TGGCC}}$ $^{G}_{}$ $^{A}_{}$ $\overline{\text{TGG}}$

Joining of multiple D's

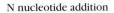
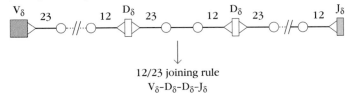

V_δ 23   12 D_δ 23   12 D_δ 23   12 J_δ

V_H 23   12 D_H 12   23 J_H

12/23 joining rule

V_δ-D_δ-D_δ-J_δ

12/23 joining rule

V_H-D_H-J_H

N nucleotide addition

V   D   J

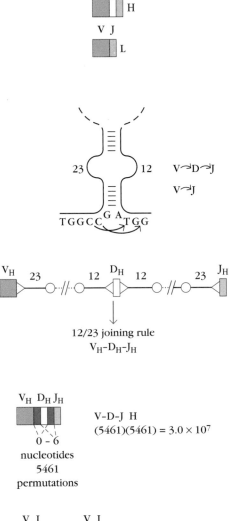

0 – 6
nucleotides
5461
permutations

V–D–D–J δ
$(5461)(5461)(5461) = 1.6 \times 10^{11}$
V–D–J β
$(5461)(5461) = 3.0 \times 10^7$
V–J α,γ
$(5461) = 5.5 \times 10^3$

V_H D_H J_H

0 – 6
nucleotides
5461
permutations

V–D–J H
$(5461)(5461) = 3.0 \times 10^7$

Somatic hypermutation

$\ominus$

V J   V J

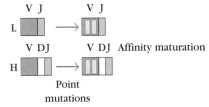

L   ⟶

V DJ   V DJ   Affinity maturation

H   ⟶

Point
mutations

Figure 10-5 Comparison of mechanisms that generate diversity for the T cell receptor and for the immunoglobulin receptor.

V_α and V_β gene segments than immunoglobulin V_H and V_κ segments, this difference is offset by the greater number of J segments in TCR germ-line DNA. Assuming that the antigen-binding specificity of a given T-cell receptor depends upon the variable region in both the α and β chains, random association of 3.75×10^3 V_α combinations with 6×10^2 V_β combinations can generate a minimum of 2.2×10^6 possible combinations for the $\alpha\beta$ TCR receptor.

The position of the heptamer/nonamer recognition signal sequences in the TCR β- and δ-chain genes permits additional diversity to be generated while the 12/23 joining rule is observed. As Figure 10-5 illustrates, it is possible for a V_β gene segment to join directly with a J_β gene segment or for one D_β to join with another D_β generating V_β-J_β combinations or V_β-D_β-D_β-J_β combinations in addition to the most common V_β-D_β-J_β combinations. Similar alternative joining also can occur in the δ-chain genes. The position of the recognition signals in immunoglobulin heavy-chain DNA prohibits formation of such alternative combinations.

The diversity generated in the TCR by means of germline V, D, J combinations is further augmented by N-region diversification. As in immunoglobulin heavy-chain gene rearrangement, this addition of nucleotides occurs at joining junctions and is catalyzed by a terminal deoxynucleotidyl transferase. Whereas N-region diversification occurs only in the immunoglobulin heavy-chain genes, it occurs in both $\alpha\beta$ and $\gamma\delta$ genes of the TCR. As many as six nucleotides can be added by this mechanism at each junction, generating up to 5461 possible combinations assuming random selection of nucleotides. The T-cell receptor gene families can also exhibit junctional diversity, resulting from flexibility in the joining process, at the V-to-D and D-to-J junctions. As with the immunoglobulin genes, this flexibility can generate many nonproductive rearrangements (see Figure 8-8), but it also increases diversity by encoding alternative amino acids at each junction. Each junctional region in a TCR gene encodes only 10–20 amino acids, and yet enormous diversity can be generated in these regions. Estimates suggest that the combined effects of N-region nucleotide addition and joining flexibility can generate as many as 10^{13} possible amino acid sequences in the TCR junctional regions alone. Unlike the immunoglobulin genes, the TCR genes do not seem to undergo somatic mutation. That is, the functional TCR genes generated during T-cell maturation in the thymus are the same as those found in the mature peripheral T-cell population.

The T-cell receptor must function to recognize both a very large number of different processed antigens and a relatively small number of self-MHC molecules. It has been suggested that the limited number of germ-like V gene segments carried by T cells may generate the diversity needed for MHC recognition, whereas the enormous diversity generated at the junctional regions facilitates recognition of antigen.

Structure of T-Cell Receptors and Rearranged TCR Genes

Amino acid sequencing analyses of $\alpha\beta$ and $\gamma\delta$ TCR heterodimers have revealed a surprising similarity to the domain structure of immunoglobulins, placing the TCRs among the members of the immunoglobulin gene superfamily (see Figure 5-16). Both chains of each TCR heterodimer exhibit marked variation in the amino-terminal amino acids but conservation in the carboxy-terminal amino acids. In addition, the sequences of the variable and constant domains share some homology with the immunoglobulin domain sequences; especially noticeable is a centrally placed cysteine intrachain disulfide loop spanning 60–75 amino acids (Figure 10-6).

The variable regions of T-cell receptors are, of course, encoded by rearranged VDJ and VJ gene segments. Because the TCR has not yet been crystallized, the three-dimensional structure of its antigen-binding site can only be inferred from its homology to immunoglobulin molecules. The variable regions are thought to be folded into β-pleated-sheet structures similar to those observed in the immunoglobulins. Three complementarity-determining regions (CDRs) which appear to be equivalent to the complementarity-determining regions in immunoglobulin light and heavy chains have been identified in both the $\alpha\beta$ and the $\gamma\delta$ chains. In TCR genes, V gene segments appear to encode the CDR1 and CDR2 equivalents, whereas junctional diversity (joining flexibility and N-region nucleotide addition) generates the CDR3 equivalent. Until the TCR is crystallized, the position of the CDRs in the antigen-binding cleft remain unknown. Rearranged TCR genes also contain a short leader (L) sequence upstream of the joined VJ or VDJ units. The amino acids encoded by the L sequence are cleaved as the nascent polypeptide enters the endoplasmic reticulum.

The constant regions of each TCR chain are encoded by a C gene segment that has multiple exons corresponding to structural domains in the protein (see Figure 10-6). The first C-region exon encodes the majority of the constant region and shows some homology to the immunoglobulin constant-region domain, including an intrachain disulfide bond. Next is a short exon encoding a hinge region, which includes a cysteine residue involved in disulfide linking of the α and β or γ and δ chains. The third exon encodes a hydrophobic trans-

Rearranged α-chain gene   αβ T-cell receptor   Rearranged β-chain gene

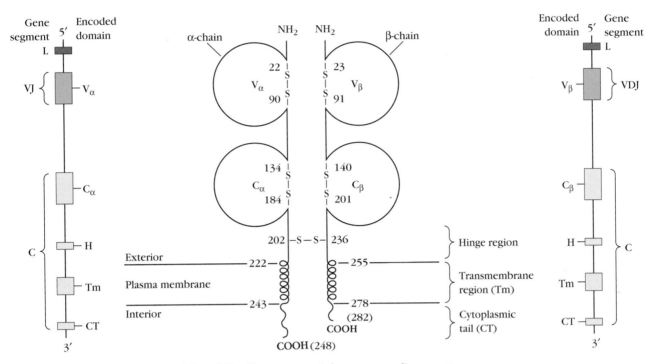

Figure 10-6 Schematic diagram of the αβ T-cell receptor and the corresponding exons (red) in the rearranged TCR genes. The variable regions, encoded by joined VJ or VDJ units, probably exhibit the immunoglobulin-fold structure and have three hypervariable regions equivalent to the CDRs in antibodies. The C gene segments contain multiple exons encoding the various constant-region domains of the α and β chains. The structure of the γδ T-cell receptor is similar. Numbers indicate residue positions in the receptor molecule. The transmembrane regions of the α and β chains contain positively charged amino acids.

membrane region of 21 or 22 amino acids, which anchors each chain in the plasma membrane. Each of the transmembrane domains contains one or two positively charged amino acids that are thought to enable the TCR to interact with negatively charged residues found in the transmembrane regions of the CD3 protein complex. Finally, each chain contains a short cytoplasmic tail, of 5–12 amino acids, at the carboxyl-terminal end. The short length of the cytoplasmic tails suggests that they are unsuitable for signal transduction, and it is thought that some other associated molecule, probably CD3, must transmit a signal from the TCR to the cytoplasm. As described in Chapter 8, differential RNA processing of the constant region in immunoglobulin heavy-chain primary transcripts produces either secreted or membrane-bound antibody. Since there is no secreted form of the T-cell receptor, such differential processing of TCR primary transcripts does not occur.

T-Cell Accessory Membrane Molecules

Although antigen-MHC recognition is mediated solely by the T-cell receptor, a variety of other membrane molecules play an important accessory role in antigen recognition and T-cell activation. Many of these accessory molecules function as adhesion molecules, strengthening the interaction between the T cell and an antigen-presenting cell or target cell. Additionally, a number of these accessory molecules transduce signals from the T-cell receptor through the membrane to the cytoplasm. Included among these accessory molecules are a number of members of the immunoglobulin gene superfamily: CD2, CD3, CD4, and CD8 (see Figure 5-16) as well as the integrin family molecule LFA-1. The association of the αβ heterodimer with these various accessory proteins is schematically diagrammed in Figure 10-7.

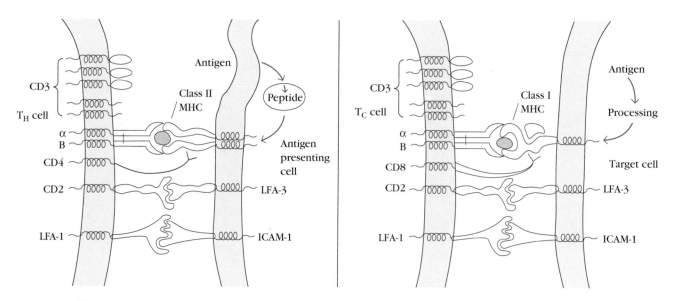

Figure 10-7 The TCR is associated on the membrane with accessory molecules that may function to transduce signals or augment MHC restriction. The roles of the molecules associated with the TCR are depicted for the interaction of a T helper cell with an antigen presenting cell and T cytotoxic cell with a target cell.

TCR-CD3 Membrane Complex

The first evidence suggesting an association of the T-cell receptor with another membrane molecule came from experiments in which fluorescent antibody to the receptor was shown to "co-cap" another membrane protein, designated CD3. Later experiments by J. P. Allison and L. Lanier demonstrated that the T-cell receptor and CD3 are located quite close together in the T-cell membrane. These researchers first treated a T-cell membrane preparation with dimethyldithio-bisproprionimidate, a cross-linking agent that spans 12 Å, and then precipitated the T-cell receptor with anti-TCR monoclonal antibody. Analysis of the precipitated T-cell receptors showed that they were cross-linked to CD3, indicating that the two proteins must be positioned within 12 Å of each other in the membrane. Subsequent experiments demonstrated not only that CD3 is closely associated with the $\alpha\beta$ heterodimer but also that its expression is required for membrane expression of $\alpha\beta$ and $\gamma\delta$ T-cell receptors. The T-cell receptor, then, exists on the membrane as a molecular complex with CD3. Mutation in either the CD3 or TCR genes results in loss of the entire molecular complex from the membrane, demonstrating the obligate requirement for coexpression of both CD3 and the T-cell receptor on the membrane.

CD3 is actually a complex of 5 polypeptides: gamma (γ), delta(δ), and epsilon(ε) complexed either to a hom-

odimer of two zeta chains ($\zeta\zeta$) or a heterodimer of zeta and eta chains ($\zeta\eta$) (Figure 10-8). About 90% of the CD3 complexes examined to date incorporate the $\zeta\zeta$ homodimer and the remainder have the $\zeta\eta$ heterodimer. The transmembrane segments of γ, δ, ε, and ζ chains each contain a negatively charged aspartic acid residue. These negatively charged groups may enable the proteins of the CD3 complex to interact with the positively charged residues within the transmembrane segment of the $\alpha\beta$ or $\gamma\delta$ heterodimers.

Once the T-cell receptor recognizes an antigen-MHC complex, the associated CD3 complex is thought to transmit a signal to the cell interior that contributes to cellular activation. Support for the role of the CD3 complex in signal transduction is strengthened by the observation that monoclonal antibody to CD3 can activate T cells in the absence of antigen-MHC recognition by the TCR. Because the monoclonal antibody to CD3 bypasses the antigen-specific T-cell receptor, all T cells are activated regardless of their antigenic specificity. Following activation, several of the CD3 proteins are phosphorylated at tyrosine or serine residues. Like other transmembrane proteins, the phosphorylation of the tyrosine or serine residues is thought to lead to the activation of second messengers involved in T cell activation. Evidence suggests that the signal transmitted by CD3 complexes incorporating the $\zeta\zeta$ homodimer may be different from the signal transmitted by CD3 complexes involving $\zeta\eta$ heterodimers.

CD4 and CD8 Accessory Molecules

T cells can be subdivided based on their expression of CD4 or CD8 membrane molecules. The CD4$^+$ T cells recognize antigen in association with class II MHC molecules and largely function as helper cells, whereas CD8$^+$ T cells recognize antigen in association with class I MHC molecules and largely function as cytotoxic cells. CD4 and CD8 are associated in the membrane with the T-cell receptor and can comigrate with the TCR-CD3 complex. Both CD4 and CD8 function as adhesion molecules; CD4 binds to class II MHC molecules, and CD8 binds to class I MHC molecules. CD4 and CD8 apparently function to increase the avidity of the interaction between a T-cell receptor and an antigen-MHC complex. For example, binding of T-cell receptors to antigen-MHC complexes has been shown to be augmented about 100-fold by the presence of CD4 or CD8 on the membrane; thus a T cell can respond to 100-fold lower levels of antigen + MHC when CD4 or CD8 is present.

CD4 is a 55-kD-membrane glycoprotein whose structure consists of four immunoglobulin-like extracellular domains, a hydrophobic transmembrane region, and a long cytoplasmic domain containing three serine residues that may be phosphorylated. CD8 is a smaller glycoprotein of approximately 32–34 kD, consisting of a single extracellular immunoglobulin-like domain, a hydrophobic transmembrane region, and a cytoplasmic domain of 25–27 residues. Like the CD4 molecule, the cytoplasmic domain contains several residues that can be phosphorylated. Unlike CD4 which exists solely as a monomer, CD8 is expressed as a homodimer, a heterodimer, or in a multimeric form.

Recently, studies have suggested that CD4 and CD8 membrane molecules do not function solely as cellular adhesion molecules but also play an additional role in signal transduction. The cytoplasmic domains of CD4 and CD8 are each associated with p56^{lck}, an *src*-related protein kinase that can phosphorylate the γ, δ, ε, and ζ chains of CD3.

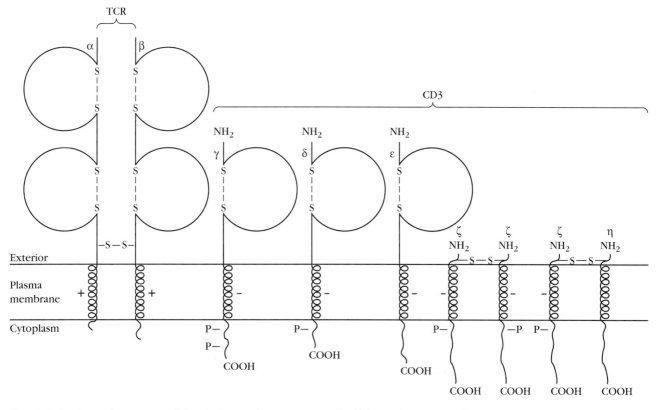

Figure 10-8 General structure of the CD3 complex containing the $\zeta\zeta$ homodimer. A small percentage of CD3 complexes contain the $\zeta\eta$ heterodimer instead of the $\zeta\zeta$ homodimer. The external domains of the γ, δ, and ε chains probably have the immunoglobulin-fold structure, which may facilitate their interaction with the T-cell receptor and with one another. Ionic interactions also may occur between the negatively charged transmembrane segments of the CD3 complex (− signs) and the positively charged transmembrane segments of the T-cell receptor. Sites that may be phosphorylated by protein kinases are indicated with a P.

Other Accessory Molecules: CD2 and LFA-1

The interaction between a T cell and an antigen-presenting cell or target cell is strengthened by two additional adhesion molecules: CD2 and LFA-1. CD2 is a 45–50-kD glycoprotein expressed on most thymocytes, all peripheral T cells, and on large granular lymphocytes. The molecule consists of two immunoglobulin-like extracellular domains, a transmembrane domain, and a long cytoplasmic domain of 116 amino acids. The physiologic ligand for CD2 is a structurally similar molecule, LFA-3, that is found on a wide variety of cells including endothelial cells and most hematopoietic cells. LFA-3 is also a member of the immunoglobulin gene superfamily, and the interaction of CD2 with LFA-3 is thought to be facilitated by the basic immunoglobulin-fold structure allowing members of this superfamily to interact across the faces of β pleated sheets. The CD2/LFA-3 interaction facilitates binding of T helper cells to antigen-presenting cells, T cytotoxic cells to their targets, and thymocytes to thymic epithelial cells. In addition to these cellular interactions the CD2 molecule on human T cells binds to a glycoprotein on sheep red blood cells that is homologous to LFA-3. Although this rosetting with SRBC has no physiologic significance, this property has been used to quantitate or separate human T cells.

CD2 also functions as a signal-transducing molecule, in some cases transducing activating signals and in other cases transducing inhibitory signals. Monoclonal antibodies to CD2 have been shown to induce resting T cells to enter the cell cycle-suggesting that CD2 may be an alternative pathway of T-cell activation. The fact that CD2 appears developmentally on thymocytes before the TCR-CD3 complex may mean that early thymocyte proliferation may be induced through the CD2 membrane molecule.

LFA-1 is another adhesion molecule that strengthens the interaction of the T cell with an antigen-presenting cell or target cell. LFA-1 is a member of the integrin family of adhesion molecules. Members of this family are heterodimers, containing two noncovalently linked α and β polypeptide chains. LFA-1 has an α chain designated as CD11a and a β chain designated CD18. Other members of this subfamily of integrin molecules share a common β chain (CD18) but are differentiated by unique α chains. This subfamily of adhesion molecules will be discussed more fully in Chapter 15.

LFA-1 binds to ICAM-1, an intercellular adhesion molecule expressed on a wide range of cells including T cells, B cells, macrophages, vascular endothelial cells, dendritic cells, and thymic epithelial cells. As T cells are activated, the avidity of LFA-1 for ICAM-1 increases, stabilizing the interaction between the T cell and the appropriate target cell or antigen-presenting cell. As will be discussed in later chapters, the increased avidity of the T cell for an antigen-presenting cell or target cell prolong the association between the interacting cells, providing time for directed secretion of various lymphokines or lytic molecules.

Signal Transduction by the TCR/CD3 Membrane Complex

Recognition of an antigen–MHC by the TCR results in T-cell activation, leading to cell proliferation and the secretion of lymphokines. The membrane events resulting in transduction of the activation signal involve the T-cell receptor together with the accessory molecules CD3 and CD4 or CD8. At least two biochemical pathways have been shown to be involved in this signal transduction (Figure 10-9). One pathway occurs after antigen-MHC recognition by a T-cell receptor complexed to CD3 incorporating the $\zeta\eta$ heterodimer. In this pathway phospholipase C (PLC) is activated and cleaves phosphatidylinositol 4,5-bisphosphate, (PIP$_2$) generating diacylglycerol (DAG) and inositol 1,4,5-trisphosphate (IP$_3$). The IP$_3$ mobilizes Ca^{2+} uptake, which serves to regulate activation of several lymphokine genes through the effect of Ca^{2+} on the calmodulin–protein kinase system. The other biochemical signal pathway follows antigen-MHC recognition by T-cell receptors complexed to CD3 incorporating the $\zeta\zeta$ homodimer. This signal activates the tyrosine kinase pathway through, as yet, unknown mechanisms. The CD4 and CD8 accessory molecules may be involved in this signal pathway, as they have both been shown to be associated with a cytoplasmic tyrosine kinase (p56^{lck}) by way of their transmembrane cytoplasmic tails.

The $\alpha\beta$ Heterodimer Alone Recognizes Antigen and MHC

With the cloning and sequencing of the $\alpha\beta$ heterodimer and the discovery of associated CD3, CD4, and CD8 membrane molecules, it became important to determine the contribution of each of these molecules to the recognition of antigen and MHC. The earlier experiment of Kappler and Marrack, described previously, had suggested that a single receptor on the T cell recognizes antigen complexed to a self-MHC molecule (see Figure 10-3). However, that experiment did not rule out the possibility that another membrane molecule, associated with the T-cell receptor, might contribute to the recognition of either antigen or MHC. A definitive experiment proving that the $\alpha\beta$ T-cell receptor alone recognizes both antigen and MHC molecules used an approach similar to that of the earlier Kappler and Marrack experiment but involved gene transfection instead of cell fusion. Functional TCR α- and β-chain genes from a T_C-cell clone specific for one hapten on H-2^d target cells were transfected into another T_C-cell clone specific for a second hapten on H-2^k target cells. The transfected cells expressed both their own T-cell receptor and the new transfected T-cell receptor. Cytolysis assays showed that the transfected cells recognized both hapten–MHC molecule complexes for which the original T_C clones were specific; however the transfected cells did not recognize either hapten when it was presented on target cells of a different MHC haplotype (Figure 10-10). In other words, transfection of the TCR genes alone transferred reactivity to both a particular antigen and particular MHC molecule.

The explanation of how the T-cell receptor recognizes antigen and MHC simultaneously may lie in the structure of class I and class II MHC molecules. As discussed in Chapter 9, most of the polymorphic amino acids in class I MHC molecules are clustered in a large groove between the membrane-distal $α_1$ and $α_2$ domains. This groove is thought to be the binding site for processed antigen (see Figure 9-10). Because of this arrangement,

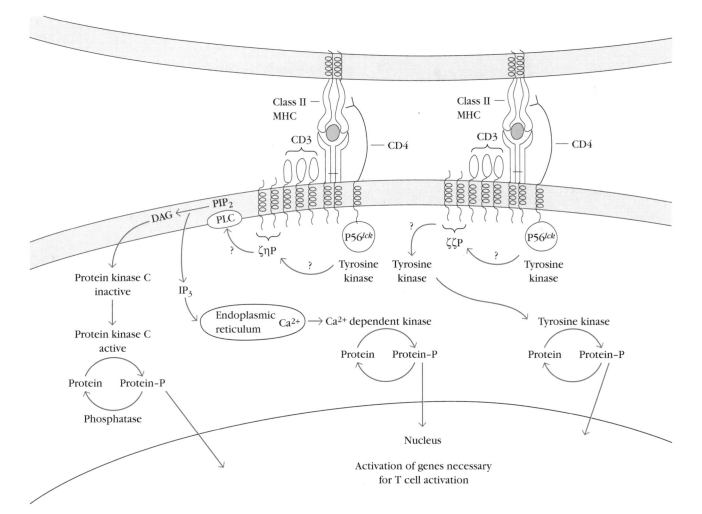

Figure 10-9 Two biochemical pathways thought to transduce the signal generated by interaction of a T_H cell with an antigen–class II MHC molecule complex. *Left:* Antigen-MHC recognition by a T-cell receptor complexed to the $ζη$ CD3 activates phospholipase C (PLC) by an as-yet-unknown mechanism. The activated PLC cleaves phosphatidylinositol 4,5-bisphosphate (PIP_2), generating diacylglycerol (DAG) and inositol 1,4,5-trisphosphate (IP_3), resulting in Ca^{2+} uptake. *Right:* Antigen-MHC recognition by a T-cell receptor complexed to the $ζζ$ CD3 activates the tyrosine kinase pathway by an unknown mechanism. A cytoplasmic tyrosine kinase (p56^{lck}) that is bound to CD4 and CD8 may play a role in this pathway. Similar pathways operate in T_C cells. [Adapted from R. H. Schwarz, 1990, *Science* **248**:1351.]

the T-cell receptor presumably can recognize epitopes on a processed antigen as well as amino acids in and near the α_1/α_2 groove of the MHC (Figure 10-11).

To determine whether T cells recognized amino acids near the groove of the class I MHC molecule, chemical mutagenesis was used to induce single amino acid changes in class I MHC molecules. The effect of these changes was then assessed on the response of various

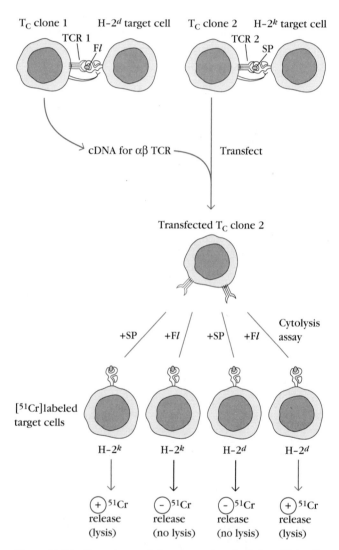

Figure 10-10   Experimental demonstration that the $\alpha\beta$ T-cell receptor alone recognizes both antigen and MHC molecules. cDNA corresponding to the $\alpha\beta$ T-cell receptor was prepared from T_C clone 1, which was specific for fluorescein (FL) on H-2^d target cells. This cDNA was transfected into T_C clone 2, specific for 3-(p-sulphophenyldiazo)-4-hydroxy-phenylacetic acid (SP) on H-2^k target cells. The transfected cells were assayed for their ability to kill H-2^d or H-2^k target cells, labeled intracellularly with [^{51}Cr], in the presence of FL or SP. The transfected cells could kill only those target cells presenting antigen associated with the original MHC restriction molecule.

T_C-cell clones. The experiments revealed that a single amino acid change in the exposed surfaces of either the α_1 or α_2 helix directly affected the ability of T_C cells to lyse target cells for which they were specific (Figure 10-12). This suggests that the T-cell receptor recognizes amino acid residues along both sides of the α_1 and α_2 helix. This is in contrast to the recognition of amino acid residues of the MHC by monoclonal antibodies, which have been shown to recognize discrete regions of the α_1 or α_2 helix but not both sides of the helix. Since the α_1 and α_2 helices form the sides of the putative antigen-binding cleft on class I MHC molecules, amino acid changes along the sides of this groove might well directly influence the ability of the T-cell receptor to interact with both antigen and MHC molecules.

Acquisition of MHC Restriction and Self-Tolerance

The specificity of the T-cell receptor for antigen in association with MHC can be achieved either by an inherent affinity in the cell's germ-line gene repertoire for molecules of the MHC or by selection in the thymus for T cells bearing receptors with a high affinity for antigen + MHC.

Inherent Affinity of Some Germ-Line TCR Genes for MHC

Most studies have failed to correlate a given TCR V_α or V_β gene segment with MHC or antigen reactivity. A number of studies have revealed T cells expressing the same V_α or V_β gene product and yet showing differences in class I or class II MHC restriction. Similarly, a number of T cells specific for the same antigen have been shown to express different V gene segments. The general consensus is that the combined three-dimensional configuration of the α- and β-chain variable-region domains generates reactivity to both antigen and MHC. There are, however, a few V gene segments which do encode gene products with an inherent affinity for MHC molecules. One example is a series of T-cell clones expressing the same germ-line β-chain V exon (V_β17a). These T-cell clones were found to bind class II IE molecules with high frequency, suggesting that the amino acid sequence encoded by this particular V gene segment has an affinity for class II MHC molecules. Such V-region genes have proven to be valuable for certain studies that are discussed later in the chapter. In general, however, most V gene segments do not have an inherent affinity for the MHC and those that do, like V_β17a are the exception and not the rule.

Selection of the T-Cell Repertoire

Given that the T cell has the potential of generating receptor diversity equal to or surpassing that of the B cell, how is this potential diversity limited so that mature peripheral T cells will only express receptors specific for antigen + self-MHC? Random gene rearrangements at the $\alpha\beta$ or $\gamma\delta$ loci combined with joining variation, nucleotide addition at the joining sites and combinatorial association of the two chains of the heterodimer can potentially generate an enormous T-cell-receptor repertoire with an estimated diversity exceeding 10^{13}. Since the T-cell germ-line gene products do not generally have inherent affinity for MHC, this process should be capable of generating receptors with specificity for soluble antigen, self MHC, or antigen + nonself MHC, in addition to the desired specificity for antigen + self MHC. In some way the enormous diversity of the germ-line repertoire must be "selected" so that only a subset of T cells bearing receptors capable of binding antigen + self-MHC is allowed to mature.

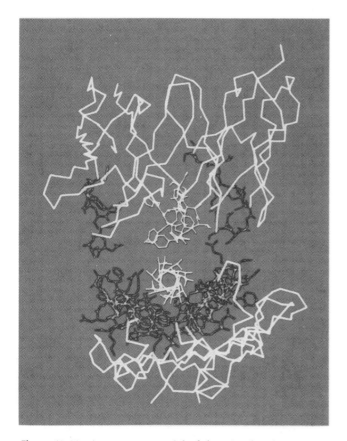

Figure 10-11 A computer model of the trimolecular complex involving a T-cell receptor, an antigenic peptide, and a MHC molecule. The foreign peptide (*middle*) contacts both the T-cell receptor (*top*) and the MHC molecule (*bottom*). The T-cell receptor can be seen to contact amino acid residues in both the peptide and the MHC molecule. [From M. M. Davis and P. J. Bjorkman, Stanford University.]

Role of the Thymus in T-Cell Maturation and Selection

As discussed briefly in Chapter 3, progenitor T cells produced in the bone marrow during hematopoiesis migrate to the thymus. Within the thymus, immature thymocytes undergo maturation and selection, yielding mature immunocompetent T_H and T_C cells that recognize antigen + self-MHC molecules (see Figure 3-12). The first step in this process is rearrangement of the germ-line TCR gene segments to produce functional $\gamma\delta$ or $\alpha\beta$ heterodimers. The immature thymocytes then begin to express the TCR/CD3 complex and to coexpress CD4 and CD8. During thymocyte maturation the microenvironment within the thymus is thought to play a selective role, so that only thymocytes whose receptors are capable of binding antigen + self-MHC are permitted to mature. Any thymocyte that fails to express a receptor owing to nonproductive rearrangement of the TCR genes is not selected. Similarly, any thymocyte whose receptor fails to recognize antigen + self-MHC is not selected. Finally, any thymocyte bearing a high-affinity receptor for self-MHC molecules alone or self-antigen + self-MHC is eliminated because it would pose the threat of an autoimmune response. It is estimated that 95–99% of all thymocyte progeny die within the thymus without maturing. This high death rate is thought to reflect the weeding out of all thymocytes whose receptors do not specifically recognize foreign antigen + self-MHC molecules.

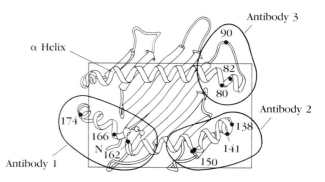

Figure 10-12 Diagrams of the α_1/α_2 domain in a class I MHC molecule showing the residues (solid black circles) at which site-directed mutagenesis affected recognition by T_C cells specific for that MHC molecule or recognition by three different anti-MHC monoclonal antibodies. Mutated MHC genes were transfected into target cells and the ability of T_C cells to kill the transfected target cells or of anti-MHC antibody to recognize them was determined. Single amino acid changes in either the α_1 or α_2 helices affected recognition by T_C cells (red outline). In contrast, recognition by each of three different monoclonal antibodies was affected by mutations in only a limited, specific region of the MHC molecule (black outlines). [Adapted from P. Ajitkumar et al. 1988. *Cell* **54**:47.]

Early evidence for the role of the thymus in selection of the T-cell repertoire came from chimeric experiments of R. M. Zinkernagel and his colleagues (Figure 10-13). These researchers implanted thymectomized and lethally irradiated F_1 (A × B) mice with a B-type thymus and then reconstituted the animals' immune system with an injection of F_1 bone marrow cells. To be certain that the thymus graft did not contain any mature T cells, it was irradiated before being transplanted. In such an experimental system, pre-T cells from the F_1 (A × B) bone marrow mature within a thymus expressing only B-type MHC molecules on its epithelial cells. Would these F_1 (A × B) T cells now be MHC-restricted for the haplotype of the thymus? To answer this question the chimeric mice were infected with LCM virus and the mature T cells were then tested for their ability to kill LCM-infected target cells from strain A or strain B mice. As shown in Figure 10-12, the T_C cells from the chimeric mice could lyse only LCM infected target cells bearing the same MHC haplotype as the implanted thymus. Apparently the implanted thymus had selected for maturation only T cells having receptors capable of recognizing antigen in association with the haplotype of the thymus.

Positive and Negative Selection

The selection of TCR specificity in the thymus is thought to involve two processes: (1) positive selection of thymocytes bearing receptors capable of binding self-MHC molecules (*MHC restriction*) and (2) negative selection by elimination of thymocytes bearing high-affinity receptors for self-MHC molecules alone or self-antigen presented by self-MHC (*self-tolerance*) (Figure 10-14). Both processes are necessary to generate mature T cells that are self-MHC restricted and self-tolerant. Thymic stromal cells, including epithelial cells, macrophages, and dendritic cells, are thought to play a role in positive and negative selection. These thymic stromal cells express high levels of class I and class II MHC molecules. Immature thymocytes expressing the TCR-CD3 complex are thought to interact with these thymic stromal cells, leading to positive and negative selection by mechanisms that are not fully understood.

Positive selection appears to involve an interaction of immature thymocytes with thymic cortical epithelial cells. Electron micrographs reveal close contact between thymocytes and epithelial cells within the thymic cortex, and there is evidence that the T-cell receptors tend to cluster at sites of contact. These immature thymocytes express the TCR-CD3 complex as well as both CD4 and CD8 accessory molecules. Because CD4 and CD8 are coexpressed on these immature thymocytes, they are referred to as "*double-positive*" thymocytes. Some researchers have suggested that the interaction of

these immature thymocytes with thymic epithelial cells, mediated by MHC-restricted T-cell receptors, might allow the T cell to receive some kind of protective signal; cells whose receptors are not MHC restricted would not

EXPERIMENT

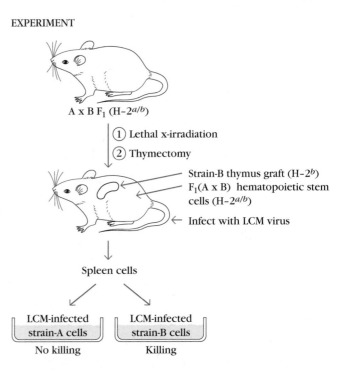

CONTROL

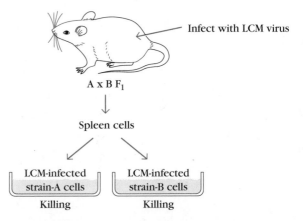

Figure 10-13 Experimental demonstration that the thymus selects only those T cells for maturation whose T-cell receptors recognize antigen presented on target cells with the haplotype of the thymus. Lethally irradiated and thymectomized F_1(A × B) mice were grafted with a strain-B thymus and reconstituted with F_1 (A × B) bone marrow cells. Following infection with the LCM virus, the CTL cells were assayed for their ability to kill [^{51}Cr] labeled strain-A or strain-B target cells infected with the LCM virus. Only strain-B target cells were lysed, suggesting that the H-2^b grafted thymus had selected for maturation only those T cells that could recognize antigen in association with H-2^b MHC molecules.

interact with the thymic epithelial cells and thus may be susceptible to the influence of various hormones, such as corticosteriods, leading to *programmed cell death* or *apoptosis*.

The MHC-restricted thymocytes bearing both high- and low-affinity receptors for self-MHC molecules then undergo negative selection. Most of the available evidence suggests that negative selection occurs within the thymic medulla, although there is also some evidence for negative selection within the thymic cortex. During negative selection, macrophages and dendritic cells bearing class I and class II MHC molecules are thought to interact with thymocytes bearing high-affinity receptors for self-antigen + self-MHC or self-MHC alone. The nature of the interaction leading to negative selection is not known. Tolerance to self-antigens would be achieved by eliminating T cells that are self-reactive and only allowing maturation of T cells specific for foreign antigen + self-MHC molecules (*altered self*). It has been very difficult to study these two processes. If one could identify and culture the pre-T-cell population, it would be possible to determine receptor specificity before and after thymic processing and thus determine the selective influence of the thymus on the T-cell repertoire, but the pre-T cell has yet to be isolated and grown in vitro.

Positive Selection: Experimental Evidence. Ada Kruis-beek obtained experimental evidence suggesting that binding of thymocytes to class I or class II MHC molecules within the thymus leads to positive selection of MHC-restricted T cells. In her experiments, mouse fetal thymic tissue was grown in tissue-culture media containing high concentrations of monoclonal antibody to either the class I or class II MHC molecules expressed by the thymic cells. Analysis of the T cells from these fetal thymic organ cultures revealed the absence of CD4$^+$ T cells in cultures grown with anti-class II monoclonal antibody and the absence of CD8$^+$ T cells in cultures grown with anti-class I monoclonal antibody. Similarly, injection of neonatal mice with anti-class II antibody prevented the development of CD4$^+$ T cells and injection of anti-class I antibody prevented the development of CD8$^+$ T cells. Thus development of these two thymocyte subpopulations correlates with the ability to recognize either class I or class II MHC molecules in the thymus. Taken together, these experiments suggest that positive selection of the CD4$^+$ or CD8$^+$ cells requires interaction of thymocytes with class I or class II MHC molecules. If the class I or class II MHC molecules are blocked by antibody, developing thymocytes cannot bind to the self-MHC molecules on the thymic stromal cells and are not positively selected.

Additional evidence that interaction with MHC molecules plays a role in positive selection came from experiments with transgenic mice (see Figure 2-9). In

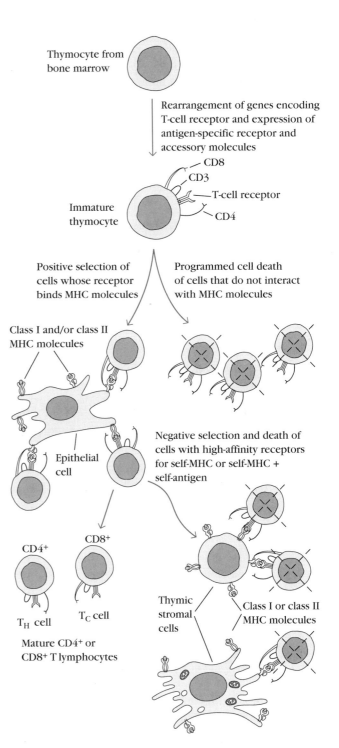

Figure 10-14 Positive and negative selection of thymocytes in the thymus. Because of thymic selection, which involves thymic stromal cells (epithelial cells, dendritic cells, and macrophages), mature T cells are both self-MHC restricted and self-tolerant.

these experiments rearranged $\alpha\beta$ TCR genes derived from a CD8$^+$ T-cell clone specific for influenza antigen + H-2^k class I MHC were injected into fertilized eggs from two different mouse strains, one with the H-2^k haplotype and one with the H-2^d haplotype. Since the receptor transgenes were already rearranged, other TCR gene rearrangements were suppressed in the transgenic mice; therefore, a high percentage of the thymocytes in the transgenic mice expressed the T-cell receptor encoded by the transgene. Thymocytes expressing the TCR transgene were found to mature into CD8$^+$ T cells only in the transgenic mice with the H-2^k class I MHC haplotype (i.e., the haplotype for which the transgene receptor was restricted). In transgenic mice with a different MHC haplotype (H-2^d), immature, double-positive thymocytes expressing the transgene were present, but these thymocytes failed to mature into CD8$^+$ T cells. These findings also suggest that interaction between T-cell receptors on immature thymocytes and self-MHC molecules is required for positive selection. In the absence of self-MHC, as in the H-2^d transgenic mice, positive selection and subsequent maturation do not occur.

Negative Selection: Experimental Evidence. Experiments by Marrack and Kappler, using monoclonal antibody to the TCR β-chain variable region encoded by the V$_\beta$17a exon, have provided evidence that thymocytes reactive with self-MHC molecules are removed during thymic processing. As noted earlier, V$_\beta$17a encodes one of the few TCR sequences shown to bind to MHC molecules, in this case to class II IE. Marrack and Kappler determined the percentage of V$_\beta$17a-bearing T cells in mice expressing IE molecules compared with the percentage in mutant mice that fail to express IE. They reasoned that if negative selection of T cells bearing high-affinity receptors for self-MHC occurs in the thymus, then a reduction in V$_\beta$17a-positive cells during thymic maturation should occur only in those mice expressing IE molecules. As shown in Figure 10-15, the percentage of immature thymocytes expressing the V$_\beta$17a exon was about the same in IE$^+$ and IE$^-$ mice. Following T-cell maturation, however, the percentage of mature thymocytes and peripheral T cells expressing the V$_\beta$17a exon decreased in IE$^+$ mice, whereas the percentage increased in IE$^-$ mice. The expression of IE appears to have selected for a T-cell repertoire lacking IE reactivity. This finding supports the theory that self-tolerance involves the deletion of thymocytes reactive with self-MHC molecules alone during T-cell maturation in the thymus.

Evidence for thymic deletion of thymocytes reactive with self-antigen has also come from analysis of thymocytes in mice containing $\alpha\beta$ TCR transgenes specific for H-Y antigen + class I MHC molecules. As in the trans-

genic experiment described in the last section, the rearranged TCR genes were obtained from a CD8$^+$ T$_c$ clone that was specific for the H-Y antigen presented by a class I D^b MHC molecule on a target cell. The H-Y antigen is encoded on the Y chromosome and therefore is expressed in male mice but not in female mice. In this experiment, the MHC haplotype of the transgenic mice was H-2^b, the same as the MHC restriction of the transgene-encoded T-cell receptor. Therefore any differences in the thymic selection of thymocytes in male and female transgenics would be related to the presence or absence of H-Y antigen. Analysis of thymocytes in the transgenic mice revealed that female mice contained thymocytes expressing the H-Y−specific TCR transgene, but male mice did not (Figure 10-16). In other words, H-Y−reactive thymocytes were self-reactive in the male mice and were eliminated. However, in female mice, which do not contain the H-Y antigen, these cells were not self-reactive and thus were not eliminated.

Unsolved Questions Regarding Thymic Selection

Many questions regarding thymic selection of the T-cell repertoire remain. The thymus must select for those T cells capable of recognizing foreign antigen + self-MHC. If positive selection selects for self-MHC−reactive T cells and then negative selection eliminates the self-MHC−reactive T cells, what keeps these two processes from completely overlapping, resulting in elimination of the

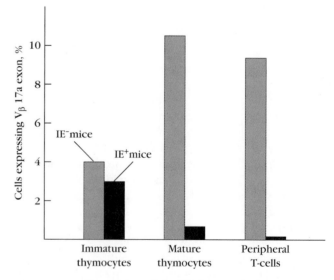

Figure 10-15   Expression of the V$_\beta$17a exon in immature thymocytes and mature T cells. The TCR sequence encoded by this exon is known to bind the class II IE MHC molecule. During thymic selection, the percentage of cells expressing V$_\beta$17a decreases in IE$^+$ mice but not in IE$^-$ mice, suggesting that thymocytes expressing T-cell receptors that react with a high affinity to self-MHC are eliminated.

entire repertoire of MHC-restricted T cells? One hypothesis suggests that differences in the affinity of T-cell receptors for self-MHC molecules prevents the thymocyte population selected by positive selection from being completely deleted by negative selection. According to this hypothesis, thymocytes bearing either high-affinity or low-affinity receptors for self-MHC molecules are selected during positive selection, whereas subsequently only those thymocytes bearing high-affinity receptors for self-MHC (or self-antigen + self-MHC) are eliminated during negative selection. In this way only thymocytes bearing low-affinity receptors for self-MHC protein would survive positive and negative selection and would leave the thymus as mature T cells with self-MHC–restricted receptors.

If this hypothesis of differential affinity for self-MHC molecules is to explain why all MHC-restricted thymocytes are not eliminated during negative selection, then there must be some mechanism that increases the ability of low-affinity receptors to bind with self-MHC molecules on thymic stromal cells during positive selection and/or that decreases their binding ability during negative selection. One possibility is that differential expression of other membrane molecules influences the avidity of thymocytes for MHC molecules at different stages during thymic processing. For example, as discussed earlier, CD4 and CD8 are known to bind to class II and class I MHC molecules, respectively. Perhaps the expression of these or other unidentified membrane molecules sufficiently increases the avidity of thymocytes bearing low-affinity receptors so that they can bind to thymic stromal cells during positive selection. The subsequent loss or lowering of these membrane molecules during subsequent development of thymocytes may lower their avidity toward self-MHC molecules, so that only thymocytes with high-affinity receptors for self-MHC (or self-MHC + self-antigen) would be able to bind to thymic stromal cells during negative selection.

Differences in the populations of thymic stromal cells involved in positive and negative selection also may influence the avidity of the thymocyte–stromal cell interaction. As noted earlier, thymic cortical epithelial cells appear to be involved in positive selection, whereas most negative selection appears to involve thymic macrophages and dendritic cells. Some researchers have suggested that thymic cortical epithelial cells express additional membrane molecules that facilitate their interaction with thymocytes bearing low-affinity receptors for self-MHC. If these membrane molecules are not expressed on thymic macrophages and dendritic cells, then thymocytes bearing low-affinity receptors for self-MHC might not bind and therefore would not be deleted.

It is not known how thymocyte recognition of self-MHC molecules is converted into a positive protective signal at one stage of thymocyte development and into a negative deleting signal at another stage. One possibility is that various thymic stromal cells secrete different factors, leading to thymocyte survival or thymocyte deletion. Another suggestion is that interaction of T-cell receptors with self-MHC molecules transmits different signals at different stages of thymocyte development. For example, this interaction may produce a signal that is transduced through the CD3 complex, leading to an increase in intracellular Ca^{2+}, which is thought to be

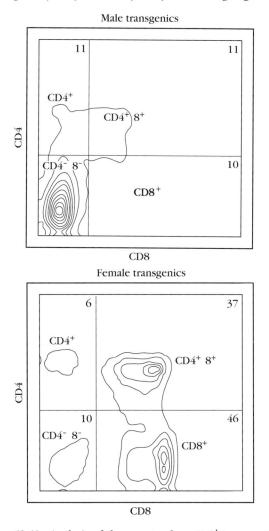

Figure 10-16 Analysis of thymocytes from H-2^b transgenic mice containing a transgene that encoded an $\alpha\beta$ T-cell receptor specific for male H-Y antigen + H-2^b class I MHC molecules. Thymocytes from male and female transgenics were analyzed with a FACS, which can separate cells that express neither CD4 or CD8, that express both accessory molecules, or that express one but not the other. As the plots show, mature CD8$^+$ T cells expressing the transgene were absent in the male mice but present in the female mice, suggesting that thymocytes reactive with a self-antigen (in this case, H-Y antigen in the male mice) are deleted during thymic selection. Numbers in quadrants refer to percentages of cells. [Adapted from H. von Boehmer and P. Kisielow, 1990, *Science* **248**:1370.]

lethal to immature thymocytes. Some workers have proposed that early in thymocyte development, the T-cell receptor and CD3 are not coupled, so that the TCR-MHC interaction would not lead to signal transduction by CD3. In this way, thymocytes may be spared from the lethal effects of high intracellular Ca^{2+} during positive selection. Later in thymocyte development, according to this proposal, the TCR is associated with CD3. As a result, interaction of thymocytes with thymic stromal cells leads to high intracellular Ca^{2+} and thymocyte destruction during negative selection.

T-Cell Development

Progenitor T cells from the bone marrow begin to migrate to the thymus at about day 11 of gestation in mice and in the eighth or ninth week of gestation in humans. The progenitor cells are attracted to the thymus by a chemotactic factor secreted by thymic epithelial cells. In a manner similar to B-cell differentiation in the bone marrow, differentiation of progenitor T cells is correlated with rearrangements of the germ-line TCR genes and expression of various surface markers. In contrast to B-cell development, however, thymocytes proliferate and differentiate along several different developmental pathways which generate functionally distinct subpopulations of mature T cells (Figure 10-17).

Changes in various membrane molecules and TCR-gene rearrangements during thymocyte development in the mouse have been studied with monoclonal antibodies and restriction-endonuclease analyses of genomic DNA. Upon entry into the thymus, progenitor T cells begin to express a membrane molecule called Thy-1, which is a marker of all thymus-derived lymphocytes in the mouse. The earliest fetal thymocytes lack detectable CD4 and CD8 and so are referred to as *double-negative* cells. These double-negative thymocytes differentiate along one of two developmental pathways. Those thymocytes which make productive rearrangements of both

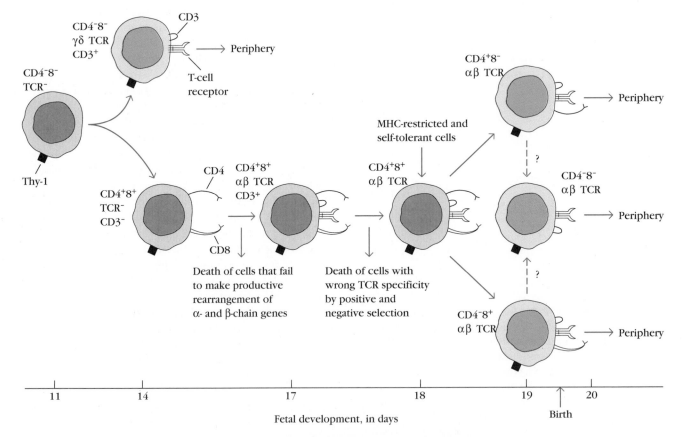

Figure 10-17   Proposed pathways for T-cell development in the thymus. Most of the immature thymocytes in the thymus die because they make an unproductive TCR-gene rearrangement or fail positive or negative selection. Four mature T-cell populations (red) are produced and move to the peripheral lymphoid organs. [Adapted from B. J. Fowlkes and D. M. Pardoll, 1989, *Adv. Immunol.* **44**:207.]

the γ- and δ-chain genes develop into double-negative, $CD3^+$ $\gamma\delta$ cells, which account for only 0.5–1.0% of thymocytes. This thymocyte subpopulation can be detected by day 14 of gestation, reaches maximal numbers between days 17 and 18, and then declines until birth. The majority of double-negative thymocytes progress down a different developmental pathway. They begin to rearrange the β-chain TCR genes and express both CD4 and CD8 membrane proteins. At day 16 of gestation these *double-positive* cells can first be detected expressing both CD4 and CD8 but not yet expressing CD3 or the $\alpha\beta$ T-cell receptor. Double-positive cells expressing both CD3 and the $\alpha\beta$ T-cell receptor begin to appear at day 17 and reach maximal levels about the time of birth. As discussed already, the vast majority of double-positive thymocytes die within the thymus. This massive cell death can be due to one of three reasons: They fail to make productive TCR-gene rearrangements, they fail to recognize MHC molecules expressed in the thymus, or they are self-reactive. Double-positive thymocytes that express the CD3–$\alpha\beta$-TCR complex and that survive thymic selection develop into either single-positive $CD4^+$ thymocytes, representing 10% of the total thymocyte population, or single-positive $CD8^+$ thymocytes, representing 5% of the total thymocyte population (Table 10-3). In addition, a small population (0.5%) of double-negative thymocytes expressing the CD3–$\alpha\beta$-TCR complex can also be detected. These cells appear late in development, usually within 5 days following birth. The origin of this population is uncertain, but it may develop from the single-positive populations through the loss of either CD4 or CD8.

Peripheral T-Cell Subpopulations

$\alpha\beta$ T Cells

As has been indicated earlier, an estimated 90–99% of peripheral T cells express the $\alpha\beta$ T-cell receptor complex. Peripheral T cells expressing the CD8 membrane marker are MHC-restricted to class I and peripheral T cells expressing the CD4 membrane marker are MHC-restricted to class II. The CD4 subpopulation generally functions as a T helper population while the CD8 subpopulation generally functions as a T cytotoxic population. Since both subpopulations express the $\alpha\beta$ heterodimer, a question that arises is whether the T cytotoxic and T helper cells express different V_α and V_β gene segments. The available evidence seems to suggest that both subpopulations can use the same pool of V_α and V_β gene segments; in one case, indeed, the same V_β gene product was identified on both class I MHC–restricted T_C cells and class II MHC–restricted T_H cells.

Table 10-3 Distribution of mouse thymocyte subpopulations characterized by the expression of the T-cell receptor (TCR), CD3, CD4, and CD8

Thymocyte subpopulations			Relative percentage
$CD4^-8^-$	TCR^-	$CD3^-$	4
$CD4^+8^+$	TCR^-	$CD3^-$	40
$CD4^-8^-$	$\gamma\delta\ TCR^+$	$CD3^+$	0.5
$CD4^+8^+$	$\alpha\beta\ TCR^+$	$CD3^+$	40
$CD4^+8^-$	$\alpha\beta\ TCR^+$	$CD3^+$	10
$CD4^-8^+$	$\alpha\beta\ TCR^+$	$CD3^+$	5
$CD4^-8^-$	$\alpha\beta\ TCR^+$	$CD3^+$	0.5

As discussed previously, functional differences between the T_H and T_C subpopulations can be established by different in vitro assay systems. The most common functional assay for T_C cells is a cell-mediated cytotoxicity assay using [^{51}Cr] labeled target cells; the amount of [^{51}Cr] released is a measure of target-cell killing by the T_C cells. Because the functions of T_H cells are diverse, this subpopulation can be assayed in various ways including activation of B cells, delayed-type hypersensitivity, induction of cytotoxic T cells, suppression of antibody production, secretion of distinct lymphokines, and in some cases cytolytic activity.

As different cloned $CD4^+$ cell lines were developed, the $CD4^+$ T cells were further subdivided by functional differences correlated with distinct panels of lymphokines released. One population, called the T_H1 subset, was found to secrete IL-2, IFN-γ, and lymphotoxin (LT). T_H1 cells helped polyclonal B-cell responses, suppressed antigen-specific B-cell responses, mediated delayed-type hypersensitivity, and mediated target-cell killing. The other subset, called the T_H2 subset, was found to secrete IL-4 and IL-5. These cells helped both specific and polyclonal B-cell responses but did not exhibit suppression, delayed-type hypersensitivity, or killing functions. There has been some controversy over whether these cloned T_H-cell subsets reflect true peripheral subsets or whether cloning itself restricts the gene expression in these cells so that they appear to differ in function and lymphokine secretion.

Recent studies with monoclonal antibodies to two differentiation antigens, designated CD45 and CDw29, have suggested that the cloned T_H1 and T_H2 subsets may reflect true peripheral T-cell subsets. One peripheral $CD4^+$ population expressed high levels of CD45 and low levels of CDw29, whereas another $CD4^+$ population expressed low levels of CD45 and high levels of CDw29. The CD45-high cells were shown to secrete IL-2 and IFN-γ but not IL-4, whereas the CDw29-high cells were shown to secrete IL-4 but not IL-2 or IFN-γ. The functional differences between these CD45-high and CDw29-high subsets also correlated with the functional differences observed for the cloned T_H1 and T_H2 subsets. Some researchers have suggested that the T_H1 and T_H2 subsets may not represent distinct developmental lineages but instead sequential stages of a single lineage, such as virgin and memory T cells. Further research is needed to clarify this area.

$\gamma\delta$ T Cells

In 1986 a small population of peripheral-blood T cells was discovered that expressed CD3 but failed to stain with monoclonal antibody specific for the $\alpha\beta$ T-cell receptor, indicating an absence of the $\alpha\beta$ heterodimer. These cells eventually were found to express the $\gamma\delta$ receptor. Such $\gamma\delta$ T cells constitute only 1–3% of the T-cell population in lymphoid organs of the mouse, but surprisingly they appear to represent a major T-cell population in the skin, intestinal epithelium, and pulmonary epithelium. Up to 1% of the epidermal cells in the skin are $\gamma\delta$ T cells, called "dendritic epidermal cells" (DEC). These cells express the Thy-1 T-cell marker and the $\gamma\delta$ T-cell receptor associated with the CD3 membrane complex but fail to express either CD4 or CD8. A second population of $\gamma\delta$ T cells has recently been identified in the intestinal epithelium of the mouse. These "intestinal epithelial lymphocytes" (IEL) also express the $\gamma\delta$ receptor associated with the CD3 membrane complex; unlike dendritic epidermal cells, these cells express CD8. Another unusual characteristic of the intestinal epithelial lymphocytes is that 25–50% of them fail to express Thy-1. Whether these cells lose the Thy-1 marker and acquire CD8 after thymic processing or whether they differentiate at a site other than the thymus remains to be determined.

Unlike $\alpha\beta$ T cells, which recirculate extensively (see Chapter 3), the $\gamma\delta$ T cells in these epithelial tissues appear not to circulate and instead remain fixed in these tissue sites. The $\gamma\delta$ T cells in different epithelial tissue sites appear to express different V_γ and V_δ gene segments. Comparison of a number of DEC clones, for example, has revealed an unusual limitation in TCR diversity. Each of the DEC clones was shown to express a restricted repertoire encoded by $V_\gamma 3J_\gamma 1$ and $V_\delta 1 D_\delta 2J_\delta 2$ gene units, with essentially no N-region diversification. In contrast, IELs were found to express $V_\gamma 5J_\gamma 1C_\gamma 1$. This selective expression of different V gene segments in different epithelial tissues may make these T cells specialized to respond to certain types of antigens that tend to be found at these sites.

The function of $\gamma\delta$ T cells is a matter of intense speculation. There are indications that some $\gamma\delta$ T cells can mediate cytotoxicity, but it is not clear whether their recognition of antigen is MHC restricted. Several re-

search reports have shown that $\gamma\delta$ T cells can mediate tumor-cell lysis in a non-MHC-restricted manner, suggesting that they may function like natural killer cells. A recent report that $\gamma\delta$ T cells respond to a mycobacterial antigen called purified protein derivative (PPD) may be an important clue regarding their function. The PPD antigen belongs to a group of highly conserved proteins, found in all organisms, called heat-shock proteins, which were so named following the observation that they are produced by cells in response to sudden increases in temperature or other environmental stresses. But heat-shock proteins are also induced by other stresses such as inflammatory responses, viral infections, and cancer. Mycobacterial PPD shows sequence homology with a mammalian heat-shock protein that is a normal component of the mitochondrial matrix. This has led to the speculation that $\gamma\delta$ T cells may be uniquely suited to respond to mammalian heat-shock proteins and may have evolved to eliminate damaged cells as well as microbial invaders.

C. A. Janeway has suggested that the $\gamma\delta$ T cell may represent the most primitive and earliest cell-mediated immune system, uniquely specialized to recognize epithelial-cell alterations outside the basement-membrane barrier. It has been proposed that these $\gamma\delta$ T cells, which may be especially suited to combat epidermal or intestinal antigens, form a surveillance system monitoring the integrity of the external epithelial cell milieu. These cells may be able to recognize heat-shock proteins or alterations caused by ultraviolet irradiation in the outer epidermal layer. DECs may be activated by epidermal keratinocytes, which have been shown to be both effective antigen-presenting cells and secretors of IL-1. Such a system would protect the epithelial-cell surfaces, preventing the spread of infection or cancer across the basement membrane into the internal milieu.

T-Cell Response to Allogeneic Histocompatibility Antigens

So far the discussion of MHC molecules has focused on their role in antigen presentation. As noted in Chapter 9, however, MHC molecules were first identified because of their role in rejection of foreign tissue. Graft-rejection reactions result from the direct response of T cells to MHC molecules, which function as *histocompatibility antigens*. Because of the extreme polymorphism of the MHC, most individuals of the same species have a unique set of histocompatibility antigens. Therefore, T cells respond even to allogeneic grafts (*alloreactivity*), and MHC molecules are considered *alloantigens*. Generally, $CD4^+$ T cells respond to class II alloantigens and $CD8^+$ T cells respond to class I alloantigens.

The alloreactivity of T cells is troubling for two reasons. First, the ability of T cells to respond to allogeneic histocompatibility antigens alone appears to contradict all the evidence indicating that T cells can respond only to foreign antigen + self-MHC molecules. For example, in the Zinkernagle and Doherty experiment discussed earlier, T cells from a virus-infected mouse could kill syngeneic target cells infected with the same virus but not allogeneic target cells infected with the same virus (see Figure 10-1). The T cells were therefore shown to be self-MHC restricted. In responding to allogeneic grafts, however, T cells recognize a foreign MHC molecule directly, instead of responding to an antigen that has been processed and presented together with a self-MHC molecule. This would appear to contradict all that we have learned about T-cell specificity. A second problem posed by the T-cell response to allogeneic MHC molecules is that the frequency of alloreactive T cells is quite high; it has been estimated that 1–5% of all T cells are alloreactive, which is far higher than the frequency of T cells reactive to antigen + self-MHC. This finding is troubling because the high frequency of alloreactive T cells appears to contradict the basic tenet of clonal selection. If 1 T cell in 20 reacts with alloantigens and if one assumes that there are on the order of 100 distinct H-2 haplotypes in mice, then there are not enough alloantigen-specific T cells to cover all the unique H-2 haplotypes, let alone foreign antigens displayed by self-MHC molecules.

One possible biologically satisfying explanation for the high frequency of alloreactive T cells is that the TCR specificity is indeed actually for antigen + self-MHC but that receptors can cross-react with certain allogeneic MHC haplotypes. In other words, if a foreign MHC molecule structurally resembles a processed peptide bound to a self-MHC molecule, T cells might respond as if the foreign MHC were altered self-MHC (Figure 10-18). Since allogeneic cells express on the order of 10^5 class I MHC molecules per cell, T cells bearing low-affinity cross-reactive receptors might be able to bind by virtue of the high density of membrane alloantigen. Foreign antigen, on the other hand, would be sparsely displayed on the membrane of an antigen-presenting cell or altered self-cell associated with class I or class II MHC molecules, limiting responsiveness to only those T cells bearing high-affinity receptors.

Experimental evidence that antigen-specific T cells can also be alloreactive has come from studies with a number of T-cell clones. For example, after immunizing an H-2^a haplotype mouse with DNP-OVA, B. Sredni and R. H. Schwarz were able to obtain a T-cell clone that responded to DNP-OVA associated with a class II IA^a molecule. This same clone, however, also responded to allogeneic cells bearing IA^s in the absence of DNP-OVA. To determine the frequency of such antigen-specific and

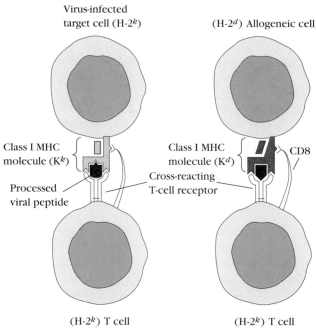

Figure 10-18 Cross-reactivity of T-cell receptors with processed foreign peptides + self-MHC molecules and with allogeneic MHC molecules may explain the observed high frequency of alloreactive T cells. As schematically illustrated, a T-cell receptor specific for the class I MHC molecule K^k(light red) associated with peptide A (black) can cross-react with an allogeneic class I MHC molecule (dark red) that structurally resembles the peptide A–K^k complex.

alloreactive T cells, Sredni and Schwarz immunized three congenic strains (B10.A, B10, and B10.S) with DNP-OVA and then isolated 20–40 antigen-specific clones from each strain. Each antigen-specific clone was then tested for alloreactivity against cells expressing different MHC haplotypes in the absence of antigen. Between 19 and 44% of the antigen-specific clones were able to respond to allogeneic cells. These findings support the hypothesis that the high percentage of alloreactive T cells reflects the existence of antigen-specific T cells whose receptor recognizes antigen + self-MHC but can cross-react with various allogeneic MHC molecules.

Summary

1. T-cell receptors, unlike antibodies, do not react with soluble antigen but rather with processed antigen associated with a self-MHC molecule on a target cell. T-cell receptors, first isolated by means of clonotypic monoclonal antibodies, are heterodimers consisting of

an α and β chain or a γ and δ chain. Like the immunoglobulin heavy and light chains, the TCR chains have constant and variable regions.

2. Germ-line TCR DNA is organized into multigene families corresponding to the α, β, γ, and δ chains. Each multigene family contains multiple variable-region gene segments (V and J in α- and γ-chain DNA and V, D, and J in β- and δ-chain DNA) and one or more constant-region C gene segments. By mechanisms similar to those used by B cells to rearrange germ-line immunoglobulin DNA, T cells rearrange the variable-region TCR gene segments to form functional genes encoding either the TCR α and β chains or γ and δ chains.

3. The mechanisms generating TCR diversity are generally similar to those generating antibody diversity. However, during rearrangement of TCR β- and δ-chain gene segments alternative joining of V, D, and J segments can occur and random nucleotides can be added at the junctions between gene segments encoding all the chains. Because of these mechanisms, the potential diversity of TCR genes is significantly greater than that of immunoglobulin genes, even though somatic mutation does not occur in TCR genes, as it does in immunoglobulin genes.

4. T-cell receptors are organized into variable and constant domains similar to those in immunoglobulins. The TCR variable-region domains are thought to be folded into the characteristic immunoglobulin-fold structure and contain three hypervariable complementarity-determining regions (CDRs), which appear to be equivalent to those in immunoglobulins. Each chain in a TCR molecule also contains a short membrane-proximal hinge region, a hydrophobic transmembrane segment, and a short cytoplasmic tail.

5. T-cell receptors, unlike membrane-bound immunoglobulins on B cells, are associated with several accessory membrane molecules, designated CD2, CD3, CD4, and CD8, which belong to the immunoglobulin superfamily. The T-cell receptors on mature T cells are complexed with CD3. Following interaction of a T-cell receptor with an antigen–MHC complex, CD3 is thought to transduce the activation signal leading to T-cell proliferation and secretion of lymphokines. CD4 and CD8 can increase the binding of T-cell receptors to antigen–MHC complexes and also may function in signal transduction CD4 bearing T cells generally function as T_H cells while CD8 bearing T cells generally function as T_C cells.

6. Recognition of antigen–MHC complexes by T cells involves only the T-cell receptor. This co-recognition appears to depend on the interaction of a T-cell receptor with epitopes on processed antigen bound to a MHC molecule and with amino acids in both the α_1 and α_2 domains of the MHC molecule.

7. Rearrangement of germ-line TCR genes during T-cell maturation in the thymus appears to produce many functional genes encoding receptors that are not specific for foreign antigen + self-MHC molecules. Thymocytes with unwanted TCR specificities are deleted in a two-step selection process. First, positive selection of all thymocytes bearing receptors that can bind a self-MHC molecule confers MHC restriction. Second, negative selection and elimination of thymocytes bearing high-affinity receptors for self-MHC alone or self-antigen + self-MHC confers self-tolerance. As a result of this thymic selection, only thymocytes that are both self-MHC restricted and self-tolerant develop into mature T cells.

8. Some 90–99% of the peripheral T cells express the $\alpha\beta$ T-cell receptor. Those T cells which express CD4 recognize antigen associated with a class II MHC molecule and generally function as T_H cells; those T cells which express CD8 recognize antigen associated with a class I MHC molecule and generally function as T_C cells. T cells expressing the $\gamma\delta$ T-cell receptor constitute only a small percentage of the total T-cell population, but they are concentrated in several epithelial tissues and may represent a primitive cell-mediated immune system that evolved to protect the integrity of external epithelial surfaces.

9. T cells respond not only to foreign antigen–self-MHC molecule complexes but also to foreign MHC molecules (histocompatibility antigens) alone. This T-cell response leads to rejection of allogeneic grafts. Some evidence suggests that this alloreactivity may result from the ability of T cells specific for antigen + self-MHC to cross-react with various allogeneic MHC molecules.

References

ALLISON, J. P., and W. L. HAVRAN. 1991. The immunobiology of T cells with invariant $\gamma\delta$ antigen receptors. *Annu. Rev. Immunol.* **9**:679.

ASHWELL, J. D., and R. D. KLAUSNER. 1990. Genetic and mutational analysis of the T cell antigen receptor. *Annu. Rev. Immunol.* **8**:139.

BIERER, B. E., B. P. SLECKMAN, S. E. RATNOFSKY, and S. J. BURAKOFF. 1989. The biologic roles of CD2, CD4 and CD8 in T cell activation. *Annu. Rev. Immunol.* **7**:579.

BLACKMAN, M., J. KAPPLER, and P. MARRACK. 1990. The role of the T cell receptor in positive and negative selection of developing T cells. *Science* **248**:1335.

DAVIS, M. M. 1990. T cell receptor gene diversity and selection. *Annu. Rev. Biochem.* **59**:475.

FINKLE, T. H., R. T. KUBO, and J. C. CAMBIER. 1991. T-cell development and transmembrane signaling: changing biological responses through an unchanging receptor. *Immunol. Today* **12**:79.

FOWLKES, B. J., and D. M. PARDOLL. 1989. Molecular and cellular events in T cell development. *Adv. Immunol.* **44**:207.

GREY, H. M., A. SETTE, and S. BUUS. 1989. How T cells see antigen. *Sci. Am.* **261**:56.

HEDRICK, S. M., D. I. COHEN, E. A. NIELSEN, and M. M. DAVIS. 1984. Isolation of cDNA clones encoding T cell-specific membrane associated proteins. *Nature* **308**:149.

MARRACK, P., and J. KAPPLER. 1986. The T cell and its receptor. *Sci. Am.* **254**:36.

MARRACK, P., and J. KAPPLER. 1987. The T cell receptor. *Science* **238**:1073.

MARRACK, P., D. LO, R. BRINSTER et al. 1988. The effect of thymus environment on T cell development and tolerance. *Cell* **53**:627.

MARUSIC-GALESIC, S., LONGO, D. L., and KRUISBEEK, A. M. 1989. Preferred differentiation of T-cell receptor specificities based on the MHC glycoproteins encountered during development: evidence for positive clone selection. *J. Exp. Med.* **169**:1619.

MATIS, L. A. 1990. The molecular basis of T cell specificity. *Annu. Rev. Immunol.* **8**:65.

RAULET, D. H. 1989. The structure, function, and molecular genetics of the γδ T cell receptor. *Annu. Rev. Immunol.* **7**:175.

SCHWARZ, R. H. 1990. A cell culture model for T lymphocyte clonal anergy. *Science* **248**:1349.

STROMINGER, J. L. 1989. Developmental biology of T cell receptors. *Science* **244**:943.

ULLMAN, K. S., J. P. NORTHROP, C. L. VERWEIJ, and G. R. CRABTREE. 1990. Transmission of signals from the T lymphocyte antigen receptor to the gene responsible for cell proliferation and immune function: the missing link. *Annu. Rev. Immunol.* **8**:421.

ZINKERNAGEL, R. M., A. ALTHAGE, E. WATERFIELD et al. 1980. Restriction specificities, alloreactivity and allotolerance expressed by T cells from nude mice reconstituted with H-2 compatible or incompatible thymus grafts. *J. Exp. Med.* **151**:376.

Study Questions

1. Indicate whether each of the following statements is true or false. If you think a statement is false, explain why.

   a. Monoclonal antibody specific for CD4 will co-precipitate the T-cell receptor along with CD4.

   b. Subtraction hybridization can be used to enrich for mRNA that is present in one cell type but absent in another cell type within the same species.

   c. Clonotypic monoclonal antibody was used to isolate the T-cell receptor.

   d. The T cell uses the same set of V, D, and J gene segments as the B cell but uses different C gene segments.

   e. The αβ heteriodimer is bivalent and has two antigen-binding sites.

2. Describe the critical experiment that proved that the αβ T-cell receptor recognizes both antigen and MHC molecules.

3. a. Which type of T-cell receptor—the αβ or the γδ heterodimer—is expressed first during thymic ontogeny?

   b. Can a single T cell express both the αβ and γδ T-cell receptor? Explain your answer.

4. Draw the basic structure of the αβ T-cell receptor indicating the polypeptide chains, domain structure, disulfide bonding, transmembrane region, cytoplasmic tails, antigen-binding site, variable region, and constant region.

5. Unlike the B-cell antigen-binding receptor, the T-cell receptor is associated on the membrane with various accessory molecules. What are these molecules and what is their role in T-cell function?

6. In the table below indicate with an X whether each property applies to the T-cell receptor (TCR) and/or B-cell immunoglobulin (Ig):

Property	TCR	Ig
Is associated with CD3		
Is monovalent		
Exists in membrane-bound and secreted forms		
Contains domains with β-pleated-sheet structures		
Is MHC restricted		
Diversity generated by imprecise joining of gene segments		
Diversity generated by somatic mutation		

7. a. In identifying the genes encoding the T-cell receptor, Hedrick and Davis made three important assumptions which proved to be correct. What were these assumptions and how did they facilitate identification of the genes encoding the T-cell receptor?

b. Suppose, instead, that Hedrick and Davis wanted to identify the genes encoding IL-4. What changes in the three assumptions should they make?

8. Mice from different inbred strains listed in the *left* column of the table below have been infected with LCM virus. Spleen cells derived from these LCM-infected mice are then tested for their ability to lyse LCM-infected [^{51}Cr] labeled target cells from the strains *listed across the top of the table.* Indicate with (+) or (−) whether you would expect to see [^{51}Cr] released from the labeled target cells.

9. In his classic chimeric-mouse experiments, Zinkernagel took bone marrow from mouse 1 and a thymus from mouse 2 and transplanted them into mouse 3, which was thymectomized and lethally irradiated. He then challenged the reconstituted mouse with LCM virus and removed its spleen cells. These spleen cells were then incubated with LCM-infected target cells with different MHC haplotypes, and the lysis of the target cells was monitored. The results of two such experiments are shown in the table below. The haplotype of strain C57Bl/6 is H-2^b and that of strain BALB/c is H-2^d.

a. Indicate the haplotype of the thymus-donor strain in the column marked "thymus donor."

b. Why were the H-2^b target cells not lysed in experiment A but were lysed in experiment B?

c. Why were the H-2^k target cells not lysed in either experiment?

For use with Question 8.

Source of spleen cells from LCM-infected mice	Release of [^{51}Cr] from LCM-Infected target cells			
	B10.D2 (H-2^d)	B10 (H-2^b)	B10.BR (H-2^k)	F$_1$ (BALB/c × B10) (H-2$^{b/d}$)
B10.D2 (H-2^d)				
B10 (H-2^b)				
BALB/c (H-2^d)				
BALB/b (H-2^b)				

For use with Question 9.

	Bone marrow donor	Thymus donor	Thymectomized, x-irradiated recipient	Lysis of LCM-infected target cells		
				H-2^d	H-2^k	H-2^b
Exp. A	C57Bl/6 × BALB/c		C57Bl/6 × BALB/c	+	−	−
Exp. B	C57Bl/6 × BALB/c		C57Bl/6 × BALB/c	−	−	+

STUDY QUESTIONS

243

10. You have cloned a T_C cell from an H-2^k mouse. This T_C-cell clone is specific for an H-2^b class I K MHC molecule. You clone the genes encoding the $\alpha\beta$ T-cell receptor from this clone and use them to prepare transgenic mice from an H-2^k and an H-2^b strain. In the table below indicate which T-cell populations would (+) and would not (−) express the transgene in each transgenic mouse. Explain your answer for each subpopulation.

T-cell population	Transgene expression	
	H-2^k strain transgenic	H-2^b strain transgenic
CD4$^+$ CD8$^+$ thymocyte (double-positive)		
CD4$^+$ T cell		
CD8$^+$ T cell		

11. You wish to isolate cDNA clones encoding various gene products using the subtractive hybridization technique. You have available clones of the following cell types:
   a. T_H cell
   b. T_C cell
   c. Macrophage
   d. IgA-secreting myeloma cell
   e. Fibroblast
   f. Neutrophil (phagocytic cell)
   g. IgG-secreting myeloma cell

In the table below, indicate which of these cell clones you would use as the source of cDNA encoding each of the listed gene products and which clone would be the best choice for preparing mRNA to use in subtractive hybridization. In the space provided give a brief explanation for your choices.

For use with Question 11.

Gene product	Source clone for cDNA	Clone supplying mRNA for subtractive hybridization	Reason
IL-2			
CD8			
J chain			
IL-1			
CD3			

12.   a.   You isolate a sample of cells from mouse thymus and stain it using the indirect immunofluorescence method. The primary antibody is goat anti-CD3 and the secondary antibody is rabbit FITC-labeled anti-goat Ig, which emits a green color. Analysis of the stained sample by flow cytometry indicates that 70% of the cells are stained. Based on this result, how many of the thymus cells in your sample are expressing antigen-binding receptors on their surface? Explain your answer. What are the remaining unstained cells likely to be?

b.   You then separate the CD3$^+$ cells with the fluorescent-activated cell sorter (FACS) and restain them. In this case, the primary antibody is hamster anti-CD4 and the secondary antibody is rabbit PE-labeled anti-hamster-Ig, which emits a red color. Analysis of the stained CD3$^+$ cells shows that 80% of them are stained. Based on this result, can you determine how many T$_C$ cells are present in this sample? If you can, then how many T$_C$ cells are there? If you cannot, what additional experiment would you perform in order to determine the number of T$_C$ cells that are present?

Cytokines

The development of an effective immune response involves lymphoid cells, inflammatory cells, and other hematopoietic cells. The complex interactions among these cells are mediated by a group of secreted low-molecular-weight proteins that are collectively designated *cytokines* to denote their role in cell-to-cell communication. Cytokines assist in regulating the development of immune effector cells and some cytokines possess direct effector functions of their own. Just as hormones serve as messengers of the endocrine system, so cytokines serve as messengers of the immune system; however, unlike endocrine hormones, which exert their effects over large distances, the cytokines generally act locally. This chapter focuses on the biological activity and structure of cytokines, their interaction with specific receptors, the mechanism by which they affect lymphocyte activation and stimulate the inflammatory response, and their role in certain diseases and possible therapeutic uses.

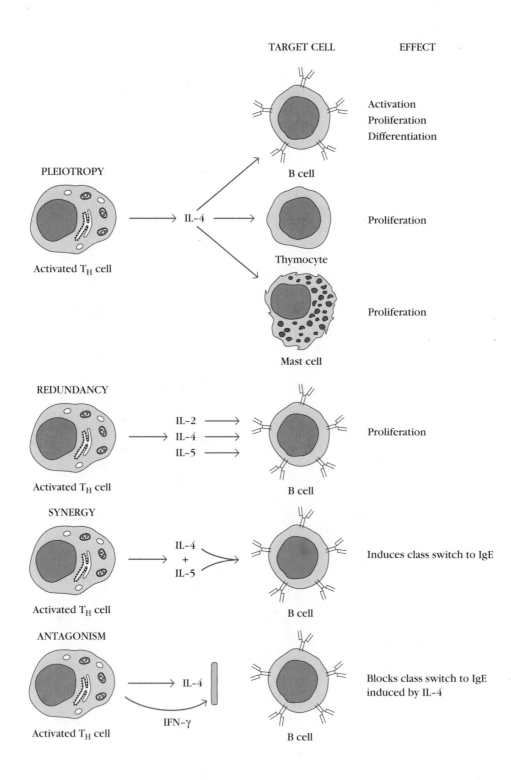

Figure 11-1 Examples of the cytokine attributes of pleiotropy, redundancy, synergism, and antagonism.

General Properties of Cytokines

Cytokines are secreted by various cells involved in the immune response and act on target cells bearing membrane receptors that are specific for a given cytokine. A particular cytokine may exhibit *autocrine* action, binding to the same cell that secreted it; it may exhibit *paracrine* action, binding to a nearby cell; in a few cases it may exhibit *endocrine* action, binding to a distant cell. Binding of a cytokine to its membrane receptor transmits a signal into the cell that leads to changes in the activation and expression of genes. Cytokines regulate the intensity and duration of the immune response by stimulating or inhibiting the proliferation of various cells or their secretion of antibodies or other cytokines.

The actions of cytokines are *pleiotropic*; that is, they elicit different biological activities from different target cells. Their actions are also *redundant*; that is, different cytokines can mediate similar functions, making it difficult to ascribe a given activity to a single cytokine. Adding to the complexity of cytokine action, two cytokines may exhibit *synergy*; that is, their combined effect on cellular activity is greater than the additive effects of the individual cytokines. In other cases cytokines exhibit *antagonism*, the effects of one cytokine inhibiting the effects of another cytokine. The attributes of pleiotrophy, redundancy, synergism, and antagonism permit cytokines to regulate cellular activity in a coordinated, interactive way (Figure 11-1). The actions of one cytokine on a responsive target cell generally regulate expression of cytokine receptors and expression of new cytokines, which in turn affect other cells. Thus the antigen-specific response of a single lymphocyte can influence the activity of a variety of cells necessary to generate an effective immune response. For example, cytokines produced by activated T_H cells can influence the activity of B cells, T_C cells, natural killer (NK) cells, macrophages, granulocytes, and hematopoietic stem cells, thereby activating an entire network of interacting cells (Figure 11-2).

It is difficult to reconcile the nonspecificity of cytokines with the established specificity of the immune system. What keeps the nonspecific cytokines from activating cells in a nonspecific fashion during the immune response? Clearly some mechanisms must operate to ensure that the specificity of the immune response is maintained. One way in which specificity is maintained is the careful regulation of the expression of cytokine receptors on cells. Often cytokine receptors are expressed on a cell only after that cell has interacted with antigen. In this way nonspecific cytokine activation is limited to antigen-primed lymphocytes. Another means of maintaining specificity may be a requirement for cell-to-cell interaction to generate effective concentrations of a cytokine at the juncture of interacting cells. In the case of the T_H cell, a major producer of cytokines, close

cellular interaction occurs when the T-cell receptor recognizes an antigen-MHC complex on an appropriate antigen-presenting cell, such as a macrophage, dendritic cell, or B lymphocyte. Cytokines secreted at the junction of these interacting cells reach concentrations high enough to affect the target cell.

Discovery and Purification of Cytokines

Recognition of the activity of cytokines began in the mid-1960s, when culture supernatants derived from in vitro cultures of allogeneic lymphocytes were found to contain biologically active factors that could regulate proliferation, differentiation, and maturation of various types of lymphoid cells and accessory cells. Soon after, it was discovered that production of these factors—now called lymphokines—by cultured lymphocytes could be induced by activation with antigen or with nonspecific mitogens (see Chapter 4).

Functional Identification

Following these early discoveries, reports of various biologically active factors generated by different in vitro culture systems rapidly accumulated. Because of slight differences in assay conditions, numerous functional responses were observed, each of which was initially attributed to a unique factor. As a consequence, the literature soon was filled with reports about different factors, each named for its biological activity and given its own acronym.

The formidable list of factors reported during this period included the following: lymphocyte-activating factor (LAF), T-cell growth factor (TCGF), B-cell growth factor (BCGF), T-cell replacing factor (TRF), B-cell differentiation factor (BDF), B-cell activating factor (BAF), mitogenic protein (MP), and thymocyte mitogenic factor (TMF). The numerous reports appearing in the literature left even experts in the field engulfed in a bewildering sea of factors and their acronyms (Table 11-1). It was not until cytokines were purified and eventually cloned that the vast array of factors generated in different biological systems could be shown to represent the activities of a limited number of cytokines.

Biochemical Purification

Biochemical isolation of cytokines was hampered by several obstacles. For one thing, a culture supernatant often contained mixtures of cytokines rather than a single cytokine, making it difficult to assign a given function to a single substance. Coupled with this was the problem

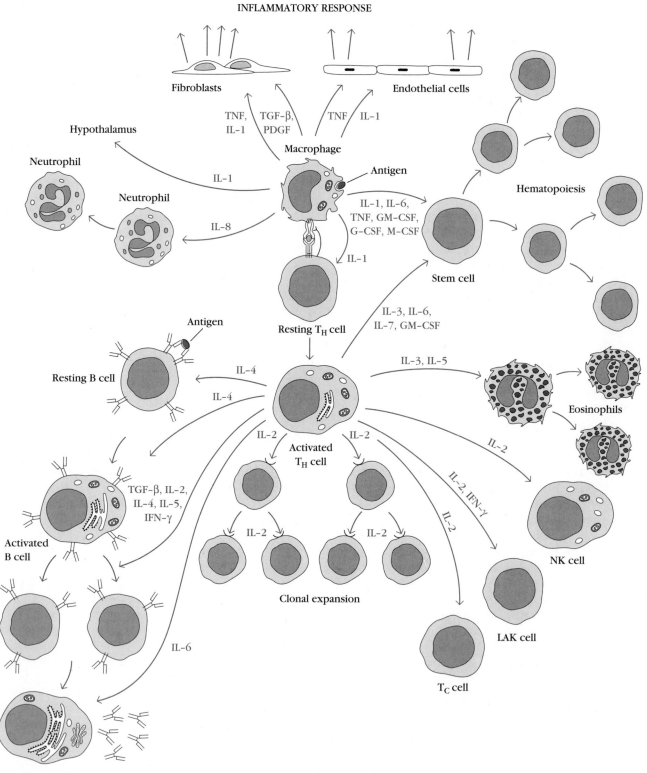

Figure 11-2 Interaction of antigen (red) with macrophages and the subsequent activation of resting T$_H$ cells leads to release of numerous cytokines, generating a complex network of interacting cells in the immune response.

Table 11-1 Some factors produced by activated lymphocytes and macrophages identified by functional assays and the purified cytokines corresponding to them

Former name based on functional assay	Acronym	Corresponding purified lymphokine
B-cell activating factor	BAF	
B-cell differentiation factor	BDF	
Endogenous pyrogen	EP	
Hematopoietin 1	HP-1	Interleukin 1
Lymphocyte-activating factor	LAF	
Mitogenic protein	MP	
Serum amyloid A inducer	SAA inducer	
T-cell replacing factor III	TRF-III	
Killer-cell helper factor	KHF	
T-cell growth factor	TCGF	Interleukin 2
Thymocyte mitogenic factor	TMF	
Burst promoting activity	BP	
Hematopoietic-cell growth factor	HPGF	
Hematopoietin 2	HP-2	
Mast-cell growth factor	MCGF	Interleukin 3
Multilineage colony-stimulating factor	Multi-CSF	
Persisting cell-stimulation factor	PSF	
B-cell differentiation factor I	BCDF-I	
B-cell growth factor I	BCGF-I	
B-cell stimulation factor I	BSF-I	Interleukin 4
Mast-cell growth factor II	MCGF-II	
T-cell growth factor II	TCGF-II	
B-cell growth factor II	BCGF-II	
Eosinophil differentiation factor	EDF	Interleukin 5
T-cell replacing factor	TRF	
B-cell differentiation factor II	BCDF-II	
B-cell stimulation factor II	BSF-2	
Hepatocyte-stimulating factor	HSF	Interleukin 6
Hybridoma-plasmacytoma growth factor	HPGF	
Interferon β_2	IFN-β_2	
Lymphopoietin 1		Interleukin 7
Monocyte-derived neutrophil chemotactic factor	MDNCF	
Neutrophil-activating factor	NAF	Interleukin 8
Neutrophil-activating peptide	NAP	
Mast-cell growth-enhancing activity	MEA	
P40		Interleukin 9
T-cell growth factor III	TCGF-III	
Cytokine-synthesis inhibitory factor	CSIF	Interleukin 10
Cachectin		Tumor necrosis factor α
Lymphotoxin		Tumor necrosis factor β

SOURCE: Adapted from D. Male, ed., 1988, *Lymphokines in Focus*, IRL Press.

that the early systems available for assaying cytokine function involved heterogeneous populations of lymphocytes, and their various responses to the cytokine being tested often gave ambiguous results. A further difficulty was that culture supernatants contained extremely low concentrations of the cytokines, with subnanomolar concentrations (10^{-10}–10^{-15} M) being biologically active.

Two developments provided a way around these obstacles and led to the biochemical characterization of cytokines. The first development was the discovery of tumor-cell lines that secreted cytokines. These tumor-cell lines provided researchers with homogeneous populations of cells, which in some cases secreted much higher concentrations of a given cytokine than did cultures of lymphoid cells. The second development was the discovery of cell lines whose growth depended on the presence of a particular cytokine. These cell lines provided researchers with a simple assay system—a homogeneous population of cells capable of proliferating in response to a given growth factor.

When the cytokines previously identified by a variety of different functions were assessed for biological activity in these defined assay systems, it soon became clear that what had seemed to be a great many cytokines, each named for its biological activity, were often just different activities of the same factor. A standardized nomenclature was developed, with most of the cytokines designated *interleukins* in reference to their role in cellular communication among leukocytes. The first to be named were interleukins 1 and 2. Interleukin 1 (IL-1) was shown to account for the biological activities previously ascribed to at least eight factors, and interleukin 2 (IL-2) accounted for the activities ascribed to four factors. In the past decade the list of defined cytokines has increased to ten interleukins and several other cytokines still named for their biological activity, and the correspondence between these purified lymphokines and previously identified factors has been clarified (see Table 11-1).

Biochemical purification of the interleukins involved a number of protein purification techniques, and usually began with cytokine-containing supernatants from cell lines producing high levels of a given cytokine. For example, leukemic monocyte lines were chosen for their production of IL-1 and various T-cell lymphomas for their production of IL-2. The cell lines were grown in large-scale cultures and were induced to produce cytokines with mitogens, phorbol esters, or other appropriate inducing agents. The secreted cytokine was then purified from several liters of culture supernatant. In most cases, the cytokine was initially concentrated by membrane filtration; further purification was achieved by such techniques as ion-exchange chromatography, repeated gel filtrations, isoelectric focusing, and high-

performance liquid chromatography (HPLC). The level of the cytokine's biological activity was determined at each step in the purification pathway.

The purification of IL-2 illustrates the general procedure. The definitive biological assay in this purification was the ability to stimulate proliferation of IL-2–dependent cell lines. The cell lines most frequently used were CTLL-2 cells, an IL-2–dependent line of mouse T_C cells, and HT-1 cells, an IL-2–dependent line of T_H cells. At each stage the purified fractions were added to the cell lines, whose proliferation was monitored by the uptake of [^{3}H] thymidine. Even with cell lines producing high levels of interleukins, biochemical purification had very poor yields. For example, from 10 L of supernatant harvested from a high IL-2–producing mouse tumor-cell line that had been induced with PHA, only 50 μg of IL-2 was recovered. As the data in Table 11-2 show, this purification achieved only a threefold increase in IL-2 specific activity, while 99% of the IL-2 was lost. Generally, biochemical purification of cytokines was unable to yield reasonable quantities of highly purified cytokines.

Cloning of Cytokine Genes

The frustrations of attempting to purify cytokines with standard biochemical techniques were overcome when the various cytokine genes were cloned using recombinant DNA techniques. The general approach used was to generate a cDNA library from appropriate cytokine-producing cell lines (see Figure 2-4) and then screen

Table 11-2   Biochemical purification of interleukin 2 (IL-2)

Purification step	Total protein recovered (mg)	Total units	Specific activity (units/mg)
10 liters crude supernatant	52.8	1.63×10^7	3.1×10^5
DEAE Sephacel	22.0	1.30×10^7	5.9×10^5
Isoelectric focusing	7.5	6.0×10^6	8.0×10^5
AcA54 gel filtration	2.0	3.5×10^6	1.75×10^6
SDS-PAGE (25K + 21K bands)	0.05	5.0×10^5	1.0×10^7

SOURCE: J. D. Watson et al., 1982, *Immunol. Ser.* **19**:52.

the library by expressing the cDNA clones in COS cells. By testing the supernatants for activity in a biological assay system (such as a cytokine-dependent cell line), any COS cells transfected with cytokine cDNA can be identified. Another technique that has been used to identify cytokine cDNA is subtractive hybridization. Since cytokines are produced only after induction with an antigen, mitogen, or other inducing agent, the mRNA of an induced cell should contain cytokine mRNA, whereas the mRNA from an uninduced cell should not. In this approach, the mRNA from induced cells is isolated and reverse-transcribed to prepare single-stranded cDNA corresponding to the genes expressed in the induced cells. By hybridizing the cDNA with mRNA from uninduced cells, it is possible to remove all cDNAs that are common to both cells, leaving unhybridized the cDNAs that are unique to induced cells and are therefore enriched in cDNA encoding the cytokines. Such enriched cDNA can be used as hybridization probes to identify cytokine mRNA, which is then converted into cDNA and transfected into bacterial or mammalian expression systems. The expressed cytokine is then assayed for biological activity. By the mid-1980s most of the genes encoding the better-known cytokines had been cloned and expressed in bacterial, yeast, insect, or mammalian tissue culture cells, so that large quantities of these proteins could be produced.

Structure and Functions of Cytokines and Their Receptors

Once the genes encoding various cytokines and their receptors had been cloned, sufficient quantities of purified preparations became available for detailed studies on the structure and function of these important proteins. Tables 11-3 and 11-4 summarize the main biological activities of the most important cytokines.

Interleukin 1 (IL-1)

The biological activity of IL-1 was first demonstrated in 1970 by I. Gery, R. K. Gershon, and B. H. Waksman. They showed that thymocytes could not ordinarily be stimulated to proliferate with the usual T-cell mitogen PHA. However, thymocytes cultured in conditioned medium from activated macrophages (adherent cells) did proliferate in response to the PHA, as indicated by the uptake of [3H] thymidine (Figure 11-3). The active macrophage-derived factor that stimulated the thymocytes was named lymphocyte-activating factor (LAF); it was eventually purified and renamed interleukin 1. Today the ability to stimulate PHA-treated thymocytes remains as the major biological assay for IL-1 activity.

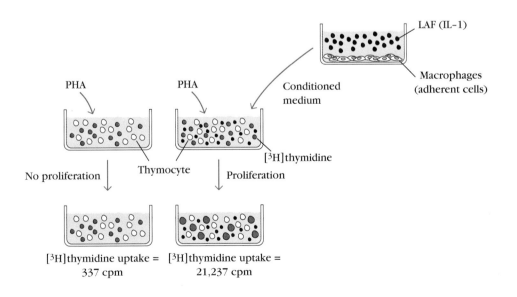

Figure 11-3 Conditioned medium from cultures of activated macrophages induce thymocyte proliferation in response to PHA. This activity led to the initial discovery of IL-1 and today is the common biological assay for this cytokine.

At first IL-1 was thought to be secreted exclusively by monocytes and macrophages. Recently, however, IL-1–like factors (identified by their ability to activate PHA-treated thymocytes) have been shown to be produced by a wide variety of cells including monocytes, macrophages, B lymphocytes, dendritic cells, fibroblasts, keratinocytes, Langerhans cells, neutrophils, astrocytes, epithelial cells, and endothelial cells. With the exception of a few transformed cell lines, IL-1 is not produced by any of these cells until they have been stimulated. Secretion of IL-1 by monocytes and macrophages can be induced with a variety of stimulants. Phagocytosis of

Table 11-3   Selected biological activities of some cytokines

Cytokine	Acronym	Secreted by	Activity
Interferon γ	IFN-γ	T_H cells, T_C cells	Enhances activity of macrophages and T_C, T_{DTH},[*] and NK cells Increases expression of MHC molecules Enhances production of IgG_{2a} Blocks IL-4–induced class switch to IgE and IgG_1
Interleukin 1	IL-1	Monocytes, macrophages, B cells, and numerous other cell types	Induces proliferation of PHA-treated thymocytes Costimulates T_H-cell activation Promotes B-cell maturation and clonal expansion Enhances activity of NK cells Chemotactically attracts neutrophils and macrophages Increases expression of ICAMs on vascular endothelial cells
Interleukin 2	IL-2	T_H cells (T_H1 subset)	Induces proliferation of antigen-primed T_H and T_C cells Supports long-term growth of antigen-specific T-cell clones Enhances activity of some NK cells and T_C cells
Interleukin 3	IL-3 (multi-CSF)	T_H cells	Supports growth and differentiation of hematopoietic cells[†] Stimulates mast-cell growth and histamine secretion
Interleukin 4	IL-4	T_H cells (T_H2 subset)	See Table 11-4
Interleukin 5	IL-5	T_H cells (T_H2 subset)	Induces B-cell proliferation and differentiation Promotes switch to IgA Acts with IL-4 to stimulate IgE production Induces eosinophil growth and differentiation[†]
Interleukin 6	IL-6	T_H cells (T_H2 subset) macrophages, monocytes, fibroblasts, and endothelial cells	Increases secretion of antibodies by plasma cells Together with IL-1, costimulates T-cell activation Aids in differentiation of myeloid stem cells[†]

certain bacteria serves as a stimulus for IL-1 production. This induction is due to a gram-negative cell-wall lipopolysaccharide (LPS), which by itself can induce IL-1 secretion. Phagocytosis of solid particles or antigen-antibody-complement complexes also stimulates IL-1 production by macrophages. Several other substances, including muramyl dipeptide (MDP), phorbol myristate acetate (PMA), certain complement components (C3a and C5a), and IFN-γ, also induce IL-1 production by macrophages. Activated T_H cells can also induce IL-1 production by macrophages, either by means of a membrane interaction between the T-cell receptor and

Table 11-3 **(Continued)** Selected biological activities of some cytokines

Cytokine	Acronym	Secreted by	Activity
Interleukin 7	IL-7	Bone-marrow stromal cells	Induces differentiation of lymphoid stem cells into progenitor B cells[†] Stimulates growth of thymocytes[†] Increases expression of IL-2 and its receptor by resting T cells
Interleukin 8	IL-8	Macrophages	Chemotactically attracts neutrophils Induces adherence of neutrophils to vascular endothelial cells and aids their migration into tissue spaces
Interleukin 9	IL-9	T_H cells (T_H2 subset)	Acts as a mitogen, inducing the proliferation of some T_H cells in the absence of antigen Promotes growth of mast cells
Interleukin 10	IL-10	T_H cells (T_H2 subset)	Suppresses cytokine production by T_H1 subset
Tumor necrosis factor α	TNF-α	Macrophages	Has cytotoxic effect on tumor cells but not on normal cells Induces numerous cell types to secrete various cytokines involved in the inflammatory response
Tumor necrosis factor β	TNF-β	T_H cells (T_H1 subset), T_C cells	Kills tumor cells and has other effects similar to those of TNF-α Enhances phagocytic activity of macrophages and neutrophils
Transforming growth factor β	TGF-β	Platelets, macrophages, lymphocytes	Chemotactically attracts monocytes and macrophages Induces increased IL-1 production by macrophages Inhibits proliferation of epithelial, endothelial, lymphoid, and hematopoietic cells Limits inflammatory response and promotes wound healing Induces class switch to IgA

* T_{DTH} cells are T cells involved with delayed-type hypersensitivity.

† See Figure 3-2 for site of action.

antigen-MHC complex on the macrophage, or by the release of certain T_H-cell cytokines, such as M-CSF, IFN-γ, or TNF-β. Following stimulation of macrophages, low levels of IL-1 can be detected in their cytoplasm within 30 min, and within 3 h of stimulation, high levels of IL-1 are secreted.

Biochemical purification of IL-1 revealed that two distinct polypeptides had IL-1 activity. Each of these polypeptides has an appropriate molecular weight of 17 kD, but they differ in their charge, so that they can be separated by isoelectric focusing. Gene cloning has confirmed these biochemical results, revealing that two independent genes (*IL-1α* and *IL-1β*) encode the two IL-1 polypeptides; the two genes have 27% sequence homology. Both proteins with IL-1 activity bind to the same IL-1 receptor on cells. It is not known how the two proteins differ in their biological activity. IL-1α also exists in a membrane-associated form (mIL-1), which may serve to activate T cells following membrane interaction.

A major function of IL-1 is its role in the activation of T_H cells, which appears to require two types of activating signals. A specific signal is generated by the interaction of T-cell receptors with processed antigen + class II MHC molecule. This signal is, in itself, insufficient to induce T_H-cell proliferation, and a second "co-stimulatory" signal is also required. The co-stimulatory signal can be delivered by the binding of either soluble IL-1 or membrane-bound IL-1 to an IL-1 receptor on the T_H-cell membrane. Together the two signals induce transcription of a number of genes in T_H cells, including those encoding IL-2, the IL-2 receptor, IL-3, IL-4, and interferon-gamma (IFN-γ). The dependence of T_H-cell activation on the IL-1 co-stimulatory signal was demonstrated by C. T. Weaver and E. R. Unanue in experiments with macrophages treated with paraformaldehyde, which makes them metabolically inactive and thus unable to produce IL-1 (Figure 11-4). In their system, macrophages were first treated with IFN-γ to induce increased expression of class II MHC molecules. Some of the macrophages then were treated with LPS to induce IL-1 production, while others were left untreated. Finally, both macrophage samples were fixed with paraformaldehyde to prevent further metabolic changes.

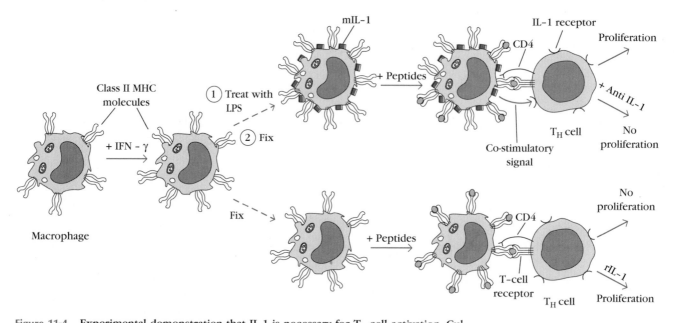

Figure 11-4   Experimental demonstration that IL-1 is necessary for T_H-cell activation. Cultured macrophages were treated with IFN-γ to induce increased expression of class II MHC molecules. The macrophages were then divided into two aliquots. One aliquot (*top*) was treated with LPS to induce production of membrane-bound IL-1 (mIL-1). The other aliquot (*bottom*) was untreated and therefore lacked mIL-1. The macrophages were then fixed with paraformaldehyde to prevent further metabolic activity. When the two aliquots were incubated with T_H cells and the antigenic peptide for which the cells were specific, only the LPS-treated macrophages induced T_H-cell proliferation. Although both macrophage samples could present the peptides and interact with the T_H cells, only the macrophages with mIL could provide the co-stimulatory signal necessary for T_H-cell activation. The role of IL-1 as a co-stimulatory signal was confirmed by the ability of anti-IL-1 to abolish the response of the LPS-treated macrophages and by the ability of recombinant IL-1 (rIL-1) to restore the response of the macrophages that were not treated with LPS.

When the two samples were incubated with a T_H-cell clone and a peptide antigen for which the clone was specific, only the macrophages that had been treated with LPS induced T_H-cell proliferation. These macrophages provided both specific and nonspecific activating signals. The specific signal resulted from interaction of T-cell receptors with the peptide–MHC complexes on the macrophages; the nonspecific signal came from the co-stimulatory mIL-1, which continued to function even after paraformaldehyde fixation. The macrophages that had not been activated with LPS lacked this co-stimulatory mIL-1 activity and thus could not activate the T_H clone.

In addition to its vital role as a co-stimulatory signal for T_H-cell activation, IL-1 has been shown to be quite pleiotrophic in its action, inducing a wide variety of effects on diverse types of cells. It promotes B-cell maturation and the clonal expansion of B cells following antigen-induced activation. It enhances NK-cell activity and influences the localized inflammatory reaction through its effects on hematopoietic cells, fibroblasts, and vascular endothelial cells. When IL-1 is administered in vivo, neutrophils are induced to leave the bone marrow, enter the circulation, and then extravasate through the capillary walls into the tissue spaces. Both neutrophils and macrophages are chemotactically attracted to IL-1, facilitating the buildup of phagocytic cells during an inflammatory reaction.

Interleukin 1 has also been shown to have far-reaching endocrine-like effects on a variety of cells and tissues. For example, it induces liver hepatocytes to produce a number of acute-phase proteins including fibrinogen, C-reactive protein, and haptoglobin, each of which contributes to host defense during an infection. IL-1 also acts upon the central nervous system via the hypothalamus, inducing fever, somnolence (drowsiness), and anorexia (decreased appetite). In addition it acts on muscle cells, inducing production of prostaglandins; this activity has been shown to lead to proteolysis, ultimately resulting in muscle wasting.

Interleukin 2 (IL-2)

In 1976 D. A. Morgan, F. W. Ruscetti, and R. Gallo observed that conditioned media from T cells activated by PHA were capable of maintaining T-cell proliferation in culture. This activity was characterized by Kendall Smith and co-workers, who made the seminal discovery that a single factor (originally called T-cell growth factor and later designated IL-2) produced by mitogen-activated T cells was responsible for the proliferative activity. The factor was shown to support long-term proliferation in cultures of normal mitogen- or antigen-activated T cells, making it possible for the first time to develop clones of normal T cells.

With the discovery of IL-2–dependent cell lines, production of IL-2 in various in vitro systems could be assayed. Treatment of IL-2–producing lymphoid clones with anti-CD4 and complement abolished IL-2 production, thus demonstrating that the T_H cell was the major producer of IL-2. Induction of IL-2 production by T_H cells is associated with their activation. As discussed in the previous section, T_H-cell activation requires two signals: one signal generated by interaction of a T_H cell with an antigen-MHC complex on an antigen-presenting cell (or with a mitogen) and a co-stimulatory signal generated by interaction with IL-1 produced by the APC. Within 24–48 h of activation, T_H cells begin to synthesize and secrete IL-2 and to express high-affinity membrane receptors for IL-2 (Figure 11-5).

Biochemical purification of IL-2 and subsequent cloning of the *IL-2* gene revealed that IL-2 is a single polypeptide whose molecular weight is generally given as 15.5 kD. Although IL-2 is encoded by a single gene, differences in post-translational glycosylation of the protein give rise to some size and charge heterogeneity. The various glycosylated forms of IL-2 do not appear to differ functionally, but some researchers have speculated that glycosylation may influence the half-life of IL-2 within the body.

Isolation and Characterization of the IL-2 Receptor

As research on lymphokines proceeded, monoclonal antibodies were produced to various membrane components on activated T_H cells. One of these monoclonal antibodies, designated anti-TAC, played an important role in the identification and subsequent isolation of the IL-2 receptor. Anti-TAC was found to inhibit the binding of radiolabeled IL-2 to activated T_H cells and to prevent activation of T_H cells with mitogen + IL-2. When anti-TAC was incubated with T_H cells, it bound to a 55-kD-membrane protein, which initially was assumed to be the IL-2 receptor. However, several unexpected findings raised questions about this conclusion. For example, although NK cells could be activated with IL-2, they failed to stain with fluorescein-labeled anti-TAC. Another odd finding was that the number of IL-2-binding sites on T_H cells did not equal the number of binding sites for anti-TAC; that is, binding studies with radiolabeled IL-2 and anti-TAC revealed that more anti-TAC molecules than IL-2 molecules bound to each activated T_H cell. Later, when the gene encoding the 55-kD putative IL-2 receptor was cloned, additional inconsistent results were obtained. When this gene was transfected into nonlymphoid cells, the transfected cells bound IL-2 only with low affinity, whereas when the gene was transfected into T_H cells, they bound IL-2 with high affinity.

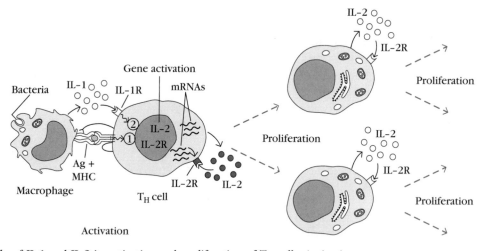

Figure 11-5   Role of IL-1 and IL-2 in activation and proliferation of T_H cells. Activation requires two signals: (1) a signal resulting from interaction of the T-cell receptor with an antigen-MHC complex on a macrophage or other antigen-presenting cell and (2) a co-stimulatory IL-1 signal. These two signals stimulate activity and stimulate expression of the genes encoding IL-2 and the high-affinity IL-2 receptor (IL-2R). IL-2 acts as an autocrine factor to stimulate T_H-cell proliferation. As antigen-MHC activation declines, the production of IL-2 and of IL-2 receptors also declines, stopping further T_H-cell proliferation. T_C-cell proliferation also is induced by IL-2.

These conflicting observations were resolved with the discovery that the membrane receptor for IL-2 actually consists of two subunits, a 55-kD α subunit (to which anti-TAC binds) and a 75-kD β subunit. Both subunits can bind IL-2 but with different affinities: The α subunit has a low affinity for IL-2; the β subunit has an intermediate affinity; and the $\alpha\beta$ heterodimer has a very high affinity (Figure 11-6). The NK cell was shown to express the 75-kD β subunit constitutively, accounting for its ability to be activated by IL-2 as well as its failure to stain with fluorescent-labeled anti-TAC. Activated T_H cells express both high-affinity and low-affinity IL-2 receptors. There are approximately 5×10^3 high-affinity receptors and ten times as many low-affinity receptors on an activated T_H cell. Thus activated T_H cells bind more anti-TAC than IL-2 molecules because of the greater number of low-affinity receptors, which bind anti-TAC, accounting for the earlier binding results.

Regulation of IL-2–Mediated Cell Proliferation

Interleukin 2 plays an essential role in triggering proliferation of antigen- or mitogen-treated T cells (both T_H and T_C cells). After binding to the high-affinity $\alpha\beta$ IL-2 receptor, IL-2 is rapidly internalized, triggering intracellular events that culminate in T-cell proliferation. Any T cell expressing the high-affinity IL-2 receptor can proliferate in response to IL-2, regardless of its antigenic specificity, but a built-in safeguard ensures that only

antigen-activated T cells will respond to IL-2. Resting T lymphocytes do not express the high-affinity receptor for IL-2 and therefore do not proliferate if IL-2 is secreted by a nearby cell. Only after a T cell is activated by antigen or a mitogen is the β subunit expressed, equipping the cell with the high-affinity IL-2 receptor. As long as a specific interaction continues between a T-cell receptor and antigen-MHC complex, expression of the high-affinity IL-2 receptor is stimulated; once this interaction stops, expression of the IL-2 receptor decreases. In this way, regulation of the expression of the high-affinity IL-2 receptor modulates the clonal expansion mediated by IL-2.

Interleukin 3 (IL-3)

Activated T_H cells secrete a number of colony-stimulating factors (CSFs) that support the growth and differentiation of various hematopoietic cells (see Figure 3-4). The earliest-acting of these factors was named multi-CSF because of its ability to stimulate hematopoietic cells of multiple lineages. This factor was cloned in 1984 and renamed interleukin 3. A 28-kD glycoprotein, IL-3 is secreted by activated T_H cells and has a number of effects that contribute to localized inflammatory reactions, including stimulation of mast-cell growth and histamine secretion.

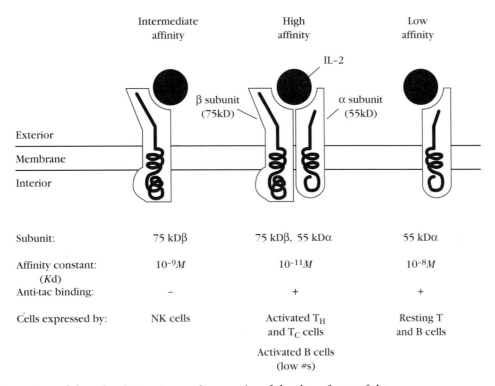

Figure 11-6 Comparison of the subunit structure and properties of the three forms of the IL-2 receptor. The α and β subunits differ in their affinity for IL-2 and the ability to bind anti-TAC antibodies. The dimer formed by noncovalent interaction of the α and β subunits has a high affinity for IL-2 and binds anti-TAC.

Interleukin 4 (IL-4)

Interleukin 4 is another cytokine possessing a broad spectrum of biological effects on several types of target cells (Table 11-4). Perhaps the best studied of its activities are those involving the activation, proliferation, and differentiation of B cells. This factor was first described by two independent research groups in separate articles in the same journal issue in 1982. One group described a T-cell–derived B-cell growth factor (BCGF-I) that activated B cells after cross-linkage of their membrane receptors by anti-IgM. The other group reported a T-cell factor that induced B-cell differentiation into plasma cells secreting IgG1. Within 4 years the gene for the differentiation factor (BCDF-I) was cloned and the two activities initially ascribed to the B-cell growth factor and B-cell differentiation factor turned out to be due to the same protein, now called interleukin 4.

Interleukin 4 has been shown to exert different effects on B cells at different stages in the cell cycle. On resting B cells, IL-4 acts as an activating factor, inducing the resting cells to enlarge in size and increase their expression of class II MHC molecules. Following activation by

Table 11-4 Biological activities of interleukin 4 (IL-4)

Target cell	Activity
B cells	Costimulates activation of resting B cells by increasing cell volume and enhancing expression of class II MHC molecules Induces proliferation and differentiation of antigen- or mitogen-activated B cells Induces class switch to IgG1 and IgE
T cells	Induces T-cell growth Stimulates proliferation of thymocytes Induces T-cell cytotoxic activity
Macrophages	Increases expression of class I and class II MHC molecules Increases phagocytic activity
Mast cells	Stimulates growth

antigen or mitogen, IL-4 acts as a growth factor, driving the B cell to replicate its DNA. Finally, in the case of proliferating B lymphocytes, IL-4 acts as a differentiation factor by regulating class switching to the IgG1 and IgE isotypes. In this role IL-4 has been termed a "switch-inducing" factor.

Interleukin 5 (IL-5)

Interleukin 5, like IL-4, has been shown to stimulate both B-cell proliferation and differentiation. This factor enhances production of IgA; it also appears to act synergistically with IL-4 to enhance production of IgE. Interleukin 5 also induces growth and differentiation of eosinophils.

Interleukin 6 (IL-6)

Activated T_H cells, macrophages, monocytes, and fibroblasts and several tumors (e.g., cardiac myxomas, cervical cancer, and bladder cancer) produce IL-6 constitutively. Several myeloma cells have been shown to secrete IL-6, which in this case functions in an autocrine manner to stimulate cell proliferation. Among the other activities of IL-6 is stimulation of immunoglobulin secretion by plasma cells and, in concert with IL-1, it acts as a costimulator of T_H-cell activation.

Interleukin 7 (IL-7)

Interleukin 7, first cloned in 1989, induces lymphoid stem cells to differentiate into progenitor B cells. This cytokine was discovered by expressing a cDNA library from bone-marrow stromal cells in Cos cells and testing the supernatants for biological activity. About 720,000 recombinants were screened before a clone possessing IL-7 activity was identified. Since its discovery, IL-7 has been shown to increase expression of IL-2 and IL-2 receptors in resting T cells, thereby inducing T-cell proliferation. In addition, IL-7 stimulates the proliferation of both fetal and adult thymocytes.

Interleukin 8 (IL-8)

Secreted primarily by monocytes, IL-8 has a variety of effects on neutrophils. For example, in the presence of IL-8 neutrophils adhere to vascular endothelial cells and emigrate from the blood into the tissue compartment toward a concentration gradient of IL-8. This cytokine is such a potent chemotactic factor for neutrophils that nanogram quantities are active.

Interleukin 9 (IL-9)

A glycoprotein secreted by certain T_H-cell clones, IL-9 supports the proliferation of T_H cells in the *absence* of antigen or antigen-presenting cells. It is produced by the T_H2 subset of long-term mouse T-cell clones and may act as an autocrine growth factor during antigen activation. Recently IL-9 has also been shown to promote the growth of mast cells.

Interleukin 10 (IL-10)

Recently an important regulatory cytokine, *cytokine-synthesis inhibitory factor* (*CSIF*), or IL-10, has been cloned and characterized. This cytokine is secreted by the T_H2 subset of long-term mouse T-cell clones and suppresses cytokine production by the T_H1 subset. The T_H1 subpopulation secretes IL-2 and IFN-γ and has been implicated in macrophage activation in the delayed-type hypersensitivity response. The T_H2 subpopulation secretes IL-4 and IL-5, triggering a predominantly humoral antibody response. The fact that IL-10 secretion by the T_H2 subpopulation suppresses cytokine production by the T_H1 subpopulation confers upon this cytokine a central role in regulating humoral and cell-mediated responses. The T_H1 and T_H2 subsets and the role of IL-10 in some diseases are discussed later in this chapter.

Interferons (IFNs)

The interferons are a family of glycpoproteins, produced by a variety of cell types, that interfere with viral replication and help to regulate the immune response. Interferon alpha (IFN-α), derived from various leukocytes, and interferon beta (IFN-β), derived from fibroblasts, were the first interferons to be characterized. Interferon gamma (IFN-γ) was discovered later and shown to be secreted by T lymphocytes following antigen or mitogen activation. All three interferons are released from virus-infected cells and confer antiviral protection on neighboring cells. Unlike IFN-α and IFN-β, which predominantly function to induce an antiviral state, IFN-γ has various pleiotrophic activities including the ability to enhance the functional activity of macrophages, T_C cells, T cells involved in delayed-type hypersensitivity (T_{DTH} cells), and NK cells. One of the most interesting effects of IFN-γ is the induction of increased class I and class II MHC expression on cells. The increased synthesis of class II MHC molecules by macrophages allows them to function as more effective antigen-presenting cells. Interferon gamma also has antagonistic activity against a number of cytokines. For example, when IFN-γ is added together with IL-4 to B cells, the class switch to IgE is blocked.

Tumor Necrosis Factors α and β

Around the turn of the century, William Coley, a surgeon, observed that when cancer patients developed certain bacterial infections, the tumors would become necrotic. In the hope that this might provide a cure for cancer, Coley began to inject cancer patients with supernatants derived from various bacterial cultures. These culture supernatants, called "Coley's toxins," induced hemorrhagic necrosis in the tumor but had numerous undesirable side effects of their own, making them unsuitable for cancer therapy. Decades later the active component of Coley's toxin was shown to be a lipopolysaccharide (endotoxin) component of the bacterial cell wall. This endotoxin does not itself induce tumor necrosis but instead induces production of a macrophage-derived serum factor, which now is called tumor necrosis factor α (TNF-α). This cytokine has a direct cytotoxic effect on tumor cells but not on normal cells (Figure 11-7). The mechanism of the tumor-specific cytotoxicity of TNF-α is unknown. Potential immunotherapeutic approaches using TNF-α for the treatment of cancer are examined in Chapter 23.

Tumor necrosis is not the only activity of TNF-α. It also plays an important role in the development of an effective inflammatory response, which serves to eliminate various invading pathogens. Together with IL-1, TNF-α acts on a variety of cells including T cells, B cells, neutrophils, fibroblasts, endothelial cells, and bone marrow cells, inducing these cells to secrete various factors necessary for the development of an effective inflammatory response.

Production of TNF-α is, however, a double-edged sword and can lead to harmful and sometimes fatal host reactions. In the 1980s Cerami and co-workers were trying to determine why some parasitic and bacterial infections and tumors induced a catabolic state leading to extensive weight loss (cachexia), sometimes resulting in shock and death. They discovered that a macrophage-derived factor was responsible for the profound wasting and called the factor cachectin. Cloning of the genes for tumor necrosis factor α and cachetin revealed that they were the same protein, now designated TNF-α. This cytokine is also involved in bacterial toxic shock, as discussed later in the chapter.

A second chemically related polypeptide, secreted primarily by activated T cells, was also shown to kill tumor cells while sparing normal cells and to elicit similar biological effects involving myriad localized inflammatory reactions. This factor, originally called lymphotoxin (LT), is now called TNF-β, indicating that it is closely related to TNF-α. Both proteins share approximately 28% sequence homology, and both are encoded by tightly linked genes within the class III region of the MHC, suggesting that the two genes evolved from a common gene by a tandem duplication event.

Transforming Growth Factor β

Transforming growth factors are small polypeptides that were first identified by their ability to induce proliferation and transformation of noncancerous cells in culture. Transforming growth factor β is produced by platelets, macrophages, T cells, and B cells. Although initially defined as a growth factor, TGF-β also inhibits proliferation of epithelial, endothelial, lymphoid, and hematopoietic cells. This cytokine is thought to play an important role in regulating the duration of the inflammatory response, allowing the healing process to proceed. It is also a potent immunomodulator, which has many pleiotrophic effects. For example, TGF-β inhibits the activity of a number of other cytokines, including IL-2, IL-4, IFN-γ, and TNF.

Secretion of Cytokines by T$_H$-Cell Subsets

As discussed in Chapter 10, two mouse CD4$^+$ T$_H$-cell subsets have recently been distinguished in vitro by the lymphokines they secrete. As shown in Table 11-5, these two subsets, designated T$_H$1 and T$_H$2, both secrete IL-3 and GM-CSF, but otherwise they differ in the lymphokines they secrete. The differences in the lymphokines secreted may reflect different biological activities of the T$_H$1 and T$_H$2 subsets. Interestingly, some of the lymphokines secreted by these subsets have opposite ef-

Table 11-5 Cytokine production by mouse T$_H$-cell subsets*

Cytokine	Subset T$_H$1	T$_H$2
IFN-γ	+	−
TNF-β (LT)	+	−
IL-2	+	−
IL-3	+	+
IL-4	−	+
IL-5	−	+
IL-6	−	+
IL-9	−	+
IL-10	−	+
GM-CSF	+	+

* Both T$_H$1 and T$_H$2 express CD4. These subsets have been observed only in long-term in vitro cultures of mouse T cells and may not exist in vivo.

SOURCE: Adapted from: T. R. Mosmann and K. W. Moore. 1991. *Immunoparisitol. Today* (March):A49.

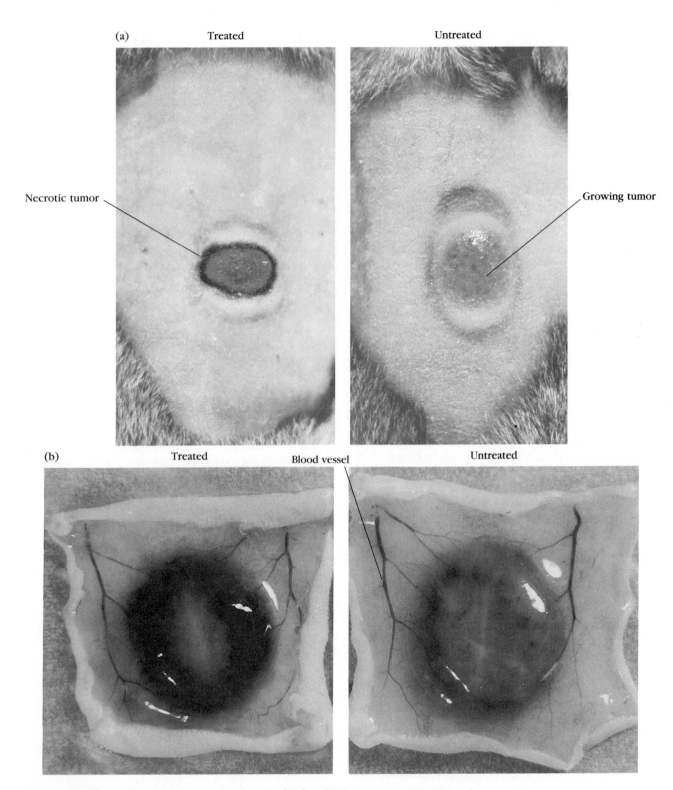

Figure 11-7   Effect of injecting bacterial endotoxin (LPS) or TNF-α on cancerous tumors in mice. (a) A cancerous tumor in a mouse injected with endotoxin (*left*) shows hemorrhagic necrosis compared with a tumor in an untreated mouse (*right*). Endotoxin is thought to induce production of TNF-α, which then acts to destroy the tumor. (b) In an untreated tumor (*right*), blood vessels, which bring nutrients to the tumor cells, are visible. Within hours after injection of TNF-α (*left*) many of the vessels within the tumor are destroyed, leading to hemorrhagic necrosis. [From L. J. Old, 1988. Tumor Necrosis Factor. *Sci. Am.* **258**:59.]

fects. For example, IL-2 (secreted by T_H1) promotes IgG2a production by B cells but inhibits IgG1 and IgE production. On the other hand, IL-4 (secreted by T_H2) promotes production of IgG1 and IgE and suppresses production of IgG2a. The T_H1 subset may be particularly suited to respond to viral infections because it secretes IL-2, which activates T_C cells and induces production of IFN-γ, which has antiviral activity. The T_H2 subset may be more suited to respond to parasitic infections and may cause allergic reactions, since IL-4 and IL-5 are known to induce IgE production and eosinophil activation, respectively. It is not known whether these T_H1 and T_H2 subsets are present in normal mice. They have

only been observed in long-term in vitro cultures, which has led some to ask whether they represent true in vivo subpopulations or whether instead they represent different maturational stages of a single lineage. There is no human counterpart for these mouse T_H-cell subsets.

Role of Cytokines in Lymphocyte Activation

Virgin, or resting, T and B lymphocytes are noncycling cells in the G_0 stage of the cell cycle. Activation drives a resting cell to enter the cell cycle, progressing through G_1 into the S phase, in which DNA is replicated. The G_1-to-S transition represents a critical restriction point in the cell cycle. Once a cell has reached S, it completes the cell cycle, moving through G_2 and into mitosis (M). After analyzing the events involved in the progression of lymphocytes from G_0 to the S phase, Ken Ichi Arai noted a number of similarities with events that had been identified in fibroblast cells. Two types of growth signals act at different stages to drive a fibroblast along a progression from G_1 to S. First, platelet-derived growth factor (PDGF) delivers to a fibroblast a *competence signal*, which drives the cell from early G_1 to late G_1 and renders the cell competent to receive the next signal. At this point insulin-like growth factor (IGF) and epidermal growth factor (EGF) act on the competent fibroblast cell, serving as *progression signals* to drive the cell through G_1 and into S. Activation of T and B lymphocytes appears to follow a similar sequence with early signals driving a resting cell from G_0 to early G_1 and rendering the cell competent to receive second-level progression signals that drive the cell from G_1 into S and ultimately to cell division and differentiation.

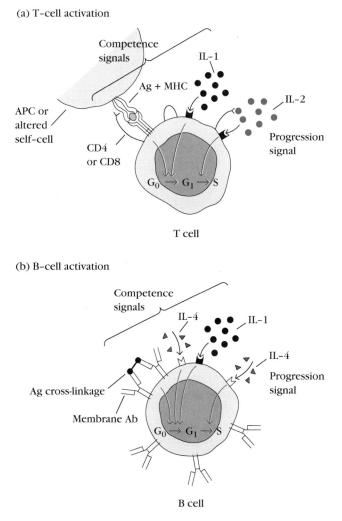

(a) T-cell activation

(b) B-cell activation

Figure 11-8   Activation of resting T and B cells in the G_0 state to the S phase of the cell cycle requires competence signals and progression signals. In both cases, the competence signals result from interaction with antigen and co-stimulatory interleukin(s). The progression signal is generated by IL-2 in T cells and IL-4 in B cells.

T-Lymphocyte Activation

Activation of resting T cells from G_0 into early G_1 is thought to require two competence signals, the first one supplied by the interaction of an antigen-MHC complex with the T-cell receptor and the second supplied by an accessory cell in the form of co-stimulatory IL-1 (Figure 11-8). These events transduce a signal across the plasma membrane that results in the transcription of a number of genes, including those encoding IL-2 and the IL-2 receptor. The subsequent binding of IL-2 to its receptor is thought to serve as a progression signal that drives a T cell from G_1 into S. There is speculation that the interaction of IL-2 and its receptor plays an important role in committing the T cell to an activated state of differentiation, because expression of IL-2 at 45 min and of the IL-2 receptor at 2 h parallels the 2-h time course required for commitment of a T cell to activation.

The biochemical events involved in activation have been studied by using a T-cell tumor line that responds to a T-cell-receptor–mediated signal and co-stimulatory IL-1 signal by producing IL-2. It is possible to replace the TCR and IL-1 signals with other agents to simplify the system. The requirement for an antigen-MHC interaction with the TCR can be replaced with mitogens such as Con A or PHA, or it can be replaced with antibody to CD3. The requirement for the co-stimulatory IL-1 signal can be replaced with agents that activate protein kinase C, such as phorbol myristate acetate (PMA). This system has revealed that the two competence signals appear to activate two synergistically acting biochemical pathways, one involving hydrolysis of phospatidylinositol leading to increased intracellular calcium and the other involving protein kinase C activation (see Figure 10-9).

Within 15 min of receiving these competence growth signals, the T cell begins to transcribe a number of genes, including several DNA-binding proteins. The cellular oncogene product *c-fos* is detected within 15 min; by 30 min another oncogene product, *c-myc*, can be detected along with several other DNA-binding proteins including NFAT-1 and NF-κB (Table 11-6). NFAT-1, NF-κB, and *c-fos* have each been shown to bind to the enhancer of the IL-2 gene, resulting in increased transcription of this gene within 45 min of activation. By 2 h after activation,

Table 11-6   Time course of gene expression by T_H cells following activation

Gene product	Function	Time mRNA expression begins	Location	Ratio of activated to nonactivated cells
		Immediate		
c-fos	Cellular oncogene Nuclear-binding protein	15 min	Nucleus	> 100
NFAT-1	Nuclear-binding protein	20 min	Nucleus	50
c-myc	Cellular oncogene	30 min	Nucleus	20
NF-κB	Nuclear-binding protein	30 min	Nucleus	> 10
		Early		
IFN-γ	Cytokine	30 min	Secreted	> 100
IL-2	Cytokine	45 min	Secreted	> 1000
c-abl	Cellular oncogene	1 h	Nuclear	10
Insulin receptor	Hormone receptor	1 h	Cell membrane	3
IL-3	Cytokine	1–2 h	Secreted	> 100
TGF-β	Cytokine	< 2 h	Secreted	> 10
IL-2 receptor	Cytokine receptor	2 h	Cell membrane	> 50
TNF-β	Cytokine	1–3 h	Secreted	> 100
Cyclin	Cell cycle protein	4–6 h	Cytoplasmic	> 10
IL-4	Cytokine	< 6 h	Secreted	> 100
IL-5	Cytokine	< 6 h	Secreted	> 100
IL-6	Cytokine	< 6 h	Secreted	> 100
c-myb	Cellular oncogene	16 h	Nuclear	100
GM-CSF	Cytokine	20 h	Secreted	?
		Late		
HLA-DR	Class II MHC molecule	3–5 days	Cell membrane	10
VLA-4	Adhesion molecule	4 days	Cell membrane	> 100
VLA-1, VLA-2, VLA-3, VLA-5	Adhesion molecules	7–14 days	Cell membrane	> 100, ?, ?, ?

SOURCE: Adapted from G. Crabtree, 1989, *Science* **243**:357.

the T cell becomes committed to an activated state of differentiation. Interestingly, the timing of this commitment parallels the expression of the IL-2 receptor, and it has been suggested that the interaction of IL-2 and its receptor serves as a progression signal, driving the cell from G_1 into the S phase of the cell cycle and thereby committing the cell to activation.

The need for two competence signals, one from the interaction of antigen-MHC with the TCR and the other from co-stimulatory IL-1, has been postulated to be due to a requirement for two interacting DNA-binding proteins for T-cell activation. The IL-1 (PMA)–induced signal induces the expression of a transcription factor, AP-1, encoded by the cellular protooncogene *c-jun*. The TCR-mediated signal generated by PHA induces expression of *c-fos*. Interestingly, *c-fos* and AP-1 have been shown to interact through a conserved set of repeated leucine residues, forming a DNA-binding protein motif called a "leucine zipper." The AP-1/*c-fos* heterodimer then interacts with a conserved AP-1 binding site in the IL-2 enhancer. This interaction could account for the need for two signals for T-cell activation; the TCR-mediated signal would induce *c-fos* and the IL-1–mediated signal would induce AP-1 (Figure 11-9).

Once a T cell is committed to activation, it begins to produce and secrete various cytokines, which mediate different effector functions (see Table 11-6). The expression of the cytokine genes appears to be regulated by complex mechanisms that have yet to be unraveled. At the present time, little is known of the mechanism by which the cell-membrane events involved in activation generate the long-term phenotypic changes corresponding to different T-cell subpopulations.

B-Lymphocyte Activation

In the primary immune response, a resting B cell is activated by antigen and various T_H-cell cytokines to progress from the G_0 state into the cell cycle; subsequent proliferation and differentiation then generate antibody-secreting plasma cells. Activation of a resting B cell requires binding of antigen to the cell's membrane-bound antibody and also co-stimulatory signals generated by IL-1 and IL-4. Activation can also be achieved with the B-cell mitogen LPS or with anti-IgM, which binds to membrane-bound IgM, again together with the co-stimulatory IL-4 signal. It has been suggested that interaction of antigen and membrane-bound antibody serves as a competence signal to drive a resting B cell from G_0 into early G_1, at which stage the cell becomes responsive to IL-4. At this point, interaction of IL-4 with the B cell acts as a competence signal, driving the cell from early G_1 to late G_1. Interleukin 4 also functions as

a progression signal that drives the B cell through the G_1 restriction point and into the S phase of the cell cycle (see Figure 11-9b). B-cell activation and the role of IL-4 and other cytokines in the proliferation and differentiation of activated B cells are described in more detail in Chapter 12.

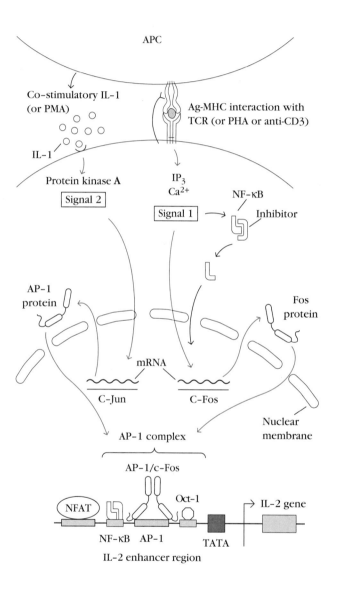

Figure 11-9 The need for two signals for T-cell activation—one from the interaction of antigen-MHC with the TCR and one from co-stimulatory IL-1—has been hypothesized as vital to the need for two interacting DNA-binding proteins. The TCR-mediated signal induces the expression of *c-fos*, while the IL-1–mediated signal induces expression of AP-1. These two DNA-binding proteins interact in a leucine zipper motif and bind to a conserved AP-1 binding site in the IL-2 enhancer, contributing to activation of the IL-2 gene.

Role of Cytokines in the Inflammatory Response

In response to infection or tissue injury, a complex cascade of nonspecific events, known as the *acute-phase response* (*APR*), is initiated that provides early protection by restricting the tissue damage to the site of infection or tissue injury. The acute-phase response involves both localized and systemic responses. The localized inflammatory response develops as plasma clotting factors are produced resulting in activation of the clotting, kinin-forming, and fibrinolytic pathways. Various cytokines have been shown to influence this localized inflammatory response by facilitating both the adherence of inflammatory cells to vascular endothelial cells and their migration through the vessel and into the tissue spaces. This results in an influx of lymphocytes, neutrophils, monocytes, eosinophils, basophils, and mast cells to the site of tissue damage, where these cells participate in clearance of the antigen.

The systemic response includes the induction of fever, increased synthesis of hormones such as ACTH and hydrocortisone, increased white blood cell production (leukocytosis), and production of a large number of hepatocyte-derived acute-phase proteins including C-reactive protein (CRP) and serum amyloid A (SAA). The increase in body temperature inhibits the growth of a number of pathogens and appears to enhance the immune response to the pathogen. C-reactive protein (CRP) is a prototype acute-phase protein whose serum levels increase by 1000-fold during an acute-phase response. It is composed of five identical polypeptides held together by noncovalent interactions. C-reactive protein binds to a wide variety of microorganisms and activates complement, resulting in the deposition of a complement component, C3b, on the surface of the microorganism. Phagocytic cells express C3b receptors and phagocytose the C3b-coated microorganisms.

The acute-phase inflammatory reaction is initiated following the activation of tissue macrophages and the release of three cytokines: TNF-α, IL-1, and IL-6. These three cytokines act synergistically to induce many of the localized and systemic changes observed in the acute-phase inflammatory response. All three cytokines act locally on fibroblasts and endothelial cells inducing coagulation and an increase in vascular permeability. Both TNF and IL-1 induce increased expression of adhesion molecules on vascular endothelial cells. TNF has been shown to induce increased expression of ELAM-1, an endothelial leukocyte adhesion molecule that selectively binds neutrophils. IL-1 induces increased expression of ICAM-1 and VCAM-1, the intercellular adhesion molecules for lymphocytes and monocytes. Circulating neutrophils, monocytes, and lymphocytes adhere to the wall of a blood vessel by recognizing these adhesion molecules and then move through the vessel wall into the tissue spaces (Figure 11-10a). IL-1 and TNF also act on macrophages and endothelial cells inducing production of IL-8. IL-8 contributes to the influx of neutrophils by increasing their adhesion to vascular endothelial cells and by acting as a potent chemotactic factor. Other cytokines also serve as chemotactic factors for various leukocyte populations. For example, IFN-γ has been shown to chemotactically attract macrophages, bringing increased numbers of phagocytic cells to a site where antigen is localized. In addition, IFN-γ and TNF activate macrophages and neutrophils, promoting increased phagocytic activity and increased release of lytic enzymes into the tissue spaces.

The combined action of IL-1, TNF, and IL-6 are also responsible for many of the systemic changes that occur during an acute-phase inflammatory response. Each of these cytokines acts on the hypothalamus to induce a fever response. Within 12–24 h of an acute-phase inflammatory response, increased levels of IL-1, TNF, and IL-6 induce hepatocyte production of acute-phase proteins. TNF also acts on vascular endothelial cells and macrophages inducing secretion of colony-stimulating factors (M-CSF, G-CSF, and GM-CSF). Production of CSFs will result in induction of hematopoiesis, resulting in transient increases in the necessary white blood cells to fight the infection.

TNF, IL-1, and IL-6 are not produced constitutively by cells. Instead synthesis of these cytokines is induced by various stimuli including certain viruses, the endotoxin component of gram-negative bacterial cell walls, as well as the cytokines themselves. Both TNF and IL-1 have been shown to induce expression of each other as well

Figure 11-10   The acute-phase inflammatory response is mediated by three principal cytokines: TNF-α, IL-1, and IL-6. (a) These three cytokines act synergistically to induce many of the events leading to an inflammatory response including increased adherence of circulating white blood cells to vascular endothelial cells and their extravasation to the tissue spaces. IL-1 induces increased expression of ICAMs on the vascular endothelial cells. IL-8 contributes to the process by inducing neutrophil adherence to the endothelial cells. IL-8 and IFN-γ exhibit chemotactic activity for neutrophils and macrophages, respectively. IFN-γ also functions to activate macrophages, increasing their phagocytotic ability and their lysosomal enzyme content. (b) TNF-α, IL-1, and IL-6 have been shown to be induced together. The molecular mechanism that coordinates the expression of these three cytokines is begining to be unraveled. In the case of the IL-6 gene, for example, both IL-1 and TNF-α have been shown to induce the expression of DNA-binding proteins that bind to the IL-6 enhancer, resulting in activation of the IL-6 gene. Thus, as IL-1 and TNF-α levels increase, IL-6 production is also increased.

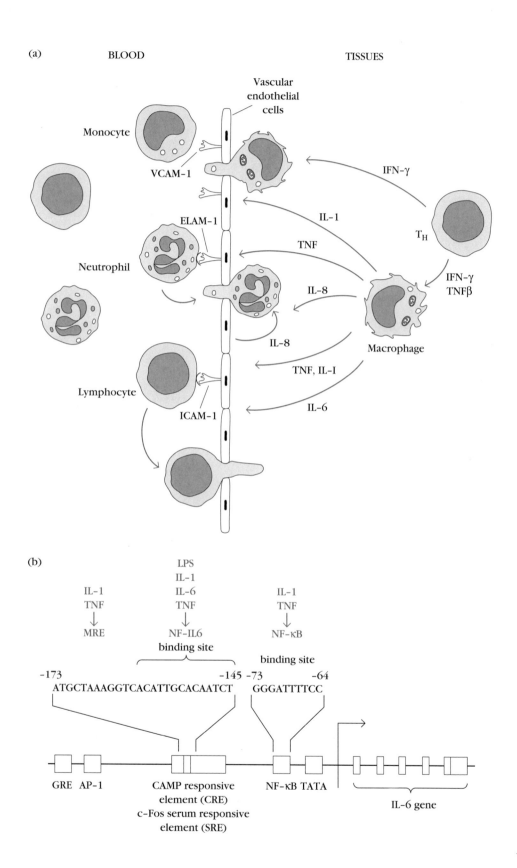

as expression of IL-6. The genes for TNF, IL-1, and IL-6 have been cloned, and nuclear factors that bind to promoter or enhancer sequences are beginning to be identified. In the case of the IL-6 gene, for example, the promoter sequence has been shown to contain several regulatory regions to which DNA-binding proteins bind (Figure 11-10b). Three of these DNA-binding proteins are the nuclear factor IL-6 (NF-IL6), the multiresponse element (MRE), and nuclear factor κB (NF-κB). All three DNA binding proteins have been shown to be induced by IL-1 and by TNF. Thus, as IL-1 or TNF levels increase, IL-6 production is also increased.

It is important that the duration and intensity of the inflammatory response be carefully regulated to control tissue damage and facilitate the tissue repair mechanisms that are necessary for wound healing. TGF-β has been shown to play an important role in limiting the inflammatory response. It also promotes accumulation and proliferation of fibroblasts and the deposition of an extracellular matrix which is required for proper tissue repair.

Cytokines and Disease

Defects in the complex regulatory networks governing the expression of cytokines and cytokine receptors have been implicated in a number of diseases. Overexpression or underexpression of an appropriate or inappropriate cytokine or cytokine receptor may contribute to a disease process. In this section, several examples of diseases resulting from cytokine abnormalities are described and the possible therapeutic uses of cytokines are discussed.

Bacterial Septic Shock

The role of cytokine overproduction in pathogenesis can be illustrated by bacterial septic shock. This condition may develop within a few hours following infection by certain gram-negative bacteria including *E. coli, Klebsiella pneumoniae, Pseudomonas aeruginosa, Enterobacter aerogenes,* and *Neisseria meningitidis.* The symptoms of bacterial septic shock, which often is fatal, include a drop in blood pressure, fever, diarrhea, and widespread blood clotting in various organs. The incidence of shock with gram-negative bacterial sepsis is quite high, and has been estimated to develop in 5 out of every 1000 patients admitted to hospitals. The mortality rate is also high and treatment with conventional antibiotics is of little benefit.

Bacterial septic shock appears to develop when bacterial cell-wall endotoxins stimulate macrophages to overproduce IL-1 and TNF-α. It is the increased levels of IL-1 and TNF-α that cause septic shock. In one study, for example, higher levels of TNF-α were found in patients who died of meningitis than in those who recovered. Furthermore, a condition resembling bacterial septic shock can be produced by injection of recombinant TNF-α in the absence of gram-negative bacterial infection. Recent reports offer some hope that neutralization of TNF-α or IL-1 activity with monoclonal antibodies or antagonists may prevent this fatal shock from developing in these bacterial infections. Monoclonal antibody to TNF-α was shown to prevent an otherwise fatal dose of endotoxin-induced shock in animal models. And another study has shown that injection of a recombinant IL-1 receptor antagonist, which can prevent IL-1 binding to the IL-1 receptor, significantly reduced the mortality due to septic shock in rabbits. It is hoped that these experimental results will have therapeutic benefit for the treatment of bacterial septic shock in humans.

Bacterial Toxic Shock and Related Diseases

A variety of microorganisms produce toxins that act as superantigens, stimulating large numbers of T cells irrespective of their antigenic specificity. As discussed in Chapter 4, superantigens bind simultaneously to a class II MHC molecule and to the V_β region of the T-cell receptor, activating all T cells bearing a particular V_β family (see Figure 4-16). Unlike conventional antigens, superantigens are not internalized, processed, and presented by antigen-presenting cells. Instead they bind directly to the class II MHC molecule, apparently binding outside of the antigen-binding cleft of the MHC molecule. Once the superantigen is bound to the class II MHC molecule, it binds to a particular part of the T-cell receptor V_β chain. Unlike the T-cell response to conventional antigens which is MHC restricted, T cells can be activated by superantigens bound to allogeneic or even xenogeneic MHC molecules. Thus, superantigens appear to violate the basic tenet of MHC restriction for T-cell activation. The interaction of the superantigen with the T-cell receptor appears to involve regions of the V_β chain that are well away from the complementarity-determining regions of the TCR, suggesting that the superantigen interacts with a site that is distinct from the conventional antigen–MHC binding site on the TCR. The superantigen is thought to bind to a region of β pleated sheet exposed on the side of the TCR. Superantigens activate large numbers of T cells. While only

$1/10^4$–$1/10^6$ T cells respond to conventional antigens, between 1/4–1/20 T cells respond to superantigens. The large number of T cells responsive to superantigens corresponds to the number of V_β genes carried in the germ line, which is about 20 V_β genes in mice. Assuming that each V_β gene is expressed with equal frequency, then one would expect each superantigen to interact with about 1/20 T cells.

A number of bacterial superantigens have been implicated as the causative agent of a number of diseases. Included among these bacterial superantigens are *Staphylococcal aureus* enterotoxins (SEA, B, C1-3, D, and E), exfoliating toxins (A and B), toxic shock syndrome toxin (TSST-1), *Streptococcal pyogenes* pyrogenic toxins (A, B, and C), and *Mycoplasma arthritidis* supernatent (MAS). The large numbers of T cells activated by these superantigens results in massive levels of cytokine production, inducing diseases such as food poisoning and fatal toxic shock. The toxic shock syndrome toxin (TSST-1) for example, has been shown to induce extremely high levels of TNF and IL-1. As discussed for bacterial septic shock, these cytokines can induce systemic reactions including fever, widespread blood clotting, and shock.

Lymphoid and Myeloid Cancers

Abnormalities in cytokine production or expression of cytokine receptors have been associated with some lymphoid and myeloid cancers. Some B-cell myelomas, for instance, secrete IL-6, which serves as an autocrine stimulator of myeloma-cell growth. When monoclonal antibodies to IL-6 are added to in vitro cultures of such myeloma cells, their growth is inhibited. Perhaps the strongest case for an association between inappropriate expression of a cytokine receptor and malignancy comes from the often-fatal adult T-cell leukemia associated with the HTLV-1 retrovirus. The leukemic T cells express the high-affinity IL-2 receptor in the apparent absence of activation by any antigen or mitogen. The molecular basis for this defect expression of the IL-2 receptor involves the tax gene of the HTLV-1 genome. This gene encodes a 40-kD protein that binds to the enhancer sequence in the long terminal repeat region of the viral genome, facilitating viral activation. The tax protein also induces expression of a cellular factor (or factors) that binds to the promoter regions of the genes encoding IL-2 and its receptor and thus activates these genes. An HTLV-1–infected cell therefore expresses IL-2 and the IL-2 receptor constitutively, in the absence of antigen or mitogen activation, rendering the cell responsive to IL-2–induced proliferation.

Chagas' Disease

The protozoan *Trypanosoma cruzi* is the causative agent of Chagas' disease, which is characterized by severe immune suppression. The ability of *T. cruzi* to mediate immune suppression can be observed by culturing peripheral-blood T lymphocytes in the presence and in the absence of *T. cruzi* and then evaluating their immune reactivity. Normally antigen, a mitogen, or an anti-CD3 monoclonal antibody activates peripheral T lymphocytes, but in the presence of *T. cruzi* T lymphocytes are not activated by any of these agents. The defect in these lymphocytes has been traced to a dramatic reduction in the 55-kD α subunit of the IL-2 receptor. When T lymphocytes were cocultured with *T. cruzi*, a 90% decrease in lymphocytes expressing the 55-kD subunit was demonstrated by a lack of staining with fluorescein-labeled anti-Tac. As noted earlier, the 55-kD α subunit is a necessary component of the high-affinity IL-2 receptor. The mechanism by which *T. cruzi* suppresses expression of the subunit remains to be determined. There is some evidence that a factor secreted by *T. cruzi* mediates this suppression because the suppression can be induced across a filter that inhibits contact between the lymphocytes and protozoa. Such a factor, once isolated, could have untold clinical applications for regulating the level of activated T cells in leukemias and autoimmune diseases.

Cytokine-Related Therapies

The availability of purified cloned cytokines and soluble cytokine receptors offers the prospect of specific clinical therapies to modulate various branches of the immune response. For example, activation and proliferation of T_H cells in response to alloantigens on organ transplants initiates T_C-cell activation and subsequent graft rejection. Various approaches have been tried experimentally to suppress T_H-cell proliferation and thereby prolong graft survival (Figure 11-11). Monoclonal antibody to the α subunit of the IL-2 receptor has been shown to block IL-2 activation of T_H cells and has prolonged the survival of heart transplants in rats. A cloned soluble form of the IL-1 receptor lacking the transmembrane and cytoplasmic domains also blocks T_H-cell activation in response to alloantigens and has prolonged heart transplants in animal models. Cytokines conjugated to various toxins, such as the β chain of diphtheria toxin, have been shown to diminish kidney- and heart-transplant rejection in animals. These conjugates selectively bind to and kill activated T_H cells. Finally, IL-2 analogs that retain their binding activity but have lost their biological

CHAPTER 11 CYTOKINES

activity have the potential of serving as antagonists that block IL-2 activity. Such analogs have been produced by site-directed mutagenesis of cloned *IL-2* genes.

In immunodeficiency diseases and in cancer, enhanced—rather than diminished—T-cell activation is desirable. Intervention with cloned IL-2, IFN-γ and TNF-α have each had some degree of clinical success.

(a)

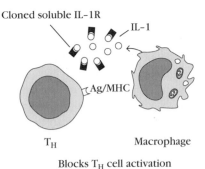

Antibodies to IL-2R

IL–2R

T$_H$ T$_C$

Blocks T$_H$ cell proliferation and T$_C$ cell activation

(b)

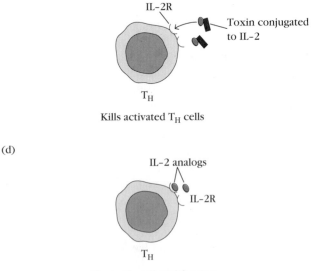

Cloned soluble IL-1R   IL-1

Ag/MHC

T$_H$ Macrophage

Blocks T$_H$ cell activation

(c)

IL–2R

Toxin conjugated to IL-2

T$_H$

Kills activated T$_H$ cells

(d)

IL-2 analogs

IL-2R

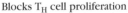

T$_H$

Blocks T$_H$ cell proliferation

Figure 11-11 Experimental approaches used to suppress T$_H$-cell activation or proliferation. These approaches make use of (a) antibodies against the IL-2 receptor (IL-2R), (b) cloned, soluble IL-1 receptors (IL-1R), (c) diphtheria toxin conjugated to IL-2, and (d) various IL-2 analogs.

Culturing of various populations of natural killer cells or T$_C$ cells in the presence of high concentrations of IL-2 has been shown to generate cells with effective antitumor properties, which are referred to as *lymphokine-activated killer* (*LAK*) cells. Their role in tumor therapy is examined in Chapter 21.

Cytokine therapy may also prove to be effective in the treatment of allergies. Given the opposing effects of IL-2 and IL-4 on isotype production, it may be possible to enhance a desired isotype selectively. Selective inhibition of IgE may benefit patients with allergies. In animal models, for example, monoclonal antibody to IL-4 has been used to decrease IgE production. Clearly these approaches have enormous clinical applications for the millions of people who suffer from allergies.

Cytokine-related therapy does have limitations, however. During an immune response, cytokines produced locally by interacting cells may achieve relatively high local concentrations that cannot be mimicked by clinical administration. In addition, cytokines often have a very short half-life, so that repeated administration may be required in order to maintain effective levels. For example, recombinant human IL-2 has a half-life of only 7–10 min when administered intraveneously. Finally, the pleiotrophic effects of many cytokines can cause unpredictable and undesirable side effects. The side effects from administration of recombinant IL-2, for instance, range from mild ones (e.g., fever, chills, diarrhea, and weight gain) to anemia, thrombocytopenia, shock, respiratory distress, and coma.

Summary

1. The complex cellular interactions involving cells of the immune, inflammatory and hematopoietic systems are mediated by a group of secreted low-molecular-weight proteins collectively called cytokines. Those secreted by lymphocytes are often referred to as lymphokines; those secreted by macrophages, as monokines. Most cytokines act on nearby target cells, although in some cases a cytokine can act on the cell that secretes it. The biological activities of cytokines exhibit pleiotrophy, redundancy, synergy, and antagonism, which contribute to the complexity of cytokine networks.

2. Biochemical purification of cytokines and subsequently the cloning of cytokine genes revealed that many activities previously attributed to different cytokines in fact were mediated by a relatively small number of multifunctional proteins. These discoveries brought some simplification to a field that was plagued by an overwhelming array of supposedly single-function factors. Today, the most important recognized cytokines include IFN-γ, interleukins 1–10, TNF-α, TNF-β, and TGF-β.

3. A particular cytokine can act on any target cell that expresses receptors for that cytokine. An important way in which the activity of cytokines is directed toward specific cells is by regulation of the expression of their receptors. For example, a T_H cell does not express the high affinity IL-2 receptor until it has interacted with an antigen-MHC complex and with IL-1. As long as the antigen-MHC-TCR interaction continues, the IL-2 receptor is expressed, but once this interaction ceases, the expression of the IL-2 receptor stops as well.

4. Several cytokines—particularly, IL-1, IL-2, and IL-4—are required for activation of B or T cells. They function as competence signals, driving the resting cell from the G_0 state into G_1 and/or act as progression signals driving the cell from G_1 into S, thus inducing cellular proliferation. Some cytokines act as differentiation factors that help to determine the final effector function of an activated T or B cell.

5. Development of an effective inflammatory response also depends on the action of numerous cytokines. These include IL-1, IL-8, and IFN-γ, which aid in the movement of leukocytes to tissue sites where antigen is located. The phagocytic activity of macrophages and neutrophils is promoted by IFN-γ and TNF-α. The inflammatory response is, in part, limited by TGF-β, which also promotes wound healing.

6. Abnormalities in the expression of cytokines or their receptors may result in various diseases including bacterial toxic shock, certain lymphoid and myeloid cancers, and Chagas' disease. Cytokine-related therapies that either increase or decrease selected parts of the immune response offer promise of reducing graft rejection, treating certain cancers and immunodeficiency diseases, and reducing allergic reactions.

References

ARAI, K., F. LEE, A. MIYAJIMA et al. 1990. Cytokines: coordinators of immune and inflammatory responses. *Annu. Rev. Biochem.* **59**:783.

BALKWILL, F. R., and F. BURKE, 1989. The cytokine network. *Immunol. Today* **10**:299.

BEUTLER, B. 1990. The tumor necrosis factors: cachectin and lymphotoxin. *Hospital Practice* (February 15):45.

CRABTREE, G. R. 1989. Contingent genetic regulatory events in T lymphocyte activation. *Science* **243**:355.

DI GIOVINE, F. S., and G. W. DUFF. 1990. Interleukin 1: the first interleukin. *Immunol. Today* **11**.

FARRAR, W. L., D. K. FERRIS, and A. HAREL-BELLAN. 1990. Lymphokine-induced molecular signal transduction. In *Immunophysiology*, Oxford Press, p. 67.

HERMAN, A., J. W. KAPPLER, P. MARRACK, and A. M. PULLEN. 1991. Superantigens: mechanism of T-cell stimulation and role in immune responses. *Annu. Rev. Immunol.* **9**:745.

KIERSZENBAUM, F., M. B. SZTEIN, and L. A. BELTZ. 1989. Decreased human IL-2 receptor expression due to a protozoan pathogen. *Immunol. Today* **10**:129.

MOSMANN, T. R., and K. W. MOORE. 1991. The role of IL-10 in crossregulation of T_H1 and T_H2 responses. *Immunoparasitology Today* (March):A49.

PAUL, W. E. 1987. Interleukin 4/B cell stimulatory factor 1: one lymphokine, many functions. *FASEB* **1**:456.

PAUL, W. E. 1989. Pleiotrophy and redundancy: T cell derived lymphokines in the immune response. *Cell* **57**:521.

SMITH, K. 1988. Interleukin-2: inception, impact and implications. *Science* **240**:1169.

SMITH, K. 1990. Interleukin-2. *Sci. Am.* **262**:50.

TANAGUCHI, T. 1988. Regulation of cytokine expression. *Annu. Rev. Immunol.* **6**:439.

Study Questions

1. Indicate whether each of the following statements is true or false. If you think a statement is false, explain why.

  a. The IL-2 receptor consists of two transmembrane proteins.

  b. The anti-TAC monoclonal antibody recognizes the IL-1 receptor on T cells.

  c. When a T_H cell is activated, it begins to express IL-2 and the high-affinity IL-2 receptor.

  d. By itself, the 55-kD α subunit of the IL-2 receptor cannot bind IL-2.

  e. Expression of the α subunit of the IL-2 receptor is indicative of T_H-cell activation.

2. When IL-2 is secreted by one T cell in a peripheral lymphoid organ, do all of the T cells in the vicinity proliferate in response to the IL-2 or only some of them? Explain.

3. You have identified a mutant T_H-cell clone that secretes IL-2 and expresses IL-2 receptors, but the clone does not proliferate and exhibits low-affinity binding of the secreted IL-2. Propose two defects that might account for these observations. How might you determine which hypothesis is correct?

4. You have generated three mutant T_H-cell clones that do not proliferate in response to antigen + a MHC molecule presented on antigen-presenting cells. In order to try to determine the reason for this lack of proliferation, you first treat each clone with antigen + MHC and then determine (1) whether IL-2 is secreted by the cells, (2) the ability of the cells to bind IL-2, and (3) whether the cells stain with anti-TAC antibody. The results of these experiments are shown in the table below.

   a. What are the possible defects in each of the clones?

   b. Defects in mutant cells sometimes are more complex than they appear. One way to assess the complexity of a mutation(s) is to try to restore the normal phenotype by repairing the obvious defect. Based on the data above, what are the simplest things you could do to try to restore the ability of clone 1, 2, and 3 to proliferate?

5. An infection usually elicits both an immune response and a localized inflammatory response at the site of the infection. An effective inflammatory response requires differentiation and proliferation of various nonlymphoid white blood cells. Explain how hematopoiesis in the bone marrow is induced by an infection.

6. The discovery of two general types of cell lines paved the way for biochemical isolation and purification of cytokines and the subsequent cloning of cytokine genes. What are the unique properties of these cell lines? Why have these cell lines been so important in cytokine research?

Clone	Proliferation	IL-2 release	IL-2 binding	Anti-TAC stain
1	−	+	Little or none	−
2	−	+	Low affinity $(K = 10^{-8}\,M)$	+
3	−	−	High affinity $(K = 10^{-11}\,M)$	+
Control	+	+	High affinity $(K = 10^{-11}\,M)$	+

Generation of the Humoral Immune Response

The humoral immune response, which is uniquely adapted to the elimination of extracellular pathogens, is characterized by the production of large numbers of antibody molecules specific for antigenic determinants (epitopes) on a foreign pathogen. The potential diversity generated by this branch of the immune system can provide $\sim 10^8–10^{11}$ different antigen-binding specificities. This enormous antigen-binding diversity is coupled with conservation of constant-region sequences, which confer biological effector functions on antibody molecules. These effector functions facilitate effective elimination of foreign pathogens from a host animal.

Antibodies protect the host in a variety of ways: antibodies can activate the complement system, resulting in lysis of the microorganism; antibodies serve as opsonins, enhancing phagocytosis of the microorganism; antibodies bind to bacterial toxins and neutralize their toxicity; antibodies bind to viruses and inhibit their ability to infect host cells; antibodies at mucous membrane surfaces bind to potential pathogens and prevent colonization; antibodies bind to Fc receptors on NK cells or macrophages in ADCC, conferring specificity for antigen on these otherwise nonspecific cells.

The significant role of humoral immunity in host defense is highlighted by individuals born with humoral immunodeficiencies. Such individuals suffer recurrent bacterial infections, which can become so severe that bacteremia, meningitis, or cellulitis develop, often with life-threatening consequences. Recurrent or chronic gastrointestinal infection is also common in patients with humoral immunodeficiencies; these can result in malabsorption of nutrients, leading to malnutrition.

The primary focus of this chapter is the cellular interactions involved in generation of an effective immune response. As discussed briefly in previous chapters, this process requires the participation of macrophages, activated T_H cells, and, of course, B cells (see Figure 1-13). The macrophage serves as an antigen-presenting cell required for activation of the T_H cell. Interaction between an antigen-specific T_H cell and a complex of antigen–class II MHC on a macrophage, along with IL-1, leads to activation and proliferation of the T_H cell. The B cell also serves as an antigen-presenting cell for the T_H cell. Unlike the macrophage which phagocytoses antigen nonspecifically, the B cell recognizes antigen specifically by its membrane immunoglobulin receptor and then internalizes the antigen through receptor-mediated endocytosis. The antigen is then processed and presented together with the class II MHC molecule on the membrane of the B cell. The activated antigen-specific T_H cell can then interact with the B cell via a trimolecular complex involving the T-cell receptor and processed antigen + class II MHC on the membrane of the B cell. This interaction releases cytokines from the T_H cell in localized concentrations necessary for the activation, proliferation, and differentiation of the B cell into antibody-secreting plasma cells and memory cells.

Kinetics of the Humoral Response

The maturation of B cells during hematopoiesis in the bone marrow is marked by the ordered progression of immunoglobulin variable-region gene rearrangements (see Figure 8-19). The outcome of this process is the generation of mature, immunocompetent B cells, all expressing IgM and IgD membrane-bound antibodies specific for a single epitope. These mature, immunocompetent B cells migrate from the bone marrow to the peripheral lymphoid organs. If a B cell encounters the antigen for which its membrane IgM and IgD are specific, the cell will be activated and will undergo clonal proliferation and differentiation. Within 24 h of activation, a B cell enlarges into a lymphoblast (see Figure 3-9), replicates its DNA, and then divides. Eight or nine rounds of cell division follow, each with an average cell-cycle time of about 12–15h. Either direct T_H-cell interaction or indirect T_H-cell participation in the form of soluble cytokines is required for these successive rounds of cell division, which culminate in differentiation of the activated B cell into plasma and memory cells. If a B cell does not encounter the antigen for which it is specific, the cell dies within a few days. Of the $\sim 10^8$ B cells in mouse peripheral lymphoid organs, nearly 90% die within a few days (Figure 12-1). These cells are continuously replaced by new virgin B cells produced in the bone marrow at the rate of about 2×10^7 immunocompetent B cells per day.

Primary Response

The first contact of an individual with an antigen generates a primary immune response, characterized by the production of antibody-secreting plasma cells and memory B cells. The kinetics of the primary response, as measured by serum antibody level, vary depending on the nature of the antigen, the route of antigen administration, the presence or absence of adjuvants, and the species or strain being immunized. The response is characterized by a lag phase, during which the B cells undergo clonal selection in response to the antigen and differentiate into plasma cells and memory cells (Figure 12-2). The lag phase is followed by a logarithmic increase in serum antibody level, which reaches a peak, plateaus for a variable time, and then declines. In the case of an antigen such as sheep red blood cells (SRBCs), the lag phase lasts 3–4 days; peak plasma-cell levels are attained within 4–5 days; and peak serum antibody levels are attained by 5–7 days. This time frame allows eight or nine successive cell divisions within the 4- to 5-day period generating plasma and memory cells. For soluble protein antigens the lag phase is a little longer, often lasting about a week, and peak plasma-cell levels are attained by 9–10 days. During a primary humoral response, IgM is secreted initially, often followed by IgG. Depending on the persistence of the antigen, a primary response can last for varying periods, sometimes only a few days and sometimes several weeks.

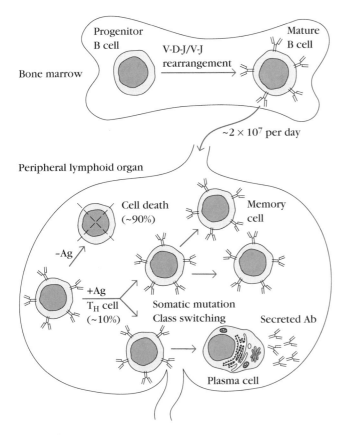

Figure 12-1 Schematic diagram of possible B-cell differentiation pathways. Random gene rearrangements of the immunoglobulin genes occurs during B-cell maturation in the bone marrow. Approximately 2×10^7 mature B cells leave the bone marrow each day. These mature B cells are carried to various peripheral lymphoid organs. In the absence of antigen activation, peripheral B cells have a short lifespan and die. In the presence of antigen and activated T_H cells, the B cells differentiate. As discussed later, somatic mutation combined with selective activation by antigen drives the response toward production of higher-affinity antibodies.

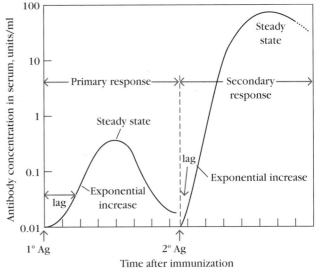

Figure 12-2 Serum antibody concentrations following primary or secondary immunization with antigen. The antibody concentrations are plotted on a logarithmic scale. The time units are not specified because the kinetics differ with the type of antigen, the route of administration, the presence or absence of adjuvants, and the species or strain of animal.

Secondary Response

The memory B cells formed during a primary response stop dividing and enter the G_0 phase of the cell cycle. These cells have variable lifespans, and some persist for the life of the individual. The existence of long-lived memory B cells accounts for a phenomenon called "original antigenic sin," which was first observed when the antibody response to influenza vaccines was monitored. Monitoring revealed that immunization with an influenza vaccine of one strain elicited an antibody response to that strain but, paradoxically, also elicited an antibody response of greater magnitude to another influenza strain that the individual had been exposed to during childhood. It was as if the memory of the first antigen exposure had left a life-long imprint on the immune system. This phenomenon can be explained by the presence of a memory-cell population, elicited by the influenza strain encountered in childhood, that is activated by cross-reacting epitopes on the vaccine strain. This process, then generates a secondary-level response, characterized by antibodies with higher affinity for the earlier viral strain.

The capacity to develop a secondary response depends on the existence of a population of memory B cells and memory T cells. Antigen activation of these memory cells results in a secondary antibody response that can be distinguished from the primary response in several ways: The response occurs more rapidly, reaches a greater magnitude, and lasts for a longer duration (see Figure 12-2). In addition, the secondary response is characterized by secretion of antibody with a higher affinity for the antigen and includes a variety of isotypes in addition to IgM. The fact that there are more memory B cells specific for the given antigen than there were virgin B cells in the primary response accounts, in part, for some of these differences (Table 12-1). It is not uncommon for a secondary response to generate antibody levels 100 to 1000 times higher than the levels attained in the primary response. The higher levels of antibody coupled with the overall higher affinity provide an effective host defense against reinfection. In addition, the change in isotype that occurs in the secondary response provides antibodies whose biological effector functions are particularly suited to eliminate a given pathogen.

Table 12-1 Comparison of primary and secondary antibody responses

Property	Primary response	Secondary response
Responding B cell	Naive "virgin" B cell	Memory B cell
Lag period following antigen administration	Generally 4–7 days	Generally 1–3 days
Magnitude of peak antibody response	7–10 days Varies depending on antigen	3–5 days Generaly 100–1000 times higher than primary response
Isotype produced	IgM predominates early in the response	IgG predominates
Antigens	Thymus-dependent and thymus-independent	Thymus-dependent
Antibody affinity	Lower	Higher

Experimental Systems

Studies of the cellular interactions required to generate a humoral immune response and of various factors that influence the response have depended on in vitro systems for generating the response and assay methods for measuring it.

In Vitro Generation of the Humoral Response

Analysis of the cellular interactions involved in the generation of the humoral response advanced with the development of in vitro culture systems by Robert Mishell and Richard Dutton and by J. Marbrook in the 1960s. In the Mishell-Dutton system, spleen cells are grown under low oxygen tension and with gentle agitation in tissue-culture media supplemented with fetal bovine serum to provide essential growth factors. Addition of SRBC antigen to the culture induces B-cell proliferation and differentiation into plasma cells. As will be seen, this system played an important role in clarifying the cellular interactions involved in the humoral response. Today the Mishell-Dutton culture technique continues to be used with minor modifications including the use of small microcultures.

In the Marbrook system, as in the Mishell-Dutton system, spleen cells are cultured in tissue-culture medium supplemented with fetal bovine serum. The culture conditions, however, differ from those of the Mishell-Dutton system in that the cells and antigen are placed in a tube that is separated from a larger flask containing the tissue-culture medium by a semipermeable membrane. The membrane enables nutrients to diffuse into the tube containing the cells and allows waste and metabolites to diffuse out where they are diluted in the larger container of media.

Hemolytic Plaque Assay

For many years the humoral immune response could be monitored only by quantifying antibody production. Development of the hemolytic plaque assay, by N. K. Jerne, A. A. Nordin, and C. Henry, permitted researchers to determine the number of plasma cells. This assay and its various modifications have played a significant role in studies of the humoral response.

The hemolytic plaque assay is similar in principle to the viral plaque assay. The original direct assay is used to measure plasma-cell numbers in mice primed with SRBCs. Spleen cells from primed mice are mixed in warm, melted agar with an excess of SRBCs (Figure 12-3a). The agar containing the cell suspension is poured into a Petri dish, whose bottom is covered with a layer of hard agar, and allowed to cool and solidify. The splenic lymphocytes thus are immobilized in the agar, surrounded by a sea of SRBCs. The Petri dish is incubated for 1 h at 37° C, during which time antibody secreted by plasma cells diffuses into the agar matrix and binds to the SRBCs in the vicinity of each antibody-secreting plasma cell. Guinea pig serum containing complement is then added. The complement reacts with the antibody bound to the SRBCs and mediates their lysis, leaving each plasma cell surrounded by a clear plaque

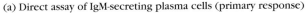

(a) Direct assay of IgM-secreting plasma cells (primary response)

(b) Indirect assay of IgM-and IgG-secreting plasma cells (secondary response)

(c) Direct assay for plasma cells secreting anti-DNP Ab

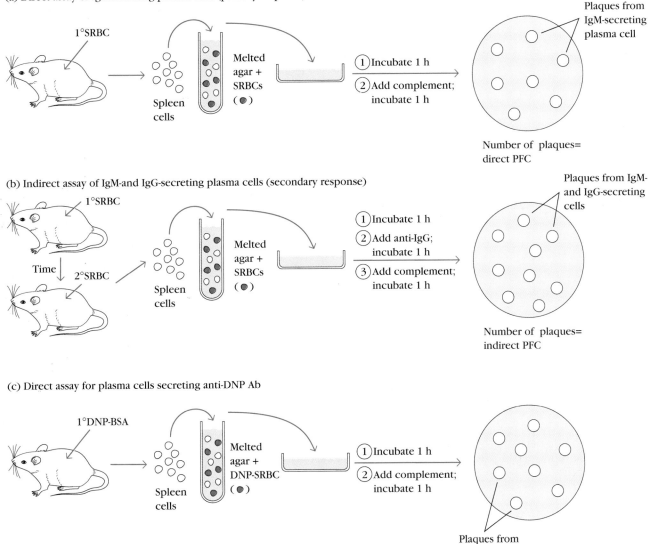

Figure 12-3 Hemolytic plaque assays. (a) A direct assay detects IgM-secreting plasma cells, which are predominant in a primary response. (b) In an indirect assay, which detects both IgM- and IgG-secreting plasma cells, antibodies against mouse IgG are added so that complement-mediated lysis of IgG-SRBC complexes will occur. By subtracting the direct PFC from the indirect PFC, the number of IgG-secreting plasma cells can be determined. In a secondary response, the indirect PFC is high and the direct PFC is low. (c) The response to immunization with antigens other than SRBCs can be determined with the hemolytic plaque assay if the immunizing protein or hapten is coupled with SRBCs.

devoid of cells (Figure 12-4). The plaques are counted, and their number is the number of plaque-forming plasma cells specific for the SRBC antigen, referred to as direct plaque-forming cells (PFC).

The hemolytic plaque assay can be adapted to determine the number of IgM-secreting plasma cells and IgG-secreting plasma cells. In the case of IgM, complement-mediated lysis is triggered by the binding of a single pentameric IgM molecule to an SRBC. However, in the case of IgG, which exists as a monomer, complement-

mediated lysis does not occur unless the Fc regions from two IgG molecules are located within 30–40 nm of each other on the membrane of an SRBC. (As discussed in Chapter 15, complement binds to the Fc region of antibody molecules.) Such close proximity of two IgG molecules does not normally result from the random binding of IgG secreted by a single plasma cell. Therefore a secondary anti-isotype antibody that reacts with the bound IgG is added to the Petri dish after the first hour of incubation and the complement is added after another

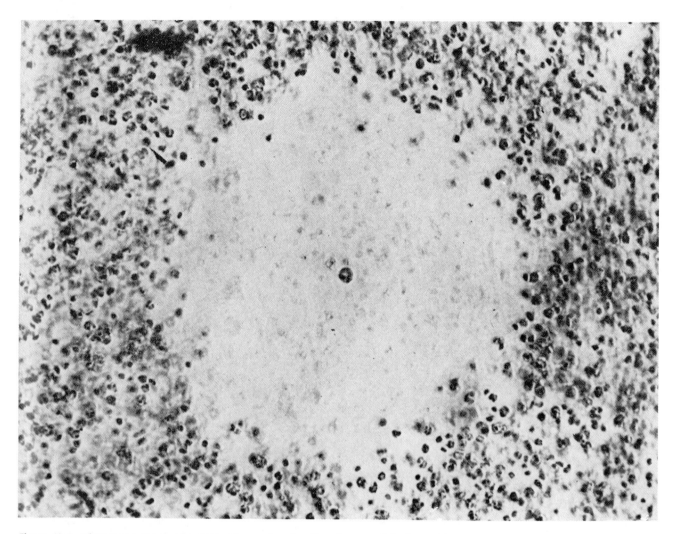

Figure 12-4 Photomicrograph of a single plaque showing the plasma cell in the center surrounded by an area of lysed SRBCs. Unlysed SRBCs are at the perimeter of the plaque. [From N. K. Jerne, 1973. The immune system. *Sci. Am.* **229**:53.]

hour (Figure 12-3b). This procedure, called the indirect hemolytic plaque assay, results in lysis of SRBCs to which IgM or IgG are bound. Subtraction of the number of plaques formed in the direct assay from the number formed in the indirect assay gives the number of IgG-secreting plasma cells, or indirect PFC. Since most of the antibody secreted during a primary response is IgM, the direct PFC is high and the indirect PFC is low. In contrast, a secondary response leads to a low direct PFC and a high indirect PFC, reflecting the switch from IgM to IgG secretion.

The hemolytic plaque assay also can be modified to quantitate plasma cells secreting antibodies specific for proteins, polysaccharides, or small haptens. In this case, the animal is immunized with the desired antigen, but before the SRBCs are mixed with the isolated spleen cells, they are coated with the immunizing antigen. The

induced antibody binds to these antigen-coated SRBCs, which are lysed when complement is added (Figure 12-3c). Uncoated SRBCs can serve as a control, since they do not lyse in response to antibody secreted from the antigen-specific plasma cells.

Recently a modification of the Jerne plaque-forming assay, called the "Elispot assay," has been developed that allows plasma cells to be quantitated without requiring SRBCs. In this modification the antigen-primed lymphocytes are incubated on a Petri dish to which antigen has been bound. As the plasma cells secrete antibody, it binds to antigen in the vicinity of the plasma cell. The bound antibody is then visualized after removal of the cells by an ELISA assay in which the dish is first incubated with enzyme-labeled anti-Ig followed by an appropriate substrate. The enzyme-substrate reaction produces a colored spot, allowing ennumeration of plasma cells.

Thymus-Independent Antigens

Most antigens that elicit a humoral immune response are thymus-dependent, because T_H-cell participation is required if they are to activate B cells. Some antigens, however, can activate B cells without the assistance of T_H cells. Included within this category of thymus-independent antigens are polymerized bacterial flagellin, lipopolysaccharide (LPS) derived from gram-negative bacterial cell walls, dextran, pneumococcal capsular polysaccharide, levan, polyvinylpyrrolidone, and ficoll.

Thymus-independent antigens have various properties in common. Many are polysaccharides and therefore cannot be displayed as peptides together with class II MHC on the membrane of the B cell. In addition, many have a polymeric structure with repeating epitopes, and many are resistant to degradation. Their polymeric structure may facilitate the cross-linkage of antigen-binding receptors on the B-cell membrane that is required for activation. Some thymus-independent antigens, at high doses, act as mitogens and are able to induce nonspecific B-cell activation, giving rise to a polyclonal response that bypasses the normal T_H-cell requirement for activation. A possible explanation of this phenomenon is that at high doses enough nonspecific binding occurs to result in polyclonal activation, whereas at lower doses only those B cells with specific receptors for a thymus-independent antigen bind enough of the antigen to be activated. These bacterial antigens induce a humoral antibody response characterized primarily by the production of IgM. Because the response to these bacterial antigens is independent of T cells, individuals born with various T-cell deficiencies generally are immune to many bacterial pathogens. Instead these individuals succumb to infection by viruses, fungi, or other pathogens capable of intracellular growth (see Chapter 20).

The humoral immune response to thymus-independent antigens is different from the response to thymus-dependent antigens. The response is generally weaker, no memory cells are formed, and only IgM is secreted. These differences highlight the important role played by the T_H-cell in generating memory B cells and in class switching to other isotypes.

Identification of Cells Required for Induction of Humoral Immunity

Experiments conducted in the 1960s and 1970s demonstrated that several types of cells must cooperate to generate a humoral immune response. Even before B and T cells were clearly defined, evidence that distinct subpopulations are required to generate an antibody response came from adoptive-transfer experiments done by Henry Claman and his co-workers in 1966. Lethally x-irradiated mice were reconstituted with syngeneic thymus cells alone, with bone marrow cells alone, or with a mixture of thymus and bone marrow cells. The mice were then immunized with SRBCs and their serum anti-SRBC levels were determined. Mice reconstituted with either thymus cells or bone marrow cells alone failed to produce any anti-SRBC antibodies, but mice reconstituted with both thymus and bone marrow cells generated a response. This early experiment demonstrated that both bone marrow cells and thymus cells were necessary for induction of the humoral response.

The development of the Mishell-Dutton in vitro culture system allowed Don Mosier to identify still another cell population required for induction of the humoral response. When spleen cells are grown in the Mishell-Dutton system, the macrophages adhere to the surface of the culture dish, whereas the lymphocytes do not. Mosier thus was able to separate macrophages from lymphocytes by carefully decanting the culture medium containing the nonadherent cells into a separate culture disk. He then determined the response of the adherent and nonadherent cells to SRBCs in the direct hemolytic plaque assay. Neither the adherent nor the nonadherent cells alone exhibited a plaque-forming response to SRBCs, but when the two populations were combined, the plaque-forming response was evident. This experiment gave the first indication that macrophages, as well as lymphocytes, are involved in generation of the humoral response.

Claman's experiments showed that both thymus and bone marrow cells are necessary to generate a humoral antibody response, but they did not identify which population produced antibodies. A now classical experiment by G. Mitchell and J. F. A. P. Miller in 1968 demonstrated that bone marrow cells were the source of antibody-producing cells. Using an adoptive-transfer system similar to that of Claman, lethally x-irradiated and thymectomized mice were reconstituted with various populations of cells and immunized with SRBC, after which the spleen cells were assayed for plaque formation (PFC) in response to SRBC. (Instead of thymus cells, Mitchell and Miller used thoracic-duct lymphocytes as an enriched source of T cells.) They showed that the duct cells and bone marrow cells in combination could generate the PFC response, confirming Claman's findings. Then they went one step further to identify the antibody-producing population by repeating the experiment with thoracic-duct lymphocytes and bone marrow cells of different MHC haplotypes. In this case, they reconstituted mice with thoracic-duct cells expressing one MHC molecule and bone marrow cells expressing another MHC molecule. With antisera specific for each MHC molecule, they could then selectively remove the thoracic duct–or bone marrow–derived population from the isolated spleen cells and determine the effect on the plaque-forming ability of the spleen cells. When reconstitution was tried initially with cells from two different allogeneic strains, no SRBC-specific plasma cells were generated. Although this finding was puzzling at the time, it made sense once the self-MHC restriction of T_H cells was demonstrated (see Figure 10-1). Mitchell and Miller then tried using semi-allogeneic cells to reconstitute thymectomized and lethally irradiated CBA(H-2^k) mice, as outlined in Figure 12-5. The mice were then reconstituted with CBA (H-2^k) bone marrow and F1 (CBA × C57BI) (H-2$^{k/b}$) thoracic-duct cells. The reconstituted mice were challenged with SRBC and after 5

days the spleen cells were assayed for PFC to SRBC. The spleen cells from these mice gave a good PFC response to the SRBC. By treating the spleen cells with antibody to the H-2^k or H-2^b MHC molecules in the presence of complement, it was possible to deplete the two populations selectively and determine the effect of each depletion on the PFC response to SRBC. Removal of H-2^k cells removed both populations and abolished the response. However, removal of the H-2^b thoracic-duct population did not affect the response. These results demonstrated that the bone marrow population, now known to contain B cells, supplied the antibody-forming cells and that the thoracic-duct population provided helper cells for generating the humoral response.

Use of Hapten-Carrier Conjugates to Study Cellular Interactions

The discovery of haptens and their use in studying antigenicity was described in Chapter 4. When animals are immunized with small organic compounds (*haptens*) conjugated to large proteins (*carriers*), the conjugate induces a humoral immune response with antibodies formed both to hapten epitopes and to unaltered epitopes on the carrier protein. Since the chemical conjugation allows multiple molecules of a single hapten to be coupled to the carrier protein and since the position of the hapten is easily accessible to the B cell's membrane-bound antibody, the hapten functions as the immunodominant B-cell epitope (see Figure 4-12). Such hapten-carrier conjugates provided immunologists with an ideal system for studying cellular interactions involved in the humoral response. Unlike complex proteins, whose B-cell epitopes are often conformational sequences dependent on the tertiary structure of the protein, a hapten constitutes a defined B-cell epitope that can be presented to B cells on different protein carriers. It was with hapten-carrier conjugates that immunologists were able to determine that the generation of a humoral antibody response requires associative recognition by T_H cells and B cells, each recognizing different epitopes on the same antigen.

A variety of different hapten-carrier conjugates have been used in immunologic research (Table 12-2). After an animal has been immunized with a hapten-carrier conjugate, the humoral response to the hapten is assessed with a modified hemolytic plaque assay, with hapten-conjugated SRBCs as the indicator cells (see Figure 12-3c). A direct hemolytic plaque assay is used to quantitate plasma cells secreting IgM antihapten antibody and an indirect assay is used to quantitate plasma cells secreting IgG antihapten antibody, an indicator of a secondary response.

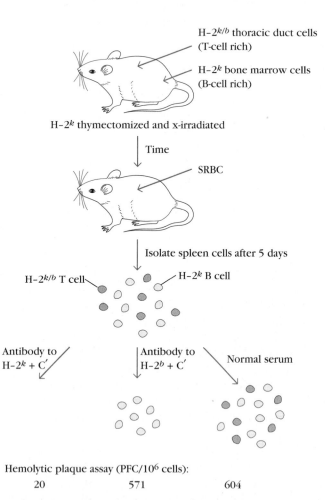

Figure 12-5 In the experimental system of Miller and Mitchell H-2^k thymectomized and X-irradiated mice were reconstituted with F$_1$ H-2$^{k/b}$ thoracic-duct lymphocytes and H-2^k bone marrow cells. The mice were challenged with SRBCs, and 5 days later the spleen cells were treated with antibody to H-2^k or H-2^b MHC antigens + complement (C). Removal of H-2^k-bearing cells eliminated the PFC response, whereas removal of H-2^b-bearing cells had no significant effect. This experiment demonstrated that bone marrow cells contain the antibody-forming population now known to be B cells.

Table 12-2 Common hapten-carrier conjugates used in immunologic research

Carrier acronym	Hapten	Carrier protein
DNP-BGG	Dinitrophenol	Bovine gamma-globulin
TNP-BSA	Trinitrophenyl	Bovine serum albumin
NIP-KLH	5-Nitrophenyl acetic acid	Keyhole limpet hemocyanin
ARS-OVA	Azophenylarsonale	Ovalbumin
LAC-HGG	Phenyllactoside	Human gamma-globulin

Table 12-3 Secondary humoral response to DNP in mice immunized with various combinations of DNP and carrier protein

Primary immunization	Secondary immunization	Secondary anti-DNP PFC
DNP − BSA	DNP − BSA	(+)
DNP + BSA	DNP + BSA	(−)
DNP − BSA	DNP + BSA	(−)
DNP − BSA	DNP − BGG	(−)
DNP − BSA + BGG	DNP − BGG	(+)

* Following the secondary immunization, spleen cells were isolated and an indirect hemolytic plaque assay was performed to determine the secondary anti-DNP PFC, using DNP-SRBCs as the indicator cells.

Recognition of Carrier Epitopes by T_H Cells

The results of early experiments using hapten-carrier conjugates to study induction of the humoral immune response were puzzling. Eventually, however, a model of T-cell and B-cell collaboration was formulated, providing a framework in which the results could be understood.

One of the earliest findings with hapten-carrier conjugates was that a hapten had to be chemically coupled to a larger carrier molecule to induce a humoral response to the hapten. If an animal was immunized with both hapten and carrier separately, no plaque-forming cells specific for the hapten were generated. A second important observation was that in order to generate a secondary plaque-forming response to a hapten, the animal had to be immunized with the same hapten-carrier conjugate used for the primary immunization. If the secondary immunization was with the same hapten but conjugated to a different, unrelated carrier, no secondary antihapten response occurred. This phenomenon, called the *carrier effect*, could be circumvented by priming the animal separately with the unrelated carrier (Table 12-3).

By repeating these experiments with an adoptive-transfer system, it was possible to demonstrate that hapten-primed cells and carrier-primed cells were distinct populations. In these experiments one mouse was primed with the DNP-BSA conjugate and another was primed with the unrelated carrier BGG, which was not conjugated to the hapten. Spleen cells from both mice were mixed and injected into a lethally irradiated syngeneic recipient. When this mouse was now challenged with DNP conjugated to the unrelated carrier BGG, there was a secondary antihapten response, as indicated by a positive hemolytic plaque assay to DNP (Figure 12-6a). Spleen cells from the BGG-immunized mice then were treated with anti-T-cell antiserum (anti-Thy-1) and complement to remove the T cells. When this T-cell–depleted sample was mixed with the DNP-BSA–primed spleen cells and injected into an irradiated mouse, no secondary antihapten response was observed. However, similar treatment of the DNP-BSA–primed spleen cells did not abolish the secondary antihapten response (Figure 12-6b,c). Later experiments, in which antisera were used to specifically deplete $CD4^+$ or $CD8^+$ T cells, showed that the removal of the $CD4^+$ T-cell subpopulation primed with the second carrier abolished the carrier effect. These experiments demonstrate that the response of hapten-primed B cells to the hapten-carrier conjugate requires the presence of carrier-primed $CD4^+$ T_H cells specific for carrier epitopes. (It is important to keep in mind that the B-cell response is not limited to the hapten determinant; in fact some B cells do react to epitopes on the carrier, but because the assay system uses hapten-conjugated SRBCs, it measures only the antihapten response.)

Because of the carrier effect, a secondary antihapten response normally occurs only if an animal has previously been primed both to the hapten and to the carrier epitopes. Under unusual experimental conditions it is possible to bypass the carrier effect by using allogeneic T cells in place of carrier-primed T cells. The allogeneic T cells recognize the MHC molecules displayed on B cells as foreign, enabling the allogeneic T cells to bind to B cells, resulting in localized cytokine production. These cytokines enable a B cell to be activated in the absence of a carrier-primed T cell. This phenomenon is called the *allogeneic effect*.

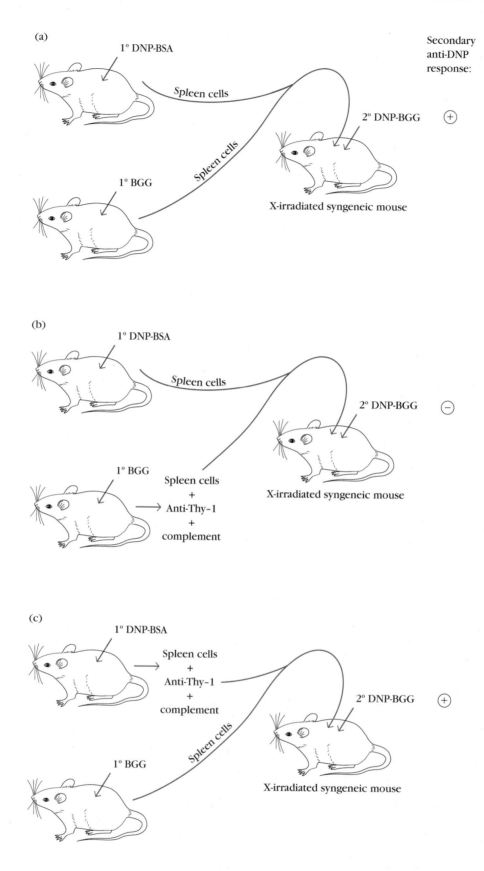

(a)

1° DNP-BSA

Spleen cells

Spleen cells

1° BGG

2° DNP-BGG

Secondary anti-DNP response:

(+)

X-irradiated syngeneic mouse

(b)

1° DNP-BSA

Spleen cells

1° BGG

Spleen cells
+
Anti-Thy–1
+
complement

2° DNP-BGG

(−)

X-irradiated syngeneic mouse

(c)

1° DNP-BSA

Spleen cells
+
Anti-Thy–1
+
complement

1° BGG

Spleen cells

2° DNP-BGG

(+)

X-irradiated syngeneic mouse

MHC Restriction in the Interaction between T_H and B Cells

Hapten-carrier systems enabled immunologists to explore various parameters affecting the collaborative response of hapten-primed B cells and carrier-primed T_H cells. Experiments by D. H. Katz and B. Benacerraf were designed to explore the influence of the MHC on the collaboration of T_H and B cells in a hapten-carrier system. The basic question they sought to answer was whether carrier-primed T cells of one MHC haplotype could cooperate with hapten-primed B cells of another MHC haplotype. To answer this question they carried out adoptive transfer of BGG-primed T cells from strain A mice into an A × B F_1 recipient, followed by the transfer of DNP-KLH–primed B cells derived from strain A or strain B mice. The mice then were immunized with DNP-BGG, and the secondary response to DNP was assessed.

One complication of this experimental design, which initially made the experiment unworkable, was the al-

logeneic effect. The transferred strain A T cells recognized the strain B allogeneic MHC antigens of the F_1 host as foreign and therefore activated the host B cells nonspecifically, making it impossible to assess the response to DNP-BGG. In order to circumvent this complication, Katz and Benacerraf exploited a previous observation that primed T cells were less susceptible to x-irradiation than unprimed T cells. Irradiation of the F_1 A × B recipient 24 h after the transfer of the BGG-primed strain A T cells eliminated the alloreactive T cells but not the BGG-primed T cells. Strain A or strain B B cells from DNP-KLH–primed mice could now be transferred into the F_1 recipient, and the secondary response to DNP-BGG could be measured (Figure 12-7).

The results revealed that carrier-primed T_H cells could assist only hapten-primed B cells sharing the same MHC haplotype. Later experiments with congenic recombinant strains revealed that allelic identity at either IA or IE MHC subregions was necessary for collaboration between T_H and B cells.

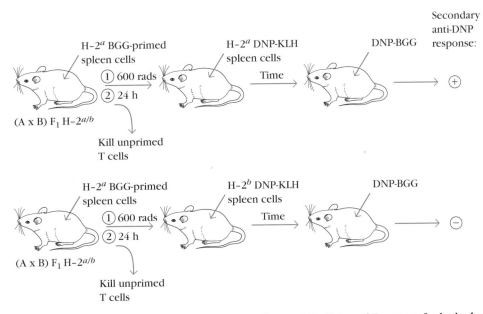

Figure 12-6 Adoptive-transfer experiments demonstrating that hapten-primed and carrier-primed cells are separate populations. (a) X-irradiated syngeneic mice reconstituted with spleen cells from both DNP-BSA–primed mice and BGG-primed mice and challenged with DNP-BGG generated a secondary anti-DNP response. (b) Removal of T cells from the BGG-primed spleen cells, by treatment with anti-Thy-1 antiserum, abolished the secondary anti-DNP response. (c) Removal of T cells from the DNP-BSA–primed spleen cells had no effect on the secondary response to DNP. These experiments show that carrier-primed cells are T cells and hapten-primed cells are B cells. The secondary anti-DNP response was measured with an indirect hemolytic plaque assay.

Figure 12-7 Katz and Benacerraf asked whether carrier primed T_H cells of one MHC haplotype could cooperate with hapten primed B cells of another MHC haplotype. F_1 (A × B) strain mice were reconstituted with strain A spleen cells from a BGG-primed animal. In order to reduce non-specific T-cell activation by allogeneic MHC expressed by the F_1 host, the adoptive recipients were X-irradiated with 600 rads. This amount of radiation had previously been shown to kill unprimed T cells but not primed T cells. In this way only the BGG-primed T cells survived. The mice were then reconstituted with strain A or strain B spleen cells from a DNP-KLH–primed mouse, and the antibody response to DNP-BGG was measured. The results revealed that the carrier-primed T_H cell and hapten-primed B cell must share the same MHC haplotype.

Associative Recognition

The experiments with hapten-carrier conjugates revealed that both T_H cells and B cells must recognize antigenic determinants on the same molecule for B-cell activation to occur. This feature of the T- and B-cell interaction in the humoral response is called *associative*, or *linked, recognition*. The conclusions drawn from hapten-carrier experiments apply generally to the humoral response. In the case of a protein such as BSA, for example, a B-cell response to epitopes on the BSA molecule takes place only if there is associative recognition by a T_H cell that is specific for distinctly different epitopes on the BSA molecule.

Early models of associative recognition based on hapten-carrier experiments envisioned a B cell binding to the hapten and a T cell binding to carrier epitopes, with the hapten-carrier conjugate serving to bridge the two cells (Figure 12-8a). Activation of the B cell was hypothesized to result from membrane interactions between the T_H and B cell and/or from the high localized concentrations of lymphokines released by the T_H cell at the junction of the interacting cells. The discovery of MHC restriction in this process meant that this simple hapten-carrier-bridge model was not sufficient and that any model of associative recognition must include a role for class II MHC molecules. That role was made clear with the discovery that B cells, like macrophages, are antigen-presenting cells. Unlike the macrophage, the B cell is antigen-specific and binds a hapten-carrier conjugate via its membrane-bound antibody. After binding, the hapten-carrier conjugate is internalized, processed in an endosomal processing pathway, and presented as a processed peptide together with a class II MHC molecule on the membrane of the B cell (Figure 12-8b). Because MHC molecules bind small peptides, often with amphipathic properties, internal peptides of the carrier are generally presented. A T_H cell recognizes the processed peptide together with the class II MHC molecule. The hapten-carrier systems highlight the important differences in epitope recognition by B and by T cells. The B cell recognizes the hapten determinant because it is accessible and hydrophilic, because it is of a size that occupies the immunoglobulin receptor, and because it is also present in multiple copies that make it the immunodominant B-cell epitope. T cells in contrast, recognize certain internal, hydrophobic residues of the carrier that are displayed following antigen processing (together with the class II MHC molecules) on the membrane of an antigen-presenting cell. B-cell activation results from membrane-mediated events and the localized release of cytokines, which together drive the B cell to proliferate and differentiate.

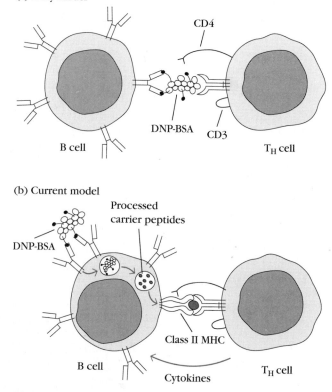

Figure 12-8 (a) Early models of associative recognition envisioned the B-cell binding to hapten determinants (black circles) and the T-cell binding to carrier determinants (open circles). In this model, MHC molecules were not involved. (b) The current model of associative recognition in which the B cell binds the hapten-carrier conjugate, internalizes and processes it, and presents carrier peptides (red circles) together with a class II MHC molecule on its membrane. The T_H cell recognizes this processed peptide together with the class II MHC molecule.

Steps in B-Cell Activation, Proliferation, and Differentiation

Activation of a B cell requires a number of sequential processes: (1) presentation of processed antigen + a class II MHC molecule by the B cell to an activated T_H cell specific for that antigen; (2) formation of a T_H-cell/B-cell conjugate involving the T-cell receptor (TCR) and antigen + MHC complex on the B-cell membrane; (3) directional release of cytokines by the T_H cell; and (4) generation of signals, by membrane-mediated events and localized cytokines, that are transduced in the B cell, causing changes in gene expression that lead to proliferation and differentiation of the B cell. The experimental demonstration of these processes and the mechanisms involved are described in this section.

Antigen Presentation by B Cells

The first experimental evidence demonstrating that B cells were major antigen-presenting cells came from an experiment of Robert Chesnut and Howard Grey in 1981. Up to that time, it had been impossible to compare the antigen-presenting capabilities of macrophages with those of B cells because macrophages take up antigen nonspecifically through phagocytosis, whereas B cells take up antigen specifically by Ig receptor-mediated endocytosis. Less than 1 B cell in 10,000 is specific for a given antigen, and it was not possible to study the response of such a small minority of antigen-presenting cells.

Chesnut and Grey bypassed this difficulty by using as the antigen rabbit antibody against mouse immunoglobulin. They chose this antigen because it binds to the Ig receptors on all B cells. This antigen binds to the Fc portion of the B-cell Ig receptors, not to the usual antigen-binding sites in the Fab portion. Nonetheless, the rabbit anti-mouse Ig is endocytosed and processed by mouse B cells like any antigen, and the processed peptides are presented with class II MHC molecules on the B-cell membrane (Figure 12-9). Using this experimental system, Chesnut and Grey showed that B cells were just as effective as macrophages in presenting antigen to T$_H$ cells.

Experiments with other systems involving antigen-specific B-cell lines have confirmed the results of Chesnut and Grey and have extended these results by showing that internalization of antigen by B cells generally requires binding of the antigen to the Ig receptor. In some cases, however, this requirement for antigen binding can be bypassed by incubating B cells in extremely high (nonphysiologic) concentrations of a particular antigen. Such *antigen-pulsed* B cells take up the antigen nonspecifically by pinocytosis (see Figure 1-5), allowing antigen processing and presentation to occur.

In all of these B-cell experimental systems it takes 30–60 min following internalization for the processed antigen to be displayed on the membrane with class II MHC molecules. Presumably this is the time required for antigen processing and binding to MHC molecules within B cells. Antigen processing in B cells as in macrophages, can be inhibited by chloroquine, suggesting that the processing pathways may be similar in the two cell types. Because a B cell recognizes antigen specifically, by way of its membrane Ig receptor, a B cell is able to present antigen to T$_H$ cells at antigen concentrations that are 1000 times lower than what is required for macrophage presentation. When antigen concentrations are high, therefore, the macrophage serves as an effective antigen-presenting cell, but as antigen levels drop, the B cell takes over as the major presenter of antigen to T$_H$ cells.

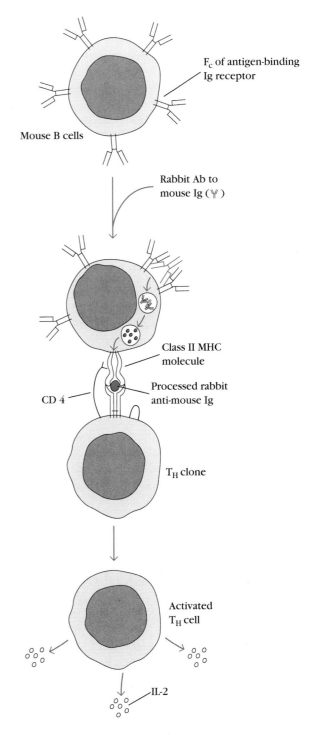

Figure 12-9 Unique experimental system used to demonstrate the antigen-binding ability of B cells. Rabbit antibody against mouse immunoglobulin binds to the Fc region of the Ig receptors on all B cells, not to specific antigen-binding sites present on just a few B cells. The rabbit anti-mouse Ig is internalized, processed, and presented like other antigens by the B cells. Addition of T$_H$ cells specific for the rabbit antibody resulted in T$_H$-cell activation, as measured by production of IL-2.

Formation of T$_H$-Cell–B-Cell Conjugate

Once a T$_H$ cell recognizes a processed antigen displayed by the class II MHC molecule on the membrane of a B cell, the two cells can interact, forming a T-B conjugate (Figure 12-10). Events occurring during this interaction were studied by observing the interaction of an antigen-specific T$_H$-cell line with antigen-pulsed B-cell hybridomas. The question asked was whether an antigen-specific T-B cell interaction would be qualitatively different from a nonspecific T-B interaction. T$_H$ cells specific for the antigen conalbumin presented on an IA^k antigen-presenting cell were incubated with either IA^k or IA^d conalbumin-pulsed B cells or with ovalbumin-pulsed IA^k B cells. Because the T$_H$ cells were MHC restricted for conalbumin and IA^k, only the conalbumin-pulsed IA^k B cells were capable of an antigen-specific interaction with the T$_H$ cells; the conalbumin-pulsed IA^d B cells and ovalbumin-pulsed IA^k B cells were nonspecific controls. To enhance their interaction, the cells were lightly pelleted by low-speed centrifugation. The pelleted cells were then gently resuspended and the interacting cell conjugates were observed in an electron microscope. Micrographs of the T-B conjugates revealed that the antigen-specific conjugates appeared to have a greater area of membrane contact than the nonspecific conjugates. What was most interesting was that the T$_H$ cells in antigen-specific conjugates exhibited a reorganization of the Golgi apparatus and the microtubular-

organizing center toward the junction with the B cell, whereas T$_H$ cells in nonspecific conjugates exhibited random orientation of the Golgi apparatus and microtubular-organizing centers. This reorganization of the Golgi apparatus may provide a mechanism for the directed release of cytokines toward the antigen-specific B cell.

Another qualitative difference between the antigen-specific T-B conjugates and the nonspecific ones is that the TCR, CD4, and LFA-1 molecules on the T$_H$-cell membrane become redistributed along the B-cell junction in antigen-specific conjugates. This clustering is seen only if the B cells are presenting both the antigen and the MHC molecule for which the T$_H$ cell is specific. Thus antigen-specific recognition, mediated by the T-cell receptor, influences the distribution of two important T$_H$-cell membrane proteins—LFA-1 and CD4—both of which are involved in cellular adhesion. As discussed in Chapter 3, LFA-1 is a member of the integrin family of receptors, which bind to intercellular adhesion molecules (ICAMs). In a T-B conjugate, LFA-1 and CD4 molecules on the T$_H$ cell bind to ICAM and class II MHC molecules on the B-cell membrane. It has been suggested that clustering of TCR, CD4, and LFA-1 molecules at the junction of an antigen-specific T-B conjugate may increase the avidity of the cellular interaction. This increased avidity would prolong the association between the T$_H$ cell and B cell, providing time for the directed secretion of various cytokines.

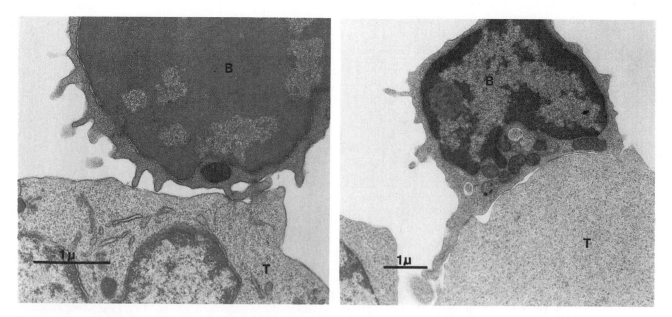

Figure 12-10   Transmission electron micrographs of T-B conjugates showing broad areas of membrane contact between the T and B cells. The bar = 1 μm. [From V. M. Sanders et al., 1986, *J. Immunol.* **137**:2395.]

Directional Release of Cytokines from T$_H$ Cells

The electron micrographs of T-B conjugates discussed in the previous section suggested that an antigen-specific interaction between T$_H$ and B cells induces a redistribution of T-cell membrane proteins and cytoskeletal elements that may result in the polarized release of lymphokines toward the interacting B cell. In an ingenious experiment, W. J. Poo and C. A. Janeway sought to determine whether cytokines are released from T$_H$ cells in a directional manner. They worked with a T$_H$-cell clone that secreted IL-4 in response to binding of a clonotypic monoclonal antibody specific for the idiotype of the T-cell receptor. This T$_H$ clone was centrifuged onto a nucleopore membrane having 3-μm pores. Since the cells were larger than 3 μm, they completely plugged the pores. The cell-packed membrane then was suspended between two chambers and monoclonal antibody specific for the T-cell receptor was added to one chamber. Measurement of IL-4 in both chambers showed that as long as low levels of antibody were used to activate the T$_H$ cells, IL-4 was released

toward the chamber containing the activating monoclonal antibody (Figure 12-11). These findings suggest that conjugate formation between antigen-specific T$_H$ and B cells results in directional release of cytokines toward the interacting B cell.

Signal Generation by Membrane Events and Cytokines

The collaborative interaction between antigen-specific T$_H$ cells and B cells ultimately results in B-cell activation, proliferation, and differentiation. Membrane events and cytokines appear to play different roles, depending on the activation state of the B cell. Resting B cells in the G$_0$ phase of the cell cycle appear to require antigen-induced receptor cross-linkage and direct T$_H$-membrane interaction. The receptor cross-linkage leads to internalization, processing, and presentation of antigen together with class II MHC molecules on the membrane of the B cell. If the antigen–class II MHC complex is recognized by an antigen-specific T$_H$ cell, a T-B conjugate is formed. The membrane events occurring during T-B

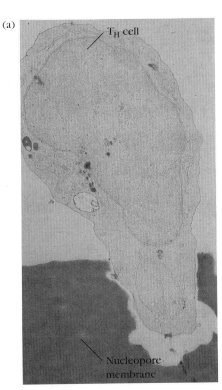
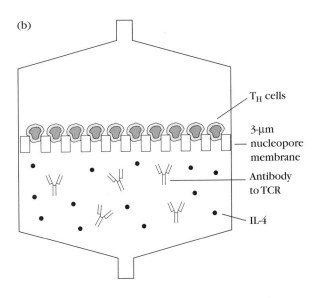

Figure 12-11 Experimental demonstration of directional release of lymphokines from T$_H$ cells. (a) Electron micrograph of T$_H$ cell centrifuged onto nucleopore membrane. Note how cell completely blocks the pore. (b) Diagram of culture system. Addition of monoclonal antibody specific for the idiotype of the T-cell receptors resulted in T$_H$-cell activation and release of IL-4 on one side of the membrane only. [From W. J. Poo et al., 1988, *Nature* **332**:378.]

conjugate formation and the relation of these events to activation signals are still largely unknown. As discussed briefly in Chapter 11, various cytokines secreted by the T_H cell act on the B cell to induce activation, proliferation, and differentiation. The nonspecific activity of cytokines can be reconciled with the highly specific nature of B-cell activation by the directional release of cytokines at the junction of conjugate formation as well as by the regulated expression of cytokine receptors only on antigen-activated B cells.

Membrane Signals

Antigen cross-linkage of the membrane IgM or IgD molecules on B cells has been shown to transmit a signal across the plasma membrane by inducing hydrolysis of phosphatidylinositol 4,5-biphosphate (PIP$_2$) to inositol 1,4,5-trisphosphate (IP$_3$) and diacylglycerol (DAG). By a pathway probably similar to that involved in T-cell activation (see Figure 10-10), IP$_3$ and DAG act as second messengers that either individually or synergistically induce a number of biochemical events eventually leading to changes in B-cell-gene expression. Because both membrane IgM and IgD receptors on the B cell extend into the cytoplasm by only three amino acids, it is thought that some other associated membrane molecule must transduce the signal from the immunoglobulin receptor into the cytoplasm. Recently a protein complex similar to the CD3 complex on the T cell has been shown to be associated with the membrane immunoglobulin receptor. This protein complex may function to transduce the signal from the immunoglobulin receptor in a manner analogous to CD3. A number of other B-cell membrane proteins may also be involved in transmembrane signaling. Cross-linkage of class II MHC molecules on the membrane of a B cell induces second messengers similar to those induced following membrane immunoglobulin cross-linkage. Thus a membrane signal may be transmitted through the class II MHC molecule as it presents antigen to a T_H cell in conjugate formation. Also, various membrane signals are induced by the binding of cytokines to their receptors. The nature of these signals and the relation of one signaling pathway to another will be an exciting area of research in the coming years.

Cytokine Signals

During activation, resting B cells in the G_0 state move into the S (DNA-synthesizing) phase of the cell cycle. This process requires two types of signals: (1) competence signals, which include antigen cross-linkage of membrane-bound IgM or IgD, co-stimulatory IL-1 and IL-4, and perhaps membrane signals associated with T-B conjugate formation; and (2) a progression signal, which is generated by interaction with IL-4 (Figure

12-12a). Subsequent to activation, additional growth factors stimulate the B cell to proliferate and differentiate.

Most of the cytokines involved in B-cell activation, proliferation, and differentiation are secreted by activated T_H cells, although IL-1 is secreted by activated macrophages. Both IL-1 and IL-4 act as co-stimulatory activation signals. Several T_H-cell lymphokines have multiple activities. For example, during activation IL-4 serves both as a competence signal and a progression signal. This cytokine also acts as a proliferation factor and differentiation factor. One of the changes observed early in B-cell activation, which is induced by IL-4, is an increase in the expression of class II MHC molecules and ICAMs on the B-cell membrane. This increase causes a B cell to function as a more effective antigen-presenting cell and increases the strength of the interaction with the T_H cell in conjugate formation.

A number of T_H-cell cytokines have been shown to act on activated B cells to induce proliferation and/or differentiation (Figure 12-12b). The precise roles of all of these cytokines have not yet been established, but some of their effects are known. Interleukin 2, for example, appears to play a role in inducing secretion of pentameric IgM. Although resting B cells do not express the IL-2 receptor and therefore cannot be activated by IL-2, IL-4 induces expression of the 75-kDa β subunit of the IL-2 receptor and IL-5 induces the 55-kDa α subunit (see Figure 11-7). Once the high-affinity receptor is expressed, a B cell can interact with IL-2. Binding of IL-2 to high-affinity receptors on activated B cells has been shown to induce J-chain expression, which is necessary for secretion of pentameric IgM (see Figure 5-11b). Cytokines have also been shown to influence which immunoglobulin class is expressed in the immune response. Interleukin 4 induces DNA-mediated class switching to the IgG1 or IgE isotypes, and TGF-β induces class switching to IgA. Cytokines also stimulate antibody secretion by activated and fully differentiated B cells. For example, IL-6 has been shown to stimulate secretion of IgM and IgG antibody by plasma cells. If monoclonal antibody to IL-6 is added to an in vitro culture, the B cells proliferate but secretion of IgG and IgM is inhibited by more than 90%.

Changes Characterizing the Secondary Humoral Response

Following a second encounter with antigen, the memory-cell response is qualitatively different from that of the primary response. Two phenomena—affinity maturation and isotype switching—characterize the secondary response and contribute to more effective elimination of foreign pathogens.

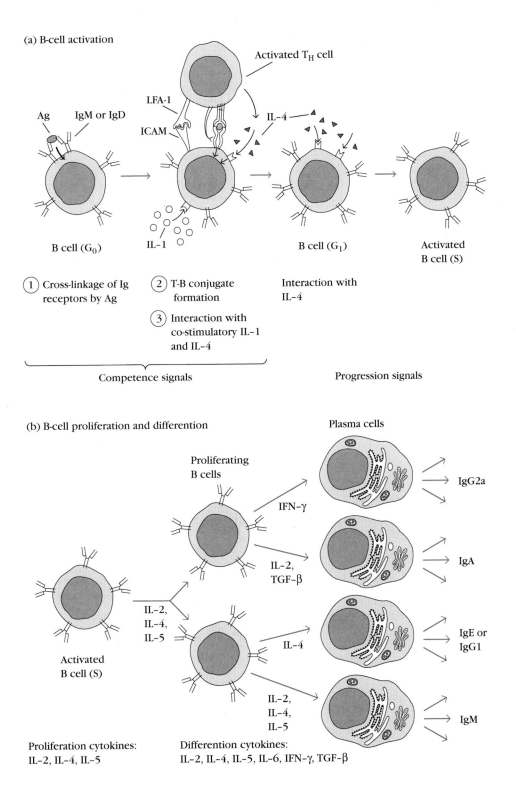

Figure 12-12 Overall pathways of B-cell activation, proliferation, and differentiation. (a) Antigen cross-linkage and interactions with IL-1 and IL-4 generate signals (arrows inside cells) that ultimately result in gene activation. The exact role of membrane interactions resulting from T-B conjugate formation in B-cell activation is still unknown. (b) Numerous cytokines participate in B-cell proliferation and differentiation. The indicated cytokine effects have been demonstrated; however, these cytokines may have other effects, and similar or identical effects may be mediated by other cytokines.

Memory Cells

A secondary humoral response is dependent on a population of memory B cells and memory T cells. Characterization of the memory B- and T- cell populations is dependent on the identification of unique cell membrane molecules to distinguish them from virgin T or B cells (Table 12-4). Unfortunately, these identifying membrane markers have eluded immunologists for years, and it is only recently that markers unique to memory cells have begun to be identified. B memory cells can be distinguished from virgin B cells by their surface immunoglobulins. While virgin B cells express IgM and IgD, memory B cells express additional isotypes, including IgG, IgA, and IgE. In addition, the level of IgD often appears to be reduced on memory B cells. Another membrane marker that appears to distinguish virgin and memory B cells is an antigen designated as Jlld. This membrane molecule is expressed in high levels on virgin B cells, whereas memory B cells express little or no Jlld. In the case of memory T cells two membrane molecules, CD44 (PgP-1) and CD45, appear to distinguish the memory cells from virgin T cells. Memory T cells express high levels of CD44 (PgP-1) and one isoform of CD45 (designated CD45R0), while virgin T cells express very low levels of CD44 (PgP-1) and express another isoform of CD45 (designated CD45R).

Little is known about the generation of the memory population. It is generally thought that memory cells originate during clonal selection as antigen-specific lymphocytes proliferate, generating both memory and effector cells. However, there is also evidence to suggest

Table 12-4   Comparison of virgin and memory T and B cells

Properties	Virgin B cell	Memory B cell
Membrane markers		
Immunoglobulin	IgM, IgD	IgM, IgD(?), IgG, IgA, IgE
Jlld	High	Low
Complement receptor	Low	High
Anatomic location	Spleen	Bone marrow, lymph node, spleen
Lifespan	Short-lived	May be long-lived
Recirculation	No	Yes
Receptor affinity	No somatic mutation	Somatic mutation increases affinity
Adhesion molecules	Low ICAM-1	High ICAM-1

Properties	Virgin T cell	Memory T cell
Membrane markers		
CD44 (Pgp-1)	Low	High
CD45R	High	Low
CD45R0	Low	High
Anatomic location	Lymph nodes, spleen	Lymph nodes, spleen
Lifespan	Short-lived	Long-lived
Recirculation	Yes	Yes, pattern altered
Activation requirements	Dendritic cell, macrophage	B cell, dendritic cell, macrophage
Receptor affinity	No somatic mutation	No somatic mutation
Cytokine secretion		
IL-2	Yes	Yes
IL-4	No	Yes
IFN-γ	Yes	Yes
Adhesion molecules		
LFA-1	Low	High
LFA-3	Low	High
MEL-14	Low	High
CD2	Low	High

SOURCE: Adapted from E. S. Vitetta, M. T. Berton, C. Burger. 1991. *Annu. Rev. Immunol.* **9**:193.

that memory cells may be a separate lineage which clonally expands following primary antigen exposure. It is not known why some antigens generate long-lasting memory while other antigens fail to do so. In some cases memory T cells have been shown to have an extremely long lifespan, residing in a resting G_0 state for up to 30 years. But, in other cases, memory cell levels may be maintained by continuous low-level cellular activation. It has been suggested that antigen trapped by follicular dendritic cells may be retained for very long periods of time, activating memory B cells, so that memory cell numbers are maintained regardless of whether the cells have a long lifespan or not.

Both B and T memory cells exhibit features that enable them to generate a more effective response. In the case of the memory B cells, they express receptors with higher affinity for antigen and therefore are activated by lower levels of antigen. Although memory T cells do not express receptors with increased affinity for antigen, they exhibit several changes that make them more responsive to antigen. In humans, memory T cells express high-affinity IL-2 receptors and therefore respond more readily to IL-2. Both memory B and memory T cells have elevated expression of cellular adhesion molecules including LFA-1 and ICAM-1 that increase the avidity of the interaction between these two cell populations. In addition, memory T cells exhibit qualitative changes in cytokine production which may enable them to be more effective activators of B cells.

Affinity Maturation

In the course of a humoral immune response, the average affinity of the antibodies produced in response to an antigen increases as much as 100- to 10,000-fold. This *affinity maturation* is the result of two processes: antigen selection of high-affinity B-cell clones and somatic mutation in the responding clones. The role played by antigen in the selection of high-affinity B-cell clones was clarified in an early experiment by H. N. Eisen and G. W. Siskind, who immunized two groups of rabbits with two different doses of DNP-BGG. Group I was immunized with 5 mg, and group II with 250 mg of DNP-BGG. The affinity of the serum anti-DNP antibodies produced in response to the antigen was then measured at 2 weeks, 5 weeks, and 8 weeks following immunization. As the data in Table 12-5 show, the average affinity of the group 1 anti-DNP antibodies increased about 140-fold from 2 weeks to 8 weeks, whereas the affinity of the group II antibodies was initially lower and did not increase. The affinity of antibody secreted by differentiated plasma cells corresponds to that of the membrane-bound antibody on the B cell from which they derive. Therefore, the nearly fivefold lower average affinity of

the group II antibodies at 2 weeks suggests that at high immunizing doses, B cells expressing both high-affinity and low-affinity membrane antibodies are activated and clonally expanded. In contrast, when the immunizing dose is low, only B cells with higher-affinity membrane-bound antibody are activated and clonally expanded (Figure 12-13). As antigen levels decline over time following immunization, competition for the available antigen increases. Now only those B cells possessing high-affinity receptors are able to bind sufficient antigen to be activated and clonally expanded. Thus, with time, the average affinity of the secreted antibody increases. In the experimental system of Eisen and Siskind, antigen concentration was never limited in group II; therefore, low-affinity B cells never had to compete with the high-affinity cells for available antigen, and the response never showed an increase in antibody affinity.

Another process that contributes to affinity maturation is somatic mutation. As discussed in Chapter 8, somatic mutation acts on the V, D, and J gene segments in rearranged functional immunoglobulin genes, introducing point mutations, deletions, and insertions. Because somatic mutation is random, it potentially can generate antibodies of higher specificity, lower specificity, or the same specificity. Contact with antigen, however, will select for those clones in which a higher-affinity receptor has been generated. Somatic mutation can first be detected late in the primary response, and it increases after a secondary contact with antigen (see Figure 8-19). The role of somatic mutation in affinity maturation has been assessed by comparing the H- and L-chain mRNA sequences of antigen-specific B-cell hybridomas at various times after antigen exposure. In one study, the secondary antibody differed from the primary antibody by 13 replacement mutations and exhibited a 100-fold higher affinity for antigen. The molecular basis

Table 12-5 Effect of immunizing dose and time on average affinity of induced anti-DNP antibodies in rabbits

Group	DNP-BGG immunizing dose (mg per animal)	K of anti-DNP antibodies* (L/mol $\times 10^6$)		
		2 weeks	5 weeks	8 weeks
I	5	0.86	14	120
II	250	0.18	0.13	0.15

* Values are averages for five animals per group and are based on binding of DNP-L-lysine with serum antibody samples obtained at indicated times after immunization.

SOURCE: Adapted from H. N. Eisen and G. W. Siskind, 1964, *Biochemistry* 3:966.

of somatic mutation remains to be determined. The finding that somatic mutations are found predominantly in secondary antibodies and in isotypes, resulting from class switching, may indicate that the mutation process is influenced by events in B-cell differentiation. Some workers have suggested, for example, that the observed increase in somatic mutation during a secondary response may result from an error-prone DNA-repair process, which would be heightened during the additional cell divisions required to generate a secondary response.

The humoral response to thymus-independent antigens exhibits very little affinity maturation. This observation suggests that T_H cells also play a role in affinity maturation, although the exact mechanism is unknown.

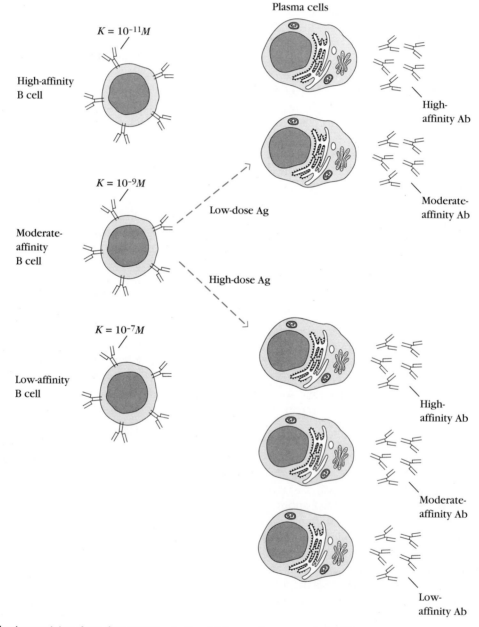

Figure 12-13   The immunizing dose determines whether high-, moderate-, or low-affinity B cells are selected for activation and hence the affinity of the antibodies secreted by the plasma cells derived from the B cells.

Class Switching

In the primary humoral response to thymus-dependent antigens, the first antibody to be secreted is IgM, followed by IgG later in the response. With secondary antigen challenge very little IgM is produced and instead IgG, IgA, or IgE appear. As noted already T_H-cell lymphokines play an important role in regulating class switching. As discussed in Chapter 8, class switching involves rearrangement of C gene segments in immunoglobulin heavy-chain genes. The data shown in Figure 8-14 suggest that IL-4–mediated class switching in B cells is a sequential process, going from C_μ to $C_\gamma 1$ to C_ε. The first switch results in replacement of IgM expression with IgG1 expression; the second switch, in loss of IgG1 and appearance of IgE. Thus activation of IgG1-positive memory B cells might give rise to IgE-secreting plasma cells. Other T_H-cell lymphokines also have been implicated in class switching. For example, IFN-γ induces LPS-activated B cells to secrete IgG2a, and TGF-β and IL-5 have been associated with IgA secretion.

Induction of the Humoral Response In Vivo

In vivo the humoral response is generated in defined anatomic sites whose structure places certain restrictions on the kinds of cellular interactions that can take place. When an antigen is introduced into the body, it becomes concentrated in several lymphoid organs. Blood-borne antigen is filtered by the spleen, whereas tissue antigen is filtered by regional lymph nodes or lymph nodules; this discussion focuses on the generation of the humoral response in lymph nodes.

A lymph node is an extremely efficient filter capable of trapping more than 90% of any antigen carried into the node by the afferent lymphatics. As antigen percolates through the cellular architecture of the node, it is either phagocytosed by macrophages or interdigitating dendritic cells within the node or is retained on the specialized follicular dendritic cells in the follicles and germinal centers. The follicular dendritic cells have long processes, along which are arrayed Fc receptors that bind antigen-antibody complexes effectively and retain the complexes for a long time on the cell membrane. Because follicular dendritic cells bind antigen that has been complexed to antibody, they are thought to be particularly important in the secondary response, when circulating-antibody levels are significant; they may have a leading role in activating memory B cells. Recent evidence has shown that follicular dendritic cells release small membrane-derived particles, 0.3–0.4 μm in diameter, which appear to originate from the beaded structures of the dendritic processes. These particles, which are heavily coated with immune complexes, are called *iccosomes*, for *i*mmune-*c*omplex *c*oating.

A model of B-cell activation, proliferation, and differentiation within lymph nodes is presented in Figure 12-14. Although some of the details are still not understood, this general scheme seems valid based on current evidence. It appears that slightly different pathways may operate during a primary and secondary response. During a secondary response, much of the tissue antigen may be complexed with circulating antibodies. Antigen or antigen-antibody complexes enter the lymph nodes via the afferent lymphatics, either alone or associated with antigen-transporting cells (e.g., Langerhans' cells or dendritic cells) and macrophages. Lymphocytes enter the lymph nodes either through the afferent lymphatic vessels or from the blood by extravasation of high endothelial cells in the postcapillary venules. Entry through the postcapillary venules enables the entering lymphocytes to migrate into the paracortical zone, a region heavily populated with T cells and antigen-presenting cells, including macrophages and interdigitating dendritic cells. Interdigitating dendritic cells express high levels of class II MHC molecules and have long processes that are estimated to contact about 200 T_H cells. Although interdigitating dendritic cells are not phagocytic, they can endocytose antigen and are thought to serve as effective antigen-presenting cells. Extensive T_H-cell activation and proliferation occurs, and the resulting activated T_H cells may then migrate from the paracortical zone to the primary follicles.

Many B cells, follicular dendritic cells, and macrophages are located within the primary follicles. Especially during a secondary response, iccosomes released from the follicular dendritic cells bind to membrane immunoglobulin receptors and are endocytosed by B cells. The endocytosed antigen may then be processed and presented together with class II MHC molecules, allowing the B cells to function as effective antigen-presenting cells for the activated T_H cells. T-B conjugate formation may then occur, resulting in B-cell activation and proliferation. As cell proliferation continues, the activated B cells migrate into the follicle, forming a dense zone of proliferating cells called the *germinal center*. (T_H cells are required for B-cell proliferation in the germinal center; in nude mice, which lack a thymus, there is no germinal-center formation.) Most of the proliferating B cells in the germinal center die, to be phagocytosed by an unusual type of macrophage, the "tingible-body" macrophage, that specializes in the phagocytosis of lymphoid cells. It is not known why such a large number of cells die at this stage, but one suggestion is that it may provide a means of eliminating any B cells with abnormal immunoglobulin-gene rearrangement.

As the surviving B cells proliferate within the germinal

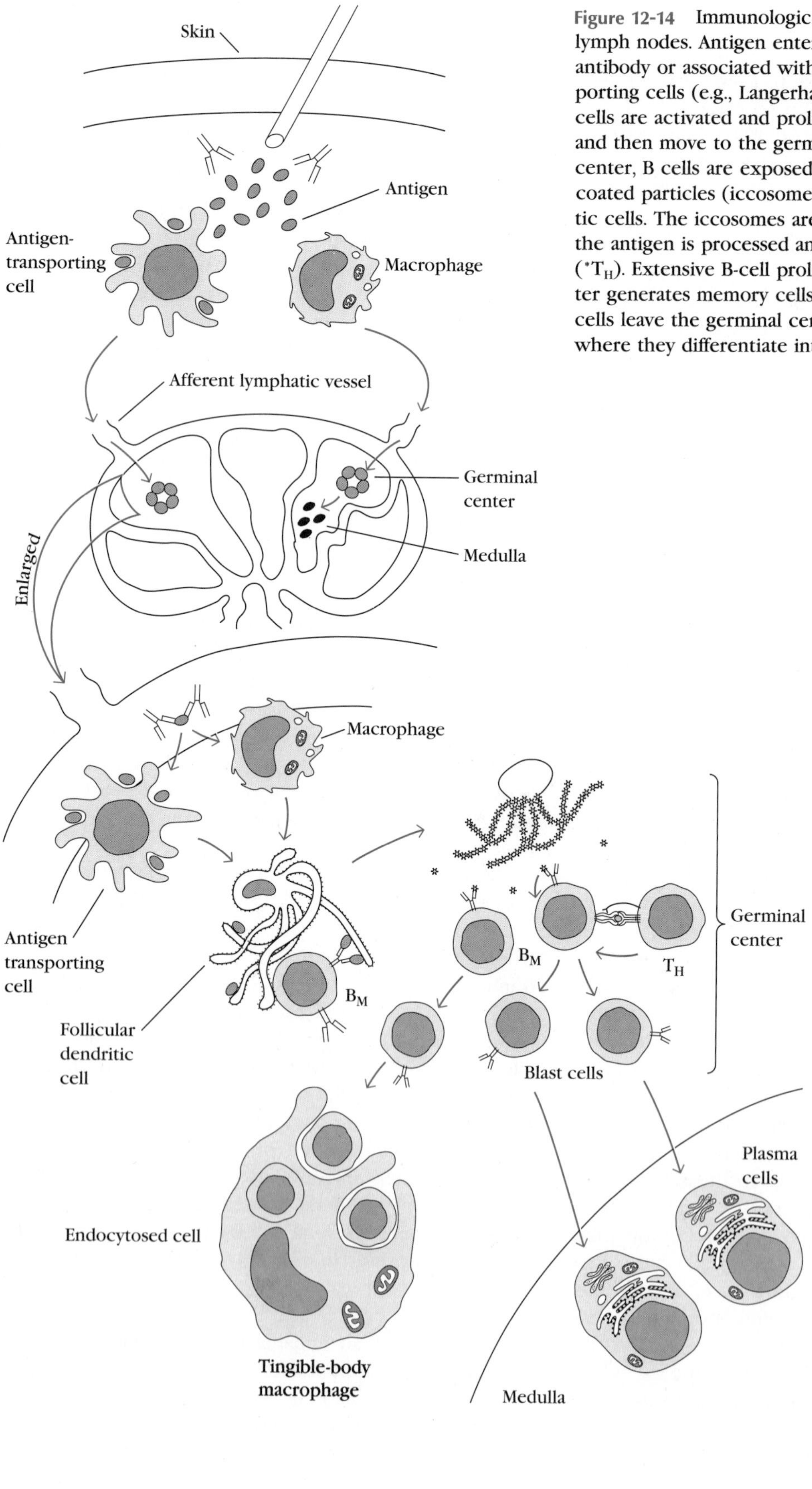

Figure 12-14 Immunologic events in the germinal center of lymph nodes. Antigen enters a node either complexed with antibody or associated with macrophages or antigen-transporting cells (e.g., Langerhans' cells or dendritic cells). T_H cells are activated and proliferate in the paracortical zone and then move to the germinal centers. Within a germinal center, B cells are exposed to small immune complex–coated particles (iccosomes) released from follicular dendritic cells. The iccosomes are endocytosed by the B cell, and the antigen is processed and presented to activated T_H cells ($^*T_H$). Extensive B-cell proliferation within the germinal center generates memory cells and large blast cells. The blast cells leave the germinal center and migrate to the medulla where they differentiate into plasma cells.

center, two types of progeny cells are formed: small lymphocytes that are thought to be memory B cells and large blast cells, which are the precursors of plasma cells. The blast cells leave the germinal centers and migrate to the medulla, where they develop into plasma cells and begin to secrete antibody molecules into the efferent lymphatics. This antibody is carried by the lymphatics to the thoracic duct, where it enters the blood. The memory B cells either remain in the follicle or leave the lymph node through the efferent lymphatic vessel and recirculate to other parts of the body.

Summary

1. Primary and secondary humoral responses show different kinetics of antibody formation. The primary response is characterized by a long lag period, a logarithmic rise in antibody formation, a short plateau, and then a relatively rapid decline. IgM is the first antibody class to be secreted, followed by IgG later in the primary response. The secondary response has a shorter lag period, a more rapid logarithmic phase, a longer plateau, and a slower decline than the primary response. Little IgM is produced in the secondary response, which is characterized by IgG or other isotypes.

2. Early adoptive-transfer experiments revealed that both B cells and T cells are required to generate a humoral immune response. The B cell was shown to be the antibody-producing cell, and the T cell was shown to function as a necessary helper cell. In vitro experiments in which adherent macrophages and nonadherent lymphocytes were separated demonstrated that macrophages also are required participants in induction of humoral immunity.

3. Studies of the humoral response to hapten-carrier conjugates revealed that both B cells and T_H cells recognize epitopes on the same conjugate molecule. The hapten serves as the immunodominant B-cell epitope, while carrier epitopes are recognized by T_H cells. These T-cell epitopes tend to be internal peptides that are exposed during antigen processing in the B cell and are presented together with class II MHC molecules on the B-cell membrane.

4. The activation, proliferation, and differentiation of B cells involves several sequential processes, starting with the uptake, processing, and presentation of antigen + class II MHC molecules by virgin B cells. Interaction of an activated antigen-specific T_H cell with an antigen-primed B cell leads to formation of a specific T-B conjugate, which exhibits close membrane interaction. The T_H cells in these conjugates undergo reorganization of the Golgi apparatus and microtubular-organizing center as well as clustering of several membrane proteins near the junction of the two cells. This redistribution of T_H-cell components may aid in the directional release of cytokines from the T_H cell toward the interacting B cell.

5. Signals generated by membrane events and cytokines are transduced into the B cell, ultimately leading to changes in gene expression. Relatively little is known about membrane signaling events in B-cell activation, proliferation, and differentiation, but the role of several cytokines have been demonstrated. Both IL-1 and IL-4 function as activation signals; IL-4 and numerous other T_H-cell lymphokines function as proliferation and differentiation signals (e.g., by inducing secretion of pentameric IgM and class switching to other isotypes).

6. As the humoral immune response proceeds, the average affinity of the induced serum antibodies increases. Such affinity maturation is thought to result from selective activation of B cells with high-affinity receptors and from somatic mutation. Affinity maturation and class switching, which also occurs during the humoral response, lead to more effective elimination of pathogens.

7. Generation of the humoral response to antigens in vivo occurs primarily in regional lymph nodes. Intense proliferation of activated B cells takes place in the germinal centers, forming small memory B cells and large B lymphoblasts. The latter migrate to the medulla where they differentiate into antibody-secreting plasma cells.

References

ABBAS, A. K. 1988. A reassessment of the mechanisms of antigen-specific T-cell-dependent B-cell activation. *Immunol. Today*:89.

CLARK, E, A., and P. J. L. LANE. 1991. Regulation of human B-cell activation and adhesion. *Annu. Rev. Immunol.* **9**:97.

DEFRANCO, A. L. 1988. Cell-cell interactions in the antibody response. *Nature* **334**:199.

FINKELMAN, F. D., J. HOLMES, I. M. KATONA et al. 1990. Lymphokine control of in vivo immunoglobulin isotype selection. *Annu. Rev. Immunol.* **8**:303.

KINCADE, P. W. 1987. Experimental models for understanding B lymphocyte formation. *Adv. Immunol.* **41**:181.

KLINMAN, N. R., and P. J. LINTON. 1990. The generation of B-cell memory: a working hypothesis. *Curr. Top. Microbiol. Immunol.* **159**:19.

KUPFER, A., S. J. SINGER, C. A. JANEWAY, and S. L. SWAIN. 1987. Coclustering of CD4 (L3T4) molecule with the T-cell receptor is induced by specific direct interaction of helper T cells and antigen-presenting cells. *Proc. Nat'l. Acad. Sci. USA* **84**:5888.

SNOW, E. C., and R. J. NOELLE. 1987. Thymus dependent antigenic stimulation of hapten-specific B lymphocytes. *Immunol. Rev.* **99**:173.

SWAIN, S., and R. W. DUTTON. 1987. Consequences of the direct interaction of helper T cells with B cells presenting antigen. *Immunol. Rev.* **99**:263.

SZAKAL, A. K., M. H. KOSCO, and J. G. TEW. 1989. Microanatomy of lymphoid tissue during humoral immune responses: structure function relationships. *Annu. Rev. Immunol.* **7**:91.

VITETTA, E. S., R. FERNANDEZ-BOTRAN, C. D. MYERS, and V. M. SANDERS. 1989. Cellular interactions in the humoral immune response. *Adv. Immunol.* **45**:1.

VITETTA, E. S., M. T. BERTON, C. BURGER et al. 1991. Memory B and T cells. *Annu. Rev. Immunol.* **9**:193.

Study Questions

1. Indicate whether each of the following statements is true or false. If you believe a statement is false, explain why.

   a. The indirect hemolytic plaque assay detects only IgG-secreting plasma cells.

   b. The B cell serves as an antigen-presenting cell to the T_H cell.

   c. IL-4 decreases IgE production by plasma cells.

   d. Immunoglobulin class switching from IgM to IgE usually is mediated by DNA rearrangements with loss of intervening DNA.

   e. Immunization with a hapten-carrier conjugate results in production of antibodies to both hapten and carrier epitopes.

   f. All the antibodies secreted by a single plasma cell have the same idiotype and isotype.

2. Four mice are immunized with antigen under the conditions listed below (a–d). In each case, indicate whether the induced serum antibodies will be heterogeneous or relatively homogeneous; have high affinity or low affinity; and be largely IgM or IgG.

   a. A primary response to a low antigen dose.

   b. A secondary response to a low antigen dose.

   c. A primary response to a high antigen dose.

   d. A secondary response to a high antigen dose.

3. Three groups of mice were immunized according to the schedule shown in the table below. Spleen cells were isolated from the immunized mice, and the number of plaque-forming cells were determined; the direct and indirect PFC counts for each group are listed in the table.

Immunization schedule	Direct PFC/10^6 spleen cells	Indirect PFC/10^6 spleen cells
(A) 1° DNP-BSA	310	343
(B) 1° DNP-BSA; 2° DNP-BSA	62	4060
(C) 1° DNP-BSA; 2° DNP-BGG	366	386

   a. Describe the assay used to measure a primary (1°) and secondary (2°) PFC response.

   b. Calculate the number of IgM-secreting and IgG-secreting plasma cells/10^6 spleen cells for each group of mice.

   c. Why is the indirect PFC so much higher than the direct PFC for group B but not for group A or C?

4. Describe the primary signals required to activate virgin B cells. What additional signals, if any, are needed to stimulate proliferation and differentiation of activated B cells?

CHAPTER

13

Cell-Mediated Immunity

The cell-mediated branch of the immune system confers immunity through the transfer of immune cells. Although antibody can also be involved, it plays a secondary role. Both antigen-specific and nonspecific cells contribute to the development of cell-mediated immunity (CMI). Specific cells include T_H/T_{DTH} cells and T_C cells; nonspecific cells include macrophages, neutrophils, eosinophils, and NK cells. Both specific and nonspecific components require localized concentrations of cytokines, which are generated by antigen-specific T cells or by the specificity conferred by binding of antibody to Fc receptors on otherwise nonspecific cells. Unlike the humoral branch of the immune system, which serves mainly to eliminate extracellular bacteria and bacterial products, the cell-mediated branch is responsible for the clearance of intracellular pathogens, virus-infected cells, tumor cells, and foreign grafts. The system is adapted to recognizing altered self-cells and eliminating them from the body.

The importance of cell-mediated immunity becomes evident when the system is defective. Children with DiGeorge syndrome, who are born without a thymus and therefore lack the T-cell component of the cell-mediated immune system, generally are able to cope with infections of extracellular bacteria but they cannot effectively eliminate intracellular pathogens. Their lack of functional cell-mediated immunity manifests itself in the form of repeated infections with viruses, intracellular bacteria, and fungi. The severity of the cell-mediated immunodeficiency in these children is such that even attenuated vaccines, capable of only limited growth in normal individuals, can produce life-threatening infections.

Cell-mediated immune responses can be divided into two major categories involving different effector populations. One group involves effector cells having direct cytotoxic activity. The second group involves a subpopulation of effector T_H cells that mediate delayed-type hypersensitivity reactions. This chapter examines the cells and effector mechanisms involved in each type of cell-mediated immune response.

Direct Cytotoxic Response

One way the immune system eliminates foreign or altered self-cells is to mount a cytotoxic reaction that results in lysis of target cells. A variety of cell-mediated cytotoxic effector mechanisms have been identified. These effector mechanisms can be subdivided into two general categories: (1) cytotoxicity involving antigen-specific cytotoxic T lymphocytes and (2) cytotoxicity involving nonspecific cells, such as natural killer cells and macrophages. The target cells to which these effector mechanisms are directed include allogeneic cells, malignant cells, virus-infected cells, and chemically conjugated cells.

Cytotoxicity Mediated by Cytotoxic T Lymphocytes

Immune activation of T cytotoxic (T_C) cells generates a population of effector cells with lytic capability called cytotoxic T lymphocytes, or CTLs. These effector cells have important roles in the recognition and elimination of altered self-cells, including virus-infected cells and

malignant cells, and in graft-rejection reactions. In general, CTLs are $CD8^+$ and are class I MHC restricted, although in rare instances $CD4^+$ class II–restricted T cells have been shown to function as CTLs. Since virtually all nucleated cells in the body express class I MHC molecules, the CTLs can recognize and eliminate almost any altered body cell.

The CTL-mediated immune response can be divided into two phases, reflecting different aspects of the cytotoxic T-cell response. The first phase—*sensitization*—involves activation and extensive proliferation of T_H cells in response to antigen presented by macrophages or other antigen-presenting cells (Figure 13-1). There is also some proliferation of T_C cells in response to recognition of an antigen–class I MHC complex on specific target cells, but this proliferation is minor compared to that of the T_H cell. The outcome of this extensive proliferation is the clonal expansion of the T_H-cell population, resulting in large increases in their secretion of IL-2. In response to interaction with an antigen–class I MHC complex *and* IL-2, the T_C cells proliferate and

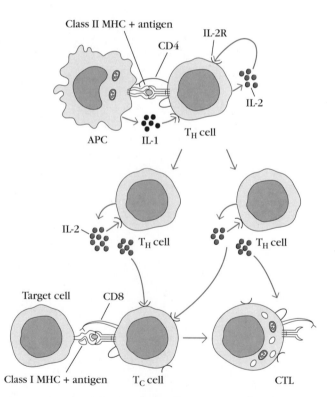

Figure 13-1   Sensitization phase of CTL-mediated immune response. Activation and extensive proliferation of T_H cells leads to localized increases in IL-2. In the presence of IL-2, T_C cells that have interacted with antigen–class I MHC complexes on the membrane of target cells are activated and differentiate into CTLs. In the subsequent effector phase of the response, CTLs destroy specific target cells.

differentiate into functional CTLs possessing lytic activity. In the second, *effector*, phase of the cytotoxic T-cell response, CTLs recognize antigen–class I MHC complexes on specific target cells, initiating a sequence of events that culminates in target-cell destruction (Figure 13-2).

Sensitization Phase

The sensitization phase of a cell-mediated cytotoxic response involves extensive proliferation of the T_H cell and production of IL-2. The sensitization phase can be measured using an in vitro mixed-lymphocyte reaction or an in vivo graft-versus-host reaction. During the sensitization phase, T_C cells undergo a sequential series of differentiation events that generate effector CTLs.

Mixed-Lymphocyte Reaction (MLR). Analysis of the mechanisms involved in CTL-mediated target-cell lysis was made possible by the development of assays to generate these cells. In 1965, X. Ginsburg and D. H. Sachs observed that when rat lymphocytes were cultured on a monolayer of mouse fibroblast cells, the rat lymphocytes proliferated and destroyed the mouse fibroblasts. In 1970 it was discovered that functional CTLs could also be generated by coculturing allogeneic spleen cells in a system termed the mixed-lymphocyte reaction (MLR). The T lymphocytes in an MLR undergo extensive blast transformation and cell proliferation. The degree of proliferation can be assessed by adding [³H] thymidine to the culture medium and monitoring uptake of label into DNA in the course of repeated cell divisions. Both populations of allogeneic T lymphocytes proliferate in an MLR unless one population is rendered unresponsive by treatment with mitomycin C or lethal x-irradiation (see Figure 9-6). In the latter system, a one-way MLR, the unresponsive population provides stimulator cells that express alloantigens foreign to the responder T cells. Within 24–48 h the responder T cells begin dividing in response to the alloantigens of the stimulator cells, and by 72–96 h a population of functional CTLs is generated. With this experimental system functional CTLs can be generated entirely in vitro, after which their activity can be assessed with various effector assays.

The significant role of T_H cells in an MLR was demonstrated by use of antibodies to the T_H-cell membrane marker CD4. In an MLR, responder T_H cells recognize allogeneic class II MHC molecules on the stimulator cells and proliferate in response to these differences. Removal of the T_H cells from the responder population with anti-CD4 antibodies plus complement abolishes the MLR and prevents generation of CTLs. (Table 13-1). In addition to the T_H cell, accessory cells such as macrophages were also shown to be necessary for the MLR. When adherent cells (largely macrophages) were removed from the

(a)

(b)

(c)

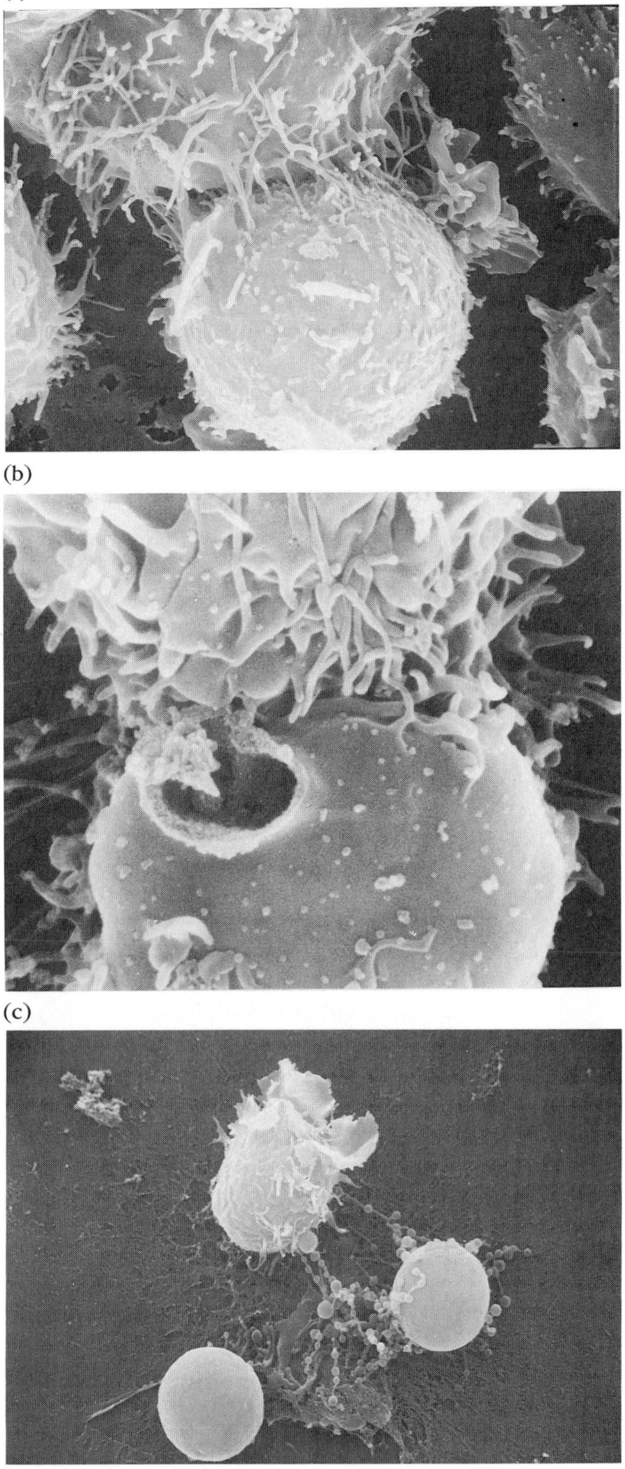

Figure 13-2 Scanning electron micrographs of tumor-cell destruction by a CTL. (a) A CTL (*top left*) makes contact with a smaller tumor cell. (b) Membrane damage to the tumor cell results in a visible cavity and allows an influx of water, resulting in cell swelling. (c) Lysis of the tumor cell has occurred leaving only cell debris and the nucleus (*right*). [From J. D. E. Young and Z. A. Cohn, 1988, *Sci. Am.* (Jan.):38.]

Table 13-1   Dependence of one-way MLR on class II MHC differences and the presence of T_H cells and macrophages

Responder population			Stimulator population			
MHC haplotype			MHC haplotype			
Class I	Class II	Treatment	Class I	Class II	Treatment	Stimulation index*
s	k	None	s	k	None	1.0
s	k	None	k	k	None	1.2
s	k	None	s	s	None	18.0
s	k	$-T_H$ cells[†]	s	s	None	1.0
s	k	None	s	s	$-$Macrophages[‡]	1.0

* Stimulation index is directly related to the uptake of [^{3}H] thymidine and is a measure of cell proliferation.

[†] T_H cells removed by treatment with anti-CD4 and complement.

[‡] When spleen cells are cultured, most of the macrophages adhere to the wall of the culture vessel; they can be removed from the stimulator population simply by decantation.

stimulator population, the proliferative response in the MLR was abolished and functional CTLs were no longer generated. Now it is known that the function of these macrophages is to activate class II MHC–restricted T_H cells whose proliferation is measured in the MLR. In the absence of T_H-cell activation, there is no proliferation.

The requirement for T_H cells in the generation of functional CTL activity in an MLR was demonstrated in a now-classical experiment by H. Cantor and E. A. Boyse. They performed one-way mixed-lymphocyte reactions with various populations of splenic lymphocytes and then assayed the cytotoxic activity generated with cell-mediated lympholysis (see Figure 9–5). The lymphocyte populations were obtained by treating spleen-cell aliquots with complement + antibodies against subpopulation membrane molecules (equivalent to CD4 or CD8) to remove T_H cells and T_C cells, respectively. Their experiment, outlined in Figure 13-3, confirmed that CD8$^+$ T cells are responsible for functional cytotoxicity, which had been demonstrated previously. In addition, they found that removal of CD4$^+$ T cells from the MLR abolished the cytotoxicity of the CD8$^+$ T cells. These results provided the first evidence that T_C cells, like B cells, require T_H cells for their activation.

Graft-versus-Host Reaction. The graft-versus-host reaction can assess cell-mediated cytotoxic reactions in vivo. The reaction develops when immunocompetent lymphocytes are injected into an allogeneic recipient whose immune system is compromised. The grafted lymphocytes begin to attack the host, and the host's com-

promised state prevents an immune response against the graft. Experimentally, these reactions develop when immunocompetent lymphocytes are transferred into a neonatal animal or an x-irradiated recipient. Graft-versus-host reactions can also develop when parental-strain lymphocytes are injected into an F_1. In humans graft-versus-host reactions often develop following transplantation of bone marrow in patients with leukemia, immunodeficiency diseases, or autoimmune anemias, or in patients requiring bone-marrow replacement following radiation exposure.

There are a number of manifestations of a graft-versus-host reaction. In animals a severe reaction results in death within a few weeks. Often the animals exhibit weight loss, which is especially noticeable in graft-versus-host disease in neonatal animals. Generally the grafted lymphocytes are carried to a number of organs, including the spleen. Here the grafted lymphocytes begin to proliferate in response to the allogeneic MHC antigens of the host. This proliferation induces an influx of host cells, which in turn display intense proliferation that results in visible spleen enlargement, or *splenomegaly*. The intensity of a graft-versus-host reaction can be assessed by calculating the spleen index as follows:

$$\frac{\text{Spleen}}{\text{index}} = \frac{\text{Weight of exp. spleen/Total body weight}}{\text{Weight of control spleen/Total body weight}}$$

A spleen index of 1.3 or greater is considered to be indicative of a positive graft-versus-host reaction.

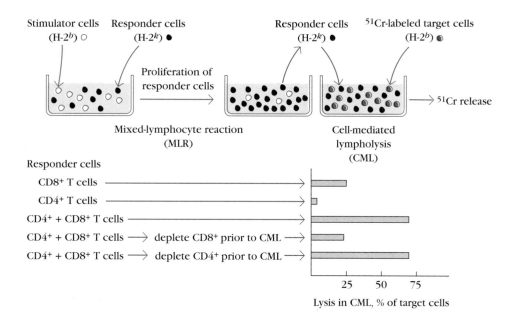

Figure 13-3 Experimental demonstration that T_H cells are necessary to generate CTLs in an MLR reaction. The responder cell population was first treated with antibodies plus complement to remove the T_H cells or T_C cells, respectively. The responder cells were then cultured with allogeneic x-irradiated stimulator cells. The cytotoxic activity of the generated CTLs was measured in a cell-mediated lympholysis (CML) assay using [^{51}Cr] labeled target cells. The amount of [^{51}Cr] released is proportional to the number of CTLs. [Based on H. Cantor and E. A. Boyse, 1975, *J. Exp. Med.* **141**:1390.]

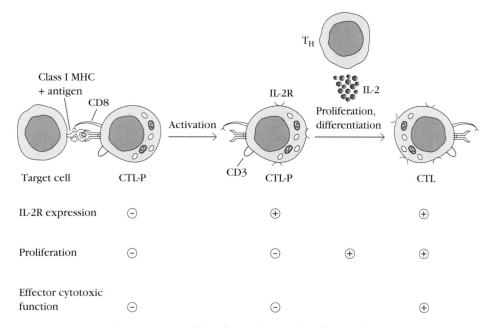

Figure 13-4 Stepwise activation of CTL precursors (CTL-P) to effector CTLs during the sensitization phase. The CTL-P lacks IL-2 receptors (IL-2R), does not proliferate, and does not have functional cytotoxic activity. Upon recognition of antigen–class I MHC complex on an appropriate target cell, a CTL-P begins to express the IL-2 receptor. In the presence of IL-2 secreted by activated T_H cells, the CTL-P proliferates and differentiates into a CTL.

Events in Activation of T_C Cells to CTLs. Until they have been activated, T_C cells are not capable of functional cytotoxic activity. Activation of these cells in the sensitization phase appears to progress in a series of stages (Figure 13-4). Initially a T_C cell, which in this context is called a *CTL precursor (CTL-P)*, does not express IL-2 receptors, does not proliferate, and does not display cytotoxic activity. Recognition of processed antigen associated with class I MHC molecules on an appropriate target cell induces a CTL-P to increase its expression of the IL-2 receptor. IL-2 produced by proliferating T_H cells binds to the IL-2 receptors on the CTL-P, inducing it to proliferate and differentiate into effector CTLs. This stepwise sequence of events during the sensitization phase ensures that only antigen-activated CTL-Ps will progress to CTLs with cytotoxic effector function. A key event in this stepwise sequence is the expression of the IL-2 receptor. The fact that the receptor is not expressed until after a CTL-P has been activated by antigen + a class I MHC molecule ensures that only antigen-specific CTL-Ps are clonally expanded by IL-2 and acquire cytotoxicity.

Effector Phase

The effector phase of a CTL-mediated cytotoxic response involves target-cell lysis by effector CTLs. A carefully orchestrated sequence of events leads to target-cell destruction by the CTL: conjugate formation, membrane attack, CTL dissociation, and target-cell destruction.

Cell-Mediated Lympholysis (CML). The development of a cell-mediated lympholysis (CML) assay was a major experimental advance that contributed to understanding of the mechanism of target-cell killing by CTL. In this assay suitable target cells are labeled intracellularly with [^{51}Cr]. Labeling is achieved by incubating the target cell in $Na_2[^{51}Cr]O_4$. The radiolabeled [^{51}Cr] diffuses into the cell. Once inside, the [^{51}Cr] binds to cytoplasmic proteins, reducing its ability to passively diffuse out of the labeled target cell. When specific activated CTLs are incubated for 1 to 4 h with these labeled target cells, the target cells lyse and the [^{51}Cr] is released. The amount of [^{51}Cr] released is directly related to the number of target cells lysed by the CTLs. By means of this assay the specificity of CTLs for allogeneic cells, tumor cells, virus-infected cells, and chemically modified cells has been demonstrated.

The T-cell subpopulation responsible for CML was identified by selectively depleting different T-cell subpopulations by means of antibody- + -complement lysis. The experiment depicted in Figure 13-3 shows that removal of CD8$^+$ T cells eliminates lysis of target cells, whereas removal of CD4$^+$ T cells has no effect on CML. The activity of CTLs exhibits class I MHC restriction. That is, CTLs can kill only target cells that express antigen presented by syngeneic class I MHC molecules (Table 13-2).

Cytotoxic T-Cell Clones. Recent technological advances have made possible the long-term culture of CTL clones. Lymphocytes from previously immunized mice are cul-

Table 13-2   Effect of CTL haplotype on ability to lyse H-2^k target cells[*]

Strain	Haplotype[†] K	IA	IE	D	[^{51}Cr] released from LCM-infected H-2^k target cells, %[‡]	Interpretation
CBA	k	k	k	k	86	Syngeneic combination works
BALB/c	d	d	d	d	18	Allogeneic combination does not work
A.TL	s	k	k	d	18	Identity at class II loci does not work
B10.A	k	k	k	d	65	Identity at class I *K* locus works
C3H.OH	d	d	d	k	57	Identity at class I *D* locus works

[*] Spleen cells containing CTLs were isolated from mice with the indicated haplotypes that had been infected with the LCM virus. Lytic ability of the spleen cells was determined in a CML assay using [^{51}Cr] labeled H-2^k target cells.

[†] The indicated alleles are for the following H-2 loci in sequence: *K, IA, IE,* and *D. K* and *D* are class I MHC loci; *IA* and *IE* are class II MHC loci.

[‡] Controls with uninfected target cells had [^{51}Cr] release ranging from 17 to 22%.

SOURCE: Adapted from J. W. Kimball, 1983, *Introduction to Immunology*, Macmillan Publishing Co.

tured with the original immunizing target cells and the differentiated CTLs are cloned in microwell cultures at limiting dilutions in the presence of high concentrations of IL-2. These cloned CTL lines have provided immunologists with large numbers of homogeneous cells with identical receptor specificity for a given target cell. With such CTL clones many of the membrane molecules and biochemical events involved in CTL-mediated target-cell destruction have been elucidated.

Mechanism of CTL-Mediated Cytotoxicity. A carefully orchestrated series of events leads to target-cell destruction by CTLs (Figure 13-5). When antigen-specific CTLs are incubated with appropriate target cells, the two cell types interact and undergo conjugate formation. Formation of a CTL–target-cell conjugate is followed within several minutes by a Ca^{2+}-dependent, energy-requiring step in which the CTL inflicts membrane damage on the target cell. Following this step the CTL cell dissociates from the target cell and goes on to bind to another target cell. Within a variable period of time (from 15 min to 3

h) after CTL dissociation, the target cell lyses. Each of the steps involved in this process have been studied in more detail with cloned CTLs.

Formation of CTL–target-cell conjugates involves antigen-MHC recognition by the CTL's antigen receptor (TCR/CD3) together with CD8. Following antigen-specific recognition, cell-to-cell adhesion takes place between the CTL and the target cell (Figure 13-6). The integrin receptor LFA-1 on the membrane of the CTL binds to intercellular cell-adhesion molecules (ICAMs) on the membrane of the target cell. This adhesion process appears to require prior activation of the CTL resulting from interaction of its TCR-CD3 complex with antigen + MHC on the target cell. Recent evidence has shown that this antigen-mediated CTL activation converts LFA-1 from a low-avidity state to a high-avidity state (Figure 13-7). Because of this phenomenon, CTLs adhere to and form conjugates only with appropriate target cells that display antigenic peptides associated with class I MHC molecules. The high-avidity LFA-1 persists for only 5–10 min after antigen-mediated activation, and

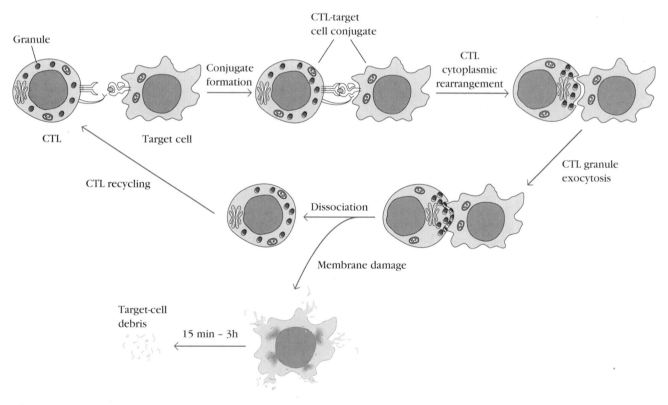

Figure 13-5 Stages in CTL-mediated killing of target cells. T-cell receptors on a CTL interact with processed antigen–class I MHC complexes on an appropriate target cell, leading to formation of a CTL–target-cell conjugate. The Golgi stacks and granules in the CTL reorient toward the point of contact with the target cell, and the granules' contents are released by exocytosis. Following dissociation of the conjugate, the CTL is recycled and the target cell is destroyed in time as the result of damage to its membrane. [Adapted from P. A. Henkart, 1985, *Annu. Rev. Immunol.* **3**:31.]

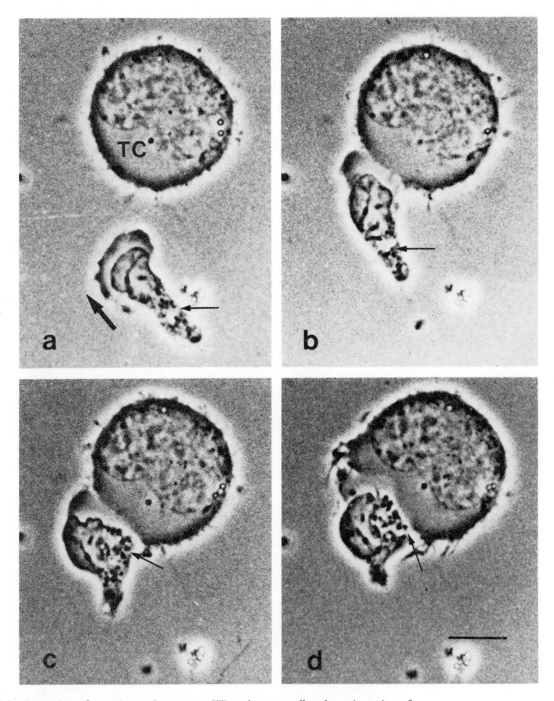

Figure 13-6   Formation of a conjugate between a CTL and target cell and reorientation of CTL cytoplasmic granules as seen by time-lapse cinematography. (a) A motile mouse CTL (*bottom*) approaches an appropriate target cell. Thick arrow indicates direction of movement. (b) Initial contact of the CTL and target cell has occurred. (c) Within 2 min of initial contact, the membrane-contact region has broadened and the rearrangement of dark cytoplasmic granules (thin arrows) is under way. (d) Further movement of dark granules toward the target cell is evident 10 min after initial contact. [From Yanelli, J. R., J. A. Sullivan, G. L. Mandell, and V. H. Engelhand. 1986. *J. Immunol.* **136**:377.]

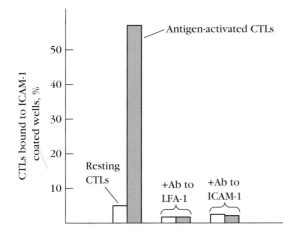

Figure 13-7 Effect of antigen activation on ability of CTLs to bind to the intercellular cell-adhesion molecule ICAM-1. Resting mouse CTLs were first incubated with anti-CD3 antibodies. Cross-linkage of CD3 molecules on the CTL membrane by anti-CD3 has the same activating effect as interaction with antigen + class I MHC on a target cell. Adhesion was assayed by binding of radiolabeled CTLs to microwells coated with ICAM-1. Antigen activation increased CTL binding to ICAM-1 more than 10-fold. The presence of excess monoclonal antibody to LFA-1 or ICAM-1 in the microwells abolished binding, demonstrating that both molecules are necessary for adhesion to occur. [Based on M. L. Dustin and T. A. Springer, 1989, *Nature* **341**:619.]

then the receptor returns to its low-avidity state. This downshift in LFA-1 avidity is thought to facilitate CTL dissociation from the target cell.

Formation of a CTL–target-cell conjugate is immediately followed by a series of events leading to target-cell membrane damage. Electron microscopy of cultured CTL clones reveals the presence of electron-dense storage granules within the cell (see Figure 13-6). Following conjugate formation the Golgi and the granules reorient within the cytoplasm of the CTL and concentrate at the region of conjugate formation. An influx of Ca^{2+} (another result of antigen-mediated activation of the CTL) induces directed exocytosis of the granules' contents at the site of conjugate formation. The importance of these granules and their contents in target-cell destruction was demonstrated when CTL granules were isolated by fractionation and shown to mediate target-cell damage by themselves.

Contained within CTL storage granules are pore-forming proteins called *perforins*, a family of six esterases called *granzymes A–F*, some high-molecular-weight proteoglycans, and various toxic cytokines such as TNF-β. CTL precursors (CTL-P) lack both cytoplasmic granules and perforin. Activation of a CTL-P results in the appearance of the cytoplasmic granules and expression of perforin within the granules. Following CTL–target-cell conjugate formation and granule exocytosis,

70-kD perforin monomers are released from the granules into the conjugate juncture, where they associate with the target-cell membrane. As the perforin molecules contact the membrane, they undergo a conformational change, exposing an amphipathic domain that inserts into the target-cell membrane; the monomers then polymerize (in the presence of Ca^{2+}) to form a cylindrical pore with an internal diameter of 5–20 nm (Figure 13-8a). A large number of perforin pores are visible on the target-cell membrane in the region of conjugate formation (Figure 13-8b). These pores are thought to facilitate entry of the various lytic substances also released from the granules, which destroy the target cell. Interestingly, perforin exhibits some sequence homology with the terminal C9 component of the complement system (see Chapter 15), and the membrane pores formed by perforin are similar to those observed in complement-mediated lysis.

One unanswered question in CTL-mediated target-cell killing is why the CTL cell itself is not killed by its own secreted perforin molecules. A single CTL cell is capable of killing multiple target cells, and yet it is not damaged in the process. Several hypotheses have been proposed to account for CTL protection. One proposal, advanced by J. D. E. Young and Z. A. Cohn, is that the CTL has a membrane protein ("protectin") that inactivates perforin either by preventing its insertion into the CTL membrane or by preventing its polymerization there. So far, however, no evidence has been adduced for such a protective protein.

A second hypothesis, proposed by P. J. Peters and coworkers, is that perforin is not released in a soluble form but rather is released within small membrane-bounded vesicles that in turn are housed in the electron-dense CTL granules. Such vesicles have in fact been observed with electron microscopy and have been shown by antibody conjugated with colloidal gold to express the TCR, CD3, and CD8 molecules of the CTL membrane (Figure 13-9). According to this hypothesis, the vesicles released from CTL granules exhibit specificity for the target cell via interaction of the TCR and CD8 with the antigen-MHC complexes on the target-cell membrane. Once the vesicles bind to the specific target cell, perforin is released and forms pores as described already. This mechanism not only would prevent self-killing of CTLs but also would prevent accidental killing of inappropriate target cells by perforin molecules that move away from the site of conjugate formation.

Other Mechanisms of CTL-Mediated Cytotoxicity. Some investigators have questioned whether perforin-mediated lysis is really the primary mechanism of CTL-mediated killing. One of the problems with the CTL lines in which cytotoxicity is studied is that they are obtained by culturing cells with high levels of IL-2. It has been suggested that such high levels of IL-2 might convert

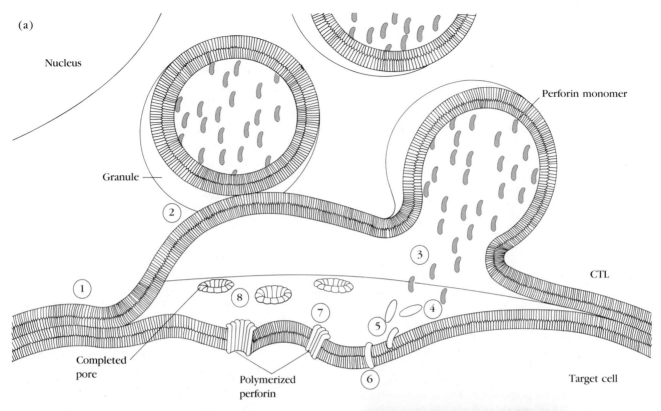

Figure 13-8 CTL-mediated pore formation in target-cell membrane. (a) In this model, a rise in intracellular Ca^{2+} triggered by CTL–target-cell interaction (1) induces exocytosis, in which the granules fuse with the CTL cell membrane (2) and release monomeric perforin into the small intracellular space between the two cells (3). The released perforin monomers undergo a Ca^{2+}-induced conformational change (4) and then bind to the target-cell membrane (5) and insert into it (6). In the presence of Ca^{2+}, the monomers polymerize within the membrane (7), forming cylindrical pores (8). (b) Electron micrograph of perforin pores on the surface of a rabbit erythrocyte target cell. [Part (a) adapted from J. D. E. Young and Z. A. Cohn, 1988, *Sci. Am.* (Jan.):38; part (b) from E. R. Podack and G. Dennert, 1983, *Nature* **301**:442.]

CTLs into NK-like cells exhibiting perforin-mediated killing that may not necessarily be the normal mechanism of CTL killing. A number of unexplained observations sharpen the controversy. Some CTL lines have been isolated that are potent target-cell killers but lack detectable perforin. Moreover, target-cell killing is accomplished by some CTL lines in the complete absence of Ca^{2+}; since Ca^{2+} is required for perforin polymerization, some other mechanism of killing must be operative in these cell lines. Another unexplained observation is that interaction of some CTLs with target cells results in a slower-than-normal killing process in which the target cells show nuclear-membrane damage and DNA fragmentation called *apoptosis*. It is not known how this process occurs, but there is come speculation that these

CTLs may induce an autolytic process within the target cells involving DNA fragmentation. Some CTL lines secrete toxic molecules, such as tumor necrosis factor β (TNF-β), which are known to activate enzymes that induce DNA fragmentation within the target-cell nucleus.

Cytotoxicity Mediated by Natural Killer Cells

Natural killer cells were discovered quite by accident when immunologists were measuring tumor-specific CTL activity in mice with tumors. Normal unimmunized mice and mice with unrelated tumors served as negative controls. Much to the consternation of the researchers,

(a)

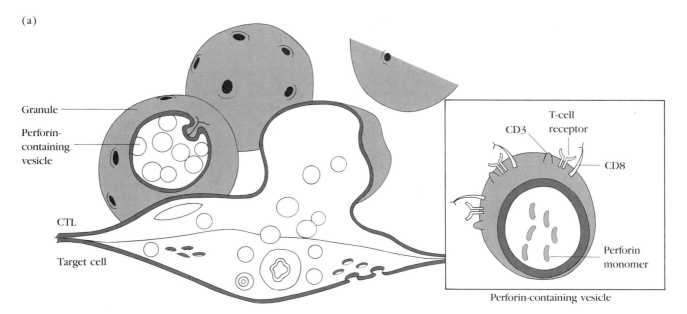

Figure 13-9   Alternative model of CTL-mediated killing in which perforin is released in small membrane-bounded vesicles. (a) Exocytosis of perforin-containing vesicles is depicted. The membrane molecules on the outer surface of these vesicles (*inset*) direct them toward the target cell where the TCR-CD3 complex and CD8 interact with antigen-class I·MHC on the target-cell membrane. (b) A more schematic illustration showing the perforin-containing vesicles thought to be derived by endocytosis of the CTL plasma membrane. Initial endocytosis results in TCR/CD3/CD8 facing inward, but subsequent membrane invagination produces smaller vesicles with TCR/CD3/CD8 facing outward. [Adapted from P. J. Peters et al., 1990, *Immunol. Today* **11**:28.]

(b)

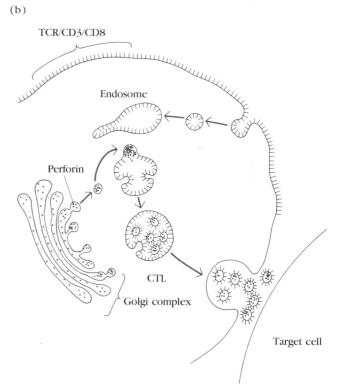

the controls showed significant tumor lysis in a CML assay. Characterization of the cells responsible for this nonspecific tumor-cell killing revealed that a population of large, granular lymphocytes was responsible. The cells, which were named natural killer (NK) cells for their nonspecific cytotoxicity make up 5% of the recirculating lymphocyte population. The lineage of NK cells remains uncertain, as they express some membrane markers of T lymphocytes and some markers of monocytes and granulocytes. Moreover, different NK cells express different sets of membrane molecules. It is not known whether this heterogeneity reflects subpopulations of NK cells or different stages in their activation or maturation. A single monoclonal antibody does bind to an IgG Fc receptor (CD16) on the membrane of more than 90% of NK cells and provides a way to monitor NK activity. This monoclonal antibody can be conjugated to a fluorescent marker, and flow cytometry can be used to separate NK cells from other cell types. The removal of CD16[+] cells has been shown to remove almost all NK-cell activity from peripheral blood.

The antitumor activity of NK cells differs from that of CTLs in several significant ways. First, NK cells do not

express antigen-specific T-cell receptors or CD3. In addition, antigen recognition by NK cells is not MHC restricted; that is, the same levels of NK cytotoxic activity are observed with syngeneic and allogeneic tumor cells. Also, although prior priming enhances CTL activity, no increase in NK activity occurs after a second injection with the same tumor cells; thus the NK response generates no immunologic memory. The nature of the NK cell's receptor and of the tumor-cell structures with which it interacts remains unknown. NK cells have also been shown to lyse some virus-infected target cells. This NK activity appears early in the response and appears to provide protection during the time required for T_C-cell activation, proliferation, and differentiation into functional CTLs. A recent report of a young woman who had normal T- and B-cell levels but completely lacked NK cells highlights their importance in viral immunity. She suffered severe varicella virus infections and a life-threatening infection with cytomegalovirus.

NK-mediated cytotoxicity appears to involve a process similar to CTL-mediated cytotoxicity. After an NK cell adheres to a target cell, degranulation of perforin-containing cytoplasmic granules occurs. The released perforin appears to damage the target cell in the same way described for the CTL. NK cells express the p75 kD component of the IL-2 receptor. The activity of NK cells is generally enhanced by IL-2 and interferon, which function synergistically to stimulate NK-cell proliferation. The resulting NK-cell population shows enhanced cytotoxicity against a wider range of target cells than untreated NK cells.

Antibody-Dependent Cell-Mediated Cytotoxicity

A number of cells that have cytotoxic potential express membrane receptors for the Fc region of the antibody molecule. When antibody is specifically bound to a target cell, these receptor-bearing cells can bind to the antibody Fc region, and thus to the target cells, and subsequently cause lysis of the target cell. Although the cytotoxic cells involved are nonspecific, the specificity of the antibody directs them to specific target cells. This type of cytotoxicity is referred to as *antibody-dependent cell-mediated cytotoxicity* (ADCC). A variety of cells have been shown to exhibit ADCC including NK cells, macrophages, monocytes, neutrophils, and eosinophils (Figure 13-10). Antibody-dependent cell-mediated killing of cells infected with the measles virus can be observed in vitro by adding antimeasles antibody together with macrophages to a culture of measles-infected cells. Similarly, cell-mediated killing of helminths, such as schistosomes or blood flukes, can be observed in vitro by incubating newly infected larvae (schistosomules) with antibody to the schistosomules together with eosinophils.

Target-cell killing by ADCC, which does not involve complement-mediated lysis, appears to involve a number of different cytotoxic mechanisms. When macrophages, neutrophils, or eosinophils bind to a target cell by way of the Fc receptor, they become more active metabolically, which leads to an increase in the lytic components in their cytoplasmic lysosomes or granules. Release of these lytic components at the site of the Fc-mediated contact may result in damage to the target cell. In addition, activated monocytes, macrophages, and NK cells

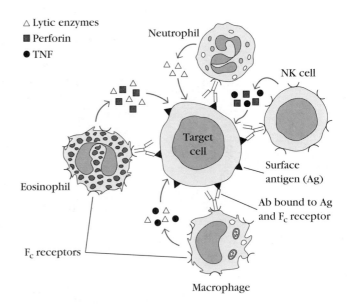

Figure 13-10 Antibody-dependent cell-mediated cytotoxicity (ADCC). Nonspecific cytotoxic cells are directed to specific target cells by binding to the Fc region of bound target-cell–specific antibodies. The target cells then are killed by the action of various substances (e.g., lytic enzymes, TNF, perforin) secreted by the nonspecific cytotoxic cells.

have been shown to secrete tumor necrosis factor, which may have a cytotoxic effect on the bound target cell. Since both NK cells and eosinophils contain perforin in cytoplasmic granules, their target-cell killing may result from perforin-mediated membrane damage similar to the mechanism described for CTL-mediated cytotoxicity.

Delayed-Type Hypersensitivity Response

When some subpopulations of activated T_H cells encounter certain types of antigens, they secrete cytokines that induce a localized inflammatory reaction called *delayed-type hypersensitivity* (DTH). The reaction is characterized by large influxes of nonspecific inflammatory cells, in which the macrophage is a major participant. Historically, this type of reaction was first described in 1890 by Robert Koch, who observed that individuals infected with *Mycobacterium tuberculosis* developed a localized inflammatory response when injected intradermally with a filtrate derived from a mycobacterial culture. He called this localized skin reaction a "tuberculin reaction." Later, as it became apparent that a variety of other antigens could induce this response, its name was changed to delayed-type hypersensitivity in reference to the delayed onset of the reaction and to the extensive tissue damage (hypersensitivity) that is

Table 13-3 Delayed type hypersensitivity

Antigens inducing response	Antigen presenting cells	T_{DTH} cells

Intracellular bacteria
  Mycobacterium tuberculosis
  Mycobacterium leprae
  Listeria monocytogenes
  Brucella abortus
Intracellular fungi
  Pneumocystis carinii
  Candida albicans
  Histoplasma capsulatum
  Cryptococcus neoformans
Intracellular parasites
  Leishmania sp.
  Schistosoma sp.
Intracellular viruses
  Herpes simplex virus
  Variola (smallpox)
  Measles virus
Contact dermatitis
  Poison oak and ivy
  Picrylchloride
  Hair dyes
  Nickel salts
	Macrophages
	Langerhans cells
	Vascular endothelial cells
		Generally $CD4^+$
		  (T_H1 subpopulation)
		Occasionally $CD8^+$
		  in response to
		  viral antigens

often associated with the reaction. The term *hypersensitivity* is somewhat misleading for it suggests that a DTH response is always detrimental. Although in some cases a DTH response does cause extensive tissue damage and is in itself pathologic, in many cases tissue damage is limited, and the response plays an important role in defense against intracellular pathogens (Table 13-3).

Phases of the DTH Response

The development of the DTH response requires an initial sensitization period of 1–2 weeks following primary contact with the antigen. During this period T_H cells are activated and clonally expanded by antigen presented together with the requisite class II MHC molecule on an appropriate antigen-presenting cell (Figure 13-11). A variety of antigen-presenting cells have been shown to be involved in the activation of a DTH response, including Langerhans' cells and macrophages. Langerhans' cells are dendritic cells found in the epidermis. These cells are thought to pick up antigen that enters through the skin and transport the antigen to the regional lymph nodes where T cells are activated to the antigen. In some species, including humans, the vascular endothelial

cells express class II MHC and also function as antigen presenting cells in the development of the DTH response.

A secondary contact with antigen induces the effector phase of the response. In the effector phase the activated T cells secrete a variety of cytokines that are responsible for the recruitment and activation of macrophages and other nonspecific inflammatory cells. Generally, the activated T cells are $CD4^+$ but in a few cases $CD8^+$ cells have also been shown to induce a DTH response. The activated T cells are often designated as T_{DTH} cells to denote their function in the DTH response, although in reality they are simply a subset of T_H cells (or in some cases T_C cells).

In general it takes an average of 24 h following secondary contact with the antigen before the DTH response becomes apparent, and the response does not generally peak until 48 to 72 h. The delayed onset of this response reflects the time required for the cytokines to induce localized influxes of macrophages and activation of these cells. Once a DTH response begins, a complex interplay of nonspecific cells and mediators is set in motion that can result in tremendous amplification. By the time the DTH response is fully developed, only about 5% of the participating cells are antigen-

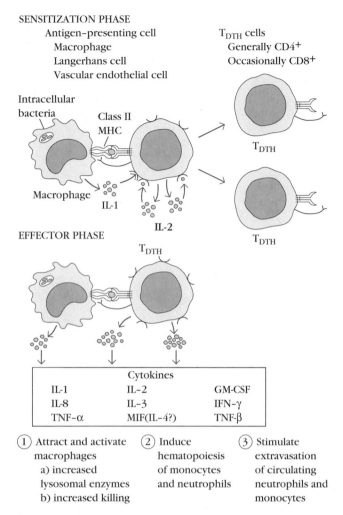

SENSITIZATION PHASE
    Antigen–presenting cell
        Macrophage
        Langerhans cell
        Vascular endothelial cell

T$_{DTH}$ cells
    Generally CD4$^+$
    Occasionally CD8$^+$

Intracellular bacteria

Class II MHC

Macrophage

IL-1

IL-2

T$_{DTH}$

T$_{DTH}$

EFFECTOR PHASE

T$_{DTH}$

T$_{DTH}$

Cytokines		
IL-1	IL-2	GM-CSF
IL-8	IL-3	IFN-γ
TNF-α	MIF(IL-4?)	TNF-β

① Attract and activate macrophages
   a) increased lysosomal enzymes
   b) increased killing

② Induce hematopoiesis of monocytes and neutrophils

③ Stimulate extravasation of circulating neutrophils and monocytes

Figure 13-11 Overview of the DTH response. In the sensitization phase following primary contact with antigen, T$_H$ cells proliferate and differentiate into T$_{DTH}$ cells. This phase takes about 1–2 weeks. In the effector phase following a secondary contact with antigen, T$_{DTH}$ cells secrete a variety of cytokines, which have three primary functions. This phase peaks about 2–3 days after secondary contact with antigen.

specific T$_{DTH}$ cells and the remainder are macrophages and other nonspecific cells. The macrophage functions as the principal effector cell of the DTH response. Cytokines elaborated by the T$_{DTH}$ cell induce blood monocytes to adhere to vascular endothelial cells and migrate from the blood into the surrounding tissues. During this process the monocytes differentiate into *activated macrophages*. These activated macrophages exhibit increased levels of phagocytosis and an increased ability to kill microorganisms. In addition, activated macrophages express increased levels of class II MHC molecules and cellular adhesion molecules and therefore function as more effective antigen-presenting cells.

The influx and activation of macrophages in the DTH response provides an effective host defense against intracellular pathogens. Generally the pathogen is rapidly

cleared with little tissue damage. However, in some cases, especially if the antigen is not easily cleared, a prolonged DTH response can itself become destructive to the host as the intense inflammatory response develops into a visible *granulomatous reaction*. A granuloma develops when continuous activation of macrophages induces the macrophages to adhere closely to one another, assuming an *epitheloid* shape and sometimes fusing to form multinucleated *giant* cells. These giant cells displace the normal tissue cells, forming palpable nodules, and cause tissue destruction by the high concentrations of lysosomal enzymes released into the surrounding tissue. In these cases the response can lead to blood-vessel damage and extensive tissue necrosis.

Cytokines Involved in DTH Reaction

Numerous cytokines play a role in generating a DTH reaction (Figure 13-12). The pattern of cytokines implicated in a DTH response suggest that T$_{DTH}$ cells may be similar to the T$_H$1 subset. IL-2 functions in an autocrine manner to amplify the population of cytokine-producing T cells. Among the cytokines produced by these cells are a number that serve to activate and attract macrophages to the site of T$_H$1 activation. IL-3 and GM-CSF induce localized hematopoiesis of the granulocyte-monocyte lineage (see Figure 3-2). IFN-γ and TNF-β (together with macrophage-derived TNF-α and IL-1) act on nearby endothelial cells, inducing a number of changes that facilitate extravasation of monocytes and other nonspecific inflammatory cells. Among the changes induced are increases in the expression of cellular-adhesion molecules including ICAMs, VCAMs, and ELAMs, changes in the shape of the vascular endothelial cells to facilitate extravasation, and secretion of IL-8 and monocyte chemotactic factor. Circulating neutrophils and monocytes adhere to the adhesion molecules displayed on the vascular endothelial cells and extravasate into the tissue spaces. Neutrophils appear early in the reaction, peaking by about 6 h and then declining in numbers. The monocyte infiltration occurs between 24 and 48 h after antigen exposure.

As the monocytes enter the tissues to become macrophages, they are drawn to the site of the DTH response by chemotactic factors such as the cytokine IFN-γ. Another cytokine, called *migration-inhibition factor* (MIF), (which may in fact be IL-4), inhibits further macrophage migration and thus prevents the macrophages from migrating from the site of a DTH reaction. As discussed later, production of MIF is the basis for a common in vitro test for the ability of an individual to generate a DTH reaction.

As the macrophages accumulate at the site of a DTH reaction, they are activated by cytokines, of which IFN-γ plays a major role. IFN-γ induces the macrophage

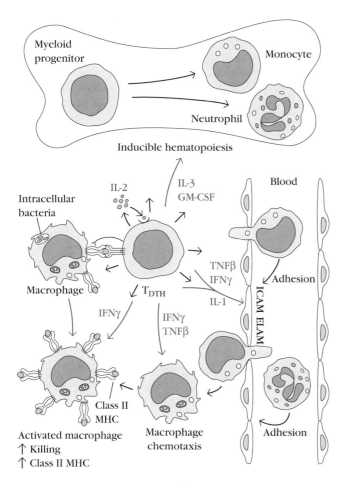

Figure 13-12 Role of cytokines in mediating a DTH tissue reaction. Cytokines secreted by T$_{DTH}$ cells are indicated in red. These cytokines act to (1) induce hematopoiesis of monocytes and neutrophils, (2) increase the expression of cell-adhesion molecules (ICAM, VCAM, and ELAM) on nearby vessel endothelial cells, (3) attract monocytes and macrophages via chemotaxis, and (4) activate macrophages. Also indicated is MIF (which may be IL-4), also secreted by T$_{DTH}$ cells, which inhibits the motility of macrophages and keeps them confined to the site of tissue activation.

this point is nonspecific, however, and often results in significant damage to healthy tissue. Generally this is the price the body pays for successful elimination of cells harboring intracellular bacterial and fungal pathogens. The importance of the DTH response in protecting the host against various intracellular pathogens is illustrated by AIDS. In this disease, CD4$^+$ T cells are severely depleted, resulting in a loss of the DTH response. Often patients suffering with AIDS develop life-threatening infections from intracellular bacteria, fungi, or protozoans that would not threaten an individual whose DTH response was intact. The immune response in AIDS patients is discussed in more depth in Chapter 21.

Another example in which delayed-type hypersensitivity plays an important role in host defense is infection by *Leishmania major*, an intracellular protozoan that causes leishmaniasis, an often fatal disease in Third-World countries. An animal model of this disease has been developed in mice. Various inbred strains infected with *L. major* show genetic differences in susceptibility to the pathogen. For example, CBA-strain mice develop small lesions at the site of inoculation and progress to a self-limited infection that renders the animals immune to further infection. Analysis of the immune response

to differentiate into activated cells, whose size, content of lysosomal enzymes, phagocytic ability, and capacity to kill intracellular pathogens are all increased compared with unactivated macrophages. Because macrophages activated by IFN-γ also express more class II MHC molecules and IL-1, they are more effective antigen-presenting cells than unactivated macrophages. Such activated macrophages can efficiently mediate activation of more T$_{DTH}$ cells, which in turn secrete more lymphokines that recruit and activate even more macrophages. This self-perpetuating response, however, is a double-edged sword, with a fine line existing between a beneficial, protective response and a detrimental response characterized by extensive tissue damage.

Protective Role of the DTH Response

Delayed-type hypersensitivity responses play an important role in defense against various intracellular bacteria and fungi. A variety of intracellular pathogens (e.g., *Mycobacterium tuberculosis, Listeria, Brucella, Candida,* and *Pneumocystis carinii*) are known to induce this type of immune response. The accumulation of activated macrophages with localized release of lysosomal enzymes results in rapid destruction of cells harboring intracellular pathogens (Figure 13-13). The response at

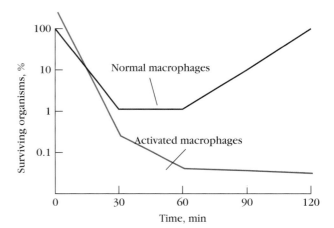

Figure 13-13 Survival of the intracellular pathogen *Listeria monocytogenes* when mixed with normal macrophages (not activated by IFN-γ) or activated macrophages in vitro. Note the logarithmic scale. The much greater ability of activated macrophages to destroy intracellular pathogens is evident.

in these mice has revealed that CD4$^+$ T cells are responsible for the immune state; the transfer of CD4$^+$ T cells from immune CBA mice was shown to confer immunity on normal syngeneic recipients. The subpopulation of CD4$^+$ T cells that confers immunity in CBA mice was shown by cytokine analysis to resemble the T$_H$1 subset of T$_H$ cells, a subpopulation that secretes IL-2, IL-3, GM-CSF, and IFN-γ. As described previously, these cytokines help mediate the DTH reaction, which results in elimination of intracellular pathogens by activated macrophages. Inbred strains of mice that do not develop immunity to *Leishmania* (e.g., BALB/c), and consequently progress to a fatal infection, mount an immune response characterized by lower levels of T$_H$1-type cells than found in immune mice. These experiments suggest that differences in T$_H$1 activity in different inbred strains determine the degree of immune protection against *Leishmania*. It has been suggested that this

animal model reflects possible differences in T$_H$-cell subpopulations that may exist in humans and may determine why some individuals are immune to certain intracellular pathogens, whereas others are susceptible. The next chapter will examine this topic in more detail.

Detection of DTH Reaction In Vivo and In Vitro

The presence of a DTH reaction can be measured experimentally by injecting antigen intradermally into an animal and observing whether a characteristic skin lesion develops at the injection site. A positive skin-test reaction indicates that the individual has a population of sensitized T$_{DTH}$ cells specific for the test antigen. In the skin test to determine whether an individual has been exposed to *Mycobacterium tuberculosis*, the per-

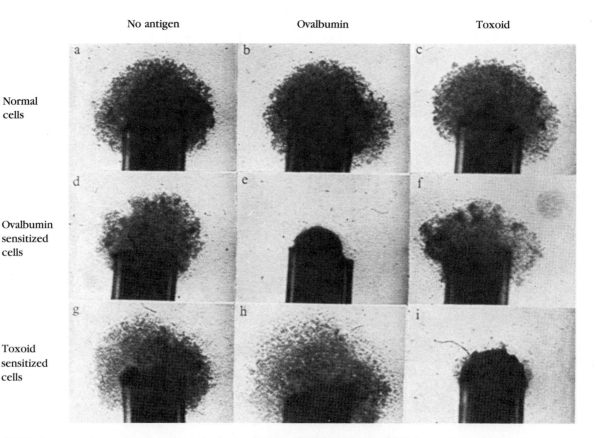

Figure 13-14   Assay for the production of macrophage migration inhibition factor (MIF) by sensitized T$_{DTH}$ cells. In the absense of MIF, macrophages migrate out of their capillary tube onto an agar matrix. In the presence of MIF, the migration of the macrophages is inhibited. [From John R. David, 1970, *Immunology*, The Upjohn Company, Kalamazoo, Mich.]

son is given an intradermal injection of PPD, a protein derived from the cell wall of the mycobacterium. Development of a red, slightly swollen, firm lesion at the site between 48 and 72 h later indicates that the individual has been exposed to *M. tuberculosis* antigens, either through direct exposure to the organism or through immunization—a procedure which is performed in some parts of the world. Development of a skin lesion in a previously sensitized individual results from the intense infiltration of cells to the site of injection during a DTH reaction; 80–90% of these cells are macrophages.

An in vitro DTH response can be detected by the presence of various cytokines whose level of activity gives some indication of the intensity of the response. For example, the secretion of MIF by lymphocytes from a sensitized animal has been shown to correlate well with the animal's ability to mount a DTH response. As mentioned earlier, MIF is thought to be secreted by activated T_{DTH} cells. Production of MIF by cultured lymphocytes exposed to antigen thus can serve as an in vitro assay for the DTH response (Figure 13-14). In this assay, lymphocytes are first cultured in the presence of antigen and appropriate antigen-presenting cells. The culture supernatant is then added together with macrophages to a glass capillary tube. The capillary tube is placed horizontally on a surface bathed in tissue-culture medium. If MIF is present, the macrophages remain in the tube, but in the absence of MIF they migrate out of the capillary tube onto the surface. Thus by monitoring macrophage migration, it is possible to determine whether significant amounts of MIF were produced in the in vitro lymphocyte culture.

Pathologic DTH Responses

In some cases the DTH response to an intracellular pathogen can cause such extensive tissue damage that the response itself is pathologic and constitutes a truly hypersensitive condition. Much of the tissue damage to the lung in tuberculosis results from the accumulation of activated macrophages whose lysosomal enzymes destroy healthy lung tissue. Delayed-type hypersensitive reactions can also develop to inappropriate antigens such as poison oak and skin-contact sensitizers. Such examples, of truly hypersensitive conditions, in which tissue damage far outweighs any beneficial effects, are discussed in Chapter 16.

Summary

1. Cell-mediated immune reactions involving direct cytotoxicity are mediated by antigen-specific cytotoxic T lymphocytes (CTLs) and nonspecific effector cells such as natural killer cells and macrophages.

2. Cytotoxicity mediated by CTLs involves a sensitization phase and an effector phase. During the sensitization phase there is extensive proliferation of T_H cells with production of IL-2. Once a cytotoxic T lymphocyte precursor (CTL-P) is activated by the recognition of antigen–class I MHC complexes, it begins to express IL-2 receptors. IL-2 produced by the proliferating T_H cells can now bind to IL-2 receptors on the CTL-P and induce cellular proliferation and differentiation into an effector CTL.

3. The effector phase of CTL-mediated cytotoxicity involves recognition of specific target cells bearing antigen and class I MHC molecules and formation of CTL–target-cell conjugates. Following conjugate formation, cytoplasmic granules within the cytoplasm of the CTL concentrate in the region of close membrane interaction with the target cell. Granule exocytosis in the zone of cellular adhesion releases the granular contents, including the protein perforin, which polymerizes and forms pores in the target-cell membrane. The CTL dissociates from the target cell, which eventually is destroyed by the membrane damage. Target-cell killing by some CTLs may depend on a slower process involving nuclear-membrane damage and DNA fragmentation.

4. Various nonspecific cells, including NK cells and macrophages, can kill target cells without having to interact with antigen-MHC complexes on the target cells. In some cases, nonspecific cytotoxic cells bind to the Fc region of antibody on target cells; such antibody-directed cell-mediated cytotoxicity (ADCC) thus directs nonspecific cytotoxic cells to specific target cells.

5. Cell-mediated immunity involving delayed-type hypersensitivity plays an important role in host defense against intracellular pathogens. T_{DTH} cells, which differentiate from activated T_H cells, secrete a number of lymphokines that cause macrophages to accumulate and to become activated. The activated macrophages are more effective killers of intracellular pathogens.

References

DUSTIN, M. L., and T. A. SPRINGER. 1989. T cell receptor cross-linking transiently stimulates through LFA-1. *Nature* **341**:619.

GROMO, G., L. INVERARDI, R. L. GELLER et al. 1987. Signal requirements in the stepwise functional maturation of cytotoxic T lymphocytes. *Nature* **327**:424.

MULLER, I., T. PEDRAZZINI, J. P. FARRELL, and J. LOUIS. 1989. T cell responses and immunity to experimental infection with *Leishmania major. Annu. Rev. Immunol.* **7**:561.

PETER, P. J., H. J. GEUZE, H. A. VAN DER DONK et al. 1989. Molecules relevant for T cell–target cell interaction are present in cytolytic granules of human T lymphocytes. *Eur. J. Immunol.* **19**:1469.

PETER, P. J., H. J. GEUZE, H. A. VAN DER DONK, and J. BORST. 1990. A new model for lethal hit delivery by cytotoxic T cells. *Immunol. Today* **11**:28.

POBER, J. S., and R. S. COTRAN. 1990. Cytokines and endothelial cell biology. *Physiol. Rev.* **70**:427.

TSCHOPP, J., and M. NABHOLZ. 1990. Perforin mediated target cell lysis by cytolytic T lymphocytes. *Annu. Rev. Immunol.* **8**:279.

YOUNG, J. D. E, and Z. A. COHN. 1988. How killer cells kill. *Sci. Am.* (Jan):38.

Study Questions

1. You have a monoclonal antibody specific for LFA-1. You perform CML assays of a CTL clone, using target cells for which the clone is specific, in the presence and absence of this antibody. Predict the relative amounts of [^{51}Cr] released in the two assays. Explain your answer.

2. You decide to coculture lymphocytes from the strains listed in the table below in order to observe the mixed-lymphocyte reaction (MLR). In each case, indicate which lymphocyte population(s) you would expect to proliferate.

Population 1	Population 2	Proliferation
C57BL/6 (H-2^b)	CBA (H-2^k)	
C57BL/6 (H-2^b)	CBA (H-2^k) mitomycin C–treated	
C57BL/6 (H-2^b)	F$_1$ (CBA × C57BL/6)	
C57BL/6 (H-2^b)	C57L (H-2^b)	

3. In the mixed-lymphocyte reaction (MLR), which cell type proliferates in response to allogeneic antigen? How would you prove the identity of the proliferating cell? Another way of assaying for the activity of this cell in the MLR is to assay IL-2 production. Why can IL-2 measurements be used to assess activity of this cell?

4. Indicate whether each of the properties listed in the table below is exhibited by T$_H$ cells and/or CTLs by placing a + or − in the appropriate columns.

Property	T$_H$ cell	CTL
Can make IL-1		
Can make IL-2		
Is class I MHC restricted		
Expresses CD8		
Is required for B-cell activation		
Is cytotoxic for target cells		
Is the main proliferating cell in an MLR		
Is the effector cell in a CML assay		
Is class II MHC restricted		
Expresses CD4		
Can respond to IL-1		
Expresses CD3		
Adheres to target cells via LFA-1		
Can express the IL-2 receptor		
Expresses the $\alpha\beta$ T-cell receptor		
Is the principal target of HIV		
Responds to soluble antigens alone		
Produces perforin molecules		

5. Mice from several different inbred strains were infected with LCM virus, and several days later their spleen cells were isolated. The ability of the primed spleen cells to lyse LCM-infected, [^{51}Cr] labeled target cells from various strains was determined. In the table below, indicate with a (+) or (−) whether the spleen cells listed in the left column would cause [^{51}Cr] release from the target cells listed across the top of the table.

6. A mouse is infected with influenza virus. How could you assess whether the mouse has T_H and T_C cells specific for influenza?

Source of primed spleen cells	[^{51}Cr] release from LCM-infected target cells			
	B10.D2 (H-2^d)	B10 (H-2^b)	B10.BR (H-2^k)	F$_1$ (BALB/c × B10) (H-2$^{b/d}$)
B10.D2 (H-2^d)				
B10 (H-2^b)				
BALB/c (H-2^d)				
(BALB/c × B10)				

Immune Regulation and Tolerance

U pon encountering an antigen the immune
system can either develop an immune response or enter a state of unresponsiveness called *tolerance.* The development of
immunity or tolerance, both of which involve
specific recognition of antigen by antigen-
reactive T or B cells, needs to be carefully regulated since an inappropriate response—whether
it be immunity to self-antigens or tolerance to a
potential pathogen—can have serious and possibly life-threatening consequences.

Regulation of the immune response takes place
in both the humoral and the cell-mediated

branch. Every time an antigen is introduced, important regulatory decisions determine the branch of the immune system to be activated, the intensity of the response, and its duration. Unfortunately, very little is yet known about these regulatory events; this lack of knowledge has made it difficult for immunologists to selectively up-regulate or down-regulate immune reactivity when such fine-tuning would be desirable. This chapter examines some of the factors known to regulate immune responsiveness and the conditions under which tolerance is induced.

Regulation of Immune Responsiveness

The nature, intensity, and duration of both the humoral and cell-mediated immune responses is influenced by prior host exposure to antigen, the nature and concentration of antigen, circulating antibodies and immune complexes, cytokines, the development of anti-idiotype antibodies, and certain T cells. Each of these factors is discussed in this section; the induction of tolerance is examined later in this chapter.

Effect of Prior Antigen Exposure

The immunologic history of an animal influences the quality and quantity of its immune response. A naive animal responds very differently from a previously primed animal to antigen challenge. Previous antigen encounter may have rendered the animal tolerant to the antigen or may have resulted in the formation of memory cells. These memory cells include distinct T_H-cell subpopulations having distinct cytokine patterns and B cells, which may have class-switched to various isotypes.

Antigen as Regulator

The nature of the antigen exerts a major effect on the type of immune response generated. Bacteria, bacterial products, and soluble protein antigens tend to induce the production of humoral antibody; intracellular bacteria and viruses induce cell-mediated immunity. Since antigen is required for immune activation, it is obvious that the clearance of antigen will diminish further immune activation and the immune response will decline.

In some cases the presence of a competing antigen can regulate the immune response to an unrelated antigen. This *antigenic competition* is illustrated by injecting mice with a competing antigen a day or two before immunization with a test antigen. As Table 14-1 reveals, the response to horse red blood cells (HRBCs)

Table 14-1   Antigenic competition between SRBCs and HRBCs

Immunizing antigen		Hemolytic plaque assay (day 8)*	
Ag1 (day 0)	Ag2 (day 3)	Test Ag	PFC/10^6 spleen cells
None	HRBC	HRBC	205
SRBC	HRBC	HRBC	13
None	SRBC	SRBC	626
HRBC	SRBC	SRBC	78

* See Figure 12-3 for assay details.

is severely reduced by prior immunization with sheep red blood cells (SRBCs) and vice versa. At the cellular level, a competing antigen may interfere with antigen presentation to and activation of T_H cells; alternatively, the immune response to the competing antigen may generate various cytokines that down-regulate a subsequent response.

Although antigen concentration is the primary regulator of the intensity of an immune response, other regulators operate at a coarse or fine level to contribute to the intensity and duration of the response. An early finding suggesting that a decline in antigen level is not solely responsible for immune regulation came from experiments of C. G. Romball and W. O. Weigle. They injected rabbits with a single dose of human IgG and then determined the number of plaque-forming plasma cells at various times. Although antigen concentrations declined in a linear fashion, the number of plasma cells generated in response to the antigen showed a cyclical response, peaking, declining, and peaking again several times (Figure 14-1). This cyclical response indicates that something other than antigen concentration must be regulating the response.

Antibody-Mediated Suppression

As in so many biochemical reactions subject to feedback inhibition by the end product, antibody exerts feedback inhibition on its own further production. If an animal is immunized with a specific antigen and is injected with preformed antibody to that same antigen just before or within 5 days after antigen priming, the immune response to the antigen is reduced as much as 100-fold. That this *antibody-mediated suppression* is not simply due to more rapid clearance of the antigen can be demonstrated if the antigen is a protein conjugated with two

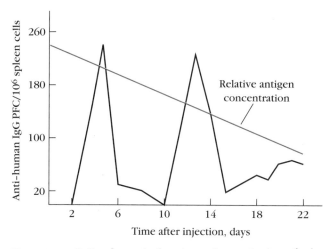

Figure 14-1 Following a single primary immunization of rabbits with human IgG, the number of splenic plasma cells secreting anti-human IgG antibodies showed a cyclical pattern despite the linear decrease in serum antigen concentration. This finding indicates that the immune response is not regulated solely by antigen concentration. [Adapted from C. G. Romball and W. O. Weigle, 1973, *J. Exp. Med.* **138**:1426.]

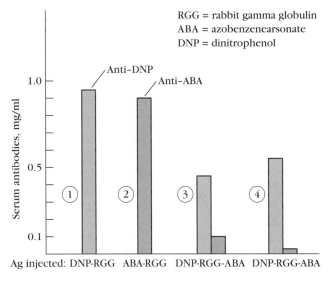

Figure 14-2 Experimental demonstration that antibody-mediated suppression is not caused only by more rapid antigen clearance. After animals were immunized with the indicated hapten-carrier conjugates, the serum concentrations of antibodies to the haptens DNP and ABA were determined. The suppression of anti-ABA production, but not of anti-DNP production, in experiment 4 indicates that antibody-mediated antigen clearance is not the sole cause of antibody-mediated suppression. [Based on data from N. I. Brody et al., 1967, *J. Exp. Med.* **126**:81.]

different haptens. For example, administration of preformed antibody to azobenzenearsonate (ABA) suppressed only the antibody response to ABA even though both ABA and DNP were presented on the same carrier and thus should have been cleared at the same rate (Figure 14-2).

One explanation for antibody-mediated suppression is that the passively administered antibody competes with antigen-reactive B cells for antigen, so that the B cells do not clonally expand. Evidence for such competition between passively administered antibody and antigen-reactive B cells comes from studies in which it took more than 10 times more low-affinity anti-DNP antibody than high-affinity anti-DNP antibody to induce comparable suppression. Furthermore, the competition for antigen between passively administered antibody and antigen-reactive B cells drives the response toward higher affinity. Only the high-affinity antigen-reactive cells can compete successfully with the passively administered antibody for the available antigen. This process is similar to affinity maturation, which occurs in the course of an immune response as the antibody formed early in the response begins to bind to the antigen, decreasing its concentration so that only the high-affinity antigen-reactive cells are stimulated later in the response (see Table 12-4).

Because of antibody-mediated suppression, certain vaccines (e.g., those for measles and mumps), are not administered to infants before the age of 1 year. The level of naturally acquired maternal IgG that the fetus acquires by transplacental transfer remains high for about 6 months after birth. If an infant is immunized with the measles or mumps vaccine while this maternal antibody is still present, the humoral response is low and the production of memory cells is inadequate to confer long-lasting immunity.

On the other hand, the down-regulation of the immune response by antibody can be used to therapeutic advantage when an Rh⁻ mother gives birth to an Rh⁺ baby. In such cases of Rh incompatibility, the mother usually is given an injection of Rhogam, an antiserum specific for the Rh antigen, within 24–48 h after delivery. This anti-Rh antibody binds to any fetal Rh antigen that may have entered the mother's blood at the time of delivery, suppressing clonal proliferation and memory-cell formation of Rh-reactive lymphocytes in the mother. This procedure substantially reduces the risk of a secondary maternal IgG response to fetal Rh⁺ blood in a subsequent pregnancy (see Chapter 16).

Immune Complexes as Regulators

Preformed antigen-antibody complexes have been shown in experiments sometimes to enhance and in other cases to suppress the immune response. These immune complexes may exert their effect by binding to Fc receptors on various cells. It has not yet been possible to predict the effect of immune-complex size on immune responsiveness. There is evidence suggesting that patients with malignant tumors often develop circulating immune complexes in which antibody is complexed with tumor antigens. These complexes have been shown to suppress the immune response in these patients.

Cytokine-Mediated Regulation

The pleiotropic, synergistic, and antagonistic effects of cytokines enable them to function as regulators of both the humoral and cell-mediated branches of the immune system. Since the early 1970s, it has been observed that humoral-antibody production and the activity of T_{DTH} cells are inversely related. More recent evidence suggests that the pattern of cytokines produced during an immune response may explain the distinction between these two functional activities.

As discussed in previous chapters, mouse T_H-cell clones derived from long-term cultures can be divided into the T_H1 and T_H2 subset, distinguished by the patterns of cytokines they secrete (see Table 11-5). The T_H1 subset functions better at mediating delayed-type hypersensitivity than activating B cells, whereas the T_H2 subset exhibits the reverse activity pattern. Furthermore, cytokines secreted by these two subsets have been shown to regulate each other. Interferon γ (IFN-γ), produced by T_H1 cells, inhibits proliferation of T_H2 cells, and interleukin 10 (IL-10), produced by T_H2 cells, inhibits cytokine production by T_H1 cells. These experimental systems illustrate the important role that the cytokine balance plays in the regulation of antibody and T_{DTH} responses, although it remains to be seen whether T cells with the T_H1 and T_H2 cytokine patterns exist as distinct subpopulations within the normal animal.

In addition to influencing whether a humoral or cell-mediated response predominates, the cytokine balance may influence susceptiblity to infection by certain pathogens. For example, as noted in the last chapter, BALB/c mice are susceptible to infection by the intracellular protozoan *Leishmania major*, whereas CBA mice are resistant. Analysis of the cytokine mRNAs from these two strains showed that the level of IFN-γ mRNA was 50- to 100-fold higher in resistant CBA mice than in susceptible BALB/c mice. Since IFN-γ plays a vital role

Table 14-2 Effects of IL-4 and IFN-γ on isotype production by LPS-activated B cells in culture

Cytokine added to culture	Isotype levels in supernatant* (ng/ml)	
	IgE	IgG1
None	1.3	1,340
IL-4	171	20,000
IL-4 + IFN-γ	4.1	3,700

* Determined after culturing cells for 7 days.

in mediating the DTH reaction, particularly macrophage recruitment and activation (see Figure 13-12), macrophages in CBA mice would be more effective than those in BALB/c mice in killing *L. major*. These results strengthen the hypothesis that T_H1-like or T_H2-like cytokine activities may regulate which branch of the immune system is activated by various antigens.

The regulatory functions of cytokines also extend to the selection of immunoglobulin isotypes. The opposing effects of IL-4 and IFN-γ illustrate how the balance of cytokines produced during an immune response can contribute to the production of very different isotypes. Class switching of LPS-activated B cells to IgG1 and IgE is induced by IL-4, but in the presence of IFN-γ the IL-4 effect is blocked (Table 14-2). In contrast, if LPS-activated B cells are cultured in the presence of IFN-γ, they secrete IgG2a; however, this effect is blocked if IL-4 is added to the culture. Thus the balance of IL-4 and IFN-γ produced during an immune response can regulate the levels of the IgG1, IgE, and IgG2a isotypes.

Idiotype Regulation: The Network Theory

The enormous diversity of antibody and T-cell receptor (TCR) specificities that can be generated by the immune system is mind-boggling. Current estimates suggest that the immune system is capable of generating on the order of 10^{11} distinct antibody specificities and $10^{15}-10^{18}$ distinct TCR specificities. Since a mouse produces only 10^8 lymphocytes per day, only a fraction of the potential repertoire is expressed during the lifetime of a mouse. Because antigen-specific antibodies and T-cell-receptors are not expressed during fetal development of the immune system, their variable-region sequences can be recognized as non-self by the immune system.

In 1973 Niels Jerne proposed a conceptual theory, called the *network theory*, that predicted the consequences of immune-system recognition of self-antibody;

(a)

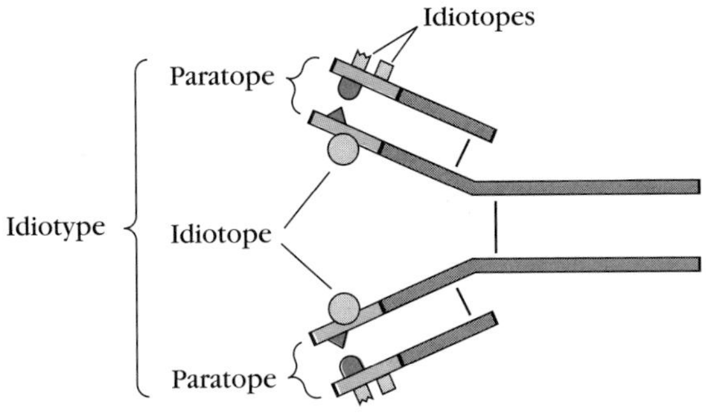

(b)

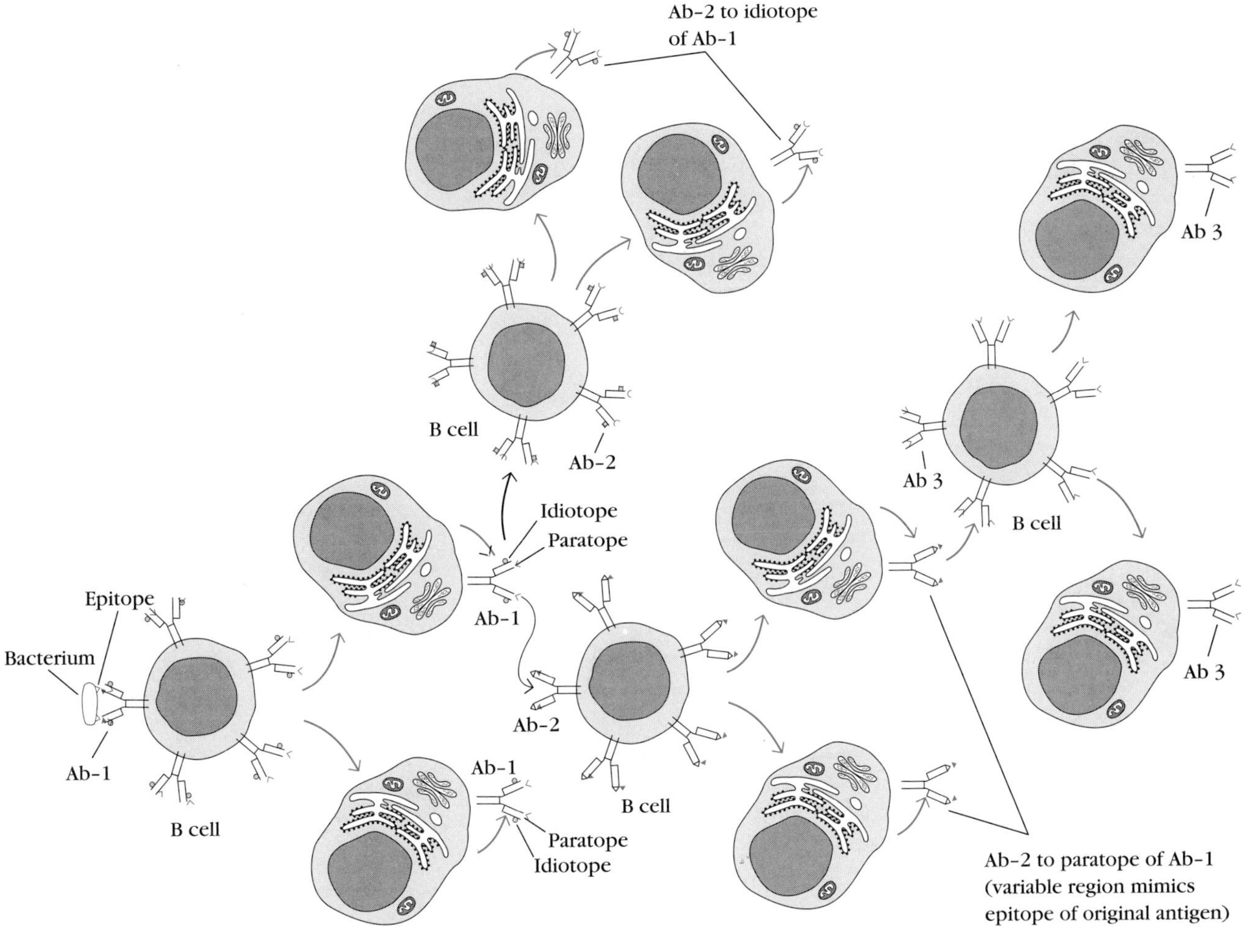

Figure 14-3 (a) Each antibody molecule expresses unique variable-region epitopes called idiotopes; the sum of the idiotopes is called its idiotype. Idiotopes may coincide with the antigen-binding site, or paratope. (b) According to the network theory, formulated by Niels Jerne, the immune response to an antigen results in the formation of anti-idiotype antibodies specific for the individual idiotopes of the primary antibody (Ab-1). These anti-idiotype antibodies (Ab-2) in turn induce the formation of anti-anti-idiotype antibodies (Ab-3). A network of interacting antibodies is thus formed that serves to regulate the immune response.

for this work, Jerne was awarded a Nobel prize in 1985. According to the network theory, as antibody is produced in response to an antigen, it in turn induces the formation of antibodies to its unique variable-region sequences. Jerne referred to each individual antigenic determinant of the variable region as an *idiotope*. Each antibody contains multiple idiotopes, and the sum of the individual idiotopes is called the *idiotype* of the antibody. In some cases, a particular idiotope and the actual antigen-combining site, which Jerne called the *paratope*, are identical; in other cases the idiotopes comprise variable-region sequences outside the antigen-binding site (Figure 14-3a). The network theory proposes that during an antibody response the antibodies formed in response to the antigen in turn induce the formation of secondary antibodies to the individual idiotopes of the first (primary) antibody. The idiotype of the primary antibody (Ab-1) activates a network of B cells whose receptors recognize the individual idiotopes of Ab-1. These B cells then differentiate into plasma cells that secrete anti-idiotype antibody (Ab-2). The individual idiotopes of Ab-2 can then further extend the network by inducing production of an anti-anti-idiotype, or Ab-3 (Figure 14-3b). This antibody often resembles idiotopes of Ab-1, and the network begins to limit itself as decreased levels of antibody are produced in each successive activation. Anti-idiotype regulation can also function within the T-cell branch of the immune system, since the $\alpha\beta$ and $\gamma\delta$ T-cell receptors have variable regions and are therefore capable of expressing an idiotope that can be recognized by other T or B cells. The idiotype network involving B and T cells represents a complex circuitry of interacting cells that functions either to enhance or to suppress immune activation. The complexity of the idiotype network has made it difficult to predict whether administration of anti-idiotype antibodies or T cells bearing anti-idiotype receptors will upregulate or downregulate immune responsiveness.

A central principle of the network theory is that some anti-idiotype antibody will be directed against the paratope and therefore will appear as the *internal image* of the original epitope. For example, if mice are immunized with anti-insulin antibody (Ab-1), they produce anti-idiotype antibody (Ab-2) to Ab-1. Some of this anti-idiotype antibody will bind to the insulin-binding paratope of Ab-1. This anti-paratope antibody will mimic the original insulin ligand; indeed this molecular mimicry is evidenced by the ability of the anti-paratope antibody to bind to the insulin receptor and induce glycolysis, just as insulin would. By re-expressing the image of the original epitope in the form of anti-paratope antibody, the immune system will continue to be activated even after the original epitope has been cleared; this may ensure that sufficient clonal proliferation and memory-cell production occurs in response to the original epitope.

The regulatory activity of anti-idiotype antibody was first observed in vivo with a system involving a myeloma protein designated TEPC-15 from BALB/c mice. Prior to the development of monoclonal antibodies immunologists depended on spontaneously occurring myelomas as sources of homogeneous antibodies. The limitation with these myeloma proteins was that the antigenic specificity was unknown and therefore researchers took on the tedious task of attempting to characterize the antigenic specificity of various myelomas. One of the myelomas characterized during this period was a BALB/c IgA myeloma designated TEPC-15, which was found to be an IgA antibody specific for phosphorylcholine (PC). Since phosphorylcholine is the major component of the pneumococcal cell-wall C polysaccharide, TEPC-15 could therefore serve as an antigen to assess anti-idiotype antibody production in mice that had been immunized with pneumococci. When BALB/c mice were immunized with pneumococci, the number of plaque-forming plasma cells was determined in two hemolytic plaque assays. The first assay detected plasma cells secreting antibody to PC by use of sheep red blood cells coated with PC as the test antigen; the second assay detected plasma cells secreting anti-idiotype antibody by use of SRBCs coated with TEPC-15. As Figure 14-4

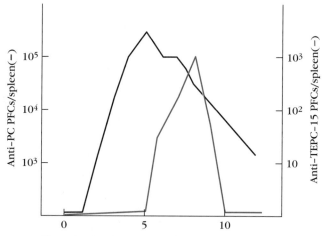

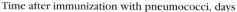

Time after immunization with pneumococci, days

Figure 14-4 Production of anti-idiotype antibodies following immunization of BALB/c mice with pneumococci. Splenic plasma cells secreting antibody to the phosphorylcholine (PC) component of the pneomococcal cell wall (black curve) were detected in a hemolytic plaque assay using PC-coated SRBCs. Splenic plasma cells secreting anti-idiotype antibody (red curve) were detected using SRBCs coated with the myeloma protein TEPC-15, which is specific for PC. [Adapted from H. Cozenza, 1976, *Eur. J. Immunol.* 6:114.]

reveals, a peak anti-PC PFC was reached about 4 days after immunization followed by a peak anti-idiotype PFC 4 days later.

Anti-idiotype antibody representing the internal image of the original antigen can potentially serve as a vaccine to induce an immune response to a pathogenic

antigen, thus avoiding immunization with the pathogen itself. For example, if mice are immunized with anti-idiotype antibody specific for the binding site of TEPC-15, they will be immune when they are later challenged with live pneumococci. Anti-idiotype vaccines have been shown to induce protective immunity in mice against hepatitis B virus (Figure 14-5), as well as rabies virus, Sendai virus, *Streptococcus pneumoniae*, *Listeria monocytogenes*, *Trypanosoma rhodesiense*, and *Schistosoma mansoni.* The development of anti-idiotype vaccines for humans holds much promise, particularly when immunization with a killed or attenuated vaccine would pose an unacceptable risk to the patient.

T-Cell–Mediated Suppression

When animals are immunized with large doses of certain antigens they become unresponsive, or tolerant, to those antigens. In the early 1970s, Richard Gershon and K. Kondo discovered that the unresponsive state could be transferred from tolerant mice to normal syngeneic mice simply by the transfer of T cells. Their experiments led to the hypothesis that there exists a population of regulatory T cells that are capable of mediating suppression of the immune response. The cells were called T suppressor (T_S) cells.

T. Tada and T. Takemori confirmed the results of Gershon and Kondo using high doses of keyhole limpet hemocyanin (KLH) to induce suppression. When KLH-primed spleen cells from suppressed mice were transferred to normal syngeneic recipients, the recipients' response to an injection of DNP-KLH, measured by a hemolytic plaque assay, was nearly abolished. However, spleen cells from mice suppressed with an unrelated antigen (BGG) had no effect on the recipients response to DNP-KLH, demonstrating that the suppressive effect is antigen-specific (Table 14-3).

Experiments with the A/J strain of mice revealed that the suppressive effect of T_S cells can be idiotype-specific in some cases. When A/J mice are immunized with KLH conjugated to the hapten azobenzenearsonate (ABA), they exhibit a limited antibody response, with most of the induced antibody expressing a single anti-ABA idiotype designated CRI_A. When A/J mice were pretreated with anti-idiotype (anti-CRI_A) serum and then were immunized with ABA-KLH, they no longer produced anti-ABA antibodies with the CRI_A idiotype. This suppressive effect also occurred when T cells from A/J mice treated with the anti-idiotype serum were transferred to normal A/J mice. When these recipient mice were immunized with ABA-KLH, they did not express anti-ABA antibody with the CRI_A idiotype, demonstrating that in this system the T_S cells are idiotype-specific.

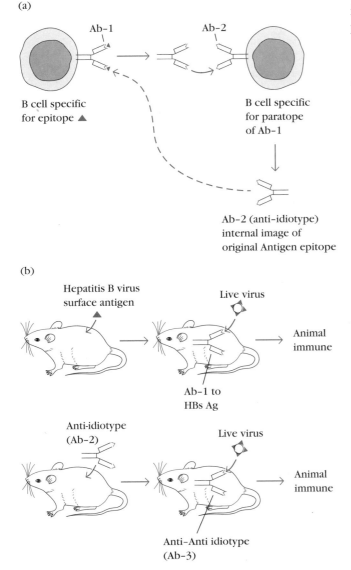

(a)

(b)

Figure 14-5 (a) The binding site on some anti-idiotype antibody (Ab-2) resembles the structure of the epitope on the original antigen. Such anti-paratope antibody can interact with B cells specific for the original antigen, thus inducing production of more antibody against the antigen. (b) Immunization with anti-idiotype antibody has been shown experimentally to protect mice against hepatitis B virus without exposing the animal to the virus. HBsAg = hepatitis B surface antigen.

Table 14-3 Transfer of immune suppression by antigen-specific T cells*

Donor spleen cells*	Immune response of recipient	
	Immunogen	Anti-DNP PFC
None	DNP-KLH	11,000
KLH-primed	DNP-KLH	89
KLH-primed with T cells removed	DNP-KLH	20,600
BGG-primed	DNP-KLH	11,600

* Donor mice were immunized with high doses of KLH or BGG, and their spleen cells were transferred to normal syngeneic mice. The recipients were then injected with DNP-KLH, and the immune response was determined in a hemolytic plaque assay using DNP-coated SRBCs as the test antigen.

SOURCE: Data from T. Tada and T. Takemori, 1974. *J. Exp. Med.* **140**:239.

In some experimental systems T suppressor cells have been shown to release suppressor factors. Unlike cytokines which are not antigen specific, some suppressor factors have been shown to be antigen-specific, some have been shown to be idiotype-specific, and some have been shown to be MHC restricted, suggesting that they may be soluble released forms of the T cell's receptor. There is speculation that suppressor factors might bind to peptides + MHC displayed on antigen-presenting cells, serving to block the interaction of the antigen-presenting cell with other T cells.

Are T$_S$ Cells A Distinct Subpopulation?

Although T-cell–mediated suppression is a very real phenomenon that has been reproduced in a variety of experimental systems, the evidence that this suppression is mediated by a distinct T-cell subpopulation has increasingly been called into question. The cells mediating suppression in the various experimental systems generally have been identified as CD8$^+$ T cells. These presumed T$_S$ cells were initially distinguished from CD8$^+$ T$_C$ cells by the presence of a membrane marker designated l-J, which purportedly mapped to the MHC I region. When the MHC was mapped by chromosome walking, however, the I-J region was shown not to exist—a finding that called into question the existence of the supposed I-J membrane marker. To date, despite the development of a large number of monoclonal antibodies specific for cell-membrane molecules, no unique membrane marker for a T$_S$-cell population has been identified.

The inability to maintain stable T-cell clones capable of transferring suppression in vivo or to clone antigen-specific suppressor factors also raises doubt about their existence. This limitation is in stark contrast to the large number of stable T$_H$ and T$_C$ clones that have been produced and the many factors that have been characterized and shown to mediate helper or cytotoxic activities in vivo. The antigen receptor on putative T$_S$ cells has also not been characterized. S. Hedrick and co-workers eval-

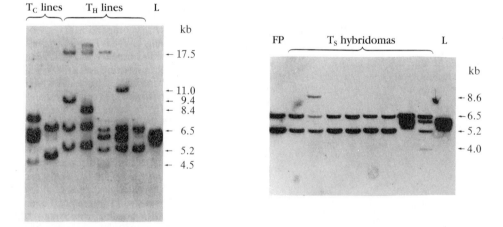

Figure 14-6 Evaluation of gene rearrangements in β-chain DNA by Southern blot analysis of TCR genes in T-cell lines functionally defined as T$_H$, T$_C$, and T$_S$ cells. DNA from each cell line was digested with restriction endonucleases; the fragments were electrophoresed, blotted onto nitrocellulose, and then identified with radiolabeled β-chain cDNA. The liver-cell DNA (L) represents unrearranged, germ-line β-chain DNA. The blot patterns for all the T$_H$ and T$_C$ lines were different from one another and from liver-cell DNA, indicating that β-chain gene rearrangement had occurred in these lines. In contrast, the T$_S$ hybridomas exhibited the same blot patterns as liver cells and the fusion partner (FP) indicating that no rearrangement of the β-chain gene DNA had occurred. [Adapted from S. Hedrick et al., 1985, *Proc. Nat'l Acad. Sci.* **82**:531.]

uated gene rearrangements of the gene encoding the β chain of the $\alpha\beta$ T-cell receptor in T-cell lines that had been defined functionally as T_H cells, T_C cells, and T_S cells. Whereas each of the different T_H and T_C lines showed unique β-chain gene rearrangements, the T_S lines did not show functional rearrangements of the β chain, suggesting that suppressor cells do not utilize the $\alpha\beta$ heterodimer as their antigen-binding receptor (Figure 14-6).

Possible Explanations for T-Cell–Mediated Suppression

The inability to characterize a T-cell subpopulation functioning as the effector cell in immune suppression has led many immunologists to question whether a distinct T_S-cell lineage actually exists. They suggest that immune suppression may be generated by existing lymphocyte subpopulations, not by a separate cell lineage. For example, in one experimental system T cells activated by Con A had been shown to suppress a mixed-lymphocyte reaction (MLR). This suppression had been attributed to T_S cells. Later experiments revealed that the suppression resulted from the absorption of IL-2 by activated T_C cells, which depleted the level of IL-2 in the culture supernatant; since IL-2 is required for the MLR, this depletion of IL-2 effectively blocked the MLR in this system. This finding suggests that some of the suppressive effects observed in other experimental systems that have been attributed to putative T_S cells may, in fact, result from depletion of IL-2, an essential cytokine in both humoral and cell-mediated immune responses.

In some experimental systems the activities attributed to T_S cells may actually result from the antagonistic effects of cytokines produced by different subpopulations of antigen-specific T_H cells. For example, IL-10 is secreted by the T_H2 subset and functions to inhibit lymphokine production in the T_H1 subset. If a particular immune response depended on IL-2–mediated activation, the production of IL-10 would suppress that response. Similarly, IL-4 has been shown to block the IL-2 signal for proliferation in a B-cell line. In an experimental system that monitored B-cell activation by IL-2, production of IL-4 by antigen-specific T_H cells might lead to the erroneous conclusion that T_S cell had suppressed the response. Similar antagonistic effects between IL-4 and IFN-γ, discussed earlier in this chapter, might also be interpreted as T_S-cell activities.

In most experimental systems, only a single response is monitored (e.g., production of IL-2; generation of plasma cells secreting a particular isotype). For this reason, what appear to be suppressive effects may, in some cases, represent diversion from one isotype to another or diversion from one type of immune response to another. For example, if an experimental system is measuring IgE production and if IFN-γ is produced, then the IgE response would be suppressed and the production of IgG2a, induced by the IFN-γ, would go undetected. In such a system, a change in the nature of the immune response would be misinterpreted as suppression. In some cases, T cell mediated suppression may be mediated by a population of T cells with cytotoxic activity. Recent evidence has demonstrated the existence of class-II MHC restricted cytotoxic T cells that are able to selectively kill antigen-presenting cells. These cytotoxic T cells have been shown to kill antigen-specific B cells which capture antigen by means of their immunoglobulin receptor and display a processed peptide together with the class II MHC on their membrane. In humans activated T_H cells also display class II MHC and there is some intriguing evidence suggesting that some of the depletion of $CD4^+$ T cells in AIDS may be due to selective killing by a population of class II restricted cytotoxic T cells. These cytotoxic T cells are thought to recognize processed peptides of a HIV envelope glycoprotein (gp120) that is taken up by uninfected $CD4^+$ T cells by receptor mediated endocytosis and displayed together with the class II MHC molecule on the membrane of the uninfected T cell. Chapter 21 will cover this topic in more detail.

The considerations discussed in this section and the previous section call into question the T_S cell as a distinct subpopulation. The observed suppression of particular immune responses in various experimental systems may, in fact, result from cytokine-mediated regulation of immune responsiveness or merely reflect changes in the pattern of cytokines present in the system, or changes in the population of effector cells that have been generated.

Tolerance Induction

Why does the immune system not respond to self-antigens? Clearly there is nothing that uniquely distinguishes self-antigens from foreign antigens. And certainly the random V-J and V-D-J gene rearrangements of the immunoglobulin genes and TCR genes are capable of generating self-reactive specificities. Therefore the immune system must become unresponsive to self-antigens. This state of specific immunologic unresponsiveness is called *tolerance*. Tolerance can develop naturally, as it does when the developing animal becomes unresponsive to self-antigens, or tolerance can be induced experimentally. Experimentally induced tolerance is defined as a state in which an animal will fail to respond to an antigen that would normally be immunogenic. Immunologic tolerance does not simply reflect the absence of an immune response, but rather an adaptive response of the immune system, one meeting the criteria of antigen specificity and memory that are the hallmarks of any immune response. It is not known whether similar mechanisms generate both naturally acquired self-tolerance and experimentally induced tolerance. What is clear, however, is that the induction of tolerance depends on a number of variables and may proceed by a number of mechanisms.

Fetal and Neonatal Induction of Tolerance

In 1945 Ray Owen made some interesting observations on nonidentical (dizygotic) twins born to cows whose twin placentas had fused at an early developmental stage, resulting in mixing of the circulating cells and antigens of the two calves. Owen observed that such twins are chimeras expressing two genetically distinct types of blood cells. Each calf was found to accept the genetically dissimilar blood cells of its twin without mounting an immune response against the cells; in other words, these calves were tolerant to each other's blood cells. In 1951 P. B. Medawar extended these observations by showing that such dizygotic twins could also accept skin grafts from each other. On the basis of these observations F. M. Burnet postulated in 1954 that "recognition of self is something that needs to be learned and is not an inherent genetic quality of an organism." He suggested that this learning takes place during embryonic development of the immune system when interaction of immune cells with self-antigens would lead to the elimination or inactivation of self-reactive lymphocyte clones. In the dizygotic twin cows, Burnet hypothesized, exposure to the blood-cell antigens during fetal development had resulted in elimination of reactive lymphocytes, allowing the nonself blood cells to be viewed as self-cells by the immune system.

To test the hypothesis that tolerance is learned by immune-system cells during early development of the immune system, R. Billingham, L. Brent, and P. B. Medawar injected strain A mice at birth with allogeneic strain B spleen cells. They discovered that as adults the neonatally injected strain A mice accepted skin grafts from the same strain B allogeneic mice while retaining the ability to reject skin grafts from other strains of mice. Exposure to strain B alloantigens when the immune system was immature had created a specific state of tolerance to these antigens. Tolerance can also be induced by injection of soluble protein antigens into fetal or neonatal animals. However, tolerance to soluble protein antigens is not as long-lived as tolerance to allogeneic cells, probably because of a difference in antigen persistence. The injection of allogeneic cells creates chimeras in which the allogeneic cells persist, whereas injected protein antigens are gradually cleared by phagocytosis.

Burnet proposed that the immune system normally learns not to respond to self-components because of their presence during fetal development. Triplett tested this hypothesis by removing the pituitary gland from embryonic tree frog larvae. He reasoned that if the pituitary gland was absent during embryonic life, the frog's immune system would not acquire self-tolerance to the antigens of the pituitary. He allowed the larvae to mature in the absence of the pituitary (maintaining the pituitary glands by implanting them in the dermis of other tadpoles until the larvae had matured). When the pituitary gland was reimplanted in its original donor, the frog rejected its own pituitary, suggesting that in the absence of the pituitary antigens self-tolerance to the pituitary had not been induced. If, however, only one half of the pituitary was removed and later reimplanted, the reimplanted part of the pituitary was accepted, suggesting that exposure of the immune system to pituitary antigens during early development had induced self-tolerance.

The induction of tolerance requires 100-fold lower concentrations of protein antigens in neonatal mice than in adult mice, supporting the idea that immature lymphocytes learn tolerance more easily than mature lymphocytes. As discussed in Chapter 10, during development of T cells within the thymus, exposure to self-antigens is thought to result in negative selection and elimination of self-reactive thymocytes (see Figure 10-15). Some similar mechanism involving exposure to self-antigens may induce tolerance in immature B cells. For example, when immature B cells, which express IgM but not IgD, were treated with anti-IgM antibody, the membrane IgM was endocytosed, presumably by the mechanism of receptor-mediated endocytosis, which is known to occur following antigen-mediated cross-linkage of B-cell membrane-bound antibody molecules. Comparison of the effect of treatment with anti-IgM on immature and mature B cells showed that the immature B cells lost more membrane IgM, and took longer to regenerate their membrane IgM, than the mature B cells. This finding led to speculation that interaction of immature B cells with self-antigens during development might induce loss of the IgM antigen-binding receptor and thus bring about self-tolerance.

Adult Induction of Tolerance

It is more difficult to induce tolerance in adult animals than in fetal or neonatal ones, but it can be done under certain experimental conditions. A number of variables influence the *tolerogenicity* of a given antigen, that is, its ability to induce tolerance. In addition, T cells and B cells differ in their susceptibility to tolerance induction.

Factors Affecting Tolerogenicity of Antigens

The route of administration, the structure of an antigen, and the dosage all affect tolerance induction by a given antigen. Generally, intravenous administration of an antigen is more likely to induce tolerance than administration by other routes. Antigens whose structure makes them difficult for macrophages to phagocytose and process tend to be good in inducing tolerance. For example, deaggregated proteins centrifuged at high speeds to remove aggregates generally are not phagocytosed well and tend to be effective tolerogens. Polymers of D-amino acids are also effective tolerogens, presumably because macrophages lack the necessary enzymes to degrade these synthetic polymers and therefore are unable to present peptides derived from these polymers together with MHC molecules.

The effect of antigen dosage on tolerogenicity was first discovered in mice when a potential vaccine for pneumococcal pneumonia was tested at two different doses. Mice were injected with 0.5 mg or 0.5 μg of the pneumococcal polysaccharide antigen and then were challenged with live pneumococci. Much to the surprise of the researchers, the mice given a high dose of the polysaccharide antigen all died after being challenged with live pneumococci, whereas the mice given the low dose were immune and survived challenge with the live organism. When this experiment was repeated, this time giving the mice an initial high dose of the polysaccharide followed by the low dose, the mice continued to show an absence of immunity and died following injection of the live organism. In other words, the high antigen dose had created a state of tolerance in these mice, so that they were no longer responsive to the 0.5-μg antigen dose that had previously induced immunity.

The relation of antigen dose to tolerance induction was studied more fully by N. A. Mitchison. He immunized groups of mice with various dosages of BSA over a 16-week period, waited 2 weeks, and then challenged the mice with a dose of BSA previously shown to be immunogenic. Serum antibody to BSA was measured, expressed as a percentage of that in control animals that had received only the final, immunogenic BSA challenge, and plotted against the BSA doses in the priming immunizations (Figure 14-7). Mitchison was surprised to find two zones of tolerance in which prior immunization inhibited the response to the immunogenic dose: a high zone above 10^{-2} g of BSA and a low zone that peaked at about 10^{-9} g of BSA. Between these two zones was an immunogenic zone, ranging from about 10^{-6} to 10^{-2} g of BSA, in which prior immunization produced immunity, evidenced by a secondary response to the final immunogenic dose of BSA. From these results Mitchison concluded that very high or very low doses of antigen are most likely to lead to a tolerant state. This

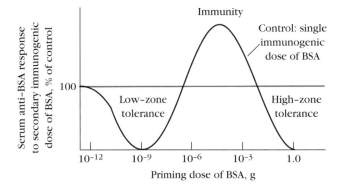

Figure 14-7 Experimental induction of tolerance at low and high doses of antigen. Mice were primed with various doses of BSA and then challenged with a known immunogenic dose. The serum anti-BSA level was less than that of controls at priming doses above 10^{-2} g (high-zone tolerance) and at low doses centered at 10^{-9} g (low-zone tolerance). Between these tolerance zones was a zone of immunity, characterized by a heightened secondary antibody response. [Adapted from N. A. Mitchison, 1964, *Proc. Royal Society (B)* **161**:275.]

principle has been applied in vaccine production, where the dosage has been shown to be critical for induction of immune status, and in allergy desensitization, where repeated low-dose injections of allergens have been shown to induce a state of tolerance to normal allergen levels (see Chapter 16).

Susceptibility of T and B Cells to Tolerance Induction

Tolerance can be induced in both B and T cells, but the two lineages differ substantially in the quantity of antigen needed to induce tolerance and in the duration of the tolerant state. In order to compare tolerance induction in T cells and B cells, J. Chiller and co-workers injected mice with deaggregated human gamma globulin (deHGG) and then removed thymus (T) and bone marrow (B) cells at various times after injection. The tolerant cells were combined with normal bone marrow or thymus cells and then injected into x-irradiated syngeneic recipients, which were later challenged with an immunogenic dose of HGG. Mice receiving either tolerant thymus cells plus normal bone marrow cells or tolerant bone marrow cells plus normal thymus cells were tolerant to the immunogenic dose of HGG. However, the kinetics of tolerance induction was fundamentally different for T cells and B cells (Figure 14-8). The thymus cells became tolerant sooner after injection of deHGG and remained tolerant longer than the bone marrow cells, indicating that immunologic tolerance is

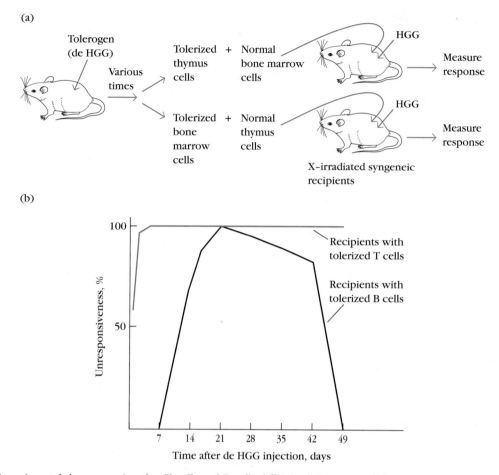

Figure 14-8 Experimental demonstration that T cells and B cells differ in their susceptibility to tolerance induction. (a) Outline of experimental protocol. At the time of this experiment there was no way to separate B cells from T cells; therefore, the thymus was used as a source of T cells and bone marrow as a source of B cells. After transfer of tolerance-induced cells plus normal cells into syngeneic, x-irradiated recipients, the response of the recipients to an immunizing dose of HGG was determined. (b) Plot of unresponsiveness of the recipients versus time after tolerogen injection when tolerance-induced cells were removed. Note that T cells became tolerant sooner and remained tolerant longer than B cells. [Adapted from J. Chiller et al., 1971, *Science* **171**:813.]

maintained more effectively by T cells than by B cells. However, since most B-cell responses require T-cell help, even if a B cell is responsive to a given antigen, antibody production will be determined by the state of responsiveness of the T cells.

Mechanisms of Tolerance Induction

The ability of the immune system to discriminate between self- and nonself-antigen implies that the system must be able to tell the difference—to make a qualitative distinction—between contact with self-antigen and contact with nonself antigen. Just how this distinction is achieved is a matter of a great deal of speculation. One long-standing hypothesis suggests that the qualitative

distinction of what constitutes a self-antigen is achieved temporally, that is, by the maturational state of a T or B cell when it contacts antigen. Immature T and B cells would be expected to contact only self-antigens. Contact of self-antigen with antigen-binding receptors on immature T and B cells may induce either death of the cell (*clonal deletion*) or an immunologically unresponsive state (*clonal anergy*) in which the antigen-reactive lymphocytes are present but are functionally inactive. Tolerance induction in immature B and T cells occurs in the primary lymphoid organs during the process of maturation. The process of B-cell maturation in the bone marrow has been difficult to study owing to the diffuse organization of this tissue, whereas T-cell maturation within the thymus has been studied extensively and was described in detail in Chapter 10.

It is difficult to imagine, however, that all possible self-

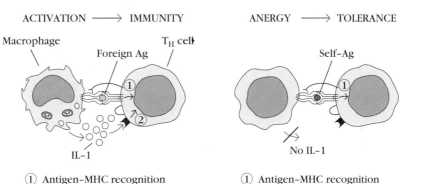

ACTIVATION ⟶ IMMUNITY   ANERGY ⟶ TOLERANCE

① Antigen–MHC recognition   ① Antigen–MHC recognition

② IL-1 co-stimulatory signal   Absence of co-stimulatory IL-1

Figure 14-9 The presence or absence of a co-stimulatory IL-1 signal may regulate whether mature peripheral T_H cells enter a state of immune activation (*left*) or a state of tolerance through clonal anergy (*right*). It has been suggested that mature peripheral T_H cells encounter self-antigens (red circle) only in the absence of co-stimulatory IL-1; antigen interaction in this case leads to functionally inactive (anergic) T_H cells and a state of tolerance. Interaction of mature B cells and T_C cells with self-antigens in the absence of their co-stimulatory signals would likewise lead to clonal anergy of these lineages. [Based on R. H. Schwartz, 1990, *Science* **248**:1349.]

antigens have access to the bone marrow and thymus during T- and B-cell maturation. Instead, it seems likely that some immunocompetent T and B cells are generated with receptors specific for self-antigens that were not present in the primary lymphoid organ during their maturation. To address this problem it has been suggested that tolerance to self-antigens may also be induced in mature peripheral lymphocytes. This is particularly important in the case of the B-cell system because a B cell's antigen-binding Ig receptor does not remain constant following maturation but is diversified in mature peripheral B cells through the process of somatic mutation. This means that self-reactive B cells might well be generated by random mutational events in mature cells. Tolerance induction in mature peripheral T and B cells again requires some mechanism for distinguishing contact with self-antigen from contact with nonself-antigen. One possibility is that antigen encountered in the presence of a co-stimulatory signal delivered by a T_H cell or an antigen-presenting cell leads to immunity, whereas antigen encountered in the absence of that co-stimulatory signal leads to tolerance. For example, if T and B cells encounter self-antigens only in an environment devoid of the necessary co-stimulatory signals required for an immune response, the lymphocytes may enter a state of clonal anergy (Figure 14-9). The following sections examine some of the experimental evidence for clonal deletion and clonal anergy during tolerance induction in immature and mature T and B cells. The development of autoimmunity, in which tolerance to self-antigens is defective, is explored in Chapter 17.

Experimental Induction of Tolerance in B Cells

A variety of transgenic systems have been developed to study tolerance induction in B cells. These systems have shown that B cells can be rendered tolerant either through clonal deletion of self-reactive B cells or through clonal anergy, in which self-reactive B cells are functionally inactivated without physical deletion.

If the lack of a second signal drives a T cell into an anergic state, then it might be possible to make use of this fact to deliberately drive T cells into an anergic state. This could have untold clinical ramifications as it might enable clinicians to turn off autoimmune T cells or allergic T cells. If, for example, an allergen is given to an allergic individual, together with agents designed to block the second signal, then it might be possible to induce the allergen-reactive cells to enter an anergic state. For this reason, immunologists are presently focusing a great deal of attention on identifying the membrane proteins that may transmit a requisite second signal for T cell activation. One such protein, called CD28, was recently identified by James Allison. If T cells are activated by antigen/MHC while CD28 is masked with monoclonal antibody, the T cells were shown to enter an anergic state. The CD28 membrane molecule was later shown by Peter Linsley to recognize a macrophage membrane molecule called B7. Interestingly, the expression of B7 is increased by adjuvants which may begin to explain the immune-potentiating effect of various adjuvants on the immune response. As more

Table 14-4 Expression of transgene encoding IgM antibody to H-2^k class I MHC molecules

Experimental animal	No. animals tested	Expression of transgene	
		As membrane Ab	As secreted Ab (μg/ml)
Nontransgenic	13	(−)	<0.3
H-2^d Transgenics	7	(+)	93.0
H-2$^{d/k}$ Transgenics	6	(−)	<0.3

SOURCE: Adapted from D. A. Nemazee and K. Burki, 1989, *Nature* **337**:562.

mechanisms of inducing clonal anergy are uncovered it will surely have a major impact on clinical medicine, especially in areas of organ transplants, autoimmunity, and allergies.

Evidence for Clonal Deletion of B Cells

In one study transgenic mice were engineered carrying a transgene encoding an IgM antibody specific for H-2^k class I MHC molecules. The development of B cells expressing the transgene was compared in H-2^d and H-2$^{d/k}$ transgenics. In the H-2^d mice 25–50% of the B cells expressed the transgene both as membrane-bound antibody and as secreted antibody. In the H-2$^{d/k}$ mice, in contrast, the transgene was not expressed either as membrane antibody or as secreted antibody (Table 14-4). This study suggests that the presence of H-2^k class I MHC molecules in the H-2$^{d/k}$ transgenic mice induced clonal deletion of those B cells expressing the transgene-encoded IgM specific for H-2^k class I MHC molecules.

Evidence for Clonal Anergy of B Cells

The presence of antigen-reactive B cells in tolerant animals has been assessed by administering radioactively labeled antigen and quantitating the number of antigen-binding B cells in tolerant mice and in normal immune mice. Most such experiments have shown that antigen-reactive B cells are not deleted in animals in which tolerance has been induced experimentally. Even in normal animals, B cells reactive to self-antigens can be shown to be present, but their activity is regulated either by the tolerant state of T$_H$ cells or by the anergic state of the B cell itself.

A recent experiment by C. C. Goodnow and co-workers suggests that B cells may be rendered self-tolerant through clonal anergy of either immature or mature B cells. Goodnow's experimental system included two groups of transgenic mice. One carried a chicken ly-

sozyme transgene linked to a metallothionine promoter, which placed transcription of the lysozyme gene under the control of zinc levels. The other group of transgenic mice carried rearranged immunoglobulin heavy- and light-chain transgenes encoding anti-lysozyme antibody. In normal mice the frequency of lysozyme-specific B cells is on the order of 1 in 10^3, but in these transgenic mice the rearranged genes inhibit random immunoglobulin-gene rearrangements so that 60–90% of the B cells express lysozyme-specific membrane-bound antibody. Goodnow mated these two groups of transgenics to produce "double transgenic" offspring carrying both the lysozyme and anti-lysozyme transgenes. The question Goodnow then asked was whether the expression of lysozyme early in development would regulate development of the B cells expressing the anti-lysozyme transgene.

The Goodnow double-transgenic system yielded several interesting findings concerning tolerance induction in B cells. One group of double transgenics produced high levels of lysozyme (17.4 ng/ml). Comparison of these double transgenics with the anti-lysozyme transgenics revealed that both expressed anti-lysozyme membrane-bound antibody on their B cells. However, the double transgenics produced very little secreted antibody against lysozyme, and hemolytic plaque assays of their spleen cells showed many fewer plaque-forming cells than in the anti-lysozyme transgenics (Figure 14-10). These results indicate that the presence of lysozyme during B-cell maturation in the double transgenics did not cause deletion of lysozyme-reactive B cells but rather rendered these B cells anergic. A second group of double transgenics, expressing low levels of lysozyme (1.4 ng/ml) also was obtained from the matings. B cells from these mice expressed membrane-bound anti-lysozyme antibody and were capable of secreting anti-lysozyme antibody. Thus the concentration, not simply the presence, of endogenously produced lysozyme influenced the development of anergy in lysozyme-reactive B cells.

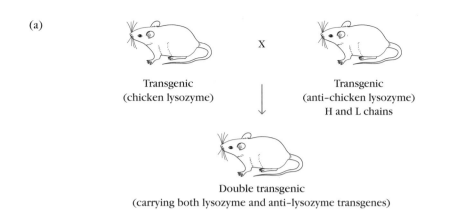

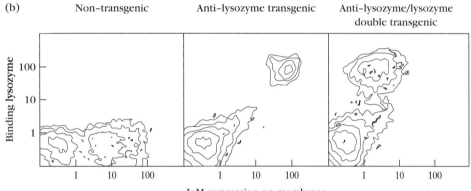

Figure 14-10 (a) Production of double transgenic mice carrying lysozyme and anti-lysozyme transgenes can be accomplished by mating lysozyme transgenic mice with anti-lysozyme transgenic mice and selecting for double transgenic progeny. B-cell development was studied in the anti-lysozyme transgenic mice and in the anti-lysozyme/lysozyme double transgenic mice. (b) FACS analysis of B cells binding to lysozyme compared to membrane IgM levels. Nontransgenics show no lysozyme binding B cells (left). Both anti-lysozyme transgenics (middle) and anti-lysozyme/lysozyme double transgenics (right) had B cells which bound lysozyme, although the level of membrane IgM shows some decrease in the double transgenics.

Table 14-5 Functional state of B cells in mice carrying a chicken lysozyme transgene and/or anti-lysozyme transgene

Experimental group	Lysozyme level (ng/ml)	Membrane anti-lysozyme Ab	Anti-lysozyme PFC/spleen[*]	Serum titer of anti-lysozyme Ab[*]
Anti-lysozyme transgenics	0	+	high	high
Anti-lysozyme + lysozyme transgenics				
Group 1	17.4	+	low	low
Group 2	1.4	+	high	high
Group 2 + Zn^{2+}	100	+	low	low

[*] Experimental animals were immunized with chicken lysozyme. Several days later hemolytic plaque assays were performed to determine the number of plasma cells secreting anti-lysozyme antibodies, and the serum anti-lysozyme titer was determined.

To determine whether the mature lysozyme-reactive B cells in the low-lysozyme double transgenics could be rendered anergic, Goodnow fed the mice zinc water, which induced expression of the lysozyme gene. Within 4 days, the concentration of lysozyme in these mice increased to 100 ng/ml. Analysis of the B cells in these zinc-induced mice showed that they had become anergic to lysozyme (Table 14-5). Goodnow has suggested that interaction of immature or mature B cells with endogenously secreted lysozyme in the absence of a second signal from T_H cells rendered the B cells anergic in both groups of transgenic mice. The development of clonal anergy in both immature and mature B cells was found to correlate with a 10- to 50-fold decrease in membrane IgM but not in membrane IgD. Whether this change in IgM expression plays a role in the inactivation of these B cells remains to be determined.

Experimental Induction of Tolerance in T Cells

Experiments studying tolerance induction in T cells have been difficult to perform because T cells bind antigen associated with MHC molecules rather than soluble antigen. Therefore, the number of antigen-specific T cells cannot be determined by the binding of radioactively labeled antigen, as is possible with B cells. Antigen-specific T cells can be assessed with clonotypic monoclonal antibody specific for the binding site of the T-cell receptor.

(a)

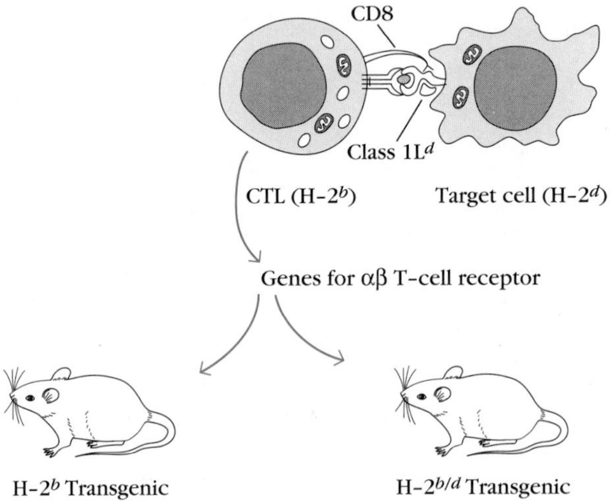

(b)

	H-2^b Transgenic	H-2$^{b/d}$ Transgenic
Expression of transgene αβ TCR	20–95% of CD8$^+$ T cells	<1% of CD8$^+$ T cells
CML assay (% ^{51}Cr released):		
L^{d+} target cells	59%	13%
L^{d-} target cells (control)	4%	13%

Figure 14-11 Experimental demonstration of clonal deletion of self-reactive T cells. (a) H-2^b and H-2$^{b/d}$ transgenic mice were produced carrying transgenes for an $\alpha\beta$ T-cell receptor derived from an H-2^b CTL. Although this particular transgene must have been specific for foreign peptides presented with self–class I MHC, it cross-reacted with allogeneic L^d class I MHC molecules. (b) T cells from the transgenic mice were analyzed by FACS to determine the presence of CD8$^+$ T cells expressing the transgenic $\alpha\beta$ T-cell receptor. The functional activity of the CD8$^+$ T cells was determined by CML assays using [^{51}Cr] labeled target cells that expressed L^d molecules. The expression of L^d in the H-2$^{b/d}$ transgenics induced clonal deletion of T cells expressing L^d-specific receptors. [Adapted from W. C. Sha et al., 1988, *Nature* **336**:73.]

Evidence for Clonal Deletion of T Cells

As discussed previously, T cells expressing a β-chain exon called $V_\beta17a$ have T-cell receptors with high reactivity to class II MHC IE molecules. In an experiment described in Chapter 10, Kappler and Marrack used monoclonal antibody to the $V_\beta17a$ gene product to assess expression of this exon in IE^+ and IE^- mice. Their results demonstrated that expression of IE molecules led to clonal deletion of IE-reactive T cells during maturation in the thymus (see Figure 10-17).

Another experimental system in which clonal deletion of self-reactive T cells has been demonstrated involves transgenic mice carrying an $\alpha\beta$-TCR transgene derived from an $H-2^b$ CTL clone specific for L^d class I MHC molecules. T cells expressing this transgene can be identified with a clonotypic monoclonal antibody. The presence of mature T cells expressing the transgene was compared in $H-2^b$ and $H-2^{b/d}$ transgenic mice (Figure 14-11). In the $H-2^b$ mice the TCR transgene was expressed on 20–95% of the peripheral T cells; most of these T cells were also $CD8^+$. Those T cells expressing the transgene were shown to be functionally capable of lysing target cells expressing L^d molecules. In the $H-2^{b/d}$ transgenic mice, expression of the transgene was eliminated, and functional T cells capable of lysing L^d targets were absent. The results indicate that the expression of L^d molecules in the $H-2^{b/d}$ transgenic mice induced clonal deletion of $CD8^+$ T cells bearing the transgene-encoded T-cell receptor specific for L^d molecules.

Evidence for Clonal Anergy of T Cells

Clonal deletion of immature T cells does not always account for the induction of T-cell tolerance, and recent experiments suggest that tolerance can be induced in mature T cells by clonal anergy. In an extension of the earlier Kappler and Marrack experiment, L. C. Burkly and co-workers used IE^- mice to produce transgenics carrying an IE transgene linked to an insulin promoter. These transgenics expressed IE molecules only on their pancreatic beta cells. Analysis of the $V_\beta17a$-positive peripheral T cells in these transgenic mice showed that they were reactive with IE molecules but were functionally anergic. In the earlier experiment (see Figure 10-17), immature T cells in the IE^+ mice encountered IE molecules on stromal cells in the thymus and were deleted. In contrast, the T cells in the transgenics were not exposed to IE in the thymus and thus were not deleted. However, the mature IE-reactive peripheral T cells in these mice presumably encountered IE molecules expressed on pancreatic beta cells. Since these cells are not antigen-presenting cells, they do not produce co-stimulatory IL-1, which is necessary to generate a T-cell response. It has been suggested that when the mature $V_\beta17a^+$ T cell encountered the IE molecule on a non-antigen-presenting cell, the lack of a co-stimulatory signal led to clonal anergy rather than to immunity.

Summary

1. Antigen, antibody, and immune complexes have each been shown to play a role in regulation of immune responsiveness. A decline in antigen levels ultimately results in diminished clonal proliferation and a decline in further humoral or cell-mediated responses. That antigen concentration is not the only regulating factor is indicated by the cyclical appearance of plasma cells that are specific for a given antigen despite a linear decline in the levels of that antigen. Antibody has been shown to suppress the immune response, possibly by binding to antigen and preventing further B-cell activation. Immune complexes have been shown to both increase and decrease the immune response to an antigen.

2. Cytokines are also important regulators of the immune response. In some cases they act synergistically, so that two cytokines together have more than an additive effect. In other cases the cytokines may act antagonistically, so that the presence of one cytokine may block the activity of another. Cytokines may also influence the type of immune response that occurs. Some cytokines have been shown to preferentially activate a cell-mediated response, such as delayed-type hypersensitivity, and other cytokines are more likely to activate a humoral antibody response.

3. The unique variable-region amino acid sequences of antibodies and T-cell receptors are recognized as antigenic determinants by the immune system. Thus the secreted antibodies and clonally expanded T-cell receptors generated in an immune response in turn elicit anti-idiotype antibodies. According to the network theory, a series (or network) of anti-idiotype antibodies are induced during an immune response; these anti-idiotype antibodies act to upregulate the immune response in some cases and to downregulate it in other cases.

4. The observed suppression of immune responsiveness by T cells, which can be transferred from a suppressed animal to a nonsuppressed one, was originally attributed to a distinct subpopulation of T cells called T_S cells. However, T_S cells expressing unique membrane markers and secreting suppression factors have not been cloned. Many researchers now believe that T-cell–mediated suppression can be explained by shifts in cytokine patterns and/or consumption in various experimental systems, resulting in changes in the nature or intensity of the immune response.

5. Immunologic tolerance is a specific state of non-responsiveness to an antigen. Tolerance develops more easily in fetal and neonatal animals than in adults, suggesting that immature T and B cells are more susceptible to the induction of tolerance. Induction of tolerance in adult animals, which can be achieved under certain circumstances, is influenced by the route of antigen administration, the dosage of antigen, and the ability of the antigen to be phagocytosed. In general, T cells are more susceptible to tolerance induction than B cells, and the tolerance of an animal probably is determined by the state of responsiveness of its T cells.

6. Induction of tolerance in both T and B cells appears to occur by two mechanisms—clonal deletion and clonal anergy—both of which have been demonstrated experimentally. In clonal deletion, immature lymphocytes are eliminated during T-cell or B-cell maturation. In clonal anergy, mature lymphocytes present in the peripheral lymphoid organs become functionally inactivated possibly by the interaction with antigen in the absence of the co-stimulatory signals necessary for generation of an immune response.

References

BATCHELOR, J. R., G. LOMBARDI, and R. I. LECHLER. 1989. Speculations on the specificity of suppression. *Immunol. Today* **10**:37.

BURKLY, L. C., D. LO, and R. A. FLAVELL. 1990. Tolerance in transgenic mice expressing major histocompatibility molecules extrathymically on pancreatic cells. *Science* **248**:1364.

COFFMAN, R. I., and J. CARTY. 1986. A T cell activity that enhances polyclonal IgE production and its inhibition by γ-interferon. *J. Immunol.* **136**:949.

COFFMAN, R., I., J. OHARA, M. W. BOND et al. 1986. B cell stimulatory factor-1 enhances the IgE response of lipopolysaccharide-activated B cells. *J. Immunol.* **136**:4538.

DAVIE, J. M., M. V. SEIDEN, N. S. GREENSPAN et al. 1986. Structural correlates of idiotopes. *Annu. Rev. Immunol.* **4**:147.

FINKELMAN, F. D., J. HOLMES, J. F. URBAN et al. 1990. Lymphokine control of in vivo immunoglobulin isotype secretion. *Annu. Rev. Immunol.* **8**:303.

FIORENTINO, D. F., M. W. BOND, and T. R. MOSMANN. 1989. Two types of mouse T helper cells: T_H2 clones secrete a factor that inhibits cytokine production by T_H1 clones. *J. Exp. Med.* **170**:2081.

GOODNOW, C. C., S. ADELSTEIN, and A. BASTEN. 1990. The need for central and peripheral tolerance in the B cell repertoire. *Science* **248**:1373.

JERNE, N. K. 1974. Towards a network theory of the Immune system. *Annals of Immun.* (Institute Pasteur) **125**C: 373.

MILLER, J. F. A. P., G. MORAHAN, J. ALLISON et al. 1989. T cell tolerance in transgenic mice expressing major histocompatibility class I molecules in defined tissues. *Immunol. Rev.* **107**:109.

ROSER, B. J. 1989. Cellular mechanisms in neonatal and adult tolerance. *Immunol. Rev.* **107**:179.

SCHWARZ, R. H. 1989. Acquisition of immunologic self-tolerance. *Cell* **57**:1073.

SCHWARZ, R. H. 1990. A cell culture model for T lymphocyte clonal anergy. *Science* **248**:1349.

VON BOEHMER, H., and P. KISIELOW. 1990. Self-nonself discrimination by T cells. *Science* **248**:1369.

Study Questions

1. Indicate whether each of the following statements is true or false. If you think a statement is false, explain why.

   a. The mature B cell is made tolerant more easily than the immature B cell.

   b. Tolerance can be induced more easily in neonatal animals than in adult animals.

   c. If mice are immunized with HRBC and then are immunized a day later with SRBC, the antibody response to the SRBC will be much higher than that achieved in control mice immunized only with SRBC.

   d. IFN-γ and IL-4 act antagonistically.

   e. Lymphokines can regulate which branch of the immune system is activated.

   f. Anti-idiotype antibody appears as the internal image of the original antigen.

   g. TEPC-15 monoclonal antibody is an anti-idiotype antibody induced in the immune response to the phosphorylcholine determinant of pneumococcal polysaccharide.

   h. The idiotype of an antibody molecule is composed of multiple idiotopes.

   i. A state of tolerance can be induced more readily with aggregated than with deaggregated antigen.

   j. Following tolerance induction by clonal anergy, antigen-binding lymphocytes are present in the tolerant animal.

   k. All T-cell tolerance occurs via clonal deletion.

2. If you wanted to use the idiotype principle to vaccinate against hepatitis B virus, what would you use to immunize the animals?

3. You have been given a mouse that is tolerant to a protein antigen A and does not produce anti-A antibodies when immunized with antigen A. How could you determine whether this tolerance results

from failure of the animal's T_H cells or B cells to respond to antigen A.

4. Define the following terms: (a) paratope, (b) epitope, (c) idiotope, and (d) agretope.

5. In the Goodnow experiment demonstrating clonal anergy of B cells, transgenic mice carrying a transgene encoding antibody against chicken lysozyme were compared with double transgenics containing the anti-lysozyme gene and a lysozyme gene linked to the zinc-activated metallothionine promoter.

   a. In both the single and double transgenics, 60–90% of the B cells expressed anti-lysozyme membrane-bound antibody. Explain why.

   b. How could you show that the membrane antibody (i.e., the Ig receptor) on these B cells is specific for lysozyme and how could you determine its isotype?

   c. Why was the metallothionine promoter used in constructing the lysozyme transgene?

   d. Design an experiment to prove that the B cells, not the T_H cells, from the double transgenics were anergic.

6. Experiments in which the expression of TCR β-chain exon $V_\beta 17a$ was assessed have provided evidence for both clonal deletion and clonal anergy of T cells. What was the major difference between these experiments that would explain why clonal deletion occurred in one and clonal anergy in the other?

7. a. What would be the consequences if a mouse strain were unable to carry out positive selection during thymic processing of its T cells.

   b. What would be the consequences if a mouse strain were unable to carry out negative selection during thymic processing of its T cells?

8. a. What is the experimental evidence showing that T cells can mediate suppression of immune responses?

   b. What experimental findings have called into question the existence of a distinct T_S subpopulation?

   c. Assuming that a distinct T_S-cell lineage does not exist, what other mechanisms could account for T-cell-mediated suppression?

9. In the transgenic experiment depicted in Figure 14-11, H-2^b and H-$2^{b/d}$ transgenic mice were produced carrying genes for the $\alpha\beta$ T-cell receptor of a H-2^b CTL clone specific for the L^d class I MHC molecule.

   a. Why did a high percentage of mature CD8$^+$ T cells express this transgene in the H-2^b mice but not in H-$2^{b/d}$ mice?

   b. Why were H-$2^{b/d}$ mice used instead of H-2^d mice in this experiment?

   c. What assay was used to assess the functional activity of the CD8$^+$ T cells?

The Complement System

T he complement system, the major effector of the humoral branch of the immune system, consists of at least 20 chemically distinct serum proteins and glycoproteins. Following initial activation, various complement components interact in a highly regulated enzymatic cascade, to generate reaction products that facilitate antigen clearance and generation of an inflammatory response. There are two pathways of complement activation—the classical pathway and the alternative pathway. The two pathways share a common terminal reaction sequence that generates a macromolecular membrane-attack complex (MAC), which lyses a variety of cells, bacteria, and viruses. The complement reaction products amplify the initial antibody-antigen reaction and convert that reaction into a more effective

Table 15-1   Characteristics of the complement proteins

Protein	Molecular weight	Serum conc. (μg/ml)	Immunologic function
Early components			
Classical pathway			
C1q	410,000	70	Structural protein: binds to Fc region of IgM and IgG antibodies
C1r	85,000	50	Serine protease: enzymatically activates C1s
C1s	85,000	50	Serine protease: enzymatically activates C4 and C2
C4	210,000	300	Structural protein: C4b binds C2b; C4a is an anaphylatoxin
C2	110,000	25	Serine protease: C2b bound to C4b acts as C3/C5 convertase to enzymatically activate C3 and C5
Alternative pathway			
Factor D	25,000	1	Serine protease: enzymatically activates factor B
Factor B	93,000	200	Serine protease: Bb subunit combined with C3b and acts as C3/C5 convertase to activate C3 and C5
Properdin	220,000	25	Binds to C3bBb (C3/C5 convertase) and stabilizes it
Both pathways			
C3	190,000	1200	Structural protein: C3b binds to Bb forming C3/C5 convertase. C3b binds C5 so that it can be activated by C5 convertase; C3a is an anaphylatoxin
Terminal components			
C5	190,000	70	Structural protein: C5b is a component of MAC that binds C6; C5a is an anaphylatoxin
C6	120,000	60	Structural protein: component of MAC that binds C7
C7	110,000	55	Structural protein: component of MAC that binds C8
C8	150,000	55	Structural protein: component of MAC that binds C9
C9	70,000	60	Structural protein: polymerizes to form MAC pore

defense mechanism. A variety of small, diffusible reaction products that are released during complement activation induce localized vasodilation and attract phagocytic cells chemotactically, leading to an inflammatory reaction. As antigen becomes coated with complement reaction products, it is more readily phagocytosed by phagocytic cells that bear receptors for these complement products. In addition, some of the complement products have been shown to play a role in the activation of B lymphocytes. Finally, the terminal components of the complement system generate the membrane-attack complex.

This chapter describes the similarities and differences in the two pathways, the regulation of the complement system, the effector functions of various complement components, and the consequences of hereditary deficiencies in some components.

Protein	Molecular weight	Serum conc. (μg/ml)	Immunologic function
Regulatory components			
Factor H	150,000	560	Blocks formation of C3 convertase in alternative pathway; serves as cofactor for factor I inactivation
Factor I	90,000	35	Cleaves C4b or C3b using MCP, CR1, factor H, or C4bBP as cofactors
Cl inhibitor (C1 Inh)	105,000	200	Dissociates C1
C4b-binding protein (C4bBP)	560,000	250	Blocks formation of C3 convertase in classical pathway; serves as cofactor for factor I inactivation
S protein	85,000	505	Binds soluble C5b67 and prevents membrane insertion
Membrane cofactor protein (MCP)	60,000	Cell-bound	Blocks C3 convertase formation in classical and alternative pathways; serves as cofactor for factor I inactivation
Decay accelerating factor (DAF)	70,000	Cell-bound	Dissociates C3 convertase in classical and alternative pathways
Homologous restriction factor (HRF)	65,000	Cell-bound	Binds to C5b678 and blocks C9 binding to autologous cells
Anaphylatoxin inactivator	310,000	35	Blocks anaphylatoxin activity

The Complement Components

The proteins and glycoproteins comprising the complement system are synthesized largely by liver hepatocytes, although significant amounts of complement components are also produced by blood monocytes, tissue macrophages, and epithelial cells of the gastrointestinal and genitourinary tracts. These components constitute 15% (by weight) of the serum globulin fraction and circulate in the serum in functionally inactive forms, many of them as proenzymes in which the enzymatically active site is masked. Activation of the proenzyme cleaves the molecule, removing an inhibitory fragment and exposing the active site. Activation of the complement system involves a sequential enzyme cascade in which the proenzyme product of one step becomes the enzyme catalyst of the next step. Each activated component has a short half-life before being inactivated.

Each complement component is designated by numerals (C1–C9), by letter symbols, or by trivial names (Table 15-1). After a component is activated, the peptide fragments are denoted by small letters, with the smaller fragment designated "a" and the larger fragment designated "b" (e.g., C3a, C3b). The larger "b" fragments bind to the target near the site of activation, and the smaller "a" fragments diffuse from the site and play a role in initiating a localized inflammatory response. The complement fragments interact with one another to form functional complexes. Those complexes that have enzymatic activity are designated by a bar over the number or symbol (e.g., $\overline{\text{C4b2b}}$, $\overline{\text{C3bBb}}$).

Initial Steps in Complement Activation

The early steps in complement activation, culminating in formation of C5b, can occur via two pathways—the classical and the alternative. The final steps leading to formation of a membrane-attack complex are the same in both pathways. The complement components involved in each pathway, and the sequence in which they take part, are outlined in Figure 15-1.

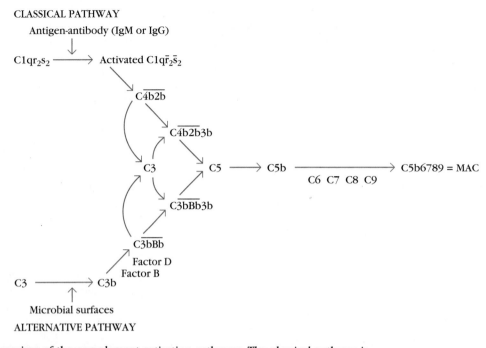

Figure 15-1   Overview of the complement activation pathways. The classical pathway is activated by the binding of C1 to antigen-antibody complexes. The alternative pathway is activated by binding of C3b to activating surfaces such as microbial cell walls. Both pathways generate C3/C5 convertases and form C5b, which is converted into a membrane-attack complex (MAC) by a common sequence of terminal reactions.

Classical Pathway

Activation of the classical complement pathway is commonly initiated by the formation of soluble antigen-antibody complexes or by the binding of antibody to antigen on a suitable target, such as a bacterial cell. IgM and certain subclasses of IgG (IgG1, IgG2, and IgG3) can activate the classical complement pathway, as can certain nonimmunologic activators. The initial stage of activation involves a sequential enzyme cascade of C1, C2, C3, and C4, which are present in plasma in functionally inactive forms. The components were named in order of their discovery and before their functional roles had been determined, so that their names do not reflect the sequence in which they react.

The complexing of antibody with antigen induces conformational changes in the Fc portion of the antibody molecule that exposes a binding site for the C1 component of the complement system. C1 exists in serum as a macromolecular complex consisting of C1q and two molecules each of C1r and C1s, held together in a Ca^{2+}-stabilized complex ($C1qr_2s_2$). The C1q molecule is composed of 18 polypeptide chains that associate to form 6 collagenlike triple helical arms, the tips of which bind to the exposed binding sites in the C_H2 domain of the antibody molecule (Figure 15-2a,b). The $C1r_2s_2$ complex

can exist in two configurations. When it is free and not bound to C1q, it assumes an S-shaped form; on binding to C1q, $C1r_2s_2$ assumes a shape similar to a figure 8 (Figure 15-2c–e). Each C1r and C1s monomer contains a catalytic domain and an interaction domain, which facilitates interaction with C1q or with each other.

Each C1 molecule must bind, via its C1q globular heads, to at least two Fc sites for a stable C1-antibody interaction to occur. When pentameric IgM is bound to antigen on a target surface, at least three binding sites for C1q are exposed. Circulating IgM, however, assumes a planar configuration in which the C1q-binding sites are not exposed (Figure 15-3). For this reason, circulating IgM cannot activate the complement cascade by itself. An IgG molecule, on the other hand, contains only a single C1q-binding site on its Fc portion, so that firm C1q binding is achieved only when two IgG molecules are within 30–40 nm of each other on a target surface or in a complex, providing two attachment sites for C1q. This difference in the structure of IgM and IgG accounts for the observation that a single molecule of IgM bound to a red blood cell is enough to activate the classical complement pathway and lyse the red blood cell, whereas some 1000 molecules of IgG are required if two molecules, randomly distributed, are to end up close enough to each other to initiate C1q binding.

(a)

(b)

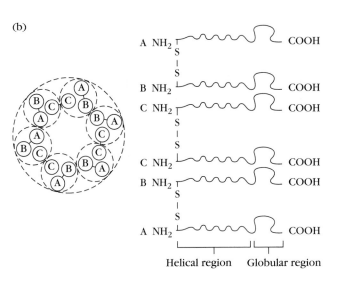

Helical region   Globular region

(c)

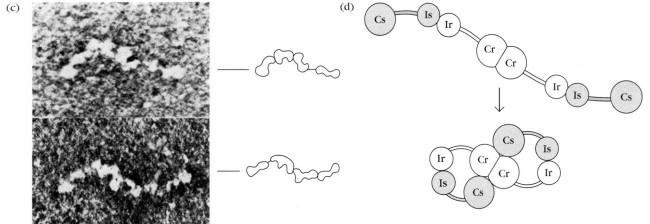

(d)

(e)

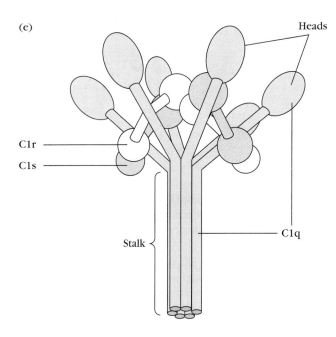

Heads

C1r

C1s

Stalk

C1q

Figure 15-2 Structure of C1q, C1r_2s_2, and the C1 macromolecular complex (C1qr_2s_2). (a) Electron micrograph of the C1q component showing stalk and six globular heads. (b) Cross-section of stalk of C1q (*left*) and schematic diagram of chain structure of two triplets (*right*). A C1q molecule consists of 18 polypeptide chains arranged into 6 triplets, each of which contains one A, one B, and one C chain. The stalk of the molecule corresponds to helical domains in the chains, and the heads correspond to globular regions. (c) Electron micrograph of free C1r_2s_2 complex showing characteristic S shape. (d) Diagram of C1r_2s_2 complex in S-shaped form (*top*) and figure-8 form (*bottom*), which it assumes on binding with C1q. Each C1r (white) and C1s (red) monomer contains a catalytic domain (C) with enzymatic activity and an interaction domain (I), which facilitates binding with C1q or with each other. (e) Diagram of C1qr_2s_2 complex. [Part (a) from H. R. Knobel, W. Villiger, and H. Isliker, 1975, *Eur. J. Immunol.* **5**:78; part (c) from J. Tschopp et al., 1980, *Proc. Nat'l. Acad. Sci. USA* **77**:7014.]

(a)

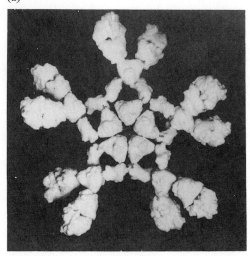

(b)

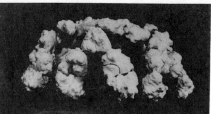

(c)   (d)   (e)   (f)

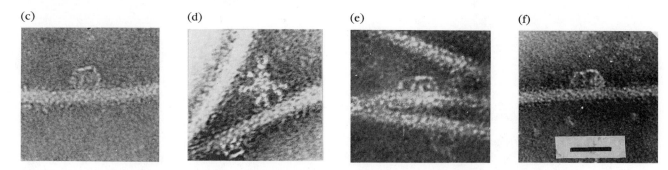

Figure 15-3 (*Above*) Models of pentameric IgM in the planar form (a), which it assumes when in solution, and in the "staple" form (b), which it assumes when bound to a solid-phase antigen. Several Fc-region binding sites are accessible for complement activation in the staple form, whereas none are exposed in the planar form. (*Below*) Electron micrographs of IgM antiflagellum antibody bound to flagella, showing the planar (c, d) and staple (e, f) forms. [From A. Feinstein, E. Munn, and N. Richardson, 1981, *Monogr. Allergy* **17**:28 and, 1981, *Ann. N. Y. Acad. Sci.* **190**:1104].

The intermediates in the classical activation pathway are depicted schematically in Figure 15-4. Binding of C1q to its Fc binding sites induces a conformational change in C1r that autocatalytically converts C1r to an active esterase enzyme. The $\overline{\text{C1r}}$ then cleaves the C1s to a similar active enzyme $\overline{\text{C1s}}$. $\overline{\text{C1s}}$ has two substrates, C4 and C2. The C4 component is a glycoprotein containing three polypeptide chains (α, β, and γ). C4 is activated when $\overline{\text{C1s}}$ hydrolyzes a small fragment (C4a) from the amino terminus of the α chain, exposing a binding site on the larger fragment, C4b. The C4b fragment attaches to the target surface in the vicinity of C1, and the C2 proenzyme then attaches to the exposed binding site on C4b, where it too is cleaved by the neighboring $\overline{\text{C1s}}$, the smaller fragment (C2a) diffuses away. The resulting $\overline{\text{C4b2b}}$ complex* is called C3/C5

convertase, referring to its role in coverting both C3 and C5 proenzymes into an enzymatically active form. The native C3 component consists of two polypeptide chains, α and β. Hydrolysis of a short fragment (C3a) from the amino terminus of the α chain by the C3/C5 convertase generates C3b (Figure 15-5). A single C3/C5 convertase molecule can generate over 200 molecules of C3b, resulting in tremendous amplification at this step

---

* The nomenclature for C2 has recently been changed. The larger fragment used to be designated as C2a but is now designated as C2b to bring the nomenclature in line with the convention of designating the larger fragment as "b." The designation C3/C5 convertase is also new. $\overline{\text{C4b2b}}$ used to be referred to as C3 convertase and $\overline{\text{C4b2b3b}}$ as C5 convertase. This has been changed since $\overline{\text{C4b2b}}$ acts as the convertase for both C3 and C5. The role of C3b is to bind C5 and alter its conformation so that the convertase can cleave it.

(a)
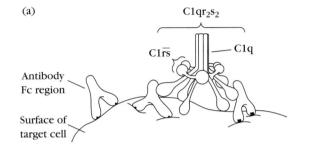

(b)
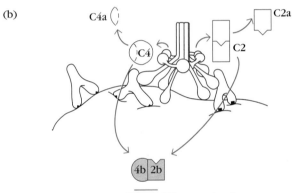

(c)
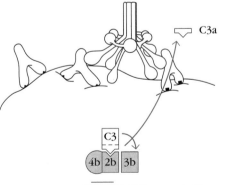

(d)
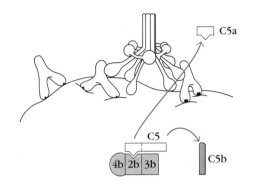

(e)
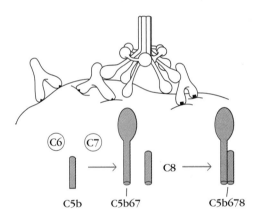

(f)
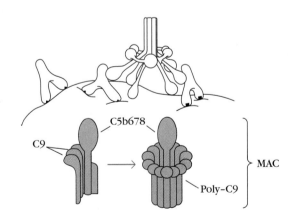

Figure 15-4 Schematic diagram of intermediates in classical pathway of complement activation. Complement complexes shaded gray are bound to the antigenic surface but do not penetrate it. Complexes shaded red can insert into the cell membrane. The completed membrane-attack complex (MAC) forms a large pore in the membrane. (See text for details).

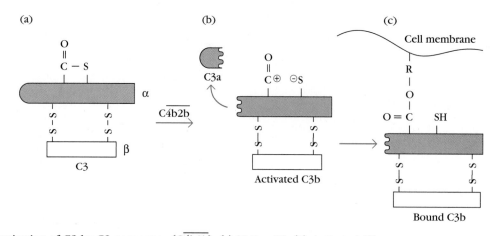

Figure 15-5   Activation of C3 by C3 convertase (C4b2b). (a) Native C3. (b) Activated C3 showing site of cleavage by C4b2b, resulting in production of the C3a and C3b fragments. (c) C3 has a labile internal thioester bond that is activated as C3b is formed, allowing the C3b fragment to bind to free —OH or —NH$_2$ groups on a cell membrane. Bound C3b exhibits various biological activities including binding of C5 and binding to C3b receptors on phagocytic cells.

of the sequence. The C3b binds to the surface of the foreign antigen and serves in turn as a binding site for the C5 component, altering its conformation so that the nearby convertase enzyme can cleave it into C5a and C5b. The bound C5b initiates formation of the membrane-attack complex in a sequence described later. The C3b also serves an important role in opsonization, because phagocytic cells have receptors for C3b and will more readily phagocytose antigen that is coated with C3b.

Alternative Pathway

Bound C5b can also be generated by a second major pathway of complement activation called the alternative pathway. The alternative pathway involves four serum proteins: C3, factor B, factor D, and properdin. Unlike the classical pathway, which generally requires antibody for its initial activation, the alternative pathway is initially activated in most cases by various cell-surface constituents that are foreign to the host (Table 15-2). For example, both gram-negative and gram-positive bacteria have cell-wall constituents that can activate the alternative pathway. The intermediates in the alternative pathway are depicted schematically in Figure 15-6.

Serum C3 contains an unstable thioester bond, which is subject to slow spontaneous hydrolysis into C3a and C3b. The C3b component can bind to foreign surface antigens (such as those on bacterial cells or viral particles) or even to the host's own cells (see Figure 15-5c). The membranes of most mammalian cells have high levels of sialic acid, which contributes to the rapid

Table 15-2   Activators of the alternative complement pathway

Pathogens and particles of microbial origin	Nonpathogens
Many strains of gram-negative bacteria	Human IgG, IgA, and IgE in complexes
Lipopolysaccharides from gram-negative bacteria	Rabbit and guinea pig IgG in complexes
Many strains of gram-positive bacteria	Cobra venom factor
Teichoic acid from gram-positive cell walls	Heterologous erythrocytes (rabbit, mouse, chicken)
Fungi and yeast cell walls (zymosan)	Anionic polymers (dextran sulfate)
Some viruses and virus-infected cells	Pure carbohydrates (agarose, inulin)
Some tumor cells (Raji)	
Parasites (trypanosomes)	

SOURCE: M. K. Pangburn, 1986, in *Immunobiology of the Complement System*, Academic Press.

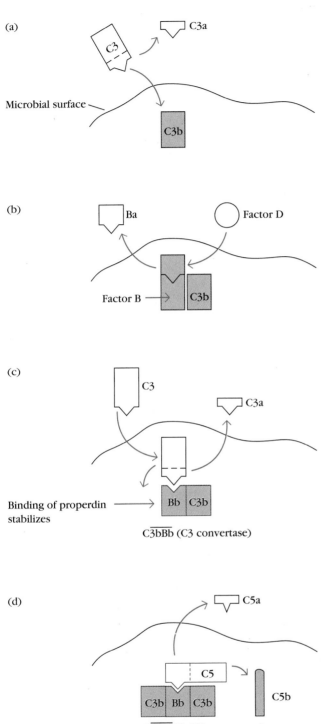

(a)

C3a

C3

Microbial surface

C3b

(b)

Ba

Factor D

Factor B → C3b

(c)

C3

C3a

Binding of properdin stabilizes → Bb C3b

C3bBb (C3 convertase)

(d)

C5a

C5

C3b Bb C3b

C5b

C3bBb3b (C5 convertase)

Figure 15-6 Schematic diagram of intermediates in formation of bound C5b by alternative pathway of complement activation. The C3bBb complex is stabilized by binding of properdin. Complexes shaded red are bound to the activating surface. Conversion of bound C5b to the membrane-attack complex occurs by the same sequence of reactions as in the classical pathway shown in Figure 15-4.

inactivation of bound C3b molecules on host cells. Because foreign antigenic surfaces such as bacterial cell walls, yeast cell walls, and certain viral envelopes have only low levels of sialic acid, C3b bound to these surfaces remains active for a longer time. Bound C3b can bind another serum protein called factor B by way of a Mg^{2+}-dependent bond. Binding to C3b exposes a site on factor B that serves as the substrate for an enzymatically active serum protein, factor D. Factor D cleaves the C3b-bound factor B, releasing a small fragment (Ba), which diffuses away, and generating C3bBb. The C3bBb complex is analogous to the C4b2b complex in the classical pathway, having both C3 and C5 convertase activity. The C3 convertase activity of C3bBb has a half-life of only 5 min unless the serum protein properdin binds to it, stabilizing it and extending the half-life of its convertase activity to 30 min.

The C3bBb generated in the alternative pathway can activate unhydrolyzed C3 to generate more C3b autocatalytically. As a result, the initial steps are repeated and amplified, so that more than 2×10^6 molecules of C3b can be deposited on an antigenic surface in less than 5 min. The C3 convertase activity of C3bBb generates the C3bBb3b complex, which exhibits C5 convertase activity, analogous to the C4b2b3b complex in the classical pathway. One of the bound C3b components in this complex can serve as an opsonin, facilitating phagocytosis; it also can serve as a binding site for C5. The C5 convertase activity of the C3bBb3b complex then hydrolyzes the bound C5 to generate C5a and C5b, which binds to the antigenic surface. Table 15-3 summarizes the components involved in formation of C3/C5 convertases in the classical and alternative pathways.

Table 15-3 Complement components in the formation of C3/C5 convertases in the classical and alternative activation pathways

	Classical pathway	Alternative pathway
Precursor proteins	C4 + C2	C3 + factor B
Activating protease	C1s	Factor D
C3 Convertase	C4b2b	C3bBb
C5 Convertase	C4b2b3b	C3bBb3b
C5-binding component	C3b	C3b

Formation of Membrane-Attack Complex

The terminal sequence of complement activation involves C5b, C6, C7, C8, and C9, which interact sequentially to form a macromolecular structure called the *membrane-attack complex (MAC)*. This complex displaces the membrane phospholipids, forming a large transmembrane channel that disrupts the membrane and enables ions and small molecules to diffuse through it freely.

As noted in the previous section, in both the classical and alternative pathways, a C3/C5 convertase cleaves C5, which contains two protein chains (α and β). Following binding of C5 to the nonenzymatic C3b component of the convertase, the amino terminus of the α chain is cleaved, generating the small C5a fragment, which diffuses away, and the large C5b fragment, which provides a binding site for the subsequent components of the membrane-attack complex (see Figure 15-4d). The C5b component is extremely labile and is inactivated within 2 min unless C6 binds with it and stabilizes its activity.

Up to this point all the complement reactions take place on the hydrophilic surface of membranes or on immune complexes in the fluid phase. As the C5b6 complex binds to C7, it undergoes a hydrophilic-amphiphilic structural transition exposing hydrophobic regions, which serve as binding sites for membrane phospholipids. If the reaction is on a target-cell membrane, the hydrophobic binding site enables the C5b67 complex to insert into the phopholipid bilayer (see Figure 15-4e). If, however, the reaction occurs on an immune complex or other noncellular activating surface, then the hydrophobic binding site cannot anchor the complex and it is released. This released C5b67 complex can bind to nearby cells and bring about "innocent-bystander" lysis. In a number of diseases in which immune complexes are produced, tissue damage results from such innocent-bystander lysis. This autoimmune process will be discussed in Chapter 16.

Binding of C8 to membrane-bound C5b67 induces a conformational change in C8, so that it too undergoes a hydrophilic-amphiphilic structural transition exposing a hydrophobic region, which interacts with the plasma membrane. The C5b678 complex creates a small pore, 10 Å in diameter; formation of this pore can lead to lysis of red blood cells but not of nucleated cells. The final step in formation of the MAC is the binding and polymerization of C9, a perforin-like molecule, to the C5b678 complex. As many as 10–16 molecules of C9 can be bound and polymerized by a single C5b678 complex. During polymerization the C9 molecules undergo a hydrophilic-amphiphilic transition, so that they also can insert into the membrane (see Figure 15-4f). The com-

(a)   (b)

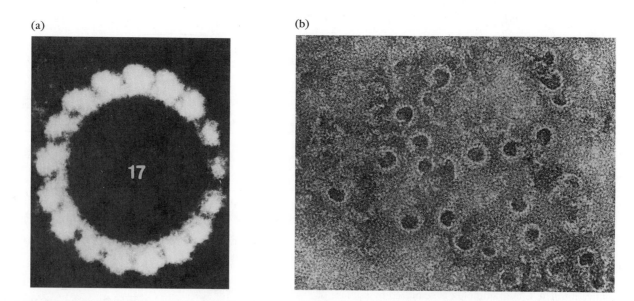

Figure 15-7   (a) Photomicrograph of poly-C9 complex formed by in vitro polymerization of C9. (b) Photomicrograph of complement-induced lesions on the membrane of a red blood cell. These lesions result from formation of membrane-attack complexes. [Part (a) from E. R. Podack, 1986, in *Immunobiology of the Complement System*, Academic Press; part (b) from J. Humphrey and R. Dourmashkin, 1969, *Adv. Immunol.* **11**:75.]

pleted MAC, which has a tubular form and functional pore size of 70–100 Å, consists of a C5b678 complex surrounded by a poly-C9 complex (Figure 15-7). Since ions and small molecules can diffuse freely through the central channel of the MAC, the cell cannot maintain its osmotic stability and is lysed by an influx of water and loss of electrolytes.

Regulation of the Complement System

Because the complement system is nonspecific and thus capable of attacking host cells as well as microorganisms, elaborate regulatory mechanisms are required to confine the reaction to designated targets. Both the classical and alternative pathways include a number of extremely labile components, which undergo spontaneous inactivation as they diffuse away from the target cells. For example, the target-binding site on C3b undergoes spontaneous hydrolysis by the time it has diffused 40 nm away from the $\overline{C4b2b}$ or $\overline{C3bBb}$ convertase enzymes. This rapid hydrolysis limits C3b binding to nearby host cells. In addition, both pathways include a series of regulatory proteins that inactivate various complement components. A glycoprotein called C1 inhibitor (C1 Inh) can form a complex with $C1r_2s_2$, causing it to dissociate from C1q and thus preventing further activation of C4 or C2 (Figure 15-8a).

The C3 convertase enzymes of the classical and alternative pathways comprise the major amplification step in complement activation, generating hundreds of molecules of C3b. The C3b generated by these enzymes can bind to nearby cells, mediating damage to the healthy cell by opsonization to phagocytic cells bearing C3b receptors or by induction of the membrane-attack complex. It is estimated that circulating red blood cells are exposed to thousands of molecules of C3b molecules each day. In order to prevent C3b-mediated damage to healthy cells, a family of regulatory proteins has evolved to regulate C3 convertase activity in the classical and alternative pathways. This family of C3 convertase regulatory proteins are related structurally by the presence of short 60–amino acid repeating sequences (or motifs) termed *short consensus repeats (SCRs)*, and they are related genetically, as they are encoded at a single chromosomal location on chromosome 1, known as the *regulators of complement activation (RCA)* gene cluster. Included within the RCA gene cluster are membrane cofactor protein (MCP or CD46), decay accelerating factor (DAF or CD55), complement receptor type 1 (CR1 or CD35), complement receptor type 2 (CR2 or CD21), C4b-binding protein (C4bBP), and factor H.

A number of RCA proteins prevent assembly of C3 convertase. In the classical pathway three structurally

different proteins act similarly to prevent assembly of C3 convertase (Figure 15-8b). These regulatory proteins include soluble C4b-binding protein (C4bBP) and two membrane-bound proteins, the type 1 complement receptor (CR1) and the membrane cofactor protein (MCP or CD46). Each of these regulatory proteins binds to C4b and prevents its association with C2b. Once C4bBP, CR1, or MCP is bound to C4b, another regulatory protein, factor I, cleaves the C4b into bound C4d and soluble C4c (see Figure 15-9a). A similar regulatory sequence occurs in the alternative pathway. In this case CR1, MCP, or a regulatory component called factor H binds to C3b and prevents its association with factor B (Figure 15-8c). Once CR1, MCP, or factor H is bound to C3b, factor I cleaves the C3b into a bound C3bi fragment and a soluble C3f fragment. Further cleavage of C3bi by factor I releases C3c and leaves C3dg bound to the membrane (Figure 15-9b).

RCA proteins also act on the assembled C3 convertase, causing it to dissociate. Included among these regulatory proteins are the previously mentioned C4bBP, CR1, and factor H, as well as an additional protein, decay-accelerating factor (DAF). DAF is a glycoprotein that is anchored covalently to a glycophospholipid membrane protein. Each of these RCA proteins accelerates decay (dissociation) of C3 convertase, releasing the enzyme (C2b or Bb) from the cell-bound component (C4b or C3b) (Figure 15-8d). Once dissociation of the C3 convertase occurs, then factor I cleaves the remaining membrane-bound C4b or C3b component to irreversibly inactivate the convertase.

Regulatory proteins also operate at the level of the membrane-attack complex. The ability of the C5b67 complex to be released and then bind to nearby cells poses a threat of innocent-bystander lysis of healthy cells. A number of serum proteins can counter this threat by binding to released C5b67 and preventing its insertion into the membrane of nearby cells. A serum protein called S protein can bind to C5b67, inducing a hydrophilic transition and thereby preventing insertion of C5b67 into the membrane of nearby cells (Figure 15-8e). The binding of the S protein to C5b67 also keeps C9 from binding to the soluble C5b67 and polymerizing, and thereby prevents the futile consumption of C9.

For a number of years it was known that complement-mediated lysis of cells was more effective if the complement was from a different species than the cells that were being lysed. The reason for this unusual finding was finally uncovered this past year with the discovery of two membrane proteins on the membrane of a wide variety of cells that block MAC formation. These two membrane proteins are homologous restriction factor (HRF) and CD59. Both membrane proteins protect cells from nonspecific complement-mediated lysis by binding to C8, preventing C9 assembly and insertion into the

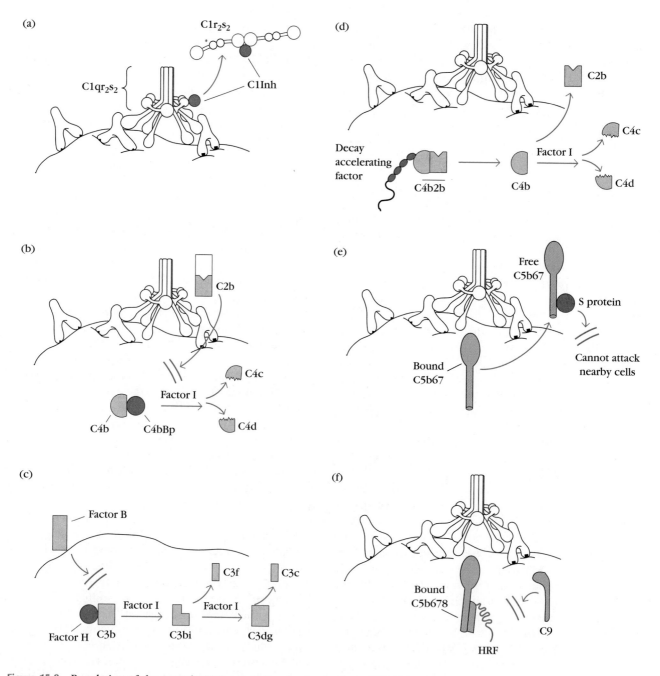

Figure 15-8 Regulation of the complement system involves a number of regulatory proteins (red), which function to inactivate various intermediates in the activation pathways. Membrane-bound intermediates are shaded gray. (a) C1 inhibitor (C1 Inh) can bind to activated C1r or C1s, causing the $C1r_2s_2$ complex to dissociate from C1q. (b) Formation of the C3 convertase in the classical pathway is blocked by the binding of C4b-binding protein (C4bBP), which prevents binding of C2b. Factor I then cleaves C4b into C4d and C4c. CR1 and membrane cofactor protein (MCP) block C3 convertase formation in a similar manner. (c) Formation of C3 convertase in the alternative pathway is blocked by binding of factor H to C3b, which prevents binding of factor B. Factor I then cleaves C3b to generate an inactive fragment C3bi, which is further degraded to yield C3c and C3dg. CR1 and MCP block C3 convertase formation in a similar manner. (d) Membrane-bound decay accelerating factor (DAF) causes dissociation of the C3 convertase enzymes (C4b2b or C3bB2). (e) S protein can bind to C5b67 that is released from the membrane, thereby preventing its insertion into nearby cells. (f) Membrane-bound homologous restriction factor (HRF) blocks MAC pore formation by binding to C5b678 and preventing binding of C9.

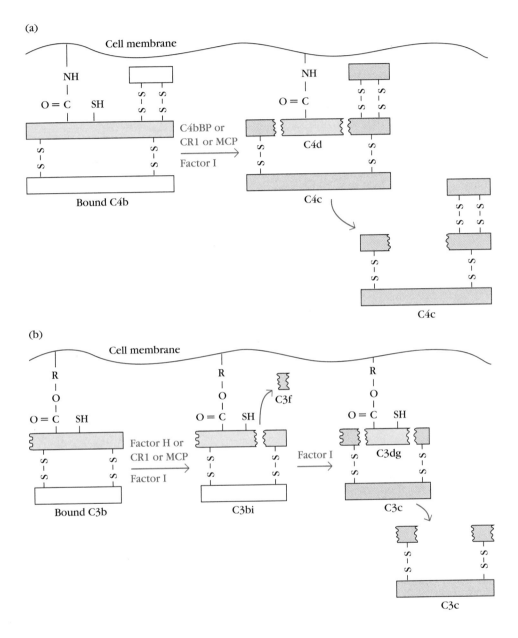

Figure 15-9 Inactivation of bound C4b and C3b by regulatory proteins of the complement system. (a) Binding of C4bBP, CR1, or MCP to C4b enable factor I to cleave C4b into a bound fragment (C4d) and a soluble fragment (C4c). (b) Binding of Factor H, CR1, or MCP to C3b enables factor I to cleave C3b into a bound fragment (C3bi) and a soluble fragment (C3f) that diffuses away. Further cleavage of C3bi by factor I generates a bound fragment (C3dg) and a soluble fragment (C3c).

plasma membrane (Figure 15-8f). In both cases the membrane proteins only block C9 assembly if the complement is from the same species as the cells, and, for this reason, they are said to display homologous restriction, for which HRF was named.

Receptors for Complement

Each of the circulating red and white blood cells express cell-membrane receptors for complement fragments. These complement receptors mediate many of the biological activities of the complement system. In addition, some complement receptors play an important role in regulating complement activity by binding biologically active complement components and degrading them into inactive products. The complement receptors and their primary ligands, which include various complement components and their proteolytic breakdown products, are listed in Table 15-4.

Type 1 Complement Receptor (CR1)

The type 1 complement receptor (CR1) is a glycoprotein having a high affinity for C3b, although it can also bind C3bi, C4b, and C4bi with lower affinity. This receptor is expressed on red blood cells, monocytes, macrophages, neutrophils, eosinophils, B cells, and some T cells. Because activation of C3 into C3a and C3b represents the major amplification step in both the classical and alternative pathways, immune complexes and particulate antigens generally become coated with C3b during complement activation. Cells expressing CR1 are able to bind both immune complexes and particulate antigens to which C3b is attached, facilitating antigen clearance. The expression of CR1 on B cells, some T cells, and dendritic cells may also enable these cells to

trap C3b-coated immune complexes in the lymph nodes and spleen, enabling the antigen to persist longer in these sites so that a more effective immune response can be generated.

As mentioned previously, CR1 also plays an important role in regulating the complement cascade. The binding of C3b or C4b to CR1 has been shown to enable proteolytic degradation by factor I (Figure 15-9). This regulatory activity is thought to be important in limiting the complement cascade so that extensive tissue damage does not occur. The following section will look at the biological role of CR1 in more detail.

Type 2 Complement Receptor (CR2)

The type 2 complement receptor (CR2) is a glycoprotein that binds several degradation products of C3b including C3d, C3dg, and C3bi. Unlike CR1, which is present on all types of circulating blood cells, CR2 expression is limited to B cells and some T cells. Interestingly, CR2 is the receptor for Epstein-Barr virus, which accounts for the susceptibility of B cells to infection by this virus. Apparently, Epstein-Barr virus has amino acid sequence homology with the C3dg degradation product, enabling it to bind to the same receptor. The function of the CR2 receptor on B cells remains unknown. There is some evidence suggesting that cross-linked C3dg binding to the CR2 receptor may play a role in B-cell activation.

Type 3 and Type 4 Complement Receptor (CR3 and CR4)

The type 3 and 4 complement receptors bind primarily the C3b degradation product C3bi. CR3 and CR4 are found on monocytes, macrophages, neutrophils, natural killer cells, and some subpopulations of T cells. These receptors are heterodimers consisting of two nonco-

Table 15-4 Ligands and cellular distribution of complement receptors

Receptor	Major ligands	Cellular distribution
CR1	C3b, C4b	Erythrocytes, neutrophils, monocytes, macrophages, B cells, some T cells, eosinophils, follicular dendritic cells
CR2	C3d, C3dg*, C3bi	B cells, some T cells
CR3 and CR4	C3bi	Monocytes, macrophages, neutrophils, natural killer cells, some T cells
C3a/C4a receptor	C3a, C4a	Mast cells, basophils, granulocytes
C5a receptor	C5a	Mast cells, basophils, granulocytes, monocytes, macrophages, platelets, endothelial cells

* Cleavage of C3dg by serum proteases generates C3d and C3g.

valently associated glycoproteins: an α and a β chain. CR3 is also known as MAC-1, and CR4 is also known as p150,95. Both are members of the integrin family of receptors along with LFA-1; these receptors generally bind cell-adhesion molecules. Each of these integrin receptors has a unique α chain but a common β chain. The α chain of CR3 and CR4 can bind C3bi. Some evidence suggests that CR3 may also bind to ICAMs and may facilitate extravasation of neutrophils from the capillary into the tissue spaces during an inflammatory reaction. Binding of complement-coated particles to CR3 triggers phagocytosis by phagocytic cells.

Receptors for C3a, C4a, and C5a

C3a, C4a, and C5a are low-molecular-weight complement fragments that diffuse away from the site of complement activation. Receptors for these fragments are present on basophils, mast cells, and granulocytes. Binding of C3a, C4a, or C5a to its receptor on a mast cell or basophil induces the cell to degranulate, releasing pharmacologically active mediators.

Biological Consequences of Complement Activation

Complement serves as an important mediator of the humoral response by amplifying the response and converting it into an effective defense mechanism for destroying invading microorganisms and viruses.

Cell Lysis

The membrane-attack complex formed by complement activation is capable of lysing a broad spectrum of microorganisms, viruses, erythrocytes, and nucleated cells. Because the alternative pathway of activation generally occurs without an initial antibody-antigen interaction, this pathway serves as an important innate system of nonspecific defense against infectious microorganisms. The requirement for an initial antibody-antigen reaction in the classical pathway supplements the nonspecific innate defense of the alternative pathway with a more specific defense mechanism.

Up to this point this text has stressed the role of cell-mediated immunity in host defense against viral infections. Nevertheless antibody and complement do play a role in host defense against viruses and are often crucial in containing viral spread during acute infection and in protecting against reinfection. Most—perhaps all—enveloped viruses are susceptible to complement-mediated lysis. The viral envelope is largely derived from the plasma membrane of the infected host cell and is therefore susceptible to pore formation via the membrane-attack complex. Among the pathogenic viruses shown to be lysed by complement-mediated lysis are herpes virus, myxoviruses, paramyxoviruses, and retroviruses.

The complement system is generally quite effective in lysing gram-negative bacteria. (Figure 15-10). In contrast, gram-positive bacteria are generally resistant to complement-mediated lysis because the thick peptidoglycan layer in their cell wall prevents insertion of the MAC into the inner membrane. A few gram-negative bacteria can develop resistance to complement-

(a) 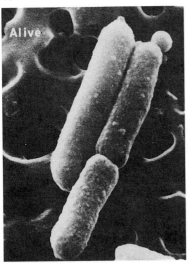   (b) 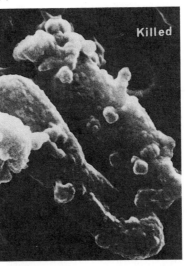   (c)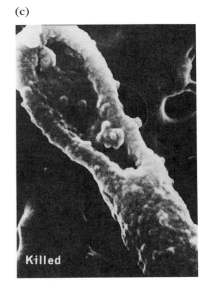

Figure 15-10 Scanning electron micrographs of *E. coli* showing (a) intact cells and (b, c) cells killed by complement-mediated lysis. Note membrane blebbing on lysed cells. [From R. D. Schreiber et al., 1979, *J. Exp. Med.* **149**:870.]

mediated lysis that correlates with the virulence of the organism. In *Escherichia coli* and *Salmonella*, resistance to complement is associated with the smooth bacterial phenotype, which is characterized by the presence of long polysaccharide side chains in the cell-wall lipopolysaccharide (LPS) component. It has been proposed that the increased LPS in the wall of resistant strains may prevent insertion of the membrane-attack complex into the bacterial membrane, so that the complex is released from the bacterial cell rather than forming a pore. Strains of *Neisseria gonorrhoeae* resistant to complement-mediated killing have been associated with disseminated gonococcal infections in humans. Some evidence suggests that the membrane proteins of resistant *Neisseria* strains undergo noncovalent interactions with the MAC that prevent its insertion into the outer membrane of the cells. These examples of resistant gram-negative bacteria are the exception; most gram-negative bacteria are susceptible to complement-mediated lysis.

Nucleated cells tend to be more resistant to complement-mediated lysis than red blood cells. Lysis of nucleated cells requires formation of multiple membrane-attack complexes, whereas a single MAC can lyse a red blood cell. Many nucleated cells, including the majority of cancer cells, can endocytose MAC. If the complex is removed soon enough, the cell can repair any membrane damage and restore its osmotic stability. This is the reason why complement-mediated lysis by monoclonal antibody specific for tumor-cell antigens is often not effective; rather, such monoclonal antibodies must be conjugated with toxins or radioactive isotopes to be effective tumor-killing agents.

Inflammatory Response

The complement cascade is often viewed in terms of the final outcome of cell lysis, and yet the events leading up to the membrane-attack complex generate important peptides with an instrumental role in the development of an effective inflammatory response (Table 15-5). As noted already, the complement "split products" C3a, C4a, and C5a, called *anaphylatoxins*, bind to receptors on mast cells and blood basophils and induce degranulation with release of histamine and other pharmacologically active mediators. The mediators induce smooth-muscle contraction and increases in vascular permeability. C3a, C5a, and C5b67 act together to induce monocytes and neutrophils to adhere to vascular endothelial cells, extravasate through the endothelial lining of the capillary, and migrate toward the site of complement activation in the tissues. C5a is most potent in mediating these processes, with picomolar quantities being effective. Activation of the complement system thus results in influxes of fluid that carries antibody and phagocytic cells to the site of antigen entry.

Table 15-5   Biological activities of complement split products that contribute to an effective inflammatory response

Substance	Biological activity
C3a	Smooth-muscle contraction Increase of vascular permeability Degranulation of mast cells and basophils with release of histamine Degranulation of eosinophils Aggregation of platelets
C3b	Opsonization of particles and solubilization of immune complexes with subsequent facilitation of phagocytosis
C3c	Release of neutrophils from bone marrow resulting in leukocytosis
C4a	Smooth-muscle contraction Increase of vascular permeability
C5a	Smooth-muscle contraction Increase of vascular permeability Degranulation of mast cells and basophils with release of histamine Degranulation of eosinophils Aggregation of platelets Chemotaxis of basophils, eosinophils, neutrophils, and monocytes Release of hydrolytic enzymes from neutrophils
Bb	Inhibition of migration and induction of spreading of monocytes and macrophages

Opsonization of Antigen

C3b is the major opsonin of the complement system. The amplification that occurs with C3 activation results in a coating of C3b on immune complexes and particulate antigens. Each of the phagocytic cells expresses complement receptors (CR1, CR3, and CR4) that bind C3b, C4b, or their degradation products (see Table 15-4). When antigen has been coated with C3b during complement activation by either pathway, the coated antigen binds to cells bearing CR1. If the cell is a phagocyte (e.g., a neutrophil, monocyte, or macrophage), phagocytosis will be enhanced (Figure 15-11). Activation

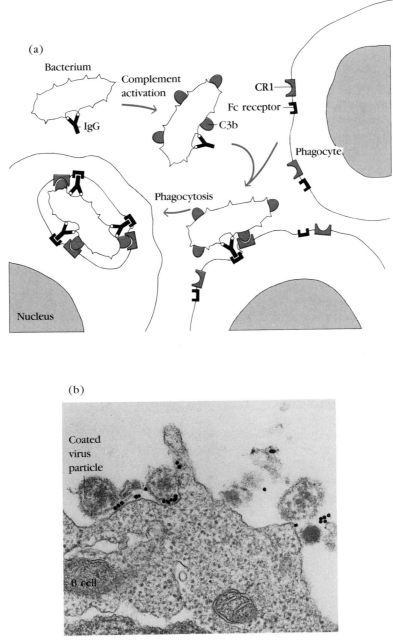

Figure 15-11 (a) Schematic representation of the role of C3b in opsonization. (b) Electron micrograph of Epstein-Barr virus coated with antibody and C3b and bound to the C3b receptors (CR1) on a B lymphocyte. [From N.R. Cooper and G. R. Nemerow, 1986, in *Immunobiology of the Complement System*, Academic Press.]

of phagocytic cells by various agents including C5a anaphylatoxin has been shown to increase the number of CR1's from 5,000 on resting phagocytes to 50,000 on activated cells, greatly facilitating their phagocytosis of C3b-coated antigen. Once C3b-coated antigen has bound to CR1, some of the C3b is degraded into C3bi and C3f. This enables the antigen to bind to CR3, which triggers phagocytosis more effectively than CR1.

Viral Neutralization

The complement system plays an important role in host defense by neutralizing viral infectivity. Some viruses (e.g., retroviruses, Epstein-Barr virus, Newcastle disease virus, and rubella virus) can activate the alternative or even the classical pathway in the absence of antibody. For most viruses, the binding of serum antibody to the repeating subunits of the viral structural proteins creates particulate immune complexes ideally suited for complement activation by the classical pathway.

The complement system mediates viral neutralization by a number of mechanisms (Table 15-6). Some degree of neutralization is achieved through the formation of larger viral aggregates, simply because these aggregates reduce the net number of infectious viral particles. Although antibody does play a role in the formation of viral aggregates, in vitro studies show that the C3b com-

ponent facilitates aggregate formation in the presence of as little as two molecules of antibody per virion. For example, polyoma virus coated with antibody is neutralized when serum is added containing activated C3. The binding of antibody and/or complement to the surface of a viral particle creates a thick protein coating that can be visualized by electron microscopy (Figure 15-12). This coating neutralizes viral infectivity by blocking attachment to susceptible host cells. The deposits of antibody and complement on viral particles also fa-

Table 15-6   Mechanisms of complement-mediated neutralization of viruses

Process	Mechanism	Requirements	Example	Biological importance
Aggregation by Ab and/or C	Reduction in net number of infectious particles as a consequence of cross-linking by bivalent Ab and/or C	Simultaneous high concentrations of virus, Ab, and/or C; high density of binding sites; high-affinity Ab and/or C interactions	Polyoma virus	Probably minor
Envelopment with Ab and/or C protein	Coating interferes with attachment or perforation	Occurs with low Ab and/or C concentrations; requires completion of the reaction sequence only through the C3 step	Influenza, EBV, and Newcastle disease viruses	Appears to be a major mechanism of viral neutralization
C-dependent viral lysis	Disruption of structure leads to irreversible loss of infectivity	Virus must be enveloped; potent activation stimulus; lipid bilayer of envelope must be accessible for C5b-9 insertion	Influenza, EBV, Newcastle disease, and Human immunodeficiency virus	Probably of minor importance except for retroviruses
Interaction with inflammatory cells via Fc and/or C receptors	Attachment to inflammatory cells leads to extracellular destruction by released mediators or to phagocytosis and intracellular destruction	Ab and/or C binding	Influenza, EBV viruses	Probably or major importance

KEY: Ab = antibody; C = complement; EBV = Epstein-Barr virus.

SOURCE: N. R. Cooper and G. R. Nemerow, 1986, in *Immunobiology of the Complement System,* Academic Press.

(a)   (b)   (c)

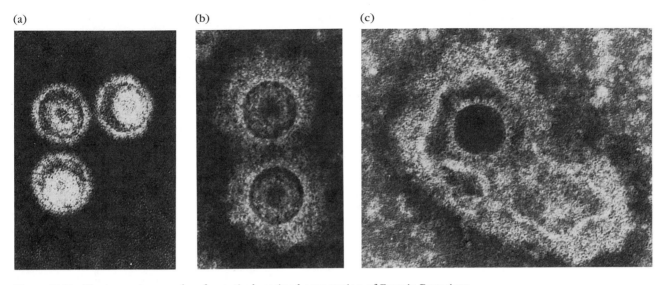

Figure 15-12 Electron micrographs of negatively stained preparation of Epstein-Barr virus. (a) Control without antibody. (b) Antibody-coated particles. (c) Particles coated with antibody and complement. [From N. R. Cooper and G. R. Nemerow, 1986, in *Immunobiology of the Complement System*, Academic Press.]

cilitate binding of the viral particle to cells possessing Fc or type 1 (CR1) complement receptors. In the case of phagocytic cells, such binding can be followed by phagocytosis and intracellular destruction of the ingested viral particle. Finally, complement is effective in lysing most, if not all, enveloped viruses, resulting in fragmentation of the envelope and disintegration of the nucleocapsid.

Solubilization of Immune Complexes

The role of the complement system in clearing immune complexes can be seen in patients with the autoimmune disease systemic lupus erythematosus (SLE). These individuals produce large quantities of immune complexes and suffer tissue damage as a result of complement-mediated lysis and the induction of type II or type III hypersensitivity (see Chapter 16). Although complement plays a significant role in the development of tissue damage in SLE, the paradoxical finding is that deficiencies in C1, C2, C4, and CR1 predispose an individual to SLE; indeed, 90% of the individuals who completely lack C4 develop SLE. The complement deficiencies are thought to interfere with effective solubilization and clearance of immune complexes; the result is the persistence of these complexes and subsequent tissue damage by the very system whose deficiency was to blame.

It is thought that the coating of soluble immune complexes with C3b facilitates their binding to CR1 on erythrocytes. Although red blood cells express lower levels of CR1 ($\sim 5 \times 10^2$ per cell) than granulocytes ($\sim 5 \times 10^4$ per cell), there are about 10^3 red blood cells for every white blood cell; therefore, erythrocytes ac-

count for about 90% of the CR1 in the blood. For this reason, erythrocytes play an important role in binding C3b-coated immune complexes and carrying these complexes to the liver and spleen, where the immune complexes are stripped from the red blood cells and are phagocytosed. In SLE patients, deficiencies in C1, C2, and C4 each contribute to reduced levels of C3b on immune complexes and hence inhibit their clearance. The lower levels of CR1 expressed on the erythrocytes of SLE patients also may interfere with the proper binding and clearance of immune complexes.

Complement Deficiencies

Genetic deficiencies have been described for each of the complement components with the exception of factor B (Table 15-7). Homozygous deficiencies in any of the early components of the classical pathway (C1q, C1r, C1s, C4, and C2) manifest similar clinical presentations, notably a marked increase in such immune-complex diseases as systemic lupus erythematosus, glomerulonephritis, and vasculitis. These deficiencies highlight the important role of the early complement reactions in generating C3b, which is critical for solubilization and clearance of immune complexes. In addition to immune-complex diseases, some of these individuals suffer from recurrent infections by such pyogenic bacteria as streptococci and staphylococci. These organisms are gram-positive and therefore resistant in any case to the lytic effects of the membrane-attack complex. Nonetheless, the early complement components ordinarily prevent

Table 15-7   Inherited complement deficiencies and associated diseases

Protein	Number of individuals with homozygous deficiencies	Clinical manifestations	
		Immune-complex diseases*	Infections
Early components			
Classical pathway			
C1q	15	14	Many with pyogenic infections
C1r/C1s	8	6	
C4	16	14	
C2	66	38	Few with pyogenic infections
Alternative pathway			
Factor B	None known	None	None
Factor D	2	None	2 (Pyogenic bacteria)
Properdin	3	None	3 (Severe *Neisseria* infections)
Both pathways			
C3	11	8	10 (Pyogenic bacteria)
Membrane-attack complex			
C5	12	1	9 (*Neisseria*)
C6	17	2	10 (*Neisseria*)
C7	14	1	6 (*Neisseria*)
C8	14	1	8 (*Neisseria*)
C9	Many	None	None
Regulatory components			
C1 Inhibitor	>500	10	Hereditary angioedema
Factor I	5	1	4 (Pyogenic bacteria)
Factor H	2	1	Hemolytic uremia syndrome

* Immune-complex diseases include systemic lupus eryhtematosus, SLE-like syndromes, glomerulonephritis, and vasculitis.

SOURCE: Adapted from J. A. Schifferti and D. K. Peters, 1983, *Lancet* **2**:957.

recurrent infection by mediating a localized inflammatory response and opsonizing the bacteria. Deficiencies in factor D and properdin—early components of the alternative pathway—appear to be associated with *Neisseria* infections but not with immune-complex disease.

C3 deficiencies have the most severe clinical manifestations, reflecting the central role of C3 in activating C5 and the membrane-attack complex in both the classical and alternative pathways. The first patient identified with a C3 deficiency was a child who suffered from frequent severe bacterial infections and was erroneously thought to have agammaglobulinemia. When tests revealed normal immunoglobulin levels, a deficiency in C3 was discovered. This case highlights the critical function of the complement system in converting a humoral an-

tibody response into an effective host-defense mechanism. The majority of patients with C3 deficiency have recurrent bacterial infections and manifest immune-complex diseases.

Individuals with homozygous deficiencies in the components involved in the membrane-attack complex manifest recurrent meningococcal and gonococcal infections caused by *Neisseria* species. In normal individuals these gram-negative bacteria are generally susceptible to complement-mediated lysis or are cleared by the opsonizing activity of C3b or C5b. Few of these individuals manifest immune-complex disease, so generally they must produce enough C3b to clear immune complexes. Interestingly, a deficiency in C9 results in no clinical symptoms, suggesting that in some cases the entire MAC is not necessary for complement-mediated lysis to occur.

Congenital deficiencies of complement regulatory proteins have also been reported. The C1 inhibitor (C1 Inh) regulates activation of the classical pathway by preventing excessive C4 and C2 activation by C1. C1-inhibitor deficiency is an autosomal dominant condition with a frequency of 1 in 1000. The deficiency gives rise to a disease called hereditary angioedema, which manifests clinically as localized edema of the tissue, often following trauma but sometimes with no known cause. The edema can be in subcutaneous tissues or within the bowel or upper respiratory tract, where it causes abdominal pain or obstruction of the airway.

A number of the membrane-bound regulatory components including decay accelerating factor (DAF) and homologous restriction factor (HRF) are anchored to the plasma membrane by glycosyl phosphatidylinisitol membrane anchors. In paroxysmal nocturnal haemoglobinuria the glycosyl phosphatidylinisitol membrane anchor is defective, resulting in an absence of DAF and HRF from the cell membrane. As a consequence of this defect, much lower levels of complement are able to lyse the red blood cells, and the individual suffers from chronic hemolytic anemia.

Summary

1. The complement system, which consists of a large group of serum proteins, can be activated by immunologic or nonimmunologic means to generate a sequential enzymatic cascade of interacting components that play an important role in antigen clearance. The two pathways of complement activation, the classical pathway and the alternative pathway, involve different complement proteins and are activated differently. The two pathways converge in a common terminal reaction sequence that generates a membrane-attack complex (MAC) responsible for cell lysis.

2. The classical pathway, activated by certain subclasses of IgG and by IgM, involves C1, C4, C2, and C3 components. The reaction sequence generates a complex of $\overline{C4b2b}$ (C3 convertase), which is able to convert C3 into C3a and C3b, and a $\overline{C4b2b3b}$ complex with C5 convertase activity. The alternative pathway is activated by a variety of microorganisms including bacteria, fungi, some viruses, and some parasites. The alternative pathway can also be activated by IgG and IgA, as well as by complexes of IgE. This pathway involves C3, factor D, factor B, and properdin. The reaction sequence generates $\overline{C3bBb}$ (C3 convertase) and $\overline{C3bBb3b}$ (C5 convertase) analogous to the convertases in the classical pathway. Both the classical and alternative pathways generate bound C5b. This component reacts sequentially with C6, C7, C8, and C9 to produce the membrane-attack complex, which mediates cell lysis by forming a large pore in the cell membrane.

3. Because of its nonspecific nature, the complement system requires elaborate regulatory mechanisms to control the reaction and prevent damage to normal tissues. Both pathways have a number of extremely labile components that lose their activity as they diffuse from the site of activation. In addition both pathways have a number of regulatory components that function to inactivate complement products and prevent excessive buildup of enzymatically active components.

4. The complement system serves as an important effector of the humoral immune response. It destroys foreign cells through the process of MAC-mediated lysis. The complement system also induces a localized inflammatory response with a buildup of fluid and inflammatory cells, and it facilitates phagocytosis of antigen through its effect as an opsonin. Binding of complement to viral particles serves to neutralize their infectivity.

5. A number of inherited complement deficiencies have been described. The consequences of these conditions depend on which complement component is deficient. C3 deficiencies, which are clinically the most severe, are often associated with immune-complex disease and susceptibility to recurrent bacterial infections. These effects reflect the central role of C3 in both the classical and alternative pathways of complement activation. Deficiency of the regulatory protein C1 inhibitor is fairly common and is associated with a localized edema called hereditary angioedema.

References

AHEARN, J. M., and D. T. FEARON. 1989. Structure and function of the complement receptors, CR1 (CD35) and CR2 (CD21). *Adv. Immunol.* **46**:183.

COOPER, N. R., and G. R. NEMEROW. 1986. Complement-dependent mechanisms of virus neutralization. In *Immunobiology of the Complement System.* Academic Press.

DAVIS, A. E. 1988. C1 inhibitor and hereditary angioneurotic edema. *Annu. Rev. Immunol.* **6**:595.

FEARSON, D. T. 1988. Complement, C receptors and immune complex disease. *Hosp. Pract.* (Aug. 15):63.

HOURCADE, D., M. HOLERS, and J. P. ATKINSON. 1989. The regulators of complement activation (RCA) gene cluster. *Adv. Immunol.* **45**:381.

JOINER, K. 1986. Role of complement in infectious diseases. In *Immunobiology of the Complement System.* Academic Press.

LACHMANN, P. J., and M. J. WALPORT. 1986. Genetic deficiency diseases of the complement system. In *Immunobiology of the Complement System*. Academic Press.

LISZEWSKI, M. K., T. W. POST, and J. P. ATKINSON. 1991. Membrane cofactor protein (MCP or CD46): newest member of the regulators of complement activation gene cluster. *Annu. Rev. Immunol* 9:431.

MULLER-EBERHARD, H. 1986. The membrane attack complex of complement. *Annu. Rev. Immunol.* 4:503.

MULLER-EBERHARD, H. J. 1988. Molecular organization and function of the complement system. *Annu. Rev. Biochem.* 57:321.

PERLMUTTER, D. H., and H. R. COLTEN. 1986. Molecular immunobiology of complement biosynthesis. *Annu. Rev. Immunol.* 4:231.

PODACK, E. R. 1986. Assembly and functions of the terminal components. In *Immunobiology of the Complement System*. Academic Press.

REID, K. B. M., and A. J. DAY. 1989. Structure-function relationships of the complement components. *Immunol. Today* 10:177.

WILSON, J. G., et al. 1987. Deficiency of the C3b/C4b receptor (CR1) of erythrocytes in systemic lupus erythematosus *J. Immunol.* 138:2706.

Study Questions

1. Indicate whether each of the following statements is true or false. If you think a statement is false, explain why.
   a. A single molecule of bound IgM can activate the C1q component of the classical complement pathway.
   b. C3a and C3b are fragments of C3.
   c. All complement components are present in the serum in a functionally inactive proenzyme form.
   d. Nucleated cells tend to be more resistant to complement-mediated lysis than red blood cells.
   e. Enveloped viruses cannot be lysed by complement because their outer envelope is resistant to pore formation by the membrane-attack complex.
   f. C4-deficient individuals have difficulty eliminating immune complexes.

2. Explain why serum IgM cannot activate complement by itself.

3. Would you expect a C1 or C3 complement deficiency to be more serious clinically. Why?

4. Some microorganisms produce enzymes that can degrade the Fc portion of antibody molecules. Why would such enzymes be advantageous for the survival of microorganisms that possess them?

5. Complement activation can occur via the classical or alternative pathway.
   a. How do the two pathways differ in the substances required for the initial activation step.
   b. How do the reaction sequences differ in the two pathways?
   c. What important biological functions do the classical and the alternate pathways share?

6. Which complement complex mediates innocent-bystander lysis? When is it likely to occur?

7. How is the complement system regulated?

8. Match each complement component(s) or reaction with its activity or description listed below.

a. _____ C3b
b. _____ C1, C4, C2, and C3
c. _____ C9
d. _____ C3, factor B, and Factor D
e. _____ C1q
f. _____ C3bBb
g. _____ C5b, C6, C7, C8, and C9
h. _____ C3 → C3a + C3b
i. _____ C3a, C5a, and C5b67
j. _____ C3a, C4a, and C5a
k. _____ C4b2b

1. Major amplification step
2. Early components of alternative pathway
3. Components of the membrane-attack complex
4. Mediates opsonization
5. Early components of classical pathway
6. Has perforin-like activity
7. Binds to Fc region of antibodies
8. Chemotatic factors
9. Has C3 convertase activity
10. Anaphylatoxins

16

Hypersensitive Reactions

An immune response evokes a battery of effector molecules that act to remove antigen by various mechanisms. Generally, these effector molecules induce a subclinical, localized inflammatory response that eliminates antigen without extensive tissue damage to the host. Under certain circumstances, however, this inflammatory response can have deleterious effects, resulting in significant tissue damage or even death. These reactions have been termed *hypersensitive*, or *allergic*, reactions. Although hypersensitivity denotes an increased response, the response is not always heightened but may, instead, reflect an inappropriate immune response to an antigen. Hypersensitive reactions may develop in the course of either humoral or cell-mediated responses.

Reactions within the humoral branch are initiated by antibody or antigen-antibody complexes and are termed *immediate hypersensitivity reactions* because the symptoms manifest within minutes or hours following an encounter with antigen by a sensitized recipient. Three types of such reactions are commonly recognized.

Reactions within the cell-mediated branch are initiated by T_{DTH} cells and are referred to as *delayed-type hypersensitivity* (DTH) reactions in reference to the delay of symptoms for days following antigen exposure. Although DTH reactions, as discussed in Chapter 13, provide an important line of defense against intracellular pathogens, they sometimes cause extensive tissue damage that is pathologic and truly hypersensitive. This chapter examines the mechanisms and consequences of the four primary types of hypersensitive reactions.

Gell and Coombs Classification

Several types of hypersensitive reactions can be distinguished, reflecting differences in the effector molecules generated in the course of the reaction. In immediate hypersensitive reactions different antibody isotypes induce different immune effector molecules. IgE antibodies, for example, induce mast cell degranulation with release of histamine and other biologically active molecules. IgG and IgM antibodies, on the other hand, induce hypersensitive reactions by activating complement: the effector molecules in these reactions are the membrane-attack complex and such complement split products as C3a, C4a, and C5a. The effector molecules in hypersensitive reactions induced by antigen-antibody complexes also are complement split products, which mediate an inflammatory reaction. In delayed hypersensitive reactions, the effector molecules are various cytokines secreted by T_{DTH} cells.

As it became clear that different immune mechanisms can give rise to hypersensitive reactions, P. G. H. Gell

Table 16-1   Gell and Coombs classification of hypersensitive reactions

Type	Descriptive name	Time course	Mechanism	Typical manifestations
			Immediate reactions	
Type I	IgE-mediated hypersensitivity	2–30 min	Ag induces cross-linkage of IgE bound to mast cells or basophils with release of vasoactive mediators	Systemic anaphylaxis Localized anaphylaxis: Hay fever Asthma Hives Food allergies Eczema
Type II	Antibody-mediated cytotoxic hypersensitivity	5–8 h	Ab directed against cell-surface antigens mediates cell destruction via complement activation or ADCC	Blood-transfusion reactions Erythroblastosis fetalis Autoimmune hemolytic anemia
Type III	Immune complex–mediated hypersensitivity	2–8 h	Ag-Ab complexes deposited in various tissues induce complement activation and an ensuing inflammatory response	Localized Arthus reaction Generalized reactions: Serum sickness Glomerulonephritis Rheumatoid arthritis Systemic lupus erythematosus
			Delayed reactions	
Type IV	Cell-mediated hypersensitivity	24–72 h	Sensitized T_{DTH} cells release cytokines that activate macrophages or T_C cells, which mediate direct cellular damage	Contact dermatitis Tubercular lesions Graft rejection

and R. R. A. Coombs proposed a classification scheme in which hypersensitive reactions are divided into four types (I, II, III, and IV), each involving distinct mechanisms, cells, and mediator molecules. These are summarized in Table 16-1. This classification scheme has served an important function in identifying the mechanistic differences among various hypersensitive reactions. But it is important to point out that a great deal more complexity exists due to a vast array of secondary effects that cross the boundaries of the classification scheme.

IgE-Mediated (Type I) Hypersensitivity

A type I hypersensitive reaction is induced by certain types of antigens, referred to as *allergens*, and has all the hallmarks of a normal humoral response. That is, an allergen induces a humoral antibody response by the same mechanisms as described previously for other soluble antigens, resulting in generation of antibody-secreting plasma cells and memory cells (see Figure

1-10). What distinguishes a type I hypersensitive response from a normal humoral response is that the plasma cells secrete IgE. This class of antibody binds with high affinity to Fc receptors on the surface of tissue mast cells and blood basophils. Such IgE-coated mast cells or basophils are said to be *sensitized*. A later exposure to the same allergen cross-links the membrane-bound IgE on sensitized mast cells and basophils, causing degranulation of these cells (Figure 16-1). The pharmacologically active mediators released from the granules exert biological effects on the surrounding tissues. The principal effects—vasodilation and smooth-muscle contraction—may be either systemic or localized, depending on the extent of mediator release.

Consequences of Type I Reactions

Type I reactions can produce conditions ranging from serious life-threatening reactions, such as systemic anaphylaxis and asthma, to hay fever and eczema, which are merely annoying.

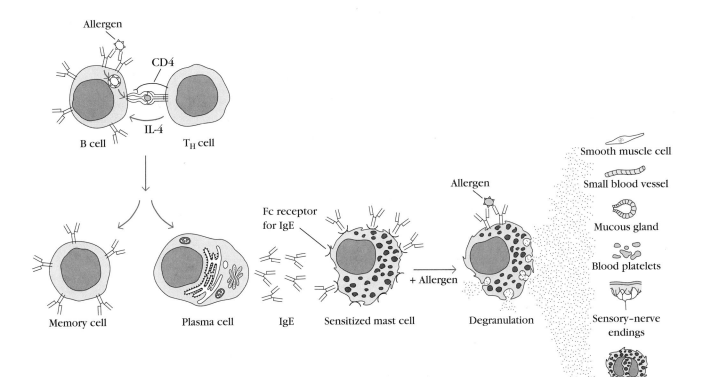

Figure 16-1 General mechanism underlying a type I hypersensitive reaction. Exposure to an allergen activates B cells to form IgE-secreting plasma cells. The secreted IgE molecules bind to IgE-specific Fc receptors on mast cells and blood basophils. Upon a second exposure to the allergen, the bound IgE is cross-linked, triggering the release of pharmacologically active mediators from mast cells and basophils. The mediators cause smooth-muscle contraction, increased vascular permeability, and vasodilation.

Systemic Anaphylaxis

Systemic anaphylaxis is a shock-like and often fatal state whose onset occurs within minutes of a type I hypersensitive reaction. This type of response was first reported in 1839 by Magendie, who noted the sudden death of dogs following repeated injections of egg albumin. This report went unnoticed until 1902 when two French physicians, Paul J. Portier and Charles R. Richet, observed a similar phenomenon. During a cruise on the yacht of the Prince of Monaco, the two physicians had been asked to develop an antitoxin to protect swimmers from the painful stings of the jellyfish, the Portuguese man-of-war. When they returned home, jellyfish were not available for their project, so they decided to use sea anemones because they also caused painful stings. While attempting to immunize dogs with a sublethal extract of sea anemone tentacles, they observed that a secondary challenge several weeks later with the same sublethal extract brought on a rapid sequence of symptoms including vomiting, bloody diarrhea, asphyxia, unconsciousness, and death. They called the response *anaphylaxis* (from Greek *ana*-against and *phylaxis*-protection) to denote that this was an inappropriate response, counter to host protective mechanisms. For his work on anaphylaxis, Richet was awarded a Nobel prize in medicine in 1913.

Systemic anaphylaxis can be induced in a variety of experimental animals and is seen occasionally in humans. Each species exhibits characteristic symptoms of anaphylaxis, which reflect differences in the distribution of mast cells as well as differences in the biologically active mediators in their mast cell granules. The animal model of choice for studying systemic anaphylaxis has been the guinea pig. Anaphylaxis can be induced in guinea pigs with relative ease, and its symptoms closely parallel those observed in humans. Active sensitization in guinea pigs is induced by a single injection of a foreign protein such as egg albumin. After an incubation period of about 2 weeks, the animal is usually challenged with an intravenous injection of the same protein. Within 1 min the animal becomes restless, its respiration becomes labored, and its blood pressure drops. As the smooth muscles of the gastrointestinal tract and bladder contract, the guinea pig defecates and urinates. Finally bronchiole constriction results in death by asphyxiation within 2–4 min of the injection. These events all stem from the systemic vasodilation and smooth-muscle contraction brought on by mediators released during the course of the reaction. Postmortem examination reveals that massive edema, shock, and bronchiole constriction are the major cause of death. The sequence of events is similar in systemic anaphylaxis in humans. A wide range of antigens have been shown to trigger this reaction in susceptible humans, including bee, wasp, hornet, and ant stings; drugs, such as penicillin, insulin, and antitoxins; and seafood and nuts. If not treated quickly, these reactions can be fatal.

Localized Anaphylaxis

In localized anaphylaxis the reaction is limited to a specific target tissue or organ, often involving epithelial surfaces at the site of allergen entry. The tendency to manifest localized anaphylactic reactions is inherited and is referred to as *atopy*. Several common conditions are associated with localized anaphylactic reactions. The most common, affecting 10% of the U.S. population, is allergic rhinitis, commonly known as *hay fever*. This results from airborne allergens reacting with sensitized mast cells in the conjunctivae and nasal mucosa to induce the release of pharmacologically active mediators from mast cells; these mediators then cause localized vasodilation and increased capillary permeability. The symptoms include watery exudation of the conjunctivae, nasal mucosa, and upper respiratory tract as well as sneezing and coughing. Asthma, another common manifestation of localized anaphylaxis, also is triggered by mast cell degranulation and mediator release but in the lower respiratory tract. The resulting constriction of the bronchioles and obstruction of the airway cause difficulty in breathing, often with wheezing. In some cases airborne or blood-borne allergens trigger an asthmatic attack (allergic asthma); in other cases an asthmatic attack can be induced by exercise or cold, apparently independent of allergen stimulation (intrinsic asthma).

Food allergens can also play a role in localized anaphylaxis. Allergen cross-linking of IgE on mast cells along the upper or lower gastrointestinal tract can induce localized smooth-muscle contraction and vasodilation and thus such symptoms as vomiting or diarrhea. Mast cell degranulation along the gut can also increase the permeability of mucous membranes, so that the allergen enters the bloodstream. Various symptoms can ensue, depending on where the allergen is deposited. For example, some individuals develop asthmatic attacks after ingesting certain foods. Others develop atopic urticaria, commonly known as hives, when a food allergen is carried to sensitized mast cells in the skin causing swollen (edematous), red (erythematous) eruptions to manifest classically known as a *wheal and flare* reaction. In atopic dermatitis (allergic eczema), which is observed most frequently in young children, the skin eruptions are filled with pus and are erythematous.

As the type I hypersensitivity reaction begins to subside, mediators released during the course of the reaction often induce a localized inflammatory reaction, called the *late-phase reaction*. The late-phase reaction begins to develop between 4–6 h following the initial type I reaction and persists for 1–2 days. The reaction is characterized by infiltration of neutrophils, eosinophils, macrophages, lymphocytes, and basophils. Of these cells, the eosinophil plays a principal role, accounting for some 30% of the cells that accumulate in the late-phase reaction. As mast cells degranulate, eosinophil chemotactic factor is released which serves to attract large numbers of eosinophils to the site. Various cytokines released at the site, including IL-3, IL-5, and GM-CSF also contribute to the growth and differentiation of the eosinophils. The eosinophils express Fc receptors for IgG and IgE isotypes and bind directly to the antibody-coated allergen. As the eosinophils are activated they degranulate, releasing a number of inflammatory mediators including leukotrienes, major basic protein, platelet-activation factor, cationic protein, and eosinophil derived neurotoxin. The release of these eosinophil-derived mediators may play a protective role in parasitic infections. However, in response to allergens, these mediators contribute to extensive tissue damage in the late-phase reaction. Neutrophils are another major participant in the late-phase reactions, accounting for 30% of the inflammatory cells. Neutrophils are attracted to the area of a type I reaction by neutrophil chemotactic factor, released from degranulating mast cells. In addition, a variety of cytokines released at the site, including IL-8, have been shown to activate neutrophils resulting in release of their granule contents including lysosomal enzymes, platelet activation factor, and leukotrienes.

Components of Type I Reactions

Allergens

The vast majority of humans mount significant IgE responses only as a defense against parasitic infections. After an individual is exposed to a parasite, serum IgE levels increase and remain high until the parasite is successfully cleared from the body. Atopic persons, however, appear to have a genetic defect affecting regulation of the IgE response. These regulatory defects allow nonparasitic antigens to stimulate inappropriate IgE production, leading to tissue-damaging type I hypersensitivity. The term *allergen* refers specifically to nonparasitic antigens capable of stimulating type I hypersensitive responses in allergic individuals.

Most allergic IgE responses occur on mucous membrane surfaces and thus in response to allergens that enter the body either by inhalation or ingestion. Of the common allergens listed in Table 16-2, relatively few have been purified and characterized. Those which have

Table 16-2 Common antigens associated with type I hypersensitivity

Proteins
Foreign serum
Vaccines

Plant Pollens
Rye grass
Ragweed
Timothy grass
Birch trees

Drugs
Penicillin
Sulfonamides
Local anesthetics
Salicylates

Foods
Nuts
Seafood
Eggs
Peas, beans

Insect venoms
Bee
Wasp
Ant

Molds

Animal hair and dander

include the allergens from rye grass pollen, ragweed pollen, codfish, birch pollen, timothy grass pollen, and bee venom. Each of these allergens has been shown to be a multiallergen system incorporating a number of allergenic components. Ragweed pollen, a major pollen allergen in the United States, is a case in point. It has been reported that a square mile of ragweed yields 16 tons of pollen in a single season. The pollen particles are inhaled, and their tough outer wall is dissolved by enzymes in the mucous secretions, releasing the allergenic substances. Chemical fractionation of ragweed has revealed a variety of substances, most of which are not allergenic but are capable of eliciting an IgM or IgG response. Of the five fractions that are allergenic (i.e., able to induce an IgE response), two evoke allergenic reactions in about 95% of ragweed-sensitive individuals and are called major allergens; these are designated the E and K fractions. The other three, called Ra3, Ra4, and Ra5, are minor allergens that induce an allergic response in only 20–30% of sensitive subjects.

What makes these agents allergens? Why are some pollens (e.g., ragweed) highly allergenic, whereas other equally abundant pollens (e.g., nettle) are rarely aller-genic? No single physicochemical property seems to distinguish the highly allergenic E and K fractions of ragweed from the less allergenic Ra3, Ra4, and Ra5 fractions and from the nonallergenic fractions. Rather, allergens as a group appear to possess diverse properties. Some allergens, including foreign serum and egg albumin, are potent antigens; others, such as plant pollens, are weak antigens. Although most allergens are proteins or protein-bound substances having a molecular weight between 15,000 and 40,000, attempts to identify some common chemical property of these antigens, one that would render them all allergenic, have failed. It appears that allergenicity is a consequence of a complex series of interactions involving not only the allergen but also the dose, the sensitizing route, sometimes an adjuvant, and—most importantly—the genetic constitution of the recipient.

Reaginic Antibody (IgE)

The first indication that some component of serum was responsible for hypersensitive reactions was C. R. Reichert's finding that he could transfer systemic anaphylaxis from primed dogs to unprimed dogs with an injection of serum from the primed dogs. The existence of a similar serum component in humans was demonstrated in 1921 by Prausnitz and Kustner. Kustner was allergic to fish, whereas Prausnitz was not. Prausnitz injected some of Kustner's serum into his skin; 24 h later he injected a boiled fish extract into the same site. Within minutes, a pronounced local wheal and flare (hive) response occurred; such a reaction came to be referred to as a *P-K reaction*. Because the serum components displayed specificity for the allergen being tested, they were assumed to be antibodies. The nature of these P-K, or *reaginic*, antibodies eluded scientists until the mid-1960s when the work of the Ishizakas suggested that reaginic antibody was a unique and as-yet-unidentified class of serum antibody (see Chapter 5). The biological activity of reaginic antibody in a P-K test could be neutralized by rabbit antisera against whole atopic human sera but not by rabbit antisera specific for the four known human immunoglobulin classes (IgA, IgG, IgM, and IgD) (Table 16-3). And when rabbits were immunized with sera from ragweed-sensitive individuals, the rabbit antiserum could inhibit (neutralize) a positive ragweed P-K test even after absorption to precipitate the rabbit antibodies specific for the known human IgG, IgA, IgM, and IgD isotypes. K. and T. Ishizaka called this new class IgE in reference to the E antigen of ragweed that they used to characterize it.

Serum IgE levels in normal individuals fall within the range of 0.1–0.4 μg/ml; even the most severely allergic individuals rarely have IgE levels greater than 1 μg/ml.

Table 16-3 Identification of IgE based on reactivity of atopic serum in P-K test*

Treatment	Allergen added	P-K reaction at skin site
None	−	−
None	+	+
Rabbit antiserum to whole atopic human serum	+	−
Rabbit antiserum minus antibodies to human IgM, IgG, IgA, and IgD	+	−

* Serum from an atopic individual was injected into rabbits to produce antiserum against human atopic serum. This was subsequently treated with human IgM, IgG, IgA, and IgD to remove antibodies to these isotypes. The remaining rabbit antiserum still neutralized the P-K reactivity of the atopic serum (last entry), indicating that a new immunoglobulin isotype was responsible for this reactivity.

SOURCE: Based on K. Ishizaka and T. Ishizaka. 1967. *J. Immunol.* 99:1187.

These low levels made physiochemical studies of IgE difficult, and it was not until the discovery of an IgE myeloma by S. G. O. Johansson and H. Bennich in 1967 that extensive chemical analysis of IgE could be undertaken. IgE was found to be composed of two heavy (ε) and two light chains with a combined molecular weight of 190,000. The increase in molecular weight over that of IgG (150,000) is due to the presence of an additional constant-region domain (see Figure 5-12). This additional domain (C_H4) contributes to an altered conformation of the Fc portion of the molecule that enables it to bind to glycoprotein receptors on the surface of basophils or mast cells.

Target Cells for IgE

The target cells for IgE were identified by incubating human leukocytes and tissue cells with either [^{125}I] labeled IgE myeloma protein or [^{125}I] labeled anti-IgE. In both cases autoradiography revealed that the labeled probe bound to blood basophils and tissue mast cells. Basophils are granulocytes that circulate in the blood of most vertebrates; in humans they account for 0.5–1.0% of the circulating white blood cells. Their granulated cytoplasm stains with basic dyes, hence the name basophil. Electron microscopy reveals a multilobed nucleus, few mitochondria, numerous glycogen granules, and electron-dense membrane-bounded granules scattered throughout the cytoplasm.

The mast cell was first described by Paul Ehrlich in 1877. The name in German means "fattening feed," a reference to the numerous granules, which were erroneously thought to have been engulfed by the cell. Mast cells are found throughout connective tissue, particularly near blood and lymphatic vessels. Some tissues, including the skin and the mucous membrane surfaces of the respiratory and gastrointestinal tract, contain high concentrations of mast cells; skin, for example, contains 10,000 mast cells per mm^3. Electron micrographs of mast cells reveal numerous membrane-bounded organelles, which contain pharmacologically active mediators, distributed throughout the cytoplasm (Figure 16-2).

IgE Fc Receptors (FcεRI and FcεRII)

The binding of radioactively labeled IgE myeloma protein or anti-IgE to the surface of mast cells and blood basophils suggested that these cells should have a receptor for IgE. When these cells were incubated with IgE, labeled with electron-dense ferritin, and examined in an electron microscope, the IgE molecules initially appeared to be distributed diffusely; subsequent treatment with anti-IgE aggregated the IgE into a patched and capped distribution. This finding suggested that the IgE receptor was a membrane molecule able to diffuse freely in the plane of the plasma membrane. Experiments revealed between 40,000 and 90,000 receptors for IgE per human basophil. Fc fragments of IgE can prevent the binding of IgE to target cells, and [^{125}I] labeled Fc fragments can bind to human basophils, whereas labeled Fab fragments fail to bind. These findings indicate that the receptor interacts with the Fc portion of an IgE molecule. The receptor displays a high affinity for IgE, with an association constant between 1 and $2 \times 10^9 \, M^{-1}$ and is designated as the FcεRI receptor. It is specific for the CH2/CH2 domain of the IgE molecule.

B cells, macrophages, and eosinophils also express a membrane Fc receptor for IgE. Unlike the FcεRI receptor of mast cells and basophils, this receptor has a much lower affinity for IgE and consequently requires much higher levels of IgE for binding. This receptor is specific for the CH3/CH3 domain of the IgE molecule and is designated as the FcεRII receptor (or CD23).

The high-affinity FcεRI IgE receptor was isolated by labeling the surface-membrane proteins on mast cells with [^{125}I] and then incubating the cells with IgE myeloma protein to saturate the receptors. The [^{125}I] receptor–IgE complexes were solubilized from the membrane in a nonionic detergent and then isolated by precipitation with anti-IgE. Analysis of the precipitates revealed an 85,000-kD glycoprotein whose hydrophobic properties suggest that it is largely embedded in the plasma membrane. The receptor contains four polypeptide chains: an α and a β chain and two indentical disulfide-linked γ chains (Figure 16-3). The α chain has two 90-aa domains that extend from the membrane and show homology to an immunoglobulin domain, placing the molecule within the immunoglobulin gene superfamily. It is by means of these two immunoglobulin-like domains that the IgE Fc receptor interacts with high affinity to the CH2/CH2 domain of the IgE molecule. The β chain spans the plasma membrane four times and is thought to link the α chain to the γ homodimers. The two γ homodimers are disulfide-linked and extend a considerable distance into the cytoplasm. They bear considerable sequence homology to the CD3 ζ chains. Like the CD3 ζ chains, the γ homodimers may be involved in signal transduction following IgE binding to the α chain of the high-affinity FcεRI receptor.

(a)   (b)   (c)

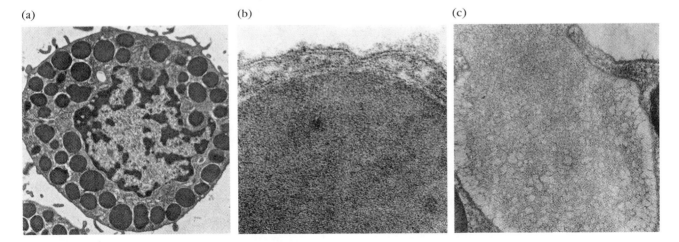

Figure 16-2 (a) Electron micrograph of a typical mast cell revealing numerous electron-dense membrane-bounded granules prior to degranulation. (b) Close-up of intact granule underlying the plasma membrane of a mast cell. (c) Granule releasing its contents during degranulation. [From S. Burwen and B. Satir, 1977, J. Cell Biol. **73**:662.]

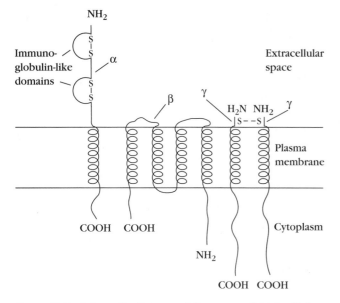

Figure 16-3   Schematic diagram of the mast cell high-affinity membrane receptor for IgE (FcεRI) showing α, β, and γ chains. The α chain has two immunoglobulin-like domains that bind to IgE. The β and γ chains are largely transmembrane and cytoplasmic and are thought to transduce the signal upon binding of IgE to its receptor. The amino acid sequence of the receptor has been determined.

Mechanism of IgE-Mediated Degranulation

The biochemical events mediating degranulation of mast cells and blood basophils have many features in common. For simplicity this section presents a general overview of mast cell degranulation mechanisms without calling attention to the slight differences between mast cells and basophils.

Receptor Cross-Linkage

IgE-mediated degranulation begins when an allergen cross-links receptor-bound (fixed) IgE on the surface of a mast cell or basophil. In itself, the binding of IgE to its receptor apparently has no effect on a target cell. It is only after cross-linkage by allergen of the fixed IgE-receptor complex that degranulation proceeds. The importance of cross-linkage is indicated by the inability of monovalent allergens, which cannot cross-link the fixed IgE, to trigger degranulation. Experimental studies with preformed IgE-allergen complexes, in which the ratio of IgE to allergen was carefully monitored, revealed that only complexes having IgE-allergen ratios of 2:1 or greater could induce degranulation. Complexes in antigen excess (having an IgE-allergen ratio of 1:2) failed

to induce degranulation because the requisite cross-linkage of receptors did not occur.

Other experiments have revealed that it is actually the cross-linkage of two or more IgE receptors—with or without IgE—that is essential for degranulation. Although cross-linkage is normally effected by the interaction of fixed IgE with divalent or multivalent allergen, it can be successfully effected by a variety of experimental means that bypass the need for allergen and in some cases even for IgE (Figure 16-4). For example, anti-IgE antibody can directly cross-link fixed IgE and induce degranulation. Chemical cross-linkage of IgE also can induce degranulation. Most significant, antibodies to the receptor itself can induce degranulation in the absence of both allergen and fixed IgE, demonstrating the crucial role of cross-linkage of the membrane receptor in initiating the subsequent biochemical events that culminate in degranulation.

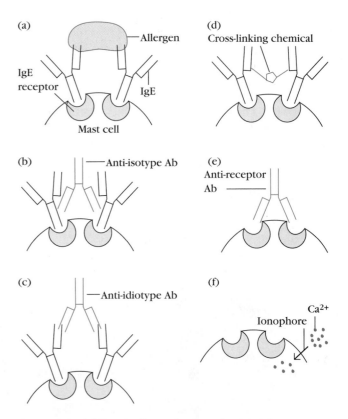

Figure 16-4   Schematic diagrams of mechanisms that can trigger mast cell degranulation. (a) Allergen cross-linkage of cell-bound IgE molecules. (b, c) Antibody cross-linkage of IgE. (d) Chemical cross-linkage of IgE. (e) Cross-linkage of IgE receptors by anti-receptor antibody. (f) Enhanced Ca^{2+} influx stimulated by an ionophore that increases membrane permeability to Ca^{2+} ions. Note that mechanisms (b), (c), and (d) do not require allergen; mechanisms (e) and (f) require neither allergen nor IgE; and mechanism (f) does not even require receptor cross-linkage.

Methylation of Membrane Phospholipids

Within 15 s after receptor cross-linkage by anti-receptor antibody, methylation of various membrane phospholipids can be observed (Figure 16-5). The cross-linkage of the IgE receptors is thought to activate a serine proesterase to form serine esterase, an enzyme that converts phosphatidylserine (PS) into phosphatidylethanolamine (PE). The cross-linkage of the IgE receptors also activates two other membrane-bound enzymes, phospholipid methyltransferase I and II (PMT I and II). PMT I faces the cytoplasmic side of the plasma membrane, and PMT II faces the exterior side. Methylation of PE to form phosphatidylcholine (PC) is achieved in two steps by the PMT enzymes. The accumulation of PC on the exterior surface of the plasma membrane causes an increase in membrane fluidity and is thought to facilitate the formation of Ca^{2+} channels. The finding that an inhibitor of methyltransferase activity (S-isobutyl-3-deazoadenosine) could inhibit both Ca^{2+} influx and the subsequent degranulation suggests that both effects depend on phospholipid methylation.

Influx of Ca^{2+}

The methylation of the phospholipids and subsequent conversion of PE to PC facilitates the opening of Ca^{2+} channels. The influx of Ca^{2+} reaches a peak within 2 min after receptor cross-linkage (see Figure 16-5). Cross-linkage of mast cells in a medium lacking Ca^{2+}

prevents degranulation unless the cells are rapidly returned to a medium containing Ca^{2+}. Experimental fusion of Ca^{2+}-containing phospholipid vesicles with the mast cell plasma membrane initiates degranulation independent even of receptor cross-linkage. Both findings demonstrate the importance of Ca^{2+} in degranulation.

The influx of Ca^{2+} has a number of effects on the mast cell. It activates the enzyme phopholipase A_2, which promotes the breakdown of PC to form lysophosphatidylcholine and arachidonic acid. Lysophosphatidylcholine further increases membrane fluidity, facilitating further Ca^{2+} influx. The arachidonic acid is converted into two classes of potent mediators, the prostaglandins and the leukotrienes, which play a vital role in allergic manifestations. The influx of Ca^{2+} also promotes the assembly of microtubules and the contraction of microfilaments, both of which are necessary for the movement of granules to the plasma membrane.

Changes in cAMP Levels

Concomitant with phospholipid methylation and Ca^{2+} influx, there is a transient increase in membrane-bound adenylate cyclase activity, with a rapid peak of cAMP reached at 15 s after IgE receptor cross-linkage. The effects of cAMP are exerted through the activation of cAMP-dependent protein kinases. These are thought to phosphorylate the granule-membrane proteins, thereby changing the granules' permeability to water and Ca^{2+}.

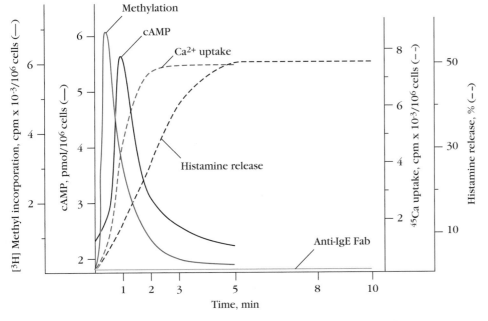

Figure 16-5 Kinetics of major biochemical events following cross-linkage of IgE on cultured human basophils with F(ab′)₂ fragments of anti-IgE. Curves are shown for phospholipid methylation (solid red), cAMP production (solid black), Ca^{2+} influx (dashed red), and histamine release (dashed black). In control experiments with anti-IgE Fab fragments, no significant changes were observed. [Adapted from T. Ishizaka et al., 1985, *Int. Arch. Allergy Appl. Immunol.* **77**:137.]

The consequent swelling of the granules appears to facilitate their fusion to the plasma membrane in degranulation. The increase in cAMP is transient: by the time Ca^{2+} influx and histamine release reach a peak after 2–3 min, the levels of intracellular cAMP have dropped to below the baseline level (see Figure 16-5). This drop in cAMP appears to be necessary for degranulation to proceed. When cAMP levels are increased by certain drugs, the degranulation process is blocked. Several of these drugs are often given to treat allergic disorders and are discussed later in the chapter.

Fusion of Granules with Plasma Membrane

The Ca^{2+} influx, transient cAMP increase and ensuing decrease, and microtubular assembly bring about the fusion of the granules with the plasma membrane and the release of the mediators from the granule. Figure 16-6 summarizes the biochemical events leading to mast cell degranulation.

Mediators of Type I Reactions

The clinical manifestations of type I hypersensitive disorders are related to the biological effects of the mediators released during mast cell or basophil degranulation. These mediators are pharmacologically active agents that act on local tissues as well as on populations of secondary effector cells including eosinophils, neutrophils, T lymphocytes, monocytes, and platelets. The mediators thus serve as an amplifying terminal effector mechanism, much as the complement system serves as an amplifier and effector of an antibody-antigen interaction. When generated in response to parasitic infection, these mediators initiate a beneficial defense process. Localized smooth-muscle contraction and the consequent vasodilation and increased vascular permeability bring an influx of plasma and inflammatory cells to attack the pathogen. On the other hand, mediator release induced by inappropriate antigens, such as allergens, results in unnecessary increases in vascular permeability and inflammation whose detrimental effects far outweigh any beneficial effect.

The mediators can be classified as either primary or secondary (Table 16-4). The primary mediators are produced before degranulation and are stored in the granules. The most significant primary mediators are histamine, proteases, eosinophil chemotactic factor, neutrophil chemotactic factor, and heparin. The secondary mediators either are synthesized after target-cell activation or are released by the breakdown of membrane phospholipids during the degranulation process. The secondary mediators include platelet-activating factor, leukotrienes, and prostaglandins. The differences in type I hypersensitivity manifestations in different species

Table 16-4   Principal mediators involved in type I hypersensitivity

Mediator	Activities
Primary	
Histamine	Increased vascular permeability; smooth-muscle contraction
Serotonin	Increased vascular permeability; smooth-muscle contraction
Eosinophil chemotactic factor (ECF-A)	Eosinophil chemotaxis
Neutrophil chemotactic factor (NCF-A)	Neutrophil chemotaxis
Proteases	Degradation of blood-vessel basement membrane; generation of complement split products
Secondary	
Platelet-activating factor	Platelet aggregation and degranulation; contraction of pulmonary smooth muscles
Leukotrienes (slow reactive substance of anaphylaxis, SRS-A)	Increased vascular permeability; contraction of pulmonary smooth muscles
Prostaglandins	Vasodilation; contraction of pulmonary smooth muscles; platelet aggregation
Bradykinin	Increased vascular permeability; smooth-muscle contraction

or different tissues depend in part on variations in primary or secondary mediators. A comparison of histamine with the leukotrienes illustrates the differences in the biological effects of the primary and the secondary mediators.

Histamine

Histamine is a major component of the mast-cell granules, accounting for about 10% of the granule weight. Because it is stored—preformed—in the granules, its biological effects are observed within minutes of mast cell degranulation. The effects are exerted when histamine binds to specific receptors on various target cells.

There are two types of histamine receptors, H_1 and H_2, which have different tissue distributions and mediate different effects when they bind histamine. The binding of histamine to H_1 receptors induces contraction of intestinal and bronchial smooth muscles, increased permeability of venules, and increased mucous secretion by goblet cells. Interaction of histamine with H_2 receptors increases vasopermeability and dilation and stimulates exocrine glands. Histamine also has a negative-feedback effect on mast cell and basophil degranulation: its binding to H_2 receptors on these cells suppresses the further release of mediators.

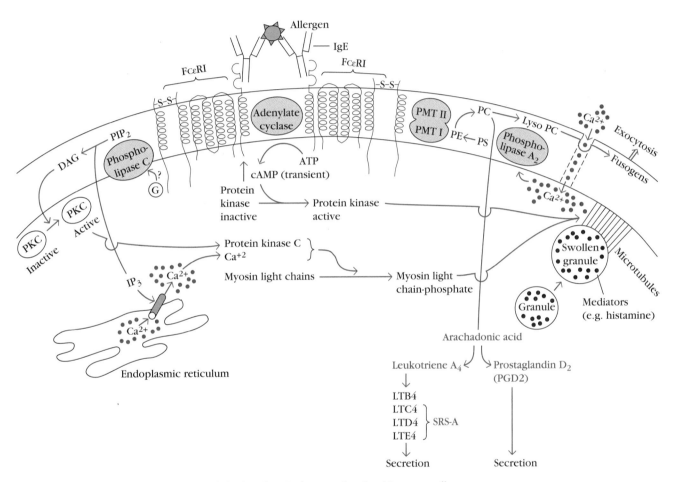

Figure 16-6 Diagrammatic overview of the biochemical events involved in mast cell activation and degranulation. Allergen cross-linkage of bound IgE activates several membrane biochemical pathways that together signal mast cell degranulation. (a) Phospholipase C mediates hydrolysis of phosphatidylinositol-4, 5-bisphosphate (PIP_2) to the second messengers, inositol trisphosphate (IP_3) and diacylglycerol (DAG). IP_3 releases Ca^{2+} from the intracellular stores. (b) Adenylate cyclase activation generates a transient increase in cAMP which mediates its second messenger effects by activating a cyclic AMP-dependent protein kinase. The protein kinase phosphorylates serine residues of selective intracellular proteins that facilitate granule swelling and contraction of the microfilaments required for granule fusion with the plasma membrane. (c) IgE/receptor cross-linkage activates methyltransferases (PMT I and II) which convert phosphatidylethanolamine to phosphatidylcholine. The phospholipid methylation is essential for a Ca^{2+} influx allowing activation of phospholipase A_2. The phospholipase A_2 acts on membrane phospholipids, producing arachidonic acid and its breakdown products: leukotriene A_4 and prostaglandin D_2. PE = phosphatidylethanolamine; PC = phosphatidylcholine; PIP_2 = phosphatidylinositol-4, 5-bisphosphate; DAG = diacylglycerol; IP_3 = inositol trisphosphate.

Leukotrienes

As secondary mediators, the leukotrienes are not formed until the mast cell undergoes degranulation and its plasma membrane is broken down. An ensuing enzymatic cascade generates the prostaglandins and the leukotrienes. It therefore takes a longer time for the biological effects of these mediators to become apparent. Their effects are more pronounced and longer-lasting, however, than those of histamine. Nanomole levels of the leukotrienes are as much as 1000 times more potent as bronchoconstrictors than histamine, and they are also more potent stimulators of mucous secretion. In humans the leukotrienes are thought to contribute to the prolonged bronchospasm and buildup of mucous seen in asthmatics.

Regulation of the Type I Hypersensitive Response

As noted earlier, the genetic constitution of an animal, the antigen dose, and the mode of antigen presentation influence the level of the IgE response (i.e., the allergenicity of an antigen). For example, inbred strains of mice have been shown to differ in their tendency to mount an IgE response. Strains such as SJL fail to produce an IgE response to appropriate allergens, whereas other strains such as BDF1, have an increased propensity for IgE production. Breeding experiments have shown that this genetic component is not linked to the MHC. A genetic component also has been shown to influence type I hypersensitive reactions in humans. When both parents are allergic, there is a 50% chance that the child will also be allergic; when only one parent is allergic, there is a 30% chance that the child will manifest some kind of type I reaction.

The effect of antigen dosage on the IgE response is illustrated by immunization of BDF1 mice. Repeated low doses of an appropriate antigen induce a persistent IgE response in these mice, but higher antigen doses result in transient IgE production and a shift toward IgG. The mode of antigen presentation also influences the development of the IgE response. For example, immunization of Lewis-strain rats with keyhole limpet hemocyanin (KLH) plus aluminum hydroxide gel or *Bordetella pertussis* as an adjuvant induces a strong IgE response, whereas injection of KLH with complete Freund's adjuvant produces a largely IgG response. Similar experimental findings have been reported in mice. Infection with the nematode *Nippostrongylus brasiliensis* (Nb), like certain adjuvants, has also been shown to convert the immune response from IgG to IgE. Nb-infected rats and mice develop higher levels of IgE specific for an unrelated antigen than do uninfected control mice (Table 16-5).

Role of Cytokines in Regulating the Type I Hypersensitivity Response

A variety of cytokines have been shown to regulate the type I hypersensitivity response at a number of levels. Cytokines have been shown to regulate isotype expression (i.e., by enhancing or suppressing class switching to IgE) or to regulate the clonal expansion of IgE-committed B cells. In addition, cytokines have been shown to influence the intensity and duration of the late-phase reaction.

Recent studies by W. E. Paul and co-workers suggest that the level of interleukin 4 (IL-4) which is secreted by activated T_H cells, regulates class switching to the IgE isotype in B cells. When normal unprimed B cells are activated in vitro with LPS, only 2% of the cells express membrane IgG1 and only 0.05% express membrane IgE. Addition of IL-4 along with the LPS to the unprimed B cells increases the percentage of B cells expressing membrane IgG1 to 40–50% and IgE to 15–25%. In an attempt to determine whether IL-4 plays a role in vivo in regulating IgE production, Paul primed Nb-infected mice with TNP-KLH in the presence or in the absence of monoclonal antibody to IL-4. The antibody to IL-4 inhibited the production of IgE specific for TNP-KLH by 99% in these Nb-infected mice compared with controls (see Table 16-5). The experiments of Sakano discussed in Chapter 8 demonstrated that IL-4 induces immunoglobulin class switching from IgM to IgG1 and IgE isotypes in the mouse (see Figure 8-13) or to IgG4 and IgE in humans.

Cytokines have also been shown to down-regulate IgE production. IFN-γ has been shown to decrease IgE production and the balance of IL-4 and IFN-γ may play an important role in determining the level of IgE produced. This would suggest that the activity of the T_H1-like and T_H2-like CD4$^+$ T-cell subsets may influence the outcome of a type I reaction. Needless to say, there is a lot of

Table 16-5 Effect of infection with *Nippostrongylus brasiliensis* (Nb) and of IL-4 on serum IgE levels in mice[*]

Treatment	Serum IgE (ng/ml)
None	0.24
N. brasiliensis	33.8
N. brasiliensis + anti-Nb antibody	35.4
N. brasiliensis + anti-IL-4 antibody	0.48

[*] Mice treated as indicated were immunized with TNP-KLH, and after an appropriate time the serum IgE level was determined.

SOURCE: F. D. Finkelman et al., 1988, *J. Immunol.* 141:2335.

interest in down-regulating IL-4 as a possible treatment for allergic individuals.

Recently evidence has revealed that, in addition to production of primary and secondary mediators, activated mast cells release various cytokines including TNF, IL-1, IL-3, IL-4, IL-5, IL-6, and GM-CSF. A number of these cytokines may contribute to some of the clinical manifestations of a type I hypersensitivity reaction. It has been suggested that high levels of TNF and IL-1 may contribute to shock in systemic anaphylaxis. (This may be similar to the role of TNF and IL-1 in bacterial septic shock and toxic shock syndrome discussed in Chapter 11). In addition, a number of the mast cell–derived cytokines may contribute to the late-phase response. Both TNF and IL-1 both have been shown to increase the expression of cellular adhesion molecules on venular endothelial cells contributing to the buildup of neutrophils, eosinophils, and monocytes in the late-phase response. In addition, IL-3, IL-5, and GM-CSF have been shown to activate eosinophils.

Regulation of IgE Production by IgE-Binding Factors

In a series of experiments, the Ishizakas identified factors secreted by T cells that enhance or suppress IgE production by IgE-committed B cells. This regulatory mechanism thus operates after class switching has occurred. The Ishizakas first cultured mesenteric lymph nodes from Nb-infected mice and isolated IgE-binding factors from the culture supernatant. These factors had an affinity for IgE and were later shown to be derived from a subset of antigen-primed T cells. Subsequent experiments also revealed that some IgE-binding factors (IgE-PF) selectively potentiate IgE production and that others (IgE-SF) suppress it. The level of potentiating or suppressing factors accounts in large part for the strain differences or adjuvant differences that have been shown to influence the IgE response. T cells in the SJL strain, a low-IgE producer, secrete IgE-SF in response to antigen, whereas T cells in the BDF1 strain, a high-IgE producer, secrete IgE-PF. Similarly, adjuvants that potentiate the IgE response induce formation of IgE-PF, and adjuvants the suppress the IgE response induce IgE-SF. T-cell–derived IgE-binding factors that suppress or potentiate IgE production have also been detected in humans.

The Ishizakas were able to isolate the mRNA encoding the IgE-binding factor from a rat T-cell hybridoma stimulated with IgE. The mRNA was used to prepare a cDNA library and the cloned DNA was transfected into COS-1 monkey kidney cells (Figure 16-7). The transfected cells produced a potentiating IgE-binding factor (IgE-PF). However, when the transfected cells were grown in tunicamycin, an inhibitor of N-linked glycosylation, the cells produced a suppressing IgE-binding factor (IgE-SF). The IgE potentiating and suppressing

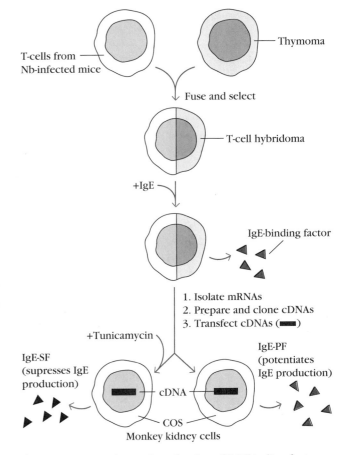

Figure 16-7 Experimental production of IgE-binding factors that either potentiate (IgE-PF) or suppress (IgE-SF) IgE production by antigen-primed spleen cells in culture. In the presence of tunicamycin, an inhibitor of glycosylation, the transfected COS cells secreted IgE-SF, whereas in the absence of this inhibitor the same cells secreted IgE-PF. Thus a single gene appears to encode both factors, and differences in glycosylation of the initial gene product generate the two factors.

factors therefore appear to be encoded by the same gene and to share a common polypeptide chain. Differences in post-translational glycosylation appear to determine whether the gene product functions as a potentiating or as a suppressing factor. Glycosylation-inhibiting factors (GIFs) inhibit the assembly of N-linked oligosaccharides to the IgE-binding factor, thereby generating IgE-SF, whereas glycosylation-enhancing factors (GEFs) promote the assembly of the oligosaccharides, thereby generating IgE-PF. The relative production of GIFs and GEFs ultimately determines whether a T cell produces IgE-SF or IgE-PF (Table 16-6).

The work of the Ishizakas suggests that different T-cell subpopulations produce glycosylation-enhancing factors (GEF) and glycosylation-inhibiting factors (GIF). Adjuvants such as *Bordetella pertussis* and alum induce CD4[+] T cells to produce GEF, whereas complete Freund's adjuvant induces CD8[+] cells to produce GIF

Table 16-6   Correlation of IgE-binding factors and glycosylation factors with level of IgE response

Experimental procedure	IgE-binding factor present	Glycosylation factor present	IgE response
Nb-infection (2 weeks)	IgE-PF	GEF	↑
Bordetella pertussis vaccine	IgE-PF	GEF	↑
KLH + alum priming	IgE-PF	GEF	↑
BDF1 mice immunized with OVA*	IgE-PF	GEF	↑
Complete Freund's adjuvant (CFA)	IgE-SF	GIF	↓
KLH + CFA priming	IgE-SF	GIF	↓
SJL mice immunized with OVA*	IgE-SF	GIF	↓

* Mice were immunized with alum-absorbed ovalbumin after ovalbumin immunization.

(Figure 16-8). As understanding of these two lympho-kines (GEF and GIF) increases, it may be possible to selectively down-regulate IgE production in allergic individuals.

Human B cells and monocytes have also been shown to secrete IgE-binding factors that regulate the IgE response. These IgE-binding factors appear to be unrelated to the T-cell–derived factors. The B-cell–derived IgE-binding factor appears to be a cleavage fragment of the low-affinity IgE FcεRII receptor (CD23) released from the cell by autoproteolytic cleavage. Release of these IgE-binding factors is induced by IL-4 and suppressed by IgE. Experiments are presently under way to determine the role of these B-cell–derived IgE-binding factors in the regulation of the IgE response.

Detection of Type I Hypersensitivity

Type I hypersensitivity is commonly identified and assessed by skin testing. Small amounts of potential allergens are introduced at specific skin sites by either intradermal injection or superficial scratching. A number of tests can be applied to sites on the forearm or back of an individual at one time. If a person is allergic to the allergen, local mast cells will degranulate and the release of histamine and other mediators produces a wheal and flare within 30 min. The advantage of skin testing is that it is relatively inexpensive to perform and allows screening of a large number of allergens in a single sitting. The disadvantage of skin testing is that it sometimes sensitizes the allergic individual to new allergens and in some rare cases may induce systemic anaphylactic shock. A few individuals also manifest a late-phase reaction, which comes 4–6 h after testing and sometimes lasts for up to

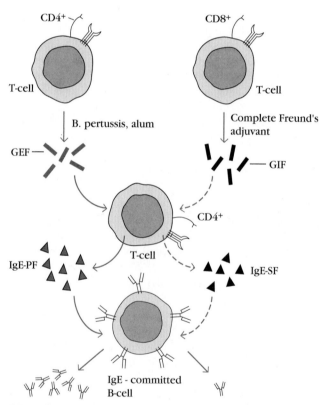

Figure 16-8   Different T-cell subpopulations produce glycosylation-enhancing factors (GEFs) or glycosylation-inhibiting factors (GIFs). These factors act on CD4$^+$ T$_H$ cells, directing production of IgE-potentiating factor (IgE-PF) or IgE-suppressing factor (IgE-SF). The action of these lymphokines on IgE-committed B cells leads to increased or decreased IgE production.

24 h. A late-phase reaction site contains an increase in eosinophils, comprising up to 30% of the cells at the site. Release of eosinophil-granule contents contributes to the tissue damage in a late-phase reaction.

Another method of assessing type I hypersensitivity is to determine the serum level of total IgE antibody by the radioimmunosorbent test (RIST). This highly sensitive technique, based on the radioimmunoassay, can determine nanogram levels of total IgE. The patient's serum is reacted with agarose beads or paper disks coated with rabbit anti-IgE. After washing the beads or discs [^{125}I] labeled rabbit anti-IgE is added. The beads or discs are counted in a gamma counter, and the radioactivity count is proportional to the level of IgE in the patient's serum (Figure 16-9a).

The similar radioallergosorbent test (RAST) detects the serum level of IgE specific for a given allergen. The allergen is coupled to beads or discs, the patient's serum is added, and unbound antibody is washed away. The amount of specific IgE bound to the solid-phase allergen is then measured by adding [^{125}I] labeled rabbit anti-IgE, washing the beads, and counting the bound radioactivity in a gamma counter (Figure 16-9b).

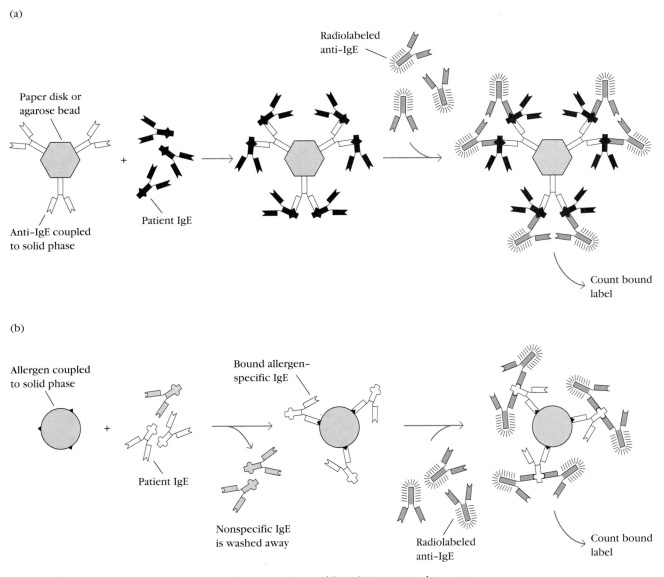

Figure 16-9 Procedures for assessing type I hypersensitivity. (a) Radioimmunosorbent test (RIST) can quantify nanogram amounts of total serum IgE. (b) Radioallergosorbent test (RAST) can quantify nanogram amounts of serum IgE specific for a particular allergen.

Therapy for Type I Hypersensitivities

Clearly the obvious first step in controlling type I hypersensitivities is to identify the offending allergen and avoid contact if possible. Often the removal of house pets, dust-control measures, or avoidance of offending foods can eliminate a type I response. Elimination of inhalant allergens (such as pollens) is a physical impossibility, however, and other means of intervention must be persued.

Immunotherapy involving repeated injections of increasing doses of allergens (hyposensitization) has been known for some time to reduce the severity of type I reactions, or even eliminate them completely, in a significant number of individuals suffering from allergic rhinitis. The introduction of allergen by subcutaneous injections appears to cause a shift toward IgG production or to induce T-cell–mediated suppression that turns off the IgE response (Figure 16-10). The IgG antibody is referred to as *blocking antibody* because it competes for the allergen, binds to it, and forms a complex that can be removed by phagocytosis, so that the allergen is not available to cross-link the fixed IgE on the mast cell membrane.

Knowledge of the mechanism of mast cell degranulation and the mediators involved in type I reactions has opened the way to therapeutic approaches based on pharmacological intervention. Antihistamines have been the most useful drugs in alleviating allergic rhinitis symptoms. These drugs act by binding to the histamine receptors on target cells and blocking the binding of histamine. The H_1 receptors are blocked by the classical antihistamines, and the H_2 receptors by a newer class of antihistamines.

A number of drugs have been shown to block mast cell degranulation by interfering with various biochemical steps in mast cell activation (Table 16-7). Disodium cromoglycate (cromolyn sodium) prevents Ca^{2+} influx into mast cells. The drug theophylline, commonly administered orally or through inhalers to asthmatics, blocks the enzyme phosphodiesterase and thus increases the level of cAMP by preventing its conversion to 5'-AMP. As noted earlier, prolonged increases in cAMP block degranulation. A number of drugs stimulate the β-adrenergic system by stimulating β receptors. Epinephrine (also known as adrenalin) is commonly administered during anaphylactic shock. It acts by binding to β receptors on bronchial smooth muscles and mast cells, elevating the cAMP levels within these cells. The increased levels of cAMP lead to relaxation of the bronchial muscles and decreased mast cell degranulation. A number of altered versions of epinephrine have been developed that bind to select β receptors and induce cAMP increases with fewer side effects than epinephrine. Cortisone and various other drugs also have been used to reduce type I reactions.

Table 16-7 Mechanism of action of some drugs used to treat type I hypersensitivity

Drug	Action
Antihistamines	Block H_1 and H_2 receptors on target cells
Cromolyn sodium	Block Ca^{2+} influx into mast cells
Theophylline	Prolongs high cAMP levels in mast cells by inhibiting phosphodiesterase, which cleaves cAMP to 5'-AMP*
Adrenalin	Stimulates cAMP production by binding to β-adrenergic receptors on mast cells*
Cortisone	Reduces histamine levels by blocking conversion of histidine to histamine Stimulates mast cell production of cAMP*

* Although cAMP rises transiently during mast cell activation, degranulation is prevented if cAMP levels remain high.

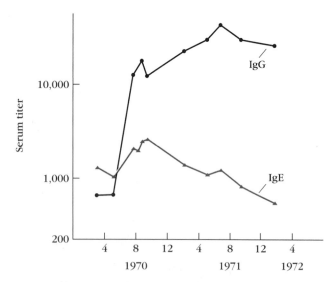

Figure 16-10 Injection of ragweed antigen continuously for 2 years into a ragweed-sensitive individual induced a gradual decrease in IgE levels and a dramatic increase in IgG. Both antibodies were measured by a radioimmunoassay. [From K. Ishizaka and T. Ishisaka, 1973, in *Asthma Physiology, Immunopharmacology and Treatment*. K. F. Austen, L. M. Lichtenstein (eds). Academic Press.]

Antibody-Mediated Cytotoxic (Type II) Hypersensitivity

Type II hypersensitive reactions involve antibody-mediated destruction of cells. This type of reaction is best characterized by blood-transfusion reactions in which host antibodies react with foreign antigens expressed by the incompatible transfused blood cells and mediate destruction of these cells. Antibody can mediate cell destruction by activating the complement system to create pores in the membrane of the foreign cell (see Figure 15-4). Antibody can also mediate cell destruction by antibody-dependent cell-mediated cytotoxicity (ADCC). As discussed in Chapter 13, cytotoxic cells with Fc receptors can bind to the Fc region of antibodies on target cells and promote killing of the cells (see Figure 13-10). Antibody bound to a foreign cell also can serve as an opsonin, enabling phagocytic cells with Fc or C3b receptors to bind and phagocytose the antibody-coated cell. Several examples to type II hypersensitive reactions will be examined.

Transfusion Reactions

A large number of proteins and glycoproteins on the RBC membrane are encoded by different genes, each of which has a number of alternative alleles. An individual possessing one allelic form of a blood-group antigen can recognize other allelic forms on transfused blood as foreign and mount an antibody response. In some cases the antibodies are acquired by natural exposure to similar antigenic determinants on a variety of microorganisms thought to be normal flora of the gut. This is the case with the A, B, O blood-group antigens (Figure 16-11a). Antibodies to the A, B, and O antigens, called *isohemagglutinins*, are usually of the IgM class. An individual with blood type A, for example, will respond to B-like epitopes on intestinal microorganisms, resulting in the production of isohemagglutinins to the B-like epitope. This same individual would not respond to A-like epitopes on the same intestinal microorganisms because these A-like epitopes are too similar to self and a state of self-tolerance to these epitopes should exist. If a type

(a)

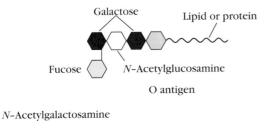
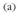

(b)

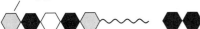

Genotype	Blood-group phenotype	Antigens on erythrocytes (*agglutinins*)	Serum antibodies (*isohemagglutinins*)
AA or AO	A	A	Anti-B
BB or BO	B	B	Anti-A
AB	AB	A and B	None
OO	O	None	Anti-A and anti-B

Figure 16-11 ABO blood group. (a) Structure of terminal sugars, which constitute the distinguishing epitopes, in the A, B, and O blood antigens. (b) ABO genotypes and corresponding phenotypes, agglutinins, and isohemagglutinins.

A individual is accidentally transfused with blood containing type B cells, the anti-B isohemagglutinins will bind to the B blood cells and mediate their destruction by means of complement-mediated lysis (Figure 16-11b). Antibodies to other blood-group antigens are acquired through repeated blood transfusions because minor allelic differences in these antigens can stimulate antibody production. These antibodies are usually of the IgG class.

Transfusion of blood into a recipient possessing antibodies to one of the blood-group antigens can result in a transfusion reaction. The clinical manifestations of transfusion reactions result from massive intravascular hemolysis of the transfused red blood cells by antibody + complement. The clinical manifestations may have immediate or delayed onset. Reactions having immediate onset are most commonly associated with ABO blood-group incompatibilities with the complement-mediated lysis triggered by the IgM isohemagglutinins. Within hours free hemoglobin can be detected in the plasma; it is filtered through the kidneys, resulting in hemoglobinuria. Some of the hemoglobin gets converted to bilirubin, which at high levels is toxic. Typical symptoms include fever, chills, nausea, clotting within blood vessels, pain in the lower back, and hemoglobin in the urine. Treatment involves prompt termination of the transfusion and maintenance of urine flow with a diuretic because the accumulation of hemoglobin in the kidney can cause acute tubular necrosis.

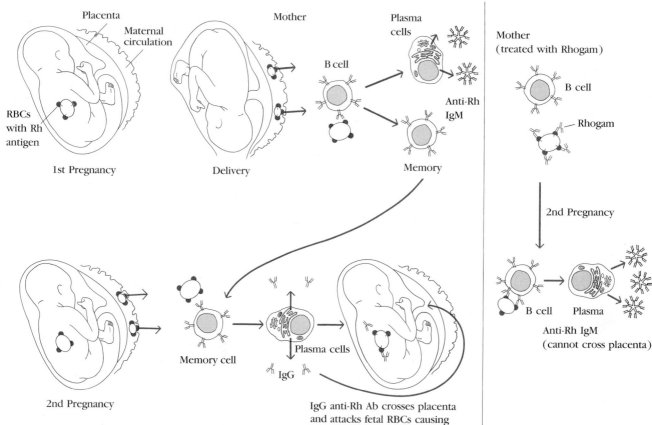

Figure 16-12 Development of erythroblastosis fetalis (hemolytic disease of the newborn) caused by Rh incompatibility between an Rh⁻ mother and Rh⁺ fetus. Generally during her first pregnancy an Rh⁻ mother is not exposed to Rh⁺ fetal red blood cells until the time of delivery when there is a great deal of placental tearing. The Rh⁻ maternal B cells will be activated in response to the fetal Rh antigen. The IgM antibody produced by the plasma cells will clear the fetal Rh antigen, but a population of long-lived memory cells will remain. During a subsequent pregnancy, release of fetal RBCs into the mother's circulation will activate these memory cells, resulting in the formation of IgG anti-Rh antibody that can cross the placenta and attack the fetal RBCs. If the mother is treated with an injection of anti-Rh antibody (Rhogam) within 24–48 h of the first delivery, the B cells will not be activated and memory B cells will not be formed. In this case the mother is more likely to produce IgM instead of IgG during subsequent pregnancies.

Delayed hemolytic transfusion reactions generally occur in individuals who have received repeated transfusions of ABO-compatible blood that is incompatible for other blood group antigens. The reactions develop between 2 and 6 days following transfusion and reflect the secondary nature of these reactions. The transfused blood induces clonal selection and production of IgG against a variety of blood-group membrane antigens. The most common blood-group antigens inducing delayed transfusion reactions are ABO, Rh, Kidd, Kell, and Duffy. Because the antibody class involved is generally IgG, RBC lysis is not complete. Instead red blood cells are destroyed at extravascular sites by agglutination, opsonization, and subsequent phagocytosis by macrophages. Symptoms include fever, low hemoglobin, increased bilirubin, mild jaundice, and anemia. Free hemoglobin is usually not detected in the plasma or urine in these reactions because RBC destruction occurs in extravascular sites. Blood-transfusion reactions can be prevented by proper cross-matching between the donor's and the recipient's blood. Cross-matching can reveal the presence of the antibodies in donor or recipient sera that can cause these reactions.

Hemolytic Disease of the Newborn

Hemolytic disease of the newborn develops when maternal IgG antibodies specific for fetal blood-group antigens cross the placenta and destroy fetal red blood cells. The consequences of such transfer can be minor, serious, or lethal. Severe hemolytic disease of the newborn, called *erythroblastosis fetalis*, is commonly caused by Rh incompatibility, which develops in Rh⁻ mothers who carry an Rh⁺ fetus (Figure 16-12). The fetal red blood cells are separated from the mother's circulation by a layer of cells in the placenta called the trophoblast. During her first pregnancy, a woman is usually not exposed to enough of these fetal red blood cells to activate Rh-specific B cells. At the time of delivery, however, separation of the placenta from the uterine wall allows larger amounts of fetal umbilical-cord blood to enter the mother's circulation. These fetal red blood cells activate Rh-specific B cells resulting in production of Rh-specific plasma cells and memory cells. The secreted antibody clears the Rh⁺ fetal red cells from the mother's circulation, but the memory cells remain, a threat to any subsequent pregnancy with an Rh⁺ fetus. Activation of these memory cells in a subsequent pregnancy results in the formation of IgG anti-Rh antibodies, which cross the placenta and damage the fetal red blood cells. Mild to severe anemia can develop, sometimes with fatal consequences. In addition, conversion of hemoglobin to bilirubin can present an additional threat to the newborn as the lipid-soluble bilirubin builds up in the brain and causes brain damage.

Hemolytic disease of the newborn caused by Rh incompatibility can be almost entirely prevented by the administration of antibodies to the Rh antigen (Rhogam) within 72 h after delivery. These antibodies bind to any fetal red blood cells that enter the mother's circulation at the time of delivery and facilitate their clearance before B-cell activation and ensuing memory-cell production can take place.

The development of hemolytic disease of the newborn caused by Rh incompatibility can be detected by testing maternal serum at intervals for antibodies to the Rh antigen. A rise in the titer of these antibodies during the pregnancy indicates that the mother has been exposed to Rh antigens and is producing increasing amounts of antibody. The presence of maternal IgG on the surface of fetal red blood cells can be detected by a *Coombs test.* Isolated fetal red cells are incubated with goat antibody to human IgG antibody (the Coombs reagent). If maternal IgG is bound to the fetal red cells, the cells agglutinate with the Coombs reagent.

Treatment of hemolytic disease caused by Rh incompatibility depends on the severity of the reaction. If the reaction is severe, the fetus can be given an intrauterine blood-exchange transfusion with Rh⁻ red blood cells. These transfusions are given every 10–21 days until delivery. In less severe cases a blood-exchange transfusion is not given until after birth, primarily to remove bilirubin; the infant is also exposed to low levels of UV light to break down the bilirubin and prevent any cerebral damage. The mother can also be treated during the pregnancy by plasmapheresis. In this procedure a cell-separation machine is used to separate the mother's blood into two fractions, cells and plasma. The plasma containing the anti-Rh antibody is discarded, and the cells are reinfused into the mother in an albumin or fresh plasma solution.

The majority of cases (65%) of hemolytic disease of the newborn have relatively minor consequences and are caused by ABO blood-group incompatibility between the mother and fetus. Type A or B fetuses carried by type O mothers most commonly develop these reactions. A type O mother is most likely to develop IgG antibody to the A or B blood-group antigens either through natural exposure or through exposure to fetal blood-group A or B antigens in successive pregnancies. Usually the fetal anemia resulting from this incompatibility is mild; the major clinical manifestation is a slight elevation of bilirubin, with jaundice. Depending on the severity of the anemia and jaundice, a blood-exchange transfusion may be required in these infants. In general the reaction is mild, however, and exposure of the infant to low levels of UV light is enough to break down the bilirubin and avoid any cerebral damage.

Drug-Induced Hemolytic Anemia

Certain antibiotics (e.g., penicillin, cephalosporin, and streptomycin) can adsorb nonspecifically to proteins on RBC membranes, forming a complex similar to a hapten-carrier complex. In some cases patients form antibodies to this drug-protein complex which can bind to the adsorbed drug on the RBC, inducing complement-mediated lysis and thus progressive anemia. When the drug is withdrawn, the hemolytic anemia disappears. Penicillin can induce all four types of hypersensitivity with various clinical manifestations (Table 16-8).

Autoimmune Type II Reactions

In a number of autoimmune diseases individuals produce autoantibody against a variety of cellular antigens. This autoantibody can mediate cellular destruction by way of a type II mechanism involving complement-mediated lysis. A few examples of these diseases are discussed here briefly; they are covered more fully in Chapter 17.

In autoimmune hemolytic anemia, autoantibody to RBC antigens mediates cell destruction. Idiopathic thrombocytopenia purpura is brought on by autoantibody to platelet antigens. As platelets are destroyed by lysis or phagocytic clearance, platelet numbers decrease and the individual may experience abnormal bleeding and clotting. In Hashimoto's thyroiditis, autoantibodies (together with a DTH response) are produced to the protein thyroglobulin, resulting in destruction of thyroid tissue and diminished production of thyroid hormones. In Goodpasture's syndrome, autoantibodies to basement-membrane antigens in the kidney and lung promote tissue damage through complement-mediated lysis; kidney biopsy samples stained with fluorescent antibodies to human IgG or C3b reveal linear deposits of antibody or complement along the basement membrane. In myasthenia gravis, autoantibodies to the acetylcholine receptor on muscles mediate receptor degradation; the resulting reduction in the number of receptors inhibits muscle stimulation by the neurotransmitter acetylcholine.

Immune Complex–Mediated (Type III) Hypersensitivity

The reaction of antibody with antigen generates immune complexes. Generally this complexing of antigen with antibody facilitates the clearance of antigen by phagocytic cells. In some cases, however, large amounts of immune complexes can lead to tissue-damaging type III hypersensitive reactions. The magnitude of the reaction depends on the quantity of immune complexes as well as their distribution within the body. Depending on where these complexes are carried, different tissue-damaging reactions can be observed. When the complexes are deposited locally (that is, very near the site of antigen entry) in tissue, a localized *Arthus reaction* develops. When the complexes are formed in the blood, a reaction can develop wherever the complexes are deposited (e.g., on blood-vessel walls, in the synovial membrane of joints, on the glomerular basement membrane of the kidney, on the choroid plexus of the brain). In any case, tissue is damaged at the site of deposition.

Type III hypersensitive reactions develop when immune complexes activate the complement system's array of immune effector molecules. The C3a, C4a, and C5a complement split products are anaphylatoxins that cause localized mast cell degranulation and consequent increase in local vascular permeability. C3a, C5a, and C5b67 are also chemotactic factors for neutrophils, which can accumulate in large numbers at the site of immune-complex deposition. Larger immune complexes are deposited on the basement membrane of blood-vessel walls or kidney glomeruli, whereas smaller complexes may pass through the basement membrane and be deposited in the subepithelium. The type of lesions that result will depend on the site of deposition of the complexes.

Much of the tissue damage in type III reactions stems from release of lytic enzymes by neutrophils as they attempt to phagocytose immune complexes. A neutrophil binds to an immune complex by means of type I complement receptors, which are specific for the C3b complement component. Because the complex is at-

Table 16-8 Penicillin-induced hypersensitive reactions

Type of hypersensitive reaction	Antibody or lymphocytes induced	Clinical manifestations
I	IgE	Urticaria, systemic anaphylaxis
II	IgM, IgG	Hemolytic anemia
III	IgG	Serum sickness, glomerulonephritis
IV	T_{DTH} cells	Contact dermatitis

tached to the basement-membrane surface, phagocytosis is impeded, allowing lytic enzymes to be released during the unsuccessful attempts of the neutrophil to ingest the adhering immune complex. Further activation of the membrane-attack mechanism of the complement system can also contribute to the tissue destruction. In addition, the activation of complement can induce aggregation of platelets, and the resulting release of clotting factors can lead to the formation of microthrombi.

Localized Type III Reactions

Injection of an antigen intradermally or subcutaneously into an animal that has high levels of circulating antibody specific for that antigen leads to formation of localized immune complexes, which mediate an acute Arthus reaction within 4–8 h (Figure 16-13). Microscopic examination of the tissue reveals neutrophils adhering to

the vascular endothelium and then migrating into the tissues at the site of immune-complex deposition. As the reaction develops, localized tissue and vascular damage results in an accumulation of fluid (edema) and red blood cells (erythema) at the site. The severity of the reaction can vary from mild swelling and redness to tissue necrosis.

Following an insect bite, a sensitive individual may have a rapid, localized type I reaction at the site. Often, some 4–8 h later, a typical Arthus reaction also develops at the site with pronounced erythema and edema. Intrapulmonary Arthus-type reactions induced by bacterial spores, fungi, or dried fecal proteins can also cause pneumonitis or alveolitis. These reactions are known by a variety of common names reflecting the source of the antigen. For example, "farmer's lung" develops after inhalation of thermophilic actinomycetes from moldy hay, and "pigeon fancier's disease," results from inhalation of a serum protein in dust derived from dried pigeon feces.

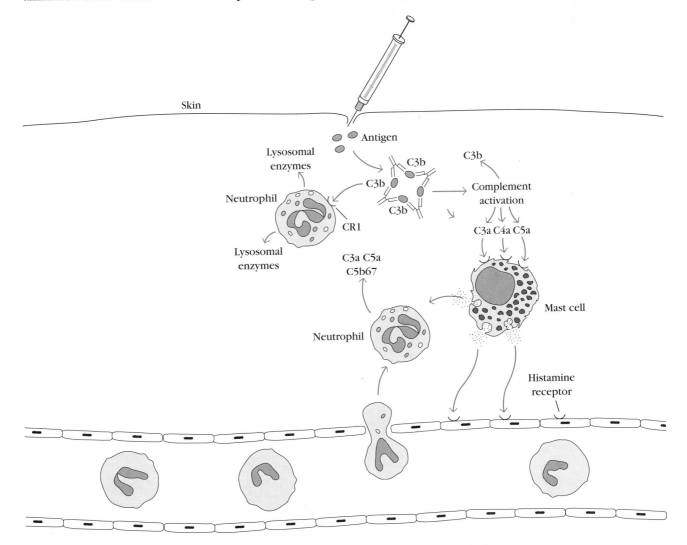

Figure 16-13 Development of a localized Arthus reaction (type III hypersensitive reaction) involves complement-mediated mast cell degranulation and release of lytic enzymes from neutrophils trying to phagocytose immune complexes. (See text for further discussion.)

Generalized Type III Reactions

When large amounts of antigen enter the bloodstream and bind to antibody, circulating immune complexes can form. If antigen is in excess, small complexes form; because these are not easily cleared by the phagocytic cells, they can cause tissue-damaging type III reactions at various sites. Historically, generalized type III reactions were often observed after the administration of antitoxins containing foreign serum, such as horse anti-tetanus or antidiphtheria serum. In such cases, the recipient of a foreign antiserum develops antibodies specific for the foreign serum proteins; these antibodies then form circulating immune complexes with the foreign serum antigens. Typically within days or weeks after exposure to foreign serum antigens, an individual begins to manifest a combination of symptoms that are called *serum sickness* (Figure 16-14). These symptoms include fever, weakness, generalized vasculitis (rashes) with edema and erythema, lymphadenopathy, arthritis, and sometimes glomerulonephritis. The precise manifestations of serum sickness depend on the quantity of immune complexes formed as well as the overall size of the complexes, which determine the site of tissue deposition.

Formation of circulating immune complexes contributes to the pathogenesis of a number of conditions other than serum sickness. These include the following:

Autoimmune Diseases

Systemic lupus erythematosus
Rheumatoid arthritis
Goodpasture's syndrome

Drug Reactions

Allergies to penicillin and sulphonamides

Infectious Diseases

Poststreptococcal glomerulonephritis
Meningitis
Hepatitis
Mononucleosis
Malaria
Trypanosomiasis

Tumors

Complexes of antibody with various bacterial, viral, and parasitic antigens have been shown to induce a variety of type III hypersensitive reactions including skin rashes, arthritic symptoms, and glomerulonephritis. Poststreptococcal glomerulonephritis, for example, develops when circulating complexes of antibody and strepto-

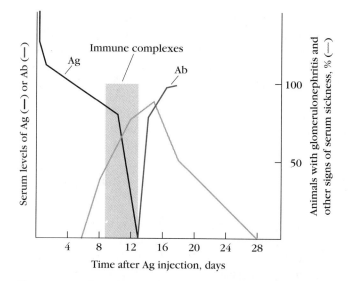

Figure 16-14   Correlation between immune-complex formation and development of symptoms of serum sickness. A large dose of antigen (BSA) was injected into a rabbit at day 0. As antibody formed, it complexed with the antigen and was deposited in the kidneys, joints, and capillaries. The symptoms of serum sickness corresponded to the peak in immune-complex formation. As the immune complexes were cleared, free circulating antibody was detected and the symptoms of serum sickness subsided. [Based on F. G. Germuth, Jr., 1953, *J. Exp. Med.* **97**:257.]

coccal antigens are deposited in the kidney and damage the glomeruli. A number of autoimmune diseases stem from circulating complexes of antibody and self-proteins, glycoproteins, or even DNA. In systemic lupus erythematosus, complexes of DNA and anti-DNA antibodies accumulate in synovial membranes, causing arthritic symptoms, or accumulate on the basement membrane of the kidney, causing progressive kidney damage. Type III reactions are also common in cancer patients, in whom complexes of antibody with shed tumor antigens can build up in the circulation, leading to skin rashes, arthritic symptoms, and/or kidney damage.

T$_{DTH}$-Mediated (Type IV) Hypersensitivity

Type IV hypersensitive reactions develop when antigen activates sensitized T$_{DTH}$ cells; these cells generally appear to be a T$_H$1 subpopulation although sometimes T$_C$ cells are involved (see Chapter 13). Activation of T$_{DTH}$ cells by antigen on appropriate antigen-presenting cells results in the secretion of various cytokines including interleukin 2 (IL-2), interferon gamma (IFN-γ), macrophage migration-inhibition factor (MIF), and tumor necrosis factor β (TNF-β) (see Figure 13-11). The overall effect of these cytokines is to draw macrophages into the area and activate them, promoting increased phagocytotic activity and increased concentrations of lysosomal enzymes for more effective killing (see Figure 13-12). As lysosomal enzymes leak out of the activated macrophages into the surrounding tissue, localized tissue destruction can ensue. These reactions typically take 48–72 h to develop, the time required from initial T$_{DTH}$-cell activation and lymphokine secretion to mediate accumulation of macrophages and the subsequent release of their lysosomal enzymes.

As discussed in Chapter 13, several lines of evidence suggest that the type IV reaction is important in host defense against parasites and bacteria that can live intracellularly. Antibodies cannot reach these organisms (because they are inside the host's cells), but the heightened phagocytotic activity and the buildup of lysosomal enzymes from macrophages in the area leads to nonspecific destruction of cells, and thus of the intracellular pathogen. When this defense process is not entirely effective, however, the continued presence of the pathogen's antigens can provoke a chronic delayed-hypersensitivity reaction, with excessive numbers of macrophages, continual release of lysosomal enzymes, and consequent tissue destruction. The granulomatous skin lesions seen with *Mycobacterium leprae* and the lung cavitation seen with *Mycobacterium tuberculosis* are both examples of the tissue damage that can result when chronic delayed-type hypersensitive reactions develop.

The reaction to an intradermal injection of an antigen can serve as a test for the presence of T$_{DTH}$ cells previously sensitized by that antigen. The use of the PPD antigen to detect previous exposure to *M. tuberculosis* was described in Chapter 13. Similar skin tests to detect previous exposure to the bacterium causing leprosy and the fungus causing coccidiomycosis utilize lepromin and coccidiodin, respectively, as test antigens. In these tests, the appearance of swelling and redness at the injection site within 48–72 h constitutes a positive reaction. In AIDS the depletion of the CD4$^+$ lymphocyte population can be monitored by repeated skin testing with any of the various antigens for which the normal T-cell population has a high percentage of positive skin-test reactivity. As AIDS progresses, the decline in T$_{DTH}$ cells is revealed by a decrease in positive skin-test reactions.

Many contact-dermatitis reactions, including the response to formaldehyde, trinitrophenol, nickel, turpentine, various cosmetics and hair dyes, poison oak, and poison ivy, are mediated by T$_{DTH}$ cells. Most of these substances are small molecules that can complex with skin proteins. This complex is internalized by antigen-presenting cells in the skin (such as Langerhans' cells), processed and presented together with the class II MHC

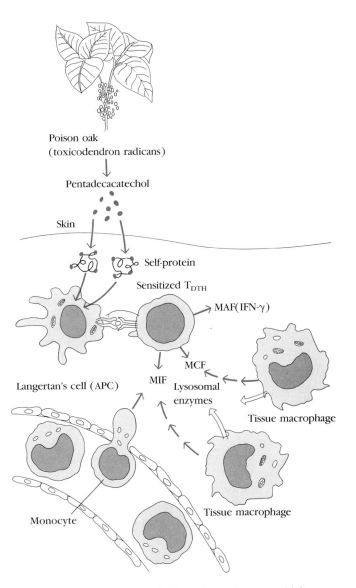

Figure 16-15 Development of delayed-type hypersensitivity reaction following second exposure to poison oak. Cytokines (MAF, MIF, and MCF) released from sensitized T$_{DTH}$ cells mediate this reaction. Tissue damage results from release of lytic enzymes from activated macrophages.

molecules, causing activation of sensitized T$_{DTH}$ cells. In the reaction to poison oak, for example, a pentadecacatechol compound from the leaves of the plant complexes with skin proteins. T$_H$ cells react with this compound appropriately expressed by local antigen-presenting cells and differentiate into sensitized T$_{DTH}$ cells. A subsequent exposure to pentadecacatechol will elicit activation of T$_{DTH}$ cells and cytokine production. Approximately 48–72 h after exposure, the secreted lymphokines cause macrophages to accumulate at the site. Activation of these macrophages and release of their lysosomal enzymes results in the redness and pustules that characterize a reaction to poison oak (Figure 16-15).

Summary

1. Hypersensitive reactions are inflammatory reactions within the humoral or cell-mediated branches of the immune system that lead to extensive tissue damage or even a fatal outcome. The differences in the reactions reflect different immune mechanisms and differences in the immune effector molecules generated.

2. A type I hypersensitive reaction is mediated by IgE antibodies, whose Fc region binds to receptors on mast cells or blood basophils. Cross-linkage by allergen of the fixed IgE initiates a sequence of intracellular events leading to mast cell or basophil degranulation and thus the release of pharmacologically active mediators. The mediators are the immune effector molecules in this reaction. The principal effects of these mediators are smooth-muscle contraction and vasodilation.

3. A type II hypersensitive reaction occurs when antibody reacts with antigenic determinants present on the surface of cells, leading to cell damage or death through complement-mediated lysis or antibody-dependent cell-mediated cytotoxicity (ADCC).

4. A type III hypersensitive reaction is mediated by the formation of immune complexes and the ensuing activation of complement. Complement split products serve as immune effector molecules that cause localized vasodilation and chemotactically attract neutrophils. Tissue damage results from the accumulation of neutrophils and their release of lytic enzymes or through the complement terminal membrane-attack complex damaging healthy tissue in the vicinity of the immune complex.

5. A type IV hypersensitive reaction involves the cell-mediated branch of the immune system. Antigen activation of sensitized T_{DTH} cells induces release of various cytokines, which serve as the immune effector molecules in this reaction. The net effect of these cytokines is to cause an accumulation and activation of macrophages, which release lysosomal enzymes that cause localized tissue damage.

References

FINKELMAN, F. D., I. M. KATONA, J. URBAN et al. 1988. IL-4 is required to generate and sustain in vivo IgE response. *J. Immunol.* **141**:2335.

GERSHWIN, L. J., and M. E. GERSHWIN. 1986. The regulation of the IgE response. *Immunol. Today* **7**:328.

ISHIZAKA, K. 1989. Regulation of immunoglobulin E biosynthesis. *Adv. Immunol* **47**:1.

ISHIZAKA, K. 1988. IgE-binding factors and regulation of the IgE antibody response. *Annu. Rev. Immunol.* **6**:513.

MYGIND, N. 1986. *Essential Allergy.* Blackwell Scientific Publications.

Study Questions

1. Indicate whether each of the following statements is true or false. If you think a statement is false, explain why.

   a. Mice infected with *Nippostrongylus brasiliensis* show decreased production of IgE.

   b. IL-4 decreases IgE production by B cells.

   c. Babies can acquire IgE-mediated allergies by passive transfer of maternal antibody.

   d. Antihistamines are effective for the treatment of type III hypersensitivity.

   e. Most pollen allergens contain a single allergenic component.

2. a. What would you expect to happen if a person were injected with (a) antibodies to IgE Fc receptors or (b) Fab fragments of such antibodies?

   b. Would the response in part (a) depend on whether or not the person was allergic? Explain.

3. Serum sickness can result when an individual is given a large dose of antiserum such as an antitoxin to snake venom. How could you take advantage of recent technological advances to produce an antitoxin that would not produce serum sickness in patients who receive it?

4. In the table below, compare and contrast the hypersensitive reactions to poison oak and ragweed pollen in terms of the characteristics listed on the left.

Characteristic	Poison oak	Ragweed pollen
Lymphocytes involved		
Other cells involved		
Mediators involved		
Mechanism		

5. What immunologic mechanisms most likely account for a person developing each of the following reactions following an insect bite?

   a. Within 1–2 min after being bitten, swelling and redness appear at the site and then disappear by 1 h.

   b. 6–8 h later swelling and redness again appear and persist for 24 h.

   c. 72 h later the tissue becomes inflamed, and tissue necrosis follows.

6. In the table on the facing page, indicate whether each immunologic event listed on the left does (+) or does not (−) occur in each type of hypersensitivity.

Immunologic event	Type I hypersensitivity	Type II hypersensitivity	Type III hypersensitivity	Type IV hypersensitivity
Ig-E–mediated degranulation of mast cells				
Lysis of antibody-coated blood cells by complement				
Tissue destruction in response to poison oak				
C3a- and C5a-mediated mast cell degranulation				
Chemotaxis of neutrophils				
Chemotaxis of eosinophils				
Activation of macrophages by IFN-γ				
Deposition of antigen-antibody complexes on basement membranes of capillaries				
Sudden death due to vascular collapse (shock) shortly after injection or ingestion of antigen				

Autoimmunity

The response of the immune system against self-components is termed *autoimmunity*. Normally the mechanisms of self-tolerance protect an individual from potentially self-reactive lymphocytes. In the 1960s it was believed that all self-reactive lymphocytes were eliminated during their development and that a failure to eliminate these lymphocytes led to auto-immune consequences. Since the late 1970s a broad body of experimental evidence has countered that belief, revealing that not all self-reactive lymphocytes are deleted during T-cell and B-cell maturation. Instead normal healthy individuals have been shown to possess mature, recirculating self-reactive lymphocytes. Since the presence of these self-reactive lymphocytes does not inevitably result in autoimmune reactions, their activity must be regulated in normal individuals through clonal anergy or clonal suppression. A breakdown in this regulation can lead to activation of self-reactive clones of T or B cells, generating humoral or cell-mediated responses against self-antigens. These reactions can cause serious damage to cells or organs, sometimes with fatal consequences. This chapter describes some common autoimmune diseases in humans and experimental animal models used to study autoimmunity. In addition various mechanisms that may contribute to induction of autoimmune reactions are discussed, as well as current and experimental therapies for treating them.

Autoimmune Diseases in Humans

Autoimmune diseases affect between 5 and 7% of the population, often causing chronic debilitating illnesses. In general, autoimmune diseases can be divided into two categories: organ-specific and systemic autoimmune disease (Table 17-1). In organ-specific autoimmune disease, the immune response is directed to a target antigen unique to a single organ or gland, so that the manifestations are largely limited to that organ. In systemic autoimmune disease, the response is directed toward a broad range of target antigens and involves a number of organs and tissues.

Organ-Specific Autoimmune Diseases

Damage to the target organs in organ-specific autoimmunity can occur as the result of direct cellular damage by humoral or cell-meditated mechanisms or by stimulating autoantibodies or blocking autoantibodies.

Diseases Mediated by Direct Cellular Damage

Autoimmune diseases involving direct cellular damage occur when lymphocytes or antibodies bind to cell-membrane antigens, causing cellular lysis and/or the buildup of inflammatory reactions in the affected organ. Gradually the cellular structure of an affected organ is replaced by connective tissue and the functon of the organ declines. A few examples of this type of autoimmune disease are briefly discussed in this section.

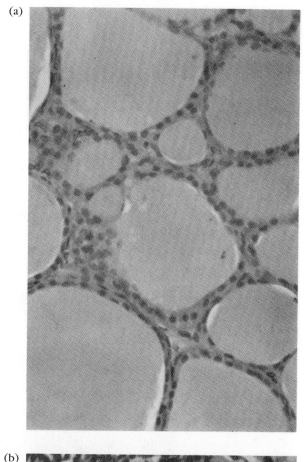

(a)

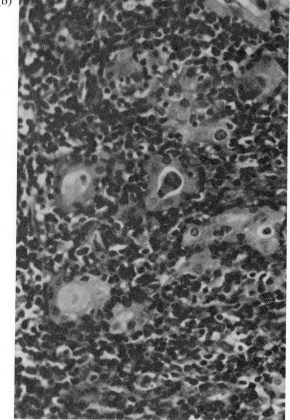

(b)

Figure 17-1 Photomicrographs of (a) normal thyroid gland and (b) gland in Hashimoto's thyroiditis showing intense lymphocyte infiltration. [From L. V. Crowley, 1983, *Introduction to Human Disease*, Wadsworth Health Sciences.]

Table 17-1 Some autoimmune diseases in humans

Disease	Self-antigen	Immune response
Organ-specific Autoimmune Diseases		
Addison's disease	Adrenal cells	Autoantibodies
Autoimmune hemolytic anemia	RBC membrane proteins	Autoantibodies
Goodpasture's syndrome	Renal and lung basement membranes	Autoantibodies
Graves' disease	Thyroid-stimulating hormone receptor	Autoantibody (stimulating)
Hashimoto's thyroiditis	Thyroid proteins and cells	T_{DTH} cells and autoantibodies
Idiopathic thrombocytopenia purpura	Platelet membrane proteins	Autoantibodies
Insulin-dependent diabetes mellitus	Pancreatic beta cells	T_{DTH} cells and autoantibodies
Myasthenia gravis	Acetylcholine receptors	Autoantibody (blocking)
Myocardial infarction	Heart	Autoantibodies
Pernicious anemia	Gastric parietal cells: (intrinsic factor)	Autoantibody
Poststreptococcal glomerulonephritis	Kidney	Antigen-antibody complexes
Systemic Autoimmune Disease		
Spontaneous infertility	Sperm	Autoantibodies
Ankylosing spondylitis	Vertebrate	Immune complexes
Multiple sclerosis	Brain or white matter	T_{DTH} and T_C cells autoantibodies
Rheumatoid arthritis	Connective tissue, IgG	Autoantibodies, immune complexes
Scleroderma	Nuclei, heart, lungs, gastrointestinal tract, kidney	Autoantibodies
Sjögren's syndrome	Salivary gland, liver, kidney, thyroid	Autoantibodies
Systemic lupus erythematosus (SLE)	DNA, nuclear protein, RBC and platelet membranes	Autoantibodies, immune complexes

Hashimoto's Thyroiditis. In this autoimmune disease, most frequently seen in middle-aged women, an individual produces autoantibodies and sensitized T_{DTH} cells specific for thyroid antigens. The response is characterized by an intense infiltration of the thyroid gland by lymphocytes, macrophages, and plasma cells, which form lymphocytic follicles and germinal centers (Figure 17-1). The ensuing inflammatory response causes a goiter, or visible enlargement of the thyroid gland. Antibodies are formed to a number of thyroid proteins, including thyroglobulin and thyroid peroxidase, both of which are involved in the uptake of iodine. Binding of the autoantibodies to these proteins interferes with iodine uptake and leads to decreased production of thyroid hormones (hypothyroidism).

Autoimmune Anemias. Autoimmune anemias include pernicious anemia, autoimmune hemolytic anemia, and drug-induced hemolytic anemia. Pernicious anemia is caused by autoantibodies to a membrane-bound intestinal protein, called intrinsic factor. Binding of intrinsic factor to vitamin B_{12} in the small intestine facilitates uptake of the vitamin. Binding of the autoantibody to intrinsic factor prevents this process, thus blocking intrinsic factor-mediated absorption of vitamin B_{12}. In the absence of vitamin B_{12}, which is necessary for proper hematopoiesis, the number of functional mature red blood cells is decreased. Pernicious anemia is treated with injections of vitamin B_{12}, thus circumventing the defect in absorption.

An individual with autoimmune hemolytic anemia makes autoantibody to RBC antigens, triggering complement-mediated lysis or antibody-mediated opsonization and thus phagocytosis of the red blood cells. The majority of autoimmune hemolytic anemias can be divided into warm and cold types. In warm hemolytic anemias the autoantibodies have optimal serologic activity at 37° C, and in cold hemolytic anemias the autoantibodies have optimal activity at 4° C but also react at 25° C and 31° C. Warm hemolytic anemias generally involve IgG autoantibodies, which often are specific for the Rh antigens. Cold hemolytic anemias generally involve IgM autoantibodies specific for the I and H RBC antigens. Clinical manifestation of cold type hemolytic anemia occurs when blood vessels, such as those in the skin of the hands of face, are exposed to the cold. The condition is reversed by warming the affected areas. The immunodiagnostic test for autoimmune hemolytic anemias generally involves a Coombs test in which the red cells are incubated with an anti-human IgG antiserum. If IgG autoantibodies are present on the red cells, the cells are agglutinated by the antiserum.

Goodpasture's Syndrome. In Goodpasture's syndrome, autoantibodies specific for certain basement-membrane antigens bind to the basement membranes of the kidney glomeruli and the alveoli of the lungs. Subsequent complement activation leads to direct cellular damage and an ensuing inflammatory response mediated by a buildup of complement split products. Damage to the glomerular and aveolar basement membranes leads to progressive kidney damage and pulmonary hemorrhage with death often within several months of the onset of symptoms. Staining of biopsies from patients with Goodpasture's

with fluorescent-labeled anti-IgG and anti-C3b reveals linear deposits of IgG and C3b along the basement membranes (Figure 17-2).

Insulin-Dependent Diabetes Mellitus. Insulin-dependent diabetes mellitus, a disease afflicting 0.2% of the population, is caused by an autoimmune attack on the pancreas. The attack is directed against specialized insulin-producing cells, called beta cells, that are located in spherical clusters (the islets of Langerhans) scattered throughout the pancreas. The autoimmune attack destroys the beta cells resulting in decreased production of insulin and consequently increased levels of blood glucose. The disease is characterized by a condition called insulitis in which large numbers of activated lymphocytes (consisting predominantly of CD8[+] T cells with some CD4[+] T cells and plasma cells) infiltrate the islets of Langerhans (Figure 17-3). A cell-mediated autoimmune response develops, resulting in beta-cell destruction. Destruction is thought to be mediated primarily by CTLs, although lymphokines produced by T_H cells may also play a role. Autoantibodies to beta cells may also contribute to cell destruction by facilitating either complement-mediated lysis or antibody-dependent cell-mediated cytotoxicity (ADCC).

Diseases Mediated by Stimulating Autoantibodies

In some autoimmune diseases antibodies act as agonists, binding to hormone receptors in lieu of the normal ligand and stimulating inappropriate activity. This usually leads to an overproduction of mediators or an increase in cell growth. This type of autoimmunity is exemplified by *Graves' disease*, which involves the thyroid gland.

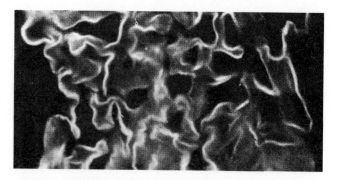

Figure 17-2   Fluorescent anti-IgG staining of a kidney biopsy from a patient with Goodpasture's syndrome reveals linear deposits of autoantibody along the basement membrane. [From J. A. Charlesworth and B. A. Pussell, 1986, in *Clinical Immunology Illustrated*, J. V. Wells and D. S. Nelson (eds.), Williams & Wilkins, p. 191.]

(a)   (b)

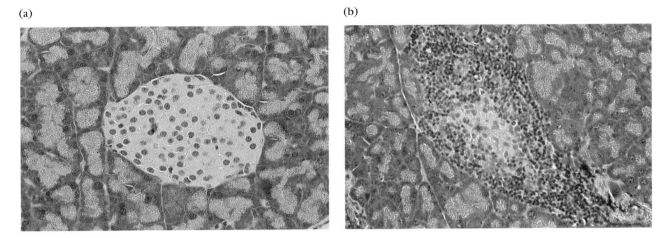

Figure 17-3   Photomicrographs of (a) islet of Langerhans in pancreas from a normal mouse and (b) in pancreas from a mouse with a disease resembling insulin-dependent diabetes mellitus. Note the lymphocyte infiltration into the islet (insulitis) in (b). [From M. A. Atkinson and N. K. Maclaren, 1990, What causes diabetes? *Sci Am.* July:62.]

The production of thyroid hormones is carefully regulated by thyroid-stimulating hormone (TSH), which is produced by the pituitary gland. Binding of TSH to a receptor on thyroid cells activates adenylate cyclase and stimulates the synthesis of two thyroid hormones, thyroxine and triiodothyronine. A patient with Graves' disease produces autoantibody to the receptor for TSH. Binding of these autoantibodies to the receptor mimics the normal action of TSH, activating adenylate cyclase and resulting in production of the thyroid hormones. Unlike TSH, however, the autoantibodies are not regulated, and consequently they stimulate the thyroid over too long a time. For this reason these autoantibodies are called *long-acting thyroid-stimulating* (LATS) antibodies (Figure 17-4a).

Diseases Mediated by Blocking Autoantibodies

In some cases of autoimmunity, autoantibodies bind to hormone receptors but act as antagonists, inhibiting receptor function. These diseases generally involve impaired secretion of mediators and gradual atrophy of the affected organ. In *myasthenia gravis*, the prototype disease of this type, autoantibodies are produced to the acetylcholine receptors on the motor end-plates of muscles. Binding of these autoantibodies to the receptors prevents binding by acetylcholine thereby inhibiting muscle activation. The antibodies also induce complement-mediated degradation of the receptor, resulting in progressive weakening of the skeletal muscles (Figure 17-4b).

Systemic Autoimmune Diseases

Autoimmune diseases with systemic manifestations reflect a generalized defect in immune regulation that results in hyperactive T cells and B cells. Tissue damage is widespread, both from cell-mediated immune responses and from direct cellular damage caused by autoantibodies or by accumulation of immune complexes.

Systemic Lupus Erythematosus (SLE). One of the best examples of a systemic autoimmune disease, SLE usually appears in women between 20 and 40 years of age and is characterized by fever, weakness, joint pain, erythematous lesions, pleurisy, and kidney dysfunction. Affected individuals may produce autoantibodies to a vast array of tissue antigens such as DNA, histones, RBCs, platelets, leukocytes, and clotting factors; interaction of these autoantibodies with their specific antigens produces various symptoms. Autoantibody specific for RBCs and platelets, for example, can lead to complement-mediated lysis, reresulting in hemolytic anemia and thrombocytopenia, respectively. When immune complexes of autoantibodies with various nuclear antigens are deposited along the walls of small blood vessels, these complexes activate the complement system and generate membrane-attack complexes, which damage the blood-vessel wall, resulting in vasculitis and glomerulonephritis.

Complement activation also generates such complement split products as C3a and C5a; serum levels of C3a and C5a may be three to four times higher in patients

(a) Stimulating autoantibodies
(Graves disease)

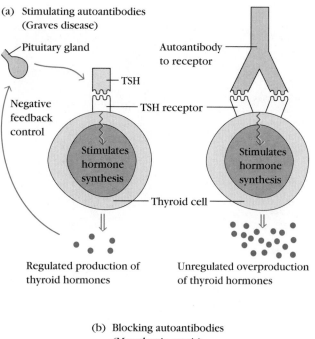

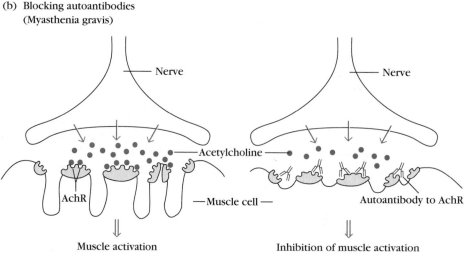

(b) Blocking autoantibodies
(Myasthenia gravis)

Figure 17-4 Autoantibodies to cell-membrane receptors can either enhance or block receptor activity. (a) In Graves' disease, autoantibody to the receptor for thyroid-stimulating hormone (TSH) induces unregulated activation of the thyroid, leading to overproduction of the thyroid hormones (red circles). (b) In myasthenia gravis, autoantibody to the acetylcholine receptor (AChR) binds to the receptor and blocks binding of acetylcholine (red circles) and subsequent muscle activation. In addition, the autoantibody induces complement activation resulting in damage to the muscle end-plate with a reduction in acetylcholine receptors as the disease progresses.

with severe SLE than in normal individuals (Figure 17-5). C5a induces increased expression of the type 3 complement receptor (CR3) on neutrophils, facilitating neutrophil aggregation and attachment to the vascular endothelium. As neutrophils attach to small blood vessels, the number of circulating neutrophils declines (neutropenia) and various occlusions of the small blood vessels develop (vasculitis). These occlusions can lead to widespread tissue damage.

Laboratory diagnosis of SLE focuses on the characteristic antinuclear antibodies, which are directed against double-stranded or single-stranded DNA, nucleoprotein, histones, and nucleolar RNA. Indirect immunofluorescent staining of serum from SLE patients produces various characteristic nuclei-staining patterns. Another diagnostic test for SLE is the LE test. When peripheral blood from SLE patients is incubated at 37° C,

the lymphocytes release their nuclei. Antibodies to nuclear antigens then react with the nuclei, and PMNs in the blood sample phagocytose the antibody-coated nuclei, forming a characteristic cell called the LE cell. Because the LE test is difficult to perform and also relatively insensitive, it is seldom used anymore to diagnose SLE.

Multiple Sclerosis (MS). Multiple sclerosis, an autoimmune disease affecting the central nervous system, is the most common cause of neurologic disability associated with disease in Western countries. Individuals with this disease produce autoreactive T cells that participate in the formation of inflammatory lesions along the myelin sheath of nerve fibers. Patients with active disease have activated T lymphocytes in their cerebrospinal fluid, which infiltrate the brain tissue and cause

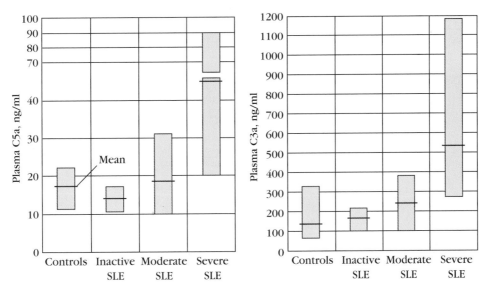

Figure 17-5 Antigen-antibody complexes produced in SLE induce complement activation with production of complement split products. Among patients with severe SLE the levels of complement split products C3a and C5a are significantly higher than in controls. [Modified from S. B. Abramson and G. Weissmann, 1988, Complement split products and the pathogenesis of SLE, *Hosp. Prac.* Dec 15:45.]

characteristic inflammatory lesions, destroying the myelin. Since myelin functions as an insulation of the nerve fibers, a breakdown in the myelin sheath leads to numerous neurologic dysfunctions.

Rheumatoid Arthritis. Rheumatoid arthritis is a common autoimmune disorder, most often affecting women from 40 to 60 years old. The major symptom is chronic inflammation of the joints, although the hematologic, cardiovascular, and respiratory systems are often affected as well. In many cases of rheumatoid arthritis a group of autoantibodies is produced that are reactive with determinants in the Fc region of IgG. These autoantibodies are call *rheumatoid factors*. The classical rheumatoid factor is an IgM antibody reactive to the Fc of IgG. Such autoantibodies bind to normal circulating IgC, forming IgM-IgG complexes that are then deposited in the joints. The immune complexes can then activate the complement cascade, resulting in a chronic inflammation of the joints.

Animal Models for Autoimmune Disease

Animal models for autoimmune diseases have contributed to our understanding of autoimmunity in humans. Autoimmunity develops spontaneously in certain inbred strains of animals; autoimmunity also can be induced by certain experimental manipulations (Table 17-2). Both types of autoimmune diseases have provided valuable insights into the mechanism of autoimmunity and into potential treatments.

Spontaneous Autoimmunity in Animals

A number of autoimmune diseases that develop spontaneously in animals have been found to have important clinical and pathologic similarities with certain autoimmune diseases in humans. Certain inbred mouse strains in particular have been valuable models for increasing understanding of the immunologic defects involved in the development of autoimmunity.

New Zealand Black (NZB) mice and F_1 hybrids of NZB and New Zealand White (NZW) mice spontaneously develop autoimmune diseases closely paralleling systemic lupus erythematosus. The NZB mice spontaneously develop autoimmune hemolytic anemia between 2 and 4 months of age and die prematurely by 18 months. Various autoantibodies can be detected, including antibodies to erythrocytes, nuclear proteins, DNA, and T lymphocytes. The autoimmune manifestations are even more severe when NZB mice are crossed with NZW mice. These F_1 (NZB × NZW) hybrids produce increased levels of anti-DNA and antinuclear antibodies and develop glomerulonephritis from immune-complex deposits in the kidney. As is true of SLE, the incidence of autoimmunity in these F_1 hybrids is greater in females, a phenomenon apparently related to estrogen levels. The effect of androgens and estrogens on development of autoimmune symptoms in these mice was studied by N. Talal. In his study, male and female F_1 (NZB × NZW) mice were castrated before puberty and then given hormone replacements. In both male and female mice that received androgens, there was a delay in the onset of autoimmunity and a reduction in its severity. Estrogens

Table 17-2 Experimental animal models of autoimmune diseases

Animal model	Possible human disease counterpart	Inducing antigen	Disease transferred by T cells
Spontaneous Autoimmune Disease			
Nonobese diabetic (NOD) mouse	Insulin-dependent diabetes mellitus (IDDM)	Unknown	Yes
F_1 (NZB × NZW) mouse	Systemic lupus erythematosus (SLE)	Unknown	Yes
Obese-strain chicken	Hashimoto's thyroiditis	Thyroglobulin	Yes
Experimentally Induced Autoimmune Disease*			
Experimental autoimmune myasthenia gravis (EAMG)	Myasthenia gravis	Acetylcholine receptor	Yes
Experimental autoimmune encephalomyelitis (EAE)	Multiple sclerosis (MS)	Myelin basic protein (MBP); proteolipid protein (PLP)	Yes
Autoimmune arthritis (AA)	Rheumatoid arthritis	M. tuberculosis (proteoglycans)	Yes
Experimental autoimmune thyroiditis (EAT)	Hashimoto's thyroiditis	Thyroglobulin	Yes

* These diseases can be induced by injecting appropriate animals with the indicated antigen in complete Freund adjuvant. Except for autoimmune arthritis, the antigens used correspond to the self-antigens associated with the human-disease counterpart. Rheumatoid arthritis involves reaction to proteoglycans, which are self-antigens associated with connective tissue.

had the opposite effect, promoting early onset of autoimmunity with increased severity.

Another important animal model is the nonobese diabetic (NOD) mouse, which spontaneously develops a form of diabetes that resembles human insulin-dependent diabetes mellitus (IDDM). Like the human disease, the NOD mouse disease begins with lymphocytic infiltration into the islets of the pancreas. Also, as in IDDM, there is a strong association between certain MHC alleles and development of diabetes in these mice. Experiments with these mice have shown that T cells from diabetic mice can transfer diabetes to nondiabetic recipients. For example, when the immune system of normal mice is destroyed by lethal x-irradiation and then the mouse is reconstituted with an injection of bone marrow cells from NOD mice, the reconstituted mice develop diabetes; conversely, when the immune system of still healthy NOD mice is destroyed by x-irradiation

and then reconstituted with normal bone marrow cells, the NOD mice do not develop diabetes. The role of $CD4^+$ and $CD8^+$ T cells in the development of diabetes has been studied in these mice. Since spleen cells from NOD mice can transfer diabetes into normal recipients, it is possible to selectively deplete either $CD4^+$ or $CD8^+$ T cells from the NOD spleen-cell suspension and then ask whether the depleted spleen cells can still transfer diabetes to normal mice. Such experiments have revealed that removal of either the $CD4^+$ or $CD8^+$ cells inhibits the transfer of diabetes, suggesting that both populations are necessary for the development of diabetes.

Several other spontaneously occurring autoimmune diseases have been discovered in animals and have served as models for similar human diseases. Among these are Obese-strain chickens, which develop both humoral and cell-mediated reactivity to thyroglobulin resembling that seen in Hashimoto's thyroiditis.

Experimentally Induced Autoimmunity in Animals

A number of experimental animal models have autoimmune dysfunctions similar to certain human autoimmune diseases (see Table 17-2). One of the first such animal models was discovered serendipitously in 1973 when rabbits were immunized with acetylcholine receptors purified from electric eels. The animals soon developed muscular weakness similar to that seen in myasthenia gravis. Soon this experimental autoimmune myasthenia gravis (EAMG) was shown to be caused when antibody to the acetylcholine receptor blocked muscle stimulation by acetylcholine in the synapse. Within a year this animal model had proved its value with the discovery that autoantibodies to the acetylcholine receptor were the cause of myasthenia gravis in humans.

Experimental autoimmune encephalomyelitis (EAE) is another animal model that has greatly improved understanding of autoimmunity. EAE can be induced in a variety of species by immunization with myelin basic protein (MBP) in complete Freund adjuvant. Within 2–3 weeks the animals develop cellular infiltration of the myelin sheaths of the central nervous system, resulting in demyelination and development of paralysis. Most of the animals die, but some recover and are now resistant to the development of disease after a subsequent injection of MBP and adjuvant. EAE is considered to be a good laboratory model for multiple sclerosis. Experimental autoimmune thyroiditis (EAT) can be induced in a number of animals by immunization with thyroglobulin in complete Freund adjuvant. Both humoral antibodies and T$_{DTH}$ cells directed against the thyroglobulin develop, resulting in thyroid inflammation. EAT appears to best mimic Hashimoto's thyroiditis. In contrast to both EAE and EAT, which are induced by immunization with self-antigens, autoimmune arthritis (AA) is induced by immunization of rats with *Mycobacterium tuberculosis* in complete Freund adjuvant. These animals develop an arthritis whose features are similar to those of rheumatoid arthritis in humans.

Role of the T$_H$ Cell, MHC, and T-Cell Receptor in Autoimmunity

The inappropriate response to self-antigens that characterizes all autoimmune diseases can involve either the humoral or the cell-mediated branch. Identifying the underlying defect in human autoimmune diseases has been difficult. Characterization of the immune defect in the various animal models has been more successful.

Surprisingly, each of the animal models has implicated the T$_H$ cell as the primary mediator of autoimmune disease. In addition, susceptibility to certain autoimmune diseases has been associated with particular MHC alleles and TCR variable-region exons.

Evidence for T$_H$-Cell Role

Autoimmune T-cell clones have been obtained from all of the animal models listed in Table 17-2 by culturing lymphocytes from the autoimmune animals in the presence of various T-cell growth factors and then inducing proliferation of specific autoimmune clones with the various autoantigens. For example, when lymph-node cells from EAE rats are cultured in vitro with myelin basic protein, clones of activated T cells emerge. When these MBP-specific T-cell clones are injected intravenously in sufficient numbers into normal syngeneic animals, the cells penetrate the blood-brain barrier and induce demyelination; EAE develops within 5 days (Figure 17-6). With a similar experimental protocol, T-cell clones specific for thyroglobulin and for *M. tuberculosis* can be isolated from EAT and AA animals, respectively. In each case the T-cell clone induces the experimental autoimmune disease in normal animals. Examination of these T cells has revealed that they bear the CD4 membrane marker. In a number of animal models for autoimmune diseases it has been possible to reverse the

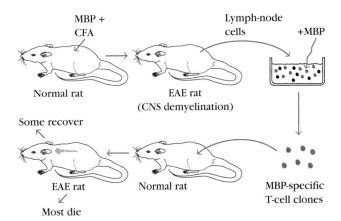

Figure 17-6 Experimental autoimmune encephalomyelitis (EAE) can be induced by injecting rats with myelin basic protein (MBP) in complete Freund's adjuvant (CFA). MBP-specific T-cell clones can be generated by culturing lymph-node cells from EAE rats with MBP. These T cells can then transfer the disease to normal animals.

autoimmunity by depleting the T-cell population with antibody directed against CD4. For example, weekly injections of anti-CD4 monoclonal antibody abolished the autoimmune symptoms in NZB × NZW mice and in mice with EAE.

Evidence for Association with MHC and T-Cell Receptor

Since T_H-cell recognition of antigen involves a trimolecular complex of an MHC molecule, peptide antigen, and T-cell receptor (TCR), the generation of self-reactive T_H cells requires that a susceptible individual possess both MHC molecules and T-cell receptors capable of binding self-antigens. A number of recent publications have revealed an association between expression of a particular MHC allele or T-cell receptor and susceptibility to autoimmunity.

Several of these studies have used the EAE animal model, whose inducing antigen—myelin basic protein (MBP)—has been well characterized and sequenced. Various MBP peptides have been assessed for their ability to activate T_H cells and elicit autoimmune encephalomyelitis reactions. The results of such experiments show that inbred mice expressing different MHC haplotypes develop EAE in response to different MBP peptides (Figure 17-7). Moreover, the same peptides that induce EAE in a given strain also induce maximal T_H-cell proliferation.

By using antibodies to type the HLA alleles expressed by individuals with various autoimmune diseases, it has been shown that some HLA alleles occur at a much higher frequency among autoimmune individuals than in the general population. The association between the expression of a given HLA allele and an autoimmune disease is expressed as the relative risk:

Relative risk =

$$\frac{\text{(patient with HLA allele) X (controls without HLA allele)}}{\text{(patients without HLA allele) X (controls with HLA allele)}}$$

A relative risk value of 1 means that the HLA allele is expressed with the same frequency in the autoimmune and control subpopulations whereas a relative risk value substantially above 1 indicates an association between the HLA allele and the autoimmune disease. However, the fact that there is an association should not be interpreted to imply that the expression of the MHC allele has caused the disease. The relationship between these MHC alleles and development of an autoimmune disease is complex. That these diseases are not inherited via simple Mendelian segregation of MHC alleles can be seen in identical twins when both inherit the MHC risk factor

but only one develops autoimmunity. This suggests that multiple genetic factors and environmental factors have roles in the development of autoimmunity, with the MHC playing an important but not exclusive role. As the antigens inducing human autoimmune diseases are identified and sequenced, it will be possible to analyze the linkage between the MHC and various diseases more fully.

Table 17-3 lists a number of human autoimmune diseases in which there is an association between a particular MHC allele and susceptibility to the disease. One difficulty in assigning an association to a particular MHC allele to autoimmunity is the genetic phenomenon of *linkage disequilibrium* in which two alleles are inherited together with a higher frequency than normally expected. Initially class I MHC alleles were shown to be associated with autoimmunity. But later most autoimmune diseases were shown to be much more strongly associated with class II MHC. The fact that some of the class I MHC alleles were in linkage disequilibrium with the class II MHC alleles made their contribution to autoimmune susceptibility appear more pronounced than it actually was.

By using the polymerase chain reaction (PCR) Hugh Mc Devitt and his co-workers analyzed the nucleotide sequences of class II MHC genes from patients with different autoimmune diseases. They found that there were short sequences within the α_1 and β_1 domains of the class II MHC that appear to play a major role in susceptibility and resistance to autoimmunity. These sequences are thought to be located within the peptide binding groove of the class II MHC molecule. In patients with insulin dependent diabetes mellitus (IDDM) and in the mouse model for diabetes (the NOD mouse) a single

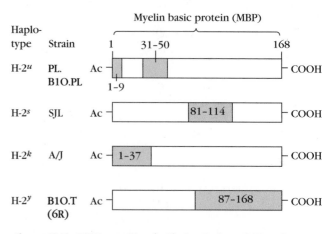

Figure 17-7 MBP peptides (red) that induce EAE and maximal T-cell proliferation in various inbred mouse strains. The haplotype of the mouse strain appears to determine which peptides are encephalitogenic.

amino acid change at residue 57 in the HLA-DQβ chain was found to correlate with resistance or susceptibility to diabetes. An aspartic residue at position 57 of the DQβ chain correlated with resistance to IDDM while a valine, serine, or alanine at this position correlated with susceptibility to IDDM. Presumably the differences in amino acids at this position influence the binding of different self-peptides to the class II MHC.

Use of particular T-cell receptor gene segments has also been linked to the development of autoimmunity. Identification of the encephalitogenic MBP peptides in different inbred strains enabled investigators to clone T cells specific for individual peptides. For example, PL- and B1O.PL-strain mice recognize two encephalitogenic peptides of MBP (peptide 35-47 and the acetylated N-terminal nonapeptide 1–9). Both peptides are recognized in association with the class II IA^u molecule. By culturing T cells from these strains with each of these peptides, T-cell clones responsive to each peptide have been obtained. Analysis of T-cell receptors in these clones has shown that both strains have an unusually high percentage of T cells in which the TCR V$_\beta$8.2 exon and V$_\alpha$4 or V$_\alpha$2.3 exons are expressed. The PL strain, for example, expresses V$_\beta$8.2 in about 80% of its T-cell clones and V$_\alpha$4 in 100% of its T-cell clones. It is thought that the preferential expression of T-cell-receptor genes in these autoimmune T-cell clones may contribute to disease susceptibility in these strains of mice. In human autoimmune diseases, evidence for selected TCR expression has been shown so far for multiple sclerosis and for myasthenia gravis.

Proposed Mechanisms of Autoimmunity

A variety of mechanisms have been proposed to account for the T-cell–mediated generation of autoimmune diseases (Figure 17-8). Evidence exists for each of these mechanisms, and it is likely that autoimmunity does not develop from a single event but rather from a number of different events.

Release of Sequestered Antigens

As discussed in Chapter 14, the induction of tolerance in self-reactive T cells is thought to occur through exposure of immature lymphocytes to self-antigens during development. Any tissue antigens that are sequestered from the circulation, and therefore are not seen by the developing immune system, will not induce self-tolerance. Exposure of mature T cells to such normally sequestered antigens at a later date might result in their

Table 17-3 HLA alleles associated with increased risk for various autoimmune diseases

Disease	HLA allele	Relative risk[*]
Ankylosing spondylitis	B27	90
Goodpasture's syndrome	DR2	16
Grave's disease	B8/DR3	3–4
Insulin-dependent diabetes mellitus	DR4/DR3 DR3/DQW8	20 100
Juvenile rheumatoid arthritis	B27/DR5	4
Multiple sclerosis	DR2	5
Myasthenia gravis	DR3	10
Pernicious anemia	DR5	5
Psoriatic arthritis (central)	B27	11
Reiter's syndrome	B27	37
Rheumatoid arthritis	Dw4/DR4	10
Sjögren's syndrome	Dw3	6
Systemic lupus erythematosus	DR3	5
Ulcerative colitis	B5	4

[*] Likelihood of developing disease compared to the general population, which is assigned a risk value of 1.

activation.

Myelin basic protein is an example of an antigen normally sequestered from the immune system, in this case by the blood-brain barrier. In the EAE model, animals are injected directly with MBP, together with adjuvant, under conditions that maximize immune exposure. In this type of animal model, the immune system is exposed to sequestered self-antigens under nonphysiologic conditions, but trauma to tissues following either an accident or a viral or bacterial infection might also release sequestered antigens into the circulation. A few tissue antigens are known to fall into this category. For example, sperm arise late in development and are sequestered from the circulation, but after a vasectomy, some sperm antigens are released into the circulation and can induce autoantibody formation in some men. Similarly the release of lens protein after eye damage or of heart-muscle antigens after myocardial infarction has been shown to lead to autoantibody formation on occasion.

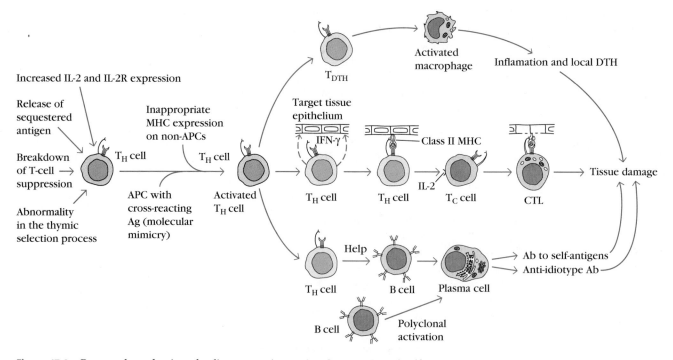

Figure 17-8 Proposed mechanisms leading to autoimmunity. Once activated self-reactive T_H cells (red) are generated, they act in various ways to mediate an autoimmune response, in this case involving tissue damage. In all likelihood, several mechanisms are involved in each autoimmune disease. See text for details. [Adapted from V. Kumar et al., 1989, *Annu. Rev. Immunol.* **7**:657.]

Cross-Reacting Antigens

A number of viruses and bacteria have been shown to possess antigenic determinants that are identical to or similar to normal host-cell components. This *molecular mimicry* appears to occur in a wide variety of organisms (Table 17-4). In one study 600 different monoclonal antibodies, specific for 11 different viruses, were tested to evaluate their reactivity with normal tissue antigens. More than 3% of the virus-specific antibodies tested also bound to normal tissue, suggesting that molecular mimicry is a fairly common phenomenon.

Molecular mimicry has been suggested as one mechanism leading to autoimmunity. One of the best examples of this type of autoimmune reaction is post-rabies encephalitis, which used to develop in some individuals who had received the rabies vaccine. In the past, the rabies virus was grown in rabbit brain-cell cultures, and preparations of the vaccine included antigens derived from the rabbit brain cells. In a vaccinated person these rabbit brain-cell antigens could induce formation of antibodies and activated T cells, which could cross-react with the recipient's own brain cells and lead to encephalitis. Cross-reacting antibodies are also thought to be the cause of heart damage in rheumatic fever, which

usually develops after a *Streptococcus* infection. In this case the antibodies are to streptococcal antigens, but they cross-react with the heart muscle.

Since the encephalitogenic MBP peptides are known, the extent to which they are molecularly mimicked by proteins from other organisms can be assessed. In one study, the sequence of the encephalitogenic MBP peptide (66–75) was compared with the known sequences of a large number of viral proteins. This computer analysis revealed sequence homologies between this MBP peptide and a number of animal viruses, including influenza, polyoma, adenovirus, Rous sarcoma, Abelson leukemia, poliomyelitis, Epstein-Barr virus, and hepatitis B. A peptide from the polymerase enzyme of the hepatitis B virus was particularly striking: a sequence of six of its 10 amino acids was homologous with a sequence in the encephalitogenic MBP peptide. To test the hypothesis of molecular mimicry as a mechanism for autoimmunity, rabbits were immunized with this hepatitis B virus peptide. The peptide was shown to induce both the formation of antibody and the proliferation of T cells that cross-reacted with MBP; in addition, central nervous system tissue from the immunized rabbits showed cellular infiltration characteristic of that seen in EAE. These findings suggest that infection with certain viruses express-

Table 17-4 Molecular mimicry between proteins of infectious organisms and human host proteins*

Protein	Residue†	Sequence‡
Human cytomegalovirus IE2	79	PDP**LGRPD**ED
HLA-DR molecule	60	VTE**LGRPD**AE
Poliovirus VP2	70	STT**KESRGT**T
Acetylcholine receptor	176	TVI**KESRGT**K
Papilloma virus E2	76	SLH**LESLKD**S
Insulin receptor	66	VYG**LESLKD**L
Rabies virus glycoprotein	147	T**KESLV**IIS
Insulin receptor	764	N**KESLV**ISE
Klebsiella pneumoniae nitrogenase	186	SR**QTDRED**E
HLA-B27 molecule	70	KA**QTDRED**L
Adenovirus 12 E1B	384	LRRGM**FRPSQ**CN
α-gliadin	206	LGQGS**FRPSQ**QN
Human immunodeficiency virus p24	160	**GVETTPS**
Human IgG constant region	466	**GVETTPS**
Measles virus P3	13	**LECIRA**LK
Corticotropin	18	**LECIRA**CK
Measles virus P3	31	**EIS**DN**LGQE**
Myelin basic protein	61	**EIS**FK**LGQE**

* In each pair, the human protein is listed second. The proteins in each pair have been shown to exhibit immunologic cross-reactivity.

† Each number indicates the position in the intact protein of the amino-terminal amino acid in the indicated peptide.

‡ Sequences are indicated by single-letter code.

SOURCE: Adapted from M. B. A. Oldstone, 1987, *Cell* **50**:819.

ing epitopes that mimic sequestered self-components may induce autoimmunity to those components. Susceptibility to this type of autoimmunity may also be influenced by the MHC haplotype of the individual, since certain class I and class II MHC molecules may be more effective than others in presenting the homologous peptide for T-cell activation.

Inappropriate Expression of Class II MHC Molecules

The beta cells of individuals with insulin-dependent diabetes mellitus (IDDM) have recently been shown to express high levels of both class I and class II MHC molecules, whereas healthy beta cells express lower levels of class I and do not express class II at all. Similarly, in Graves' disease thyroid acinar cells have been shown to express class II MHC molecules on their membranes. This inappropriate expression of class II MHC molecules, which are normally expressed only on antigen-

presenting cells, may serve to sensitize T$_H$ cells to peptides derived from the beta cells or thyroid cells, allowing activation of B cells or T$_C$ cells or sensitization of T$_{DTH}$ cells against self-antigens.

Other evidence suggests that certain agents can induce some cells that should not express class II MHC molecules to express them. For example, the T-cell mitogen phytohemagglutinin (PHA) has been shown to induce thyroid cells to express class II molecules. In vitro studies reveal that interferon gamma (IFN-γ) also induces increases in class II MHC molecules on a wide variety of cells, including pancreatic beta cells, intestinal epithelial cells, melanoma cells, and thyroid acinar cells. M. Feldman and G. F. Bottazzo have hypothesized that trauma or viral infection in an organ may induce a localized inflammatory response, and thus increased concentrations of IFN-γ, in the affected organ. If IFN-γ induces class II MHC expression on non-antigen-presenting cells, inappropriate T$_H$-cell activation might follow, with autoimmune consequences. It is noteworthy that SLE patients with active disease have higher serum titers of IFN-γ than patients with inactive disease. Feldman and Bottazzo suggested that the increase in IFN-γ in these patients may lead to inappropriate expression of class II MHC molecules and thus to T-cell activation against a variety of autoantigens.

In one experiment the role of inappropriate class II MHC expression was studied in transgenic mice. By injecting DNA carrying special promoters, one can limit the expression of the transgene to certain tissues where the promoter is activated. By such means transgenic mice were developed in which expression of class II MHC genes was controlled by the insulin promoter. In these mice the class II MHC genes were expressed at high levels in pancreatic beta cells but not in other tissues. The mice became diabetic and suffered degeneration of their beta cells, suggesting a link between inappropriate class II MHC expression and diabetes in these mice. One puzzling aspect of this experiment, however, was that lymphocytes and inflammatory cells were not observed to penetrate the pancreas in these mice. Might, then, the diabetes observed in these mice be due to some other component of the transgenic system and not to autoimmunity? For example, the abnormally high levels of class II MHC molecules in these transgenic mice may in itself inhibit the normal secretory functions of the pancreatic beta cell and decrease insulin secretion. Or class II MHC molecules may actually bind to insulin and reduce its activity, giving rise to diabetes without autoimmunity. Although the actual mechanism of diabetes in these class II MHC transgenic mice has not been established, the association between inappropriate class II MHC expression and autoimmunity is intriguing.

Lymphokine Imbalance

Increased production of interleukin 2 (IL-2) or an increased responsiveness to IL-2 has been observed in a number of autoimmune diseases. The Obese chicken, an animal model for Hashimoto's thyroiditis, shows increased IL-2 production and increased levels of the IL-2 receptor on T-cells. Elevated IL-2 serum levels have also been observed in active SLE patients and in patients with multiple sclerosis, and increased expression of the IL-2 receptor has been observed in multiple sclerosis and myasthenia gravis patients.

G. Kroemer and G. Wick have suggested that perturbations in the regulation of expression of IL-2 and its receptor (IL-2R) may have several possible consequences that could lead to autoimmune manifestations (Figure 17-9). Increased expression of IL-2 and IL-2R, for example, could promote T-cell activation, resulting in production of other lymphokines and possibly leading to various effector functions that might cause tissue damage. Overproduction of IL-2 or other lymphokines

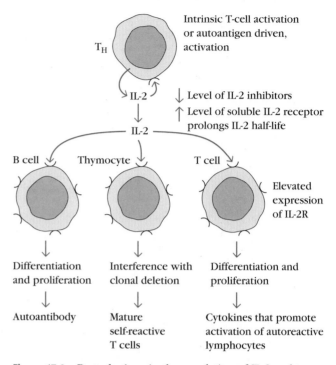

Figure 17-9   Perturbations in the regulation of IL-2 and IL-2R expression have been postulated to lead to autoimmune consequences. [Adapted from G. Kroemer and G. Wick, 1989, *Immunol. Today* **10**:246.]

from activated T$_H$ cells also could result in excessive B-cell activation and autoantibody production. Finally, increased IL-2—IL-2R expression on thymocytes might allow some of the thymocytes to escape clonal deletion within the thymus.

An interesting transgenic mouse system that implicates lymphokines in autoimmunity was developed by Nora Sarvetnik. In this system the IFN-γ transgenic was genetically engineered with the insulin promoter, so that the mice secreted IFN-γ from their pancreatic beta cells. Since IFN-γ upregulates class II MHC expression, these mice also express class II MHC molecules on their pancreatic beta cells. The mice developed diabetes, which (in contrast to the class II transgenic system previously described) was associated with cellular infiltration of lymphocytes and inflammatory cells similar to the infiltration seen in autoimmune NOD mice and in patients with insulin-dependent diabetes mellitus (Figure 17-10). Since IFN-γ induces class II MHC expression, inappropriate class II MHC expression on the beta cells may be involved in the autoimmune reaction. At the same time, other factors may also be involved in the development of autoimmunity in this system. For example, IFN-γ is also known to induce production of several other lymphokines, including IL-1 and TNF. Therefore, the development of autoimmunity in this transgenic system

(a)

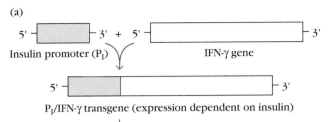

P$_I$/IFN-γ transgene (expression dependent on insulin)

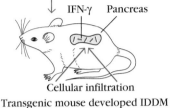

Transgenic mouse developed IDDM

Figure 17-10 Insulin-dependent diabetes mellitus (IDDM) in transgenic mice. Production of transgenic mice containing IFN-γ transgene linked to the insulin promoter (P$_I$). The transgenics, which expressed the P$_I$/IFN-γ transgene only in the pancreas, developed symptoms characteristic of IDDM. (b) Pancreatic islets of Langerhans from a normal BALB/c mouse (*left*) and from P$_I$/IFN-γ transgenics at 3 weeks (*center*) and 6 weeks (*right*) showing infiltration of inflammatory cells. [Part (b) from N. Sarvetnick et al., 1988, *Cell* **52**:773.]

(b)

may involve antigen presentation by class II MHC molecules on the pancreatic beta cells, together with a co-stimulatory signal, such as IL-1, that may activate self-reactive T cells. There is also some evidence to suggest that IL-1 may itself damage beta cells.

Dysfunction of the Idiotype Network Regulatory Pathways

As discussed in Chapter 14, production of anti-idiotype antibody that presents an internal image of a foreign antigen is thought to enhance the immune response and thus contribute to host defense (see Figure 14-3). However, production of anti-idiotype antibodies to self-proteins may contribute to autoimmune reactions in some cases.

The first evidence linking anti-idiotype antibody and autoimmunity was discovered serendipitiously. B. F. Er-

langer and colleagues were studying the acetylcholine analog Bis Q, a potent agonist of the acetylcholine receptor (AChR), whose molecular structure is complementary to the combining site of the AChR. They immunized rabbits with Bis Q to make anti-Bis Q. When other rabbits were immunized with anti-Bis Q, they developed signs of myasthenia gravis (Figure 17-11). In later experiments hybridomas secreting monoclonal anti-idiotype antibodies (anti-anti-Bis Q) were produced. When these hybridomas were injected into the peritoneal cavity of three female and three male mice, all the female mice developed myasthenia gravis.

In Graves' disease antibodies are produced to the receptor for thyroid-stimulating hormone (TSH). These antibodies bind to the receptor and stimulate the thyroid inappropriately (see Figure 17-4a). Experimentally it is possible to make antibody specific for TSH and then make antibody to this antibody (anti-idiotype). This anti-idiotype antibody has been shown to stimulate the TSH

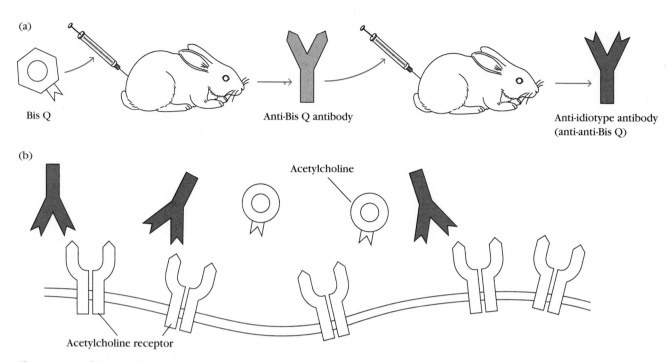

Figure 17-11   (a) Induction of experimental myasthenia gravis in rabbits by immunization with antibodies to Bis Q, an acetylcholine analog. The antibodies to Bis Q induce production of anti-idiotype antibodies (red) in these rabbits. (b) Some of the anti-idiotype antibody binds to the acethycholine receptor, blocking binding of acetylcholine and causing symptoms of myasthenia gravis.

receptor. So far, one patient with Graves' diseases has been shown to have developed an idiotype-anti-idiotype network of antibodies that participate in the autoimmune response.

Dysfunction of T-Cell–Mediated Immune Regulation

Studies of immune dysfunction in NZB mice have revealed a loss of T-cell mediated suppression activity that parallels the development of autoimmunity. As noted earlier, these mice exhibit hyperactive B-cell and T-cell responses to numerous self-proteins, mimicking SLE. When thymocytes from NZB mice 1–3 months old are injected into older NZB mice, there is a delay in the onset of the usual spontaneous autoimmune disease, suggesting that the young thymocytes have restored the immune imbalance in the NZB mouse. The Obese chicken also shows less T-cell–mediated suppression activity than control populations. When thymocytes from normal chickens were added to an in vitro culture of CTLs specific for thyroglobulin-coated chicken CRBCs, the thymocytes suppressed the cytotoxic response. However, when thymocytes from 3-week-old Obese chickens were added to the in vitro culture, there was no such suppression of cytotoxicity. The development of autoimmune thyroiditis in these young chickens may therefore reflect a decrease in their T-cell

suppression activity. Patients with a systemic autoimmune disease (e.g., systemic lupus erythematosus, rheumatoid arthritis, multiple sclerosis) also appear to have a general regulatory T-cell defect that causes hyperactivity of both B cells and T cells.

Work with experimental autoimmune encephalomyelitis (EAE) has suggested that restoration of the regulatory T-cell subpopulation can reverse autoimmunity. EAE can be induced in rats by injection of myelin basic protein (MBP) in adjuvant or of T-cell lines activated in vitro with MBP (see Figure 17-6). Some rats recover spontaneously and are resistant to further attempts to induce EAE by injection of MBP in adjuvant. There is a great deal of interest in understanding the immune state of these resistant rats. In one study female rats were injected with a male MBP-reactive T-cell line activated in vitro with MBP. As expected, these rats developed EAE and some of them recovered and became resistant to EAE induction by MBP. Months later two populations of thymocytes were isolated from the thymus of these resistant rats. One population bore the male karyotype of the original MBP-reactive T-cell line, which must have survived in the thymus of the resistant female rats. The other population of thymocytes was derived from the resistant female rats and was shown to specifically suppress the MBP-reactive T cells in vitro. This finding suggests that the presence of a low number of autoimmune MBP-specific T cells within the thymus had induced a population of T cells capable of specifically suppressing the autoimmune T cells and thus inducing resistance to EAE. Analysis of these T cells revealed that they were T_H1 cells: apparently a restoration of the balance of T_H1 cells had reversed the autoimmune disease.

Autoimmunity and Heat Shock Proteins

Heat shock proteins are a family of proteins produced by mammalian cells in response to elevated temperatures or other cellular stresses. This protein family is not unique to mammalian cells and is found in a wide variety of bacterial and parasitic pathogens. What makes this protein family interesting is their remarkable evolutionary conservation; mammalian and microbial heat shock proteins share more than 50% sequence identity. Despite their sequence homology, these proteins have been shown to serve as major immunodominant antigens in a variety of bacterial and parasitic infections. This finding is paradoxical, since one would expect that a state of immunologic tolerance should exist to foreign proteins that mimic self-components so closely. What keeps the immune response to microbial heat shock proteins from reacting with self–heat shock proteins and inducing an autoimmune response?

Recently, an immune response to heat shock proteins has been implicated in a number of autoimmune diseases. Individuals suffering from rheumatoid arthritis have been shown to have T cells responsive to mycobacterial heat shock protein (hsp65), suggesting that there may be some relationship between an immune response to this family of proteins and autoimmunity. In NOD mice, about two months prior to the onset of autoimmune destruction of the pancreatic beta cells, antibodies to hsp65 can be detected. In addition, T cells clones reactive to hsp65 have been isolated from prediabetic NOD mice. When these T cell clones are injected into an H-2 compatible, nondiabetic strain, the nondiabetic strain develops diabetes. These findings implicate an immune response to heat shock proteins to the development of rheumatoid arthritis and diabetes.

What is perplexing is that when normal individuals are immunized with killed Mycobacteria, 8 out of 9 individuals produce T cells that have been activated to hsp65. Why doesn't the response to hsp65 result in the development of autoimmunity in each of these individuals? Several proposals have been suggested. One hypothesis is that the MHC allelic products may determine which peptides of hsp65 are presented to immune T cells. Some MHC alleles may favor the presentation of microbial heat shock peptides that are likely to cross-react with self-proteins, whereas other MHC alleles may bind a different set of peptides. Another hypothesis has suggested that an immune response to heat shock pro-

teins occurs naturally but that is normally kept in check by a regulatory population of anti-idiotype T cells specific for the anti-hsp T cells.

Polyclonal B-Cell Activation

A number of viruses and bacteria can induce nonspecific polyclonal B-cell activation. Gram-negative bacteria, cytomegalovirus, and Epstein-Barr virus (EBV) are all known to be such activators, inducing the proliferation of numerous clones of B cells that secrete IgM in the absence of T_H cells. If B cells reactive to self-antigens are activated by this mechanism, autoantibodies can appear. During infectious mononucleosis, which is caused by EBV, a variety of autoantibodies are produced, including autoantibodies reactive to T and B cells, rheumatoid factors, and antinuclear antibodies. Similarly, lymphocytes from patients with SLE produce large quantities of IgM in culture, suggesting that they have been polyclonally activated. Many AIDS patients also show high levels of nonspecific antibody and autoantibodies to RBCs and platelets. These patients are often co-infected with other viruses such as EBV and cytomegalovirus, which may induce the polyclonal B-cell activation that results in autoantibody production.

Treatment of Autoimmune Diseases

Ideally, treatments for autoimmune diseases should be aimed at reducing only the autoimmune response while leaving the rest of the immune system intact. To date, this ideal has not been reached.

Current Therapies

Current treatments for autoimmune diseases are not cures but merely palliatives, aimed at reducing symptoms to provide the patient with an acceptable quality of life. For the most part these treatments aim at nonspecific suppression of the immune system, and their nonspecific nature often results in adverse side effects. Immunosuppressive drugs (e.g., corticosteroids, azathioprine, and cyclophosphamide) are often given with the intent of slowing proliferation of lymphocytes in general. By depressing the immune response in general, such drugs can reduce the severity of autoimmune symptoms. The general reduction in immune responsiveness, however, puts the patient at greater risk for infection or the development of cancer.

Another therapeutic approach that has had some success with some autoimmune diseases, such as myasthenia gravis, is removal of the thymus. Because patients with this disease often have thymic abnormalities (e.g., thymic hyperplasia or thymomas), adult thymectomy often increases the likelihood of remission of symptoms.

Plasmapheresis is a process in which plasma is removed from a patient's blood by continuous-flow centrifugation. The red blood cells are then resuspended in a suitable medium and returned to the patient. This process has been beneficial to patients with autoimmune diseases involving antigen-antibody complexes, which are removed with the plasma. Removal of the complexes, although only temporary, can result in a short-term reduction in symptoms. Patients with Graves' disease, myasthenia gravis, rheumatoid arthritis, and systemic lupus erythematosus are among those who have experienced short-term benefits from plasmapheresis.

Experimental Therapeutic Approaches

Studies with experimental autoimmune animal models have provided evidence that it is indeed possible to induce specific immunity to the development of autoimmunity.

T-Cell Vaccination

I. R. Cohen and his co-workers have been pioneers in T-cell vaccination. His research group found that animals injected with low doses ($< 10^4$) of cloned T cells specific for MBP did not develop symptoms of EAE and instead were resistant to the development of EAE when later challenged with a lethal dose of activated MBP-specific T cells or MBP in adjuvant. Later findings revealed that the efficacy of these autoimmune T-cell clones as a vaccine can be enhanced by cross-linking the cell-membrane components with formaldehyde or glutaraldehyde. When these cross-linked T cells were injected into animals with active EAE, permanent remission of symptoms was observed. The cross-linked T-cell clones apparently elicit both CD4 and CD8 anti-idiotype T cells of the recepient that recognize the clustered receptors on the autoimmune clones. Presumably these anti-idiotype T cells act to suppress the T cells that mediate EAE.

The effectiveness of the vaccine approach in animal models has led to clinical testing in human autoimmune disease. For example, a 42-year-old woman with severe progressive multiple sclerosis has been injected subcutaneously with T cells that had been isolated from her own cerebrospinal fluid, cloned in vitro, and cross-linked with formaldehyde. The progression of her disease is currently being monitored. If this approach works, it represents a specific therapy that reduces only a specific

autoimmune response without affecting overall immune responsiveness.

Monoclonal-Antibody Treatment

Monoclonal antibodies have been used successfully to treat autoimmune disease in several animal models. For example, a high percentage of F_1 (NZB × NZW) mice given weekly injections of high doses of monoclonal antibody specific for the CD4 membrane molecule recovered from their autoimmune lupus-like symptoms (Figure 17-12). Similar positive results were observed in NOD mice, in which treatment with an anti-CD4 monoclonal led to disappearance of the lymphocytic infiltration and diabetic symptoms. Because anti-CD4 monoclonals block or deplete all T_H cells, regardless of their specificity, they can threaten the overall immune responsiveness of the recipient. One remedy for this disadvantage is to try to block antigen-activated T_H cells, since these cells are involved in the autoimmune state. To do this, researchers have used monoclonal antibody directed against the high-affinity IL-2 receptor. Since only antigen-activated T_H cells express this membrane molecule and since the high-affinity receptor is involved in IL-2–mediated T_H-cell proliferation, monoclonal antibody against this receptor might specifically block antigen-activated T_H cells. This approach was tested in adult rats injected with activated MBP-specific T cells in the presence or absence of monoclonal antibody specific for the IL-2 receptor. All the control rats died of EAE, whereas six of the nine treated with the monoclonal antibody had no symptoms, and the symptoms in the other three were mild.

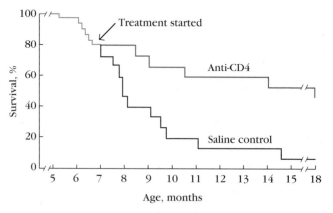

Figure 17-12 Effect of weekly injections of anti-CD4 monoclonal antibody on survival of F_1 (NZB × NZW) mice exhibiting autoimmune lupus-like symptoms. [From D. Wofsy, 1988, Treatment of autoimmune diseases with monoclonal antibodies, in *Monoclonal Antibody Therapy*, Prog. Allergy, H. Waldmann (ed.)]

The association of autoimmune disease with restricted TCR expression in a number of mouse models has prompted researchers to see if blockage of the preferred receptors with monoclonal antibody might be therapeutic. Injection of PL mice with monoclonal antibody specific for the $V_\beta 8$ T-cell receptor prevented EAE induction with MBP in adjuvant. What was even more exciting was the finding that the anti-$V_\beta 8$ monoclonal antibody could also reverse the symptoms of autoimmunity in mice manifesting induced EAE (Figure 17-13) and that these mice manifested long-term remission. Clearly, the use of monoclonal antibodies as a treatment for human autoimmune diseases presents exciting possibilities.

Similarly, the association of various MHC alleles with autoimmunity as well as the evidence for increased or inappropriate MHC expression in some autoimmune diseases has prompted some researchers to suggest that development of autoimmunity might be retarded with monoclonal antibodies specific for an appropriate MHC allelic product. Since antigen-presenting cells express many class II MHC molecules, it might be possible to selectively block an MHC molecule that is associated with autoimmunity, while sparing the other class II MHC molecules. In one study, injection of mice with monoclonal antibodies to class II MHC molecules prior to injection of myelin basic protein blocked the development of EAE. If, instead, the antibody was given after the injection of myelin basic protein, development of EAE was delayed but not prevented. In nonhuman primates, monoclonal antibodies to HLA-DR and HLA-DQ have been shown to reverse EAE.

Summary

1. Human autoimmune diseases can be divided into organ-specific and systemic diseases. The organ-specific diseases involve an autoimmune response directed primarily against a single organ or gland. In contrast, the systemic diseases are directed against a broad spectrum of tissues and have manifestations in a variety of organs.

2. There are both spontaneous and experimental animal models for autoimmune diseases. Spontaneous models include a disease in NZB and NZB × NZW F_1 mice that parallels systemic lupus erythematosus, a thyroiditis seen in Obese-strain chickens that parallels Hashimoto thyroiditis, and a diabetes in NOD mice that resembles human insulin-dependent diabetes mellitus. Several experimental animal models have been developed by immunizing animals with self-antigens in the presence of adjuvant. In experimental autoimmune myasthenia gravis (EAMG), the antigen is the acetylcholine receptor; in experimental autoimmune encephalomyelitis (EAE), the antigen is myelin basic protein; in experimental autoimmune thyroiditis (EAT), the antigen is thyroglobulin.

3. The experimental autoimmune animal models have revealed a central role for the T_H cell in the development of autoimmunity. In each of the experimentally induced autoimmune diseases, autoimmune T-cell clones can be isolated that induce the autoimmune disease in normal animals. The MHC haplotype of the experimental animal determines the ability to present various autoantigens to T_H cells. In addition, some autoimmune animals utilize a restricted repertoire of TCR genes, which may predispose the animal toward T-cell activity in response to a given self-antigen.

4. A variety of mechanisms have been proposed for autoimmunity, including release of sequestered antigens, molecular mimicry, inappropriate class II MHC expression on cells, a lymphokine imbalance, a dysfunction of the idiotype network, a dysfunction of T-cell–mediated suppression, and polyclonal activation of lymphocytes. Evidence exists for each of these mechanisms, reflecting the many different pathways leading to autoimmune reactions.

5. Current therapies for autoimmune diseases include treatment with immunosuppressive drugs, thymectomy, and plasmapheresis for diseases involving immune complexes. These therapies, which are relatively nonspecific, may have significant side effects. Two general types of

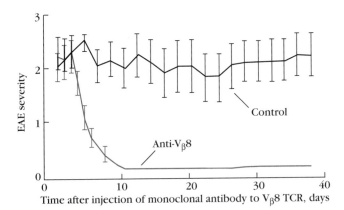

Figure 17-13 Effect of injection of monoclonal antibody to the $V_\beta 8$ T-cell receptor on PL mice exhibiting EAE symptoms. EAE was induced by injecting mice with MBP-specific T-cell clones. EAE severity scale: 3 = total paralysis of lower limbs; 2 = partial paralysis of lower limbs; 1 = limp tail; 0 = normal (no symptoms). [Adapted from H. Acha-Orbea, L. Steinman, and H. O. McDevitt. 1989. T cell receptors in murine autoimmune diseases. *Ann. Rev. Immunol.* 7:371.]

more specific therapy have shown some success in various animal models for autoimmune diseases. These approaches are vaccination with T cells specific for a given self-antigen and administration of monoclonal antibodies that react with some component specifically involved in an autoimmune reaction.

References

ACHA-ORBEA, H., L. STEINMAN, and H. O. MCDEVITT. 1989. T cell receptors in murine autoimmune diseases. *Annu. Rev. Immunol.* 7:37.

COHEN, I. R. 1989. T cell vaccination against autoimmune disease. *Hosp. Prac.* (Feb. 15):57.

COHEN, I. R. 1991. Autoimmunity to chaperonins in the pathogenesis of arthritis and diabetes. *Annu. Rev. Immunol.* 9:567.

HASKINS, K., and M. MCDUFFIE. 1990. Acceleration of diabetes in young NOD mice with a CD4$^+$ islet-specific T cell clone. *Science* 249:1433.

KANTOR, F. S. 1988. Autoimmunities: diseases of "dysregulation." *Hosp. Prac.* (July 15):75.

KROEMER, G., and G. WICK. 1989. The role of interleukin 2 in autoimmunity. *Immunol. Today* 10:246.

KRONENBERG, M. 1991. Self-tolerance and autoimmunity. *Cell* 65:537.

KUMAR, V., D. H. KONO, J. L. URBAN, and L. HOOD. 1989. The T cell receptor repertoire and autoimmune diseases. *Annu. Rev. Immunol.* 7:657.

OKSENBERG, J. R., et al. 1989. T cell receptor V$_\alpha$ and C$_\alpha$ alleles associated with multiple sclerosis and myasthenia gravis. *Proc. Nat'l. Acad. Sci. USA.* 86:988.

SEBOUN, E., et al. 1989. A susceptibility locus for multiple sclerosis is linked to the T cell receptor β^- chain complex. *Cell* 57:1095.

SINHA, A. A., M. T. LOPEZ, and H. O. MCDEVITT. 1990. Autoimmune diseases: the failure of self-tolerance. *Science* 248:1380.

WALDMAN, H. 1989. Manipulation of T cell responses with monoclonal antibodies. *Annu. Rev. Immunol.* 7:407.

WOFSY, D. 1988. Treatment of autoimmune diseases with monoclonal antibodies. *Prog. Allergy* 45:106.

ZAMVIL, S. S., and L. STEINMAN. 1990. The T lymphocyte in experimental allergic encephalomyelitis. *Annu. Rev. Immunol.* 8:579.

Study Questions

1. Match each of the following autoimmune diseases with their appropriate characteristics:

1. Experimental autoimmune encephalitis (EAE)
2. Goodpasture syndrome
3. Graves' disease
4. Systemic lupus erythematosus (SLE)
5. Insulin-dependent diabetes mellitus (IDDM)
6. Rheumatoid arthritis
7. Hashimoto's thyroiditis
8. Experimental autoimmune myasthenia gravis (EAMG)
9. Myasthenia gravis
10. Pernicious anemia
11. Multiple sclerosis
12. Autoimmune hemolytic anemia

a. Autoantibodies to intrinsic factor block vitamin B_{12} absorption
b. Autoantibodies to acetylcholine receptor
c. T_{DTH}-cell reaction to thyroid antigens
d. Autoantibodies to RBC antigens
e. T-cell response to myelin
f. Induced by injection of myelin basic protein + complete Freund adjuvant
g. Autoantibody to IgG
h. Autoantibodies to receptor for thyroid-stimulating hormone
i. Autoantibodies to basement membrane
j. Autoantibodies to DNA and DNA-associated protein
k. Induced by injection of acetylcholine receptors
l. T_{DTH}-cell response to pancreatic beta cells

2. Experimental autoimmune encephalitis (EAE) has proved to be a useful animal model of autoimmunity.
   a. Discuss how this animal model is generated.
   b. What is unusual about the animals that recover from EAE?
   c. How has this animal model indicated a role for T cells in the development of autoimmunity?

3. Molecular mimicry is one mechanism proposed to account for the development of autoimmunity. How has induction of EAE with myelin basic protein contributed to understanding of molecular mimicry in autoimmune disease?

4. Describe at least three different mechanisms by which a localized viral infection might contribute to the development of organ-specific autoimmune disease.

5. In a system developed by Sarvetnik, transgenic mice expressing the IFN-γ transgene linked to the insulin promoter developed diabetes.
   a. Why was the insulin promoter used?
   b. What is the evidence that the diabetes in these mice is due to autoimmune damage?

c. What is unusual about MHC expression in this system?

d. How might this system mimic events that might be caused by a localized viral infection in the pancreas?

6. In patients with multiple sclerosis, elevated expression of IL-2 and the IL-2R is often observed. How might this contribute to the development of this autoimmune disease?

7. Monoclonal antibodies have been administered for therapy in various autoimmune animal models. What monoclonal antibodies have been used and what is the rationale for these approaches?

18

Vaccines

The discipline of immunology has its roots in the early vaccination trials of Edward Jenner and Louis Pasteur. Since these early beginnings, vaccines have been developed for many diseases that were once major afflictions of mankind. The incidence of diseases such as diphtheria, measles, mumps, pertussis (whooping cough), rubella (German measles), poliomyelitis, and tetanus has been dramatically reduced with vaccines. The World Health Organization's Expanded Programme for Immunization estimates that, as of the late 1980s, approximately 60% of children in Third-World countries had been immunized compared with only 5% in 1974. Despite this progress it is shocking to realize that more than 5 million infants worldwide continue to die every year from diseases that could be avoided by existing vaccines. Among them are 2 million deaths from measles and 800,000 from neonatal tetanus, both of which can be completely avoided by immunization. Clearly, vaccination is a cost-effective weapon for disease prevention. Perhaps in no case have its benefits been as dramatically evident as in the eradication by the smallpox vaccine of one of mankind's long-standing and most terrible scourges. Since October of 1977 there has not been a single naturally acquired case of smallpox anywhere in the world.

Unfortunately, either for economic reasons or because of scientific obstacles, there remain diseases for which vaccines are either nonexistent or not readily available. More than 250 million people are chronically infected with hepatitis B virus (HBV); malaria infects another 200 million every year, resulting in from 1–2 million deaths; estimates suggest that 10–20 million people are infected with the human immunodeficiency virus (HIV); and the common cold and influenza continue to afflict millions of people every year.

Recent advances in immunology have led to the development of new and promising vaccine strategies. Knowledge of the differences in epitopes recognized by T cells and B cells has enabled immunologists to begin to design vaccines to maximize activation of the humoral or cell-mediated branch of the immune system. As differences in antigen-processing pathways became evident, scientists began to design vaccines to maximize antigen presentation with class I or class II MHC molecules. Genetic engineering techniques can be used to develop vaccines to maximize the immune response to selected epitopes. This chapter focuses on some of the existing vaccine strategies as well as on some experimental designs that may become the vaccines of the future.

Active and Passive Immunization

Immunity to infectious microorganisms can be achieved by active or passive immunization. In each case, immunity can be acquired by natural processes or by artificial means involving injection of antibodies or vaccines (Table 18-1).

Passive Immunization

Passive immunization, in which preformed antibodies are transferred to a recipient, can occur naturally by transplacental transfer of maternal antibodies to the developing fetus. Maternal antibodies to diphtheria, tetanus, streptococci, rubeola, rubella, mumps, and poliovirus all afford passively acquired protection to the developing fetus.

Passive immunization also can be achieved by injecting a recipient with preformed antibodies. Passive immunization is used to provide immediate protection to individuals who have been exposed to an infectious organism and are suspected of lacking active immunity to that organism. As an example, individuals with wounds who have not received up-to-date active immunization against tetanus are given an injection of horse antiserum to tetanus toxin. The preformed horse antibody neutralizes any tetanus toxin produced by *Clostridium*

Table 18-1   Immunity can be acquired through passive and active immunization

Type	Acquired through
Passive immunization	Artificial immune serum
	Natural maternal antibody
Active immunization	Artificial infection:
	Attenuated organisms
	Inactivated organisms
	Purified microbial
	macromolecules
	Cloned microbial antigens
	(alone or in vectors)
	Synthetic peptides
	Anti-idiotype antibodies
	Multivalent complexes
	Natural infection

Table 18-2   Common agents used for passive immunization

Disease	Agent
Black widow spider bite	Horse antivenin
Botulism	Horse antitoxin
Diphtheria	Horse antitoxin
Hepatitis A and B	Pooled human immune gamma globulin
Measles	Pooled human immune gamma globulin
Rabies	Pooled human immune gamma globulin
Snake bite	Horse antivenin
Tetanus	Pooled human immune gamma globulin or horse antitoxin

tetani in the wound. Passive immunization is routinely administered to individuals exposed to botulism, tetanus, diphtheria, hepatitis, measles, and rabies (Table 18-2). Passively administered antiserum is also administered to provide protection from snake bites and black widow spider bites.

Passive immunization should only be given when necessary because certain risks are associated with the injection of preformed antibody. If the anitbody was produced in another species, such as a horse, the recipient can mount a strong response to the isotypic determinants of the foreign antibody. This anti-isotype response can lead to certain complications. Some individuals, for example, produce IgE antibody specific for a passive antibody. Immune complexes of this IgE bound to the passively administered antibody can mediate systemic mast-cell degranulation, leading to systemic anaphylaxis. Other individuals produce IgG or IgM antibodies specific for the foreign antibody, which form complement-activating immune complexes. The deposition of these complexes in the tissues can lead to type III hypersensitive reactions. Even when human gamma globulin is administered passively, the recipient can generate an anti-allotype response to the human immunoglobulin, although its level is usually much lower than that of an anti-isotype response.

Active Immunization

Active immunization can be achieved through natural infection with a microorganism, or it can be acquired artificially through vaccination. In active immunization, as the name implies, the immune system plays an active role, with proliferation of antigen-reactive T or B cells resulting in memory-cell formation. Active immunization with various types of vaccines has played an important role in the reduction of deaths from infectious diseases, especially among children.

Active immunization of children is begun at about 2 months of age. A prescribed program of childhood immunizations, outlined in Table 18-3, includes the diphtheria-pertussis tetanus (DPT) combined vaccine, trivalent oral polio vaccine (OPV), measles-mumps-rubella (MMR) combined vaccine, and the recently developed *Hemophilus influenzae* (Hib) vaccine. Childhood immunization has brought about a marked reduction in various childhood diseases in the United States (Figure 18-1). As long as widespread, effective immunization programs are maintained, the incidence of these childhood diseases should remain low.

As indicated in Table 18-3, childhood immunization often requires multiple boosters at appropriately timed intervals to achieve effective immunity. One reason for this is the persistence of maternal antibodies in the

Table 18-3 Routine immunization schedule for infants and children

Age	Vaccine
2 months	Diphtheria-pertussis-tetanus (DPT) Poliomyelitis (OPV)
4 months	Diphtheria-pertussis-tetanus Poliomyelitis
6 months	Diphtheria-pertussis-tetanus
15 months	Measles-mumps-rubella (MMR)
15–24 months	Diphtheria-pertussis-tetanus Poliomyelitis
18 months–5 years	*Hemophilus influenzae* type b conjugate (Hib)
4–6 years	Diphtheria-pertussis-tetanus Poliomyelitis Measles-mumps-rubella
14–16 years	Diphtheria-tetanus

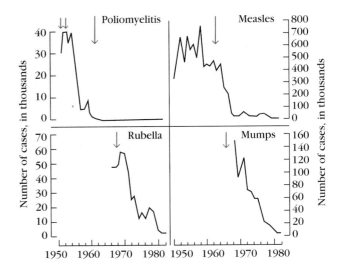

Figure 18-1 Reported annual number of cases of poliomyelitis, measles, rubella (German measles), and mumps in the United States (1950–1980) as reported by the Centers for Disease Control. The effect of introduction of vaccines (indicated by small arrows) on the incidence of these diseases is obvious. [Data from Centers for Disease Control, adapted from C. A. Mims and D. O. White, 1984, *Viral Pathogenesis and Immunology*, Blackwell Scientific.]

Table 18-4 Classification of common vaccines for humans

Disease or pathogen	Type of vaccine
Whole Bacterial Cell	
Cholera	Inactivated
Pertussis	Inactivated
Plague	Inactivated
Tuberculosis	Attenuated BCG*
Capsular Polysaccharide	
Meningitis	
Pneumococcal pneumonia	14 antigenically distinct polysaccharides
Hemophilus influenzae type b	Polysaccharide-protein carrier
Toxoids	
Diphtheria	Recombinant toxoid
Tetanus	Recombinant toxoid
Whole Viral Particles	
Influenza	Inactivated
Measles	Attenuated
Mumps	Attenuated
Rubella	Attenuated
Polio (Salk)	Inactivated
Polio (Sabin)	Attenuated
Rabies	Inactivated
Yellow Fever	Attenuated
Viral Antigens	
Hepatitis B	Recombinant surface antigen

* Bacillus Calmette-Guerin.—an avirulent strain of *Mycobacterium bovis.*

young infant. For example, passively acquired maternal antibodies bind to epitopes on the DPT vaccine and block adequate immune-system activation; therefore, this vaccine must be given several times after the maternal antibody has been catabolized to achieve adequate immunity. Passively acquired maternal antibody also interferes with the effectiveness of the measles vaccine; for this reason, the MMR vaccine is not given before 15 months of age. In Third-World countries, however, the measles vaccine is administered at 9 months, even though maternal antibodies are still present, because 30–50% of young children in these countries contract the disease before 15 months of age. Multiple immunizations with the oral polio vaccine are required to ensure that an adequate immune response is generated to each of the three strains of poliovirus that make up the vaccine.

Adult immunization policies vary depending on the risk group. Vaccines for meningitis, pneumonia, and influenza are often given to groups living in close quarters (e.g., military recruits) or to individuals with reduced immunity (e.g., the elderly). International travelers are also routinely immunized against such endemic diseases as cholera, yellow fever, plague, typhoid, hepatitis, typhus, and polio. Some of the commonly administered active immunization agents are listed in Table 18-4.

Vaccination is not 100% effective. Instead, with any vaccine a small percentage of recipients will respond poorly and therefore will not be adequately protected. This is not a serious problem if the majority of the population is immune to an infectious agent. In this case the probability of a susceptible individual contacting an infected individual is so low that the susceptible individual is not likely to become infected. This phenomenon is known as *herd immunity*. The appearance of measles epidemics among college students and unvaccinated preschool-age children in the United States during the mid- to late-1980s resulted partly from an overall decrease in vaccinations among the population that has lowered the herd immunity of the population (Figure 18-2). Among preschool-age children, 88% of those who developed measles were unvaccinated. Most of the college students who contracted measles had been vaccinated as children; the failure of the vaccine to protect them may have resulted from the presence of passively acquired maternal antibodies that reduced their overall response to the vaccine. This increase in the incidence of measles has prompted the Immunization Practices Advisory Committee of the Centers for Disease Control to recommend that children receive two immunizations with the combined measles-mumps-rubella vaccine, one at 15 months of age and one at entry to kindergarten.

Designing Vaccines for Active Immunization

Several factors must be kept in mind in developing a successful vaccine. First and foremost, the development of an immune response does not necessarily mean that a state of immunity has been achieved. Often the branch

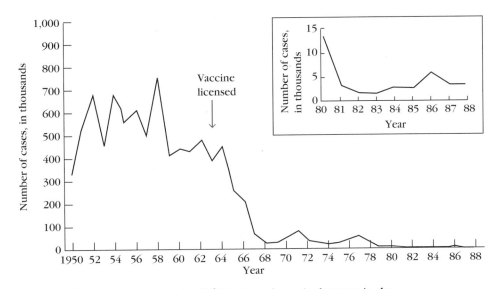

Figure 18-2 Introduction of the measles vaccine in 1962 led to a dramatic decrease in the annual incidence of this disease in the United States. Occasional outbreaks of measles in the 1980s (*inset*) occurred mainly among unvaccinated young children and among college students; most of the latter had been vaccinated, but only once, when they were young. [Data from Centers for Disease Control.]

of the immune system that is activated is critical, and therefore vaccine design must recognize the important differences between activation of the humoral and cell-mediated branches. A second factor is the development of immunologic memory. For example, a vaccine may induce a primary response that is protective but may fail to induce memory-cell formation, leaving the host unprotected after the primary response to the vaccine subsides. The role of memory cells in immunity depends, in part, on the incubation period of the pathogen. In the case of influenza virus, which has a very short incubation period of less that 3 days, disease symptoms are already under way by the time memory cells are activated. Effective protection against influenza therefore depends on maintaining high levels of neutralizing antibody by repeated reimmunizations. For pathogens with a longer incubation period, demonstrable neutralizing antibody at the time of infection is not necessary. The poliovirus, for example, has a long incubation period, requiring more than 3 days to begin to infect the central nervous system. An incubation period of this length provides the necessary time for memory B cells to respond with production of high levels of serum antibody. The vaccine for polio is therefore designed to induce high levels of immunologic memory. Following immunization with the Salk vaccine, serum antibody levels peak within 2 weeks and then decline, but the memory response continues to climb, reaching maximal levels at 6 months and persisting for years (Figure 18-3). If the individual is later exposed to the poliovirus, these memory cells will respond by differentiating into plasma cells that produce

high levels of serum antibody, which protect the individual from infection.

Vaccines designed to induce humoral antibody production must display epitopes that are accessible to the immunoglobulin receptor on B cells. As discussed in Chapter 4, B cells generally recognize epitopes that are hydrophilic and that display segmental mobility on x-ray crystallographic analysis. Many of these epitopes are

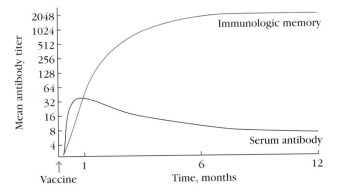

Figure 18-3 Immunization with a single dose of the Salk polio vaccine induces a rapid increase in serum antibody levels, which peak by 2 weeks and then decline. Induction of immunologic memory follows a slower time course, reaching maximal levels 6 months after vaccination. The persistence of the memory response for years following primary vaccination is responsible for immunity to poliomyelitis. [From M. Zanetti, E. Sercarz, and J. Salk, 1987, *Immunol. Today* **8**:18.]

not sequential and thus require the native structure of the protein to generate their conformation (see Figure 4-6). Inactivated or attenuated bacterial or viral vaccines often display native epitopes and thus induce humoral antibody production. Purified proteins and polysaccharides are also effective inducers of humoral immunity. Vaccination intended to produce humoral immunity also must take into account the location of the potential pathogen and the ability of different antibody isotypes to get to that location and neutralize the pathogen. In designing a vaccine for gonorrhea, for example, one of the major stumbling blocks has been the need to induce production of secretory IgA antibodies, which can block bacterial attachment to host mucous membrane cells. When vaccines are administered by injection, they tend to induce production of IgM and IgG but not secretory IgA. What is needed is a means of administering the vaccine at mucous membrane sites and keeping the vaccine at these sites long enough to induce a secretory IgA response.

For some infectious agents—notably viruses, bacteria, protozoa, and fungi that are intracellular pathogens—a cell-mediated immune response is necessary to confer immunity. A vaccine designed to induce this type of response must activate T cells as strongly as possible. Unlike B cells, which recognize epitopes on native antigen, T cells recognize antigen that has been processed and is presented along with MHC molecules. T-cell epitopes tend to be internal, hydrophobic, and linear peptides that are not revealed until the protein is denatured and unfolded in the course of antigen processing (see Table 4-5). These requirements place certain constraints on potential vaccines: To activate T_H cells, a vaccine must be processed by antigen-presenting cells and presented in association with class II MHC molecules; to activate T_C cells, a vaccine must be capable of replicating in host cells where its peptides can associate with class I MHC molecules. For this reason attenuated vaccines that permit some limited viral replication or bacterial growth within host cells are most effective for the induction of cytotoxic activity. In addition to the differences in processing routes for class I and for class II MHC presentation (see Figure 9-15), potential vaccines for inducing a cell-mediated response are limited by constraints arising from the preferential interaction of MHC molecules with different peptides (see Table 9-4). Therefore, an immunodominant T-cell epitope for one individual may not serve as an immunodominant T-cell epitope for another individual who expresses a different set of MHC antigen-presenting molecules.

In the remainder of this chapter, various approaches to the design of vaccines—both currently used vaccines and experimental ones—are described and examined in terms of their ability to induce humoral and cell-mediated immunity and memory-cell production.

Whole-Organism Vaccines

As Table 18-4 indicates, many of the common vaccines currently in use consist of inactivated (killed) or live but attenuated (avirulent) bacterial cells or viral particles. The primary characteristics of these two types of vaccines are compared in Table 18-5.

Attenuated Viral or Bacterial Vaccines

In some cases microorganisms can be *attenuated* so that they lose their pathogenicity while retaining their capacity for transient growth within an inoculated host. Attenuation can often be achieved by growing a pathogenic bacterium or virus for prolonged periods under abnormal culture conditions. The prolonged growth under conditions that are not normal selects mutants that are better suited to growth in the abnormal culture conditions and are therefore less capable of growth in the original host. For example, an attenuated strain of *Mycobacterium bovis* called Bacillus Calmette-Guerin (BCG) was developed by growing *M. bovis* on a medium containing increased concentrations of bile. After 13 years the bacteria had adapted to growth with increased bile and had become attenuated so that it could now serve as a vaccine for tuberculosis. The Sabin polio vaccine and the measles vaccine consist of viral strains that have been successfully attenuated and now serve as successful vaccines. The poliovirus used in the Sabin vaccine was attenuated by growth in monkey kidney epithelial cells. The measles vaccine contains a strain of rubella virus that was grown in duck embryo cells and later in human cell lines.

Attenuated vaccines have some advantages and some disadvantages. Because of their capacity for transient growth, such vaccines provide prolonged immune-system exposure to the individual epitopes on the attenuated organisms, resulting in increased immunogenicity and memory-cell production. As a consequence these vaccines often require only a single immunization, eliminating the need for repeated boosters. This is a major advantage in Third-World countries where epidemiologic studies have shown that roughly 20% of individuals fail to return for each subsequent booster. The ability of many attenuated vaccines to replicate within host cells makes them particularly suitable to induce a cell-mediated response.

The Sabin polio vaccine, consisting of three attenuated strains of poliovirus, is administered orally to children on a sugar cube or in sugar liquid. The attenuated viruses colonize the intestine and induce protective immunity to all three strains of virulent poliovirus. The ability of the attenuated Sabin vaccine to colonize the intestines enables it to induce production of secretory IgA, which

Table 18-5 Comparison of attenuated (live) and inactivated (killed) vaccines

Characteristic	Attenuated	Inactivated
Production	Virulent pathogen is grown under abnormal culture conditions to select for avirulent organisms	Virulent pathogen is inactivated by chemicals or γ-irradiation
Booster requirement	Generally requires only a single booster	Requires multiple boosters
Relative stability	Less stable	More stable (advantageous for Third-World countries where refrigeration is limited)
Type of immunity induced	Produces humoral and cell-mediated immunity	Produces mainly humoral immunity
Reversion tendency	May revert to virulent form	Cannot revert to virulent form

serves as an important defense against naturally acquired poliovirus. Unlike most attenuated vaccines that require a single immunizing dose, the Sabin polio vaccine requires boosters because the three strains of attenuated poliovirus in the vaccine interfere with one another's replication in the intestine. With the first immunization, one strain will predominate in its growth, inducing immunity to that strain. With the second immunization, the immunity generated by the previous immunization will limit the growth of the previously predominant strain, enabling one of the two remaining strains to predominate and induce immunity. Finally with the third immunization, immunity to all three strains is achieved.

The major disadvantage of attenuated vaccines is the possibility of their reversion to a virulent form. The rate of reversion of the Sabin polio vaccine leading to subsequent paralytic disease is about one case in four million doses of vaccine. Another concern with attenuated vaccines is the presence of other viruses as contaminants. In 1960 it was discovered that the oncogenic virus SV-40 had contaminated some monkey kidney cultures used in production of the Sabin vaccine; as a result more stringent vaccine testing was required to eliminate this contaminant.

Genetic engineering techniques provide a way to attenuate a virus irreversibly by selectively removing genes that are necessary for virulence. This has been done with a herpes virus vaccine for pigs, in which the thymidine kinase gene was removed. Because thymidine kinase is required for the virus to grow in certain types of cells (e.g., neurons), removal of this gene rendered the virus incapable of causing disease. It is possible that similar genetic engineering techniques could eliminate the risk of reversion of the attenuated polio vaccine. One strategy for developing an AIDS vaccine involves research on HIV variants in the hope of developing an irreversibly attenuated strain.

Inactivated Viral or Bacterial Vaccines

Another common approach in vaccine production is to inactivate the pathogen by heat or chemical means so that the pathogen is no longer capable of replication in the host. It is critically important to maintain the structure of epitopes on surface antigens during inactivation. Heat inactivation generally is unsatisfactory because it causes extensive protein denaturation; thus any epitopes that depend on higher orders of protein structure are likely to be altered. Chemical inactivation with formaldehyde or various alkylating agents has had success. The Salk polio vaccine and the pertussis (whooping cough) vaccine both depend on formaldehyde inactivation. In contrast with attenuated vaccines, whose immunogenicity is increased by their transient growth, killed vaccines tend to require repeated boosters to maintain the immune status of the host. In addition, killed vaccines induce a predominantly humoral antibody response; they are less effective than attenuated vaccines in inducing cell-mediated immunity.

Even though they contain killed pathogens, inactivated whole-organism vaccines still are associated with certain risks. A serious complication with the first Salk vaccines was inadequate formaldehyde killing of the vi-

Table 18-6   Risks versus benefits of the pertussis vaccine for whooping cough

	Risk of occurrence after	
Problem	Vaccination	Disease
Seizures	1:1750	1:25−1:50
Encephalitis	1:110,000	1:1000−1:4000
Severe brain damage	1:310,000	1:2000−1:8000
Death	1:1,000,000	1:200−1:1000

SOURCE: I. Tizard, *Immunology: An introduction,* 2d ed., Saunders.

rus in two vaccine lots, which caused paralytic polio in a high percentage of recipients. The pertussis vaccine highlights another problem that can arise with a complex whole-organism vaccine. Encephalitis-type reactions occur in a small percentage of infants receiving this vaccine (Table 18-6), and it has not been possible to establish just what components of the organism are responsible for these reactions.

Purified Macromolecules as Vaccines

Some of the risks of vaccines based on attenuated or killed microorganisms can be avoided with vaccines that consist of specific, purified macromolecules. The vaccines for meningococcal meningitis and pneumococcal pneumonia use a mixture of purified capsular polysaccharides as the immunogen. One of the limitations with polysaccharide vaccines is their inability to activate T_H cells. They activate B cells in a T-independent manner, resulting in IgM but no IgG production. One method that has been utilized to bypass this limitation is to conjugate the polysaccharide antigen to some sort of protein carrier. This method had been employed for the vaccine for *Haemophilus influenzae* type b, the major cause of bacterial meningitis in children under 5 years of age. In this case the type b capsular polysaccharide is covalently linked to a protein carrier, tetanus toxoid. The polysaccharide-protein conjugate is considerably more immunogenic than the polysaccharide alone, and because it activates T_H cells, it enables class switching from IgM to IgG.

One of the problems encountered with vaccines containing purified surface macromolecules is the difficulty of obtaining large-enough quantities of the purified com-

ponent. This limitation can be overcome with recombinant DNA techniques whereby a gene encoding an immunogenic protein is expressed in bacterial, yeast, or insect cells. Diphtheria and tetanus vaccines, for example, can be made by purifying the recombinant bacterial exotoxin and then inactivating the toxin with formaldehyde to form a *toxoid*. Vaccination with the toxoid induces antitoxoid antibodies, which are also capable of binding to the toxin and neutralizing its toxic effect. In production of toxoid vaccines the conditions must be closely controlled to achieve detoxification without excessive modification of the epitope structure.

Recombinant Antigen Vaccines

DNA encoding antigenic determinants can be isolated and cloned in bacteria, yeast, or mammalian cells. A number of genes from viral, bacterial, and protozoan pathogens have been successfully cloned and are presently being developed as vaccines. The DNA encoding the relevant antigen can be cloned in bacterial, yeast, insect or mammalian expression systems. The first successful recombinant vaccine was developed for the major antigen (VP1) of the foot-and-mouth disease virus. In this case, viral RNA encoding the VP1 surface antigen was transcribed into cDNA using reverse transcriptase. The VP1 cDNA was then inserted into an *Escherichia coli* plasmid and cloned in *E. coli* (see Figure 2-4). This procedure allowed production of large quantities of the VP1 antigen, which was then purified and used as a vaccine in animals.

The first recombinant antigen vaccine approved for human use was the hepatitis B vaccine. This vaccine was developed by cloning the gene for the major surface antigen of hepatitis B virus (HBsAg) in yeast cells. The recombinant yeast cells are grown in large fermenters and HBsAg accumulates intracellularly in the cells. The yeast cells are harvested and disrupted by high pressure, releasing the recombinant HBsAg, which is then purified by conventional biochemical techniques. The recombinant hepatitis B vaccine has been administered to over 8000 individuals and has been shown to induce the production of protective antibodies. This vaccine has a great deal of promise for the 250 million carriers of chronic hepatitis B worldwide!

Several recombinant vaccines for human immunodeficiency virus are presently being assessed in volunteers as potential vaccines for AIDS (see Chapter 21). Other recombinant vaccines that are being developed in animal models include the β subunit of cholera toxin, the enterotoxin of *E. coli*, the circumsporozoite protein of the malaria parasite, and a glycoprotein membrane antigen from Epstein-Barr virus. Animals immunized with these recombinant vaccines have in some cases mounted a protective immune response to a subsequent challenge with the live pathogen. One disadvantage of recombinant protein or glycoprotein vaccines is that they are processed as exogenous antigens and therefore do not tend to induce much activation of class I MHC–restricted T_C cells.

Recombinant Vector Vaccines

It is possible to introduce genes encoding major antigens of especially virulent pathogens into attenuated viruses or bacteria. The attenuated organism serves as a vector, replicating within the host and expressing the gene product of the pathogen. A number of organisms have been used for vector vaccines including vaccinia virus, attenuated poliovirus, adenoviruses, attenuated strains of *Salmonella*, and the BCG strain of myobacterium tuberculosis.

Vaccinia virus, the attenuated vaccine used to eradicate smallpox, has been widely employed as a vector vaccine. It is estimated that this large, complex virus, with a genome of about 200 genes, could be engineered to carry several dozen foreign genes without impairing its capacity to infect host cells and replicate. A genetically engineered vaccinia expresses high levels of the inserted gene product, which can then serve as a potent immunogen in an inoculated host (Figure 18-4). Enzo Paoletti has inserted genes from hepatitis B virus, herpes simplex, and influenza into vaccinia virus. Vaccine trials in the laboratory have shown that this engineered vaccinia induces antibodies to all three engineered gene products. Like the smallpox vaccine, genetically engineered vaccinia can be administered simply by dermal scratching, causing a limited localized, infection in host cells. If the foreign gene product expressed by the vaccinia is a viral envelope protein, it is inserted into the membrane of the infected host cell, inducing development of T-cell–mediated immunity as well as antibody-mediated immunity. Vaccinia virus engineered with the envelope glycoproteins of the human immunodeficiency virus (HIV) is currently being assessed both in chimpanzees and in human volunteers as a potential vaccine for AIDS. There are questions, however, about the suitability of a vaccinia vector vaccine for individuals with AIDS. In the early 1980s, an individual infected with HIV developed disseminated vaccinia after being vaccinated for smallpox with vaccinia. In healthy individuals an attenuated vaccine has only limited growth, but in individuals with immune deficiency even an attenuated vaccine can be potentially fatal.

Other attenuated vector vaccines may prove to be safer than the vaccinia vaccine. An attenuated strain of *Salmonella typhimurium* has been engineered with genes from the bacterium that causes cholera. The advantage of this vector vaccine is that Salmonella infects cells of the mucosal lining of the gut and therefore will induce secretory IgA production. For a number of diseases, including cholera and gonorrhea, increased levels of secretory IgA at mucous membrane surfaces is necessary for immunity. The Sabin vaccine strain of poliovirus is another candidate for a safe and effective vector vaccine. In this case the poliovirus vector is genetically engineered so that a portion of the gene encoding the outer capsid protein of poliovirus is replaced by DNA encoding the epitope of choice. The resulting poliovirus chimera will express the desired epitope in a highly accessible presentation protruding from the poliovirus nucleocapsid. A chimeric poliovirus vector vaccine expressing epitopes from the envelope glycoproteins of HIV has been shown to induce high levels of neutralizing antibodies specific for HIV in animal models.

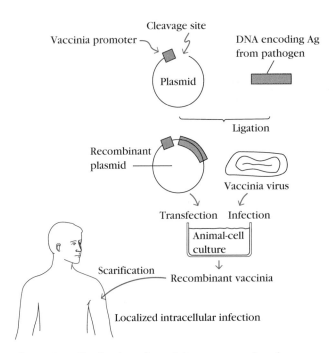

Figure 18-4 Production of vaccinia vector vaccine. A gene from a pathogenic microorganism (red) is introduced into vaccinia. Like the smallpox vaccine, the genetically engineered vaccinia can be administered by dermal scratching (scarification), resulting in a limited localized infection that allows the foreign gene to be expressed in host cells. The vaccine induces both humoral and cell-mediated immunity.

Synthetic Peptide Vaccines

The discovery that peptides can function as vaccines dates to the 1960s, when F. A. Anderer observed that a short hexapeptide fragment isolated from the tobacco mosaic virus, coupled to BSA as a protein carrier, induced a humoral response that protected against infection with the whole virus. Until the 1980s the potential of peptides as vaccines was relatively unexplored because it was widely believed that peptides were not likely to represent epitopes of native proteins and therefore would not induce humoral immunity. Although it is true that B-cell epitopes largely depend on tertiary protein configuration because they are composed of noncontiguous sequences, experiments by Richard A. Lerner revealed that this does not exclude linear peptides as vaccines. He found that almost any linear peptide could induce antibodies capable of binding to a native protein provided that the peptide represented a sequence of accessible amino acids on the surface of the native protein. In other words, a nonimmunodominant epitope on the native protein can be converted into an immunodominant epitope when it is presented to the immune system as a linear peptide sequence. And antibody produced to this linear peptide sequence can bind to the same sequence on the native protein (albeit sometimes with lower affinity). These findings led to speculation that synthetic peptides coupled to immunogenic carrier proteins might serve as effective vaccines. One advantage of this approach is that it is technically much simpler to chemically synthesize peptides than to clone proteins in genetically engineered bacteria or yeasts, as is done in producing recombinant DNA vaccines. Chemical synthesis of peptides representing various sequences in an antigen became feasible with the development of gene-cloning and DNA-sequencing techniques, since the amino acid sequence can be predicted from the corresponding nucleotide sequence.

Construction of synthetic peptides for use as vaccines to induce either humoral or cell-mediated immunity requires an understanding of the nature of T-cell and B-cell epitopes. Potential B-cell epitopes of a protein antigen can be identified by examining its structure for peptide sequences representing sites that are accessible, hydrophilic, and mobile. However, x-ray crystallographic analysis has not been performed on most proteins, B-cell epitopes are generally chosen by identifying strongly hydrophilic sequences. The assumption is that strongly hydrophilic sequences are most likely to represent accessible surface regions that constitute B-cell epitopes. Ideally, vaccines for inducing humoral immunity should include peptides composing immunodominant B-cell epitopes. Such epitopes can be identified by determining the dominant antibody in the sera of individuals who are recovering from a disease and then testing peptides for their ability to react with that antibody with a high affinity. In one such experiment, two linear synthetic peptides representing potential B-cell epitopes of HBsAg were tested for their affinity in binding to pooled antisera from individuals who had recovered from hepatitis B. It was found that a synthetic peptide consisting of cyclical repeats of amino acids 139–147 had a 10-fold higher affinity ($2.1 \times 10^7/M^{-1}$) than cyclical repeats of amino acids 124–137 ($2.5 \times 10^6/M^{-1}$). The cyclical peptide 139–147 was therefore chosen as a potential candidate for a synthetic hepatitis B vaccine.

An effective memory response for both humoral and cell-mediated immunity requires generation of a population of memory T_H cells. A successful vaccine must therefore include immunodominant T-cell epitopes. With synthetic peptide vaccines it is difficult to identify those epitopes owing to the role, unpredictable as yet, of the MHC in influencing immunodominance for the T-cell system. T cells recognize processed peptides that, in the majority of cases, appear to represent internal amphipathic peptides. As discussed in Chapter 4, these peptides must have a site (the agretope) that enables them to interact with MHC molecules as well as a site (the epitope) that enables them to interact with the T-cell receptor. MHC molecules differ in their ability to present peptides to T cells. In one experiment congenic and recombinant congenic strains of mice were tested for their ability to recognize synthetic peptides of an internal core protein (nucleoprotein) of the influenza virus. As the data in Table 18-7 show, mouse strains with different MHC haplotypes recognized and responded to different peptides. To determine whether the K or D class I MHC molecules were responsible for peptide recognition in these strains, the class I MHC genes from each strain were transfected individually into L cells. The transfected fibroblasts were incubated with the various peptides and tested for their ability to activate a CTL response with influenza-primed T_C cells from the corresponding strain. The D^b molecule was the restriction element in the C57BL/6 strain, the K^k molecule was the restriction element in the CBA strain, and the K^d molecule was the restriction element in the BALB/c strain (see Table 18-6). These results highlight the important differences among MHC molecules in peptide presentation. The MHC polymorphism within a species will therefore influence the level of T-cell responsiveness by different individuals to different peptides.

Moreover, different subpopulations of T cells probably recognize different epitopes. Experiments by E. Sercarz have identified some peptides that induce a strong helper response and other peptides that induce immunologic suppression. These helper and suppressor peptides generally represent different, nonoverlapping

Table 18-7 Effect of MHC on recognition of influenza-virus nucleoprotein peptides by inbred mouse strains

Strain	MHC haplotype	Peptide producing response in vivo*	CML response in vitro with transfected class I MHC alleles[†]	
			D	K
C57BL/6	H-2^b	365–380	+	−
CBA	H-2^k	50–63	−	+
BALB/c	H-2^d	147–161	−	+

* Mice from each strain were injected with the various peptides conjugated to a carrier protein. Only the indicated peptides induced a T-cell response as measured by a CML response.

[†] The D and K alleles from each strain were transfected individually into fibroblast L cells. The transfected cells were then incubated with the appropriate peptide and antigen-primed T$_C$ cells from the corresponding strain and the CML response was measured.

SOURCE: Based on D. C. Wraith, 1987, *Immunol. Today* **8**:239.

amino acid sequences. For example, immunization with the amino-terminal residues (1–17) of hen egg-white lysozyme suppressed the response to native lysozyme. By identifying suppressing peptides and eliminating them from synthetic vaccines, it might be possible to generate enhanced immunity. These suppressing peptides may also be valuable in situations where it is desirable to decrease the immune response, as in treating autoimmune diseases.

In designing synthetic peptide vaccines against viruses, the current approach is to look for invariant regions, whose amino acid sequence is highly conserved. Some regions of the hemagglutinin (HA) molecule of influenza virus, for example, display high levels of amino acid variation, which generate the type and subtype differences enabling the virus to escape the immune system. But invariant regions, which mediate essential biological functions, also are present in the HA molecule. For example, the sialic acid–binding site on HA allows the virus to bind to sialic acid residues on cell surfaces. Although this region on the intact viral particle does not normally induce antibody formation, synthetic peptide vaccines of this conserved region were found to neutralize viral infectivity against a number of different influenza types and subtypes. These studies provide optimism for a long-awaited influenza vaccine, which is discussed in Chapter 19. Synthetic peptide vaccines are being evaluated for hepatitis B virus, the malaria parasite, diphtheria toxin, and various proteins and glycoproteins of HIV.

Multivalent Subunit Vaccines

One of the limitations with synthetic peptide vaccines and recombinant protein vaccines is that these vaccines tend to be poorly immunogenic; in addition, they tend to induce humoral antibody production but are less able to induce a cell-mediated response. What is needed is some method of structuring a vaccine to contain immunodominant B-cell *and* T-cell epitopes. Furthermore, if a CTL response is desired, it is also necessary to be able to deliver the vaccine intracellularly so that the peptides can be processed and presented together with class I MHC molecules. A number of innovative techniques are currently being employed to develop multivalent vaccines that can present multiple copies of a given peptide or a mixture of peptides to the immune system.

One approach is to prepare solid matrix-antibody-antigen (SMAA) complexes by attaching monoclonal antibodies to particulate solid matrices and then saturating the antibody with the desired antigen. The resulting complexes are then used as vaccines. By attaching different monoclonal antibodies to the solid matrix, it is possible to bind a mixture of peptides or proteins, composing immunodominant epitopes for both T cells and B cells, to the solid matrix (Figure 18-5a). These multivalent complexes have been shown to induce vigorous humoral and cell-mediated responses. Their particulate nature contributes to their increased immunogenicity by facilitating phagocytosis by phagocytic cells.

(a)

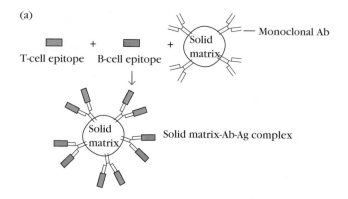

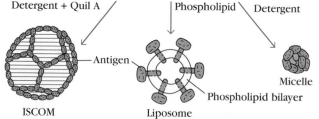

(b) Detergent extracted membrane antigens or antigenic peptides

Figure 18-5 Multivalent subunit vaccines. (a) Solid matrix-antibody-antigen complexes can be designed to contain synthetic peptides representing both T-cell epitopes (red) and B-cell epitopes (gray). (b) Protein micelles, liposomes, and immunostimulating complexes (ISCOMs) can all be prepared with extracted antigens or antigenic peptides (red). In each case, the hydrophilic residues of the antigen are oriented outward.

Another means of obtaining a multivalent vaccine is to utilize detergent to incorporate protein or peptide antigens into lipid vesicles (called liposomes), into immunostimulating complexes (called ISCOMs) or into protein micelles. (Figure 18-5b). Micelles are formed by mixing proteins in detergent and then removing the detergent. The individual proteins will orient themselves with the hydrophilic residues oriented toward the aqueous environment and the hydrophobic residues at the center so as to exclude their interaction with the aqueous environment. Liposomes containing protein antigens are prepared by mixing the proteins with a suspension of phospholipids under conditions that form vesicles bounded by a bilayer. The proteins are incorporated into the bilayer with the hydrophilic residues exposed. ISCOMs are prepared by mixing protein or peptide antigens with detergent and a glycoside called Quil A, which forms micelles that interact with the antigen. The peptide or protein is expressed as a multivalent complex on the surface of the micelle. Membrane proteins from different pathogens including influenza

virus, measles virus, hepatitis B virus, and HIV have been incorporated into micelles, liposomes, and ISCOMs and are currently being assessed as potential vaccines. In addition to their increased immunogenicity, liposomes and ISCOMs appear to deliver the antigen into cells and therefore are able to induce cell-mediated immunity.

Anti-Idiotype Vaccines

The discovery that an anti-idiotype antibody can in effect serve as the internal image of an antigen (see Figure 14-5) opened the door to the potential introduction of anti-idiotype antibodies as vaccines. What they promise, of course, is the generation of an effective immune response to a dangerous pathogen without exposure of the vaccinated individual to any form of the pathogen. One anti-idiotype vaccine currently being developed for protection against HIV is designed to bind to a conserved region on the gp120 envelope glycoprotein that is required for binding to the CD4 membrane molecule on host cells. Table 18-8 lists some of the anti-idiotype vaccines that have been evaluated.

Summary

1. A state of immunity can be induced by passive or active immunization. Passive immunization involves transfer of preformed antibodies and provides short-term protection without the requirement for an active immune response. Active immunization induces clonal selection and results in memory-cell formation.

2. The current vaccines for humans are attenuated (avirulent) microorganisms, inactivated (killed) microorganisms, or purified macromolecules. Attenuated vaccines have the advantage of transient growth and therefore stimulate a more pronounced immune response and memory-cell production without the requirement for additional boosters. Inactivated vaccines require repeated boosters but pose no risk of reversion to a pathogenic state. The use of purified macromolecules, which are less complex than whole-organism vaccines, avoids certain complications due to unknown side effects. By applying recombinant DNA techniques, it is possible to produce large quantities of a defined antigen for immunization.

3. In developing a vaccine, the branch of the immune system to be activated must be considered. To induce humoral immunity, epitopes must be accessible to B-cell immunoglobulin receptors and should represent immunodominant epitopes of the infectious agent. To induce cell-mediated immunity, a vaccine capable of

Table 18-8 Evaluation of some anti-idiotype vaccines

Infectious agents	Nature of anti-idiotype vaccine[*]	Species tested	Adjuvant	Protection[†]
Viruses				
Hepatitis	P/M	Mice	+	+
Rabies	P	Mice	+	ND
Tobacco mosaic	P	Mice	+	ND
Polio type II	M	Mice	−	−
Venezuelan equine E. myelitis	P	Mice	+	ND
Reovirus	M	Mice	−	ND
Sendai	M	Mice	−	+
Bacteria				
Streptococcus pneumoniae	M	Mice	−	+
Escherichia coli	M	Mice	+	+
Listeria monocytogenes	M	Mice	+	+
Parasites				
Trypanosoma rhodesiense	M	Mice	−	+
Schistosoma mansoni	M	Rats	−	+
Trypanosoma cruzi	P	Mice	+	ND

[*] P = polyclonal antibody; M = monoclonal antibody.

[†] ND = not done.

SOURCE: M. Zanetti, E. Sercarz, and J. Salk, 1987, *Immunol. Today* **8**:18.

transient intracellular growth is desirable to maximize the presentation of antigens with MHC molecules.

4. Vaccinia virus can be engineered to carry multiple genes from infectious microorganisms. An advantage of this vector approach is that there is some replication of the engineered vaccinia virus in host cells, which serves to maximize cell-mediated immunity to the expressed antigens.

5. Peptides can be synthesized that represent immunodominant T- or B-cell epitopes. This approach has enabled immunologists to produce defined vaccines that may make possible the selective activation of the humoral or cell-mediated branches of the immune system.

6. Anti-idiotype vaccines offer the possibility of achieving a state of immunity without having to expose the recipient to the uncertainties of vaccines derived from whole organisms or even purified macromolecules.

References

BLOOM, B. 1989. Vaccines for the third world. *Nature* **342**:115.

EVANS, D. J., J. McKEATING, J. M. MEREDITH et al. 1989. An engineered poliovirus chimaera elicits broading reactive HIV-1 neutralizing antibodies. *Nature* **339**:385

HENDERSON, D. A. 1976. the eradication of smallpox. *Sci. Am.* **235**:25.

MILCH, D. R. 1989. Synthetic T and B cell recognition sites: implications for vaccine development. *Adv. Immunol.* **45**:195.

RANDALL, R. E. 1989. Solid matrix-antibody-antigen (SMAA) complexes for constructing multivalent subunit vaccines. *Immunol. Today* **10**:336.

STEWARD, M. W., and C. R. HOWARD. 1987. Synthetic peptides: a next generation of vaccines? *Immunol. Today* **8**:51.

STOVER, C. K., V. FDELA CRUG, T. R. FUERSTETAL. 1991. New use of BCG for recombinant vaccines. *Nature* **351**:456.

TAKAHSHI, H., et al., T. TAKESHITA, B. MOREINA. 1990. Induction of CD8$^+$ cytotoxic T cells by immunization with purified HIV-1 envelope protein in Iscoms. *Nature* **344**:873.

ZANETTI, M., E. SERCARZ, and J. SALK. 1987. The immunology of new generation vaccines. *Immunol. Today* **8**:18.

ZUCKERMAN, A. J. (ed.). 1989. *Recent Developments in Prophylactic Immunization.* Immunology and Medicine Series Vol. 12. Kluwer Academic Publishers.

Study Questions

1.   Indicate whether each of the following statements is true or false. If you think a statement is false, explain why.

 a.   Transplacental transfer of maternal IgG to measles confers short-term immunity on the fetus.

 b.   Attenuated vaccines are more likely to induce cell-mediated immunity than killed vaccines are.

 c.   Hydrophilic peptides are more likely to represent immunodominant B-cell epitopes than hydrophobic peptides.

 d.   Macromolecules generally contain a large number of potential epitopes.

2.   What are the advantages and disadvantages of using attenuated organisms as vaccines?

3.   A child who had never been immunized to tetanus stepped on a rusty nail and got a deep puncture wound. The doctor cleaned out the wound and gave the child an injection of tetanus antitoxin. Why was antitoxin given instead of a booster shot of tetanus toxoid? If the child receives no further treatment and steps on a rusty nail again 3 years later, will he be immune to tetanus?

4.   What are the advantages of the Sabin polio vaccine compared to the Salk vaccine?

5.   In an attempt to prepare a synthetic peptide vaccine you have analyzed a protein for (a) amphipathic peptides and (b) mobile peptides. How might each of these peptides be used as a vaccine to induce different immune responses?

6.   You have developed a synthetic peptide vaccine representing an immunodominant T-cell epitope for strain-A mice. When the vaccine is tested in strain-B mice, no T-cell response occurs. What is the most likely explanation for this finding? How could you test this hypothesis?

7.   Explain the relationship between the incubation period of a pathogen and the active immunization strategy for achieving effective host protection.

8.   The Salk polio vaccine has been recommended for use by HIV-infected children instead of the Sabin polio vaccine. Why do you think this recommendaton was made?

CHAPTER 100

Immune Response to Infectious Diseases

In order for a pathogen to establish an infection in a susceptible host, a series of coordinated events is required to circumvent the specific and nonspecific host defenses. Generally, pathogens use a variety of strategies to escape immune destruction. Many pathogens reduce their own antigenicity either by growing within host cells, where they are sequestered from immune attack, or by shedding their membrane antigens. Other pathogens mimic host-cell membrane molecules, either by expressing molecules with similar sequences or by acquiring a covering of host membrane molecules. In some cases pathogens are able to selectively suppress the immune response or regulate the response to generate a branch of immune activation that is ineffective. Continual variation in surface antigens is another strategy that enables a pathogen to elude the immune system. This antigenic variation may occur by the gradual accumulation of mutations (antigenic drift), or it may involve an abrupt change in surface antigens (antigenic shift).

In this chapter the concepts discussed in earlier chapters, such as antigenicity (Chapter 4), immune effector mechanisms (Chapter 6, 13, and 16), immune regulation (Chapter 14), and vaccine development (Chapter 18) are applied to selected infectious diseases caused by viruses, bacteria, protozoa, and helminths—the four major types of pathogens.

Viral Infections

A number of specific immune effector mechanisms, together with nonspecific defense mechanisms, are called into play to eliminate an infecting virus (Table 19-1). At the same time the virus acts to subvert one or more of these mechanisms in order to prolong its own survival. The outcome of the infection will depend on how effectively the host's defense mechanisms resist the offensive tactics of the virus.

Viral Neutralization by Humoral Antibody

Antibodies specific for viral surface antigens are often crucial in containing the spread of a virus during acute infection and in protecting against reinfection. Most viruses express surface receptor molecules that enable them to initiate infection by binding specifically to host-cell membrane molecules. For example, influenza virus binds to sialic acid residues in cell-membrane glycoproteins and glycolipids; rhinovirus binds to intercellular adhesion molecules (ICAMs); and Epstein-Barr virus binds to type 2 complement receptors on B cells. If antibody is produced to the viral receptor, it can block infection altogether by preventing binding of viral particles to host cells. Secretory IgA in mucous secretions plays an important role in host defense against viruses by blocking viral attachment to mucosal epithelial cells. The advantage of the attenuated oral polio vaccine, discussed in Chapter 18, is that it induces production of secretory IgA, which effectively blocks attachment of poliomyelitis along the gastrointestinal tract.

Viral neutralization by antibody sometimes involves other mechanisms, which operate following viral attachment to host cells. In some cases antibodies may block viral penetration by binding to epitopes that are necessary to mediate fusion of the viral envelope with the plasma membrane. If the induced antibody is of a complement-activating isotype, lysis of enveloped virions can ensue. Antibody or complement can also agglutinate viral particles and function as an opsonizing agent to facilitate Fc or C3b receptor-mediated phagocytosis of the viral particles.

Cell-Mediated Antiviral Mechanisms

Although antibodies have an important role in containing the spread of a virus in the acute phases of infection, they are not usually able to eliminate the virus once infection has occurred—particularly if the virus is capable of entering a latent state in which its DNA is integrated into host chromosomal DNA. Once an infection is established, cell-mediated immune mechanisms are most important in host defense. Activated T_H cells produce a number of cytokines that serve, either directly or indirectly, to defend against viruses. Interferon γ (IFN-γ) acts directly by inducing an antiviral state in cells. Indirect antiviral activity can develop IL-2 and IFN-γ activate NK cells, which play an important role in host defense during the first days of many viral infections until a specific CTL response develops.

In most viral infections specific CTL activity arises within 3–4 days after infection, peaks by 1 week, and then declines. CTLs specific for the virus eliminate virus-infected self-cells and thus eliminate potential sources of new viral production. The role of CTLs in defense against viruses is demonstrated by the ability of virus-specific CTLs to confer protection on unimmunized adoptive-tranfer recipients.

Viral Evasion of Host-Defense Mechanisms

A number of viruses escape immune attack by constantly changing their antigens. In the case of the influenza virus, which is discussed more fully later, continual antigenic variation results in the frequent emergence of new infectious strains of the virus. The absence of protective immunity to these newly emerging strains leads to repeated epidemics of influenza. Antigenic variation among rhinoviruses, the causative agents of the common cold, is responsible for the inability to produce an effective vaccine for colds. Nowhere is antigenic variation greater than in the human immunodeficiency virus

Table 19-1 Mechanisms of humoral and cell-mediated immune responses to viruses

Response type	Effector molecule or cell	Activity
Humoral	Antibody (especially secretory IgA)	Blocks binding of virus to host cells, thus preventing infection or reinfection
	Antibody	Blocks fusion of viral envelope with host-cell plasma membrane
	IgG and IgM antibody	Enhances phagocytosis of viral particles (opsonization)
	IgM antibody	Agglutinates viral particles
	Complement activated by IgG or IgM antibody	Mediates opsonization by C3b and lysis of enveloped viral particles by membrane-attack complex
Cell-mediated	IFN-γ secreted by T_H or T_C cells	Has direct antiviral activity
	Cytotoxic T lymphocytes (CTLs)	Kill virus-infected self-cells
	NK cells and macrophages	Kill virus-infected cells by ADCC

(HIV), the causative agent of AIDS. Estimates suggest that HIV accumulates mutations at a rate 65-times faster than influenza virus. Because of the importance of AIDS, Chapter 21 is devoted in its entirety to this disease.

A large number of viruses evade the immune response by causing generalized immunosuppression. Among these are the paramyxovirus causing mumps, Epstein-Barr virus (EBV), cytomegalovirus, and HIV. In some cases immunosuppression is caused by direct viral infection of lymphocytes or macrophages. The virus can then directly destroy the immune cells by cytolytic mechanisms or alter the function of these cells. In other cases immunosuppression occurs as a result of a cytokine imbalance. A recent report, for example, has shown that an EBV gene is homologous to the IL-10 gene. Since IL-10 suppresses cytokine production by the T_H1 subset resulting in decreased levels of IL-2 and IFN-γ, the homologous EBV gene product may act in a similar manner.

Influenza

The influenza virus infects the upper respiratory tract and major central airways in humans, horses, birds, pigs, and even seals. It has been responsible for some of the worst pandemics (worldwide epidemics) in human history, one of which killed more than 20 million people in 1918–1919, a toll surpassing the number of casualties in World War 1. Some areas, such as Alaska and the Pacific Islands, lost more than half of their population during this pandemic.

Properties of the Influenza Virus

Influenza viral particles, or virions, are roughly spherical or ovoid in shape, with an average diameter of 90–100 nm. The virions are surrounded by an outer envelope, a lipid bilayer acquired from the plasma membrane of the infected host cell during the process of budding. Inserted into the envelope are two glycoproteins, *hemagglutinin* (HA) and *neuraminidase* (NA), which form radiating projections that are visible in electron micrographs (Figure 19-1). The hemagglutinin projections, in

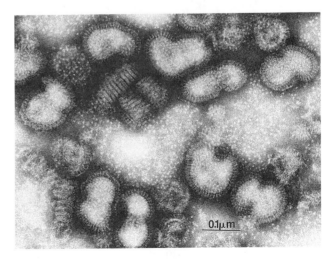

Figure 19-1 Electron micrograph of influenza virus reveals roughly spherical viral particles enclosed in a lipid bilayer with protruding hemagglutinin (HA) and neuraminadase (NA) glycoprotein spikes. [Courtesy of G. Murti, Department of Virology, St. Jude Children's Research Hospital, Memphis, TN.]

the form of trimers, are responsible for the attachment of the virus to host cells. There are approximately 1000 hemagglutinin projections per influenza virion. The hemagglutinin trimer binds to sialic acid groups on host-cell glycoproteins and glycolipids by way of a conserved amino acid sequence that forms a small groove in the hemagglutinin molecule. Neuraminidase, as its name indicates, cleaves *N*-acetylneuramic (sialic) acid from nascent viral glycoproteins and host-cell membrane glycoproteins, an activity that presumably facilitates viral budding from the infected host cell. Within the envelope an inner layer of matrix protein surrounds the nucleocapsid, which consists of eight different strands of ssRNA associated with protein and RNA polymerase (Figure 19-2). Each RNA strand encodes a different influenza protein.

Three basic types of influenza (A, B, and C) can be distinguished by differences in their nucleoprotein and matrix proteins. Type A is the most common and is responsible for the major human pandemics. Antigenic variation in hemagglutinin and neuraminidase has allowed type A influenza virus to be subtyped. According

Table 19-2 Some influenza A strains and their hemagglutinin (H) and neuraminidase (N) subtype

Species	Virus strain designation	Antigenic subtype
Human	A/Puerto Rico/8/34	H0N1
	A/Fort Monmouth/1/47	H1N1
	A/Singapore/1/57	H2N2
	A/Hong Kong/1/68	H3N2
	A/USSR/80/77	H1N1
	A/Brazil/11/78	H1N1
	A/Bangkok/1/79	H3N2
	A/Taiwan/1/86	H1N1
Swine	A/Sw/Iowa/15/30	H1N1
	A/Sw/Taiwan/70	H3N2
Horse (Equine)	A/Eq/Prague/1/56	H7N7
	A/Eq/Miami/1/63	H3N8
Birds	A/Fowl/Dutch/27	H7N7
	A/Tern/South America/61	H5N3
	A/Turkey/Ontario/68	H8N4

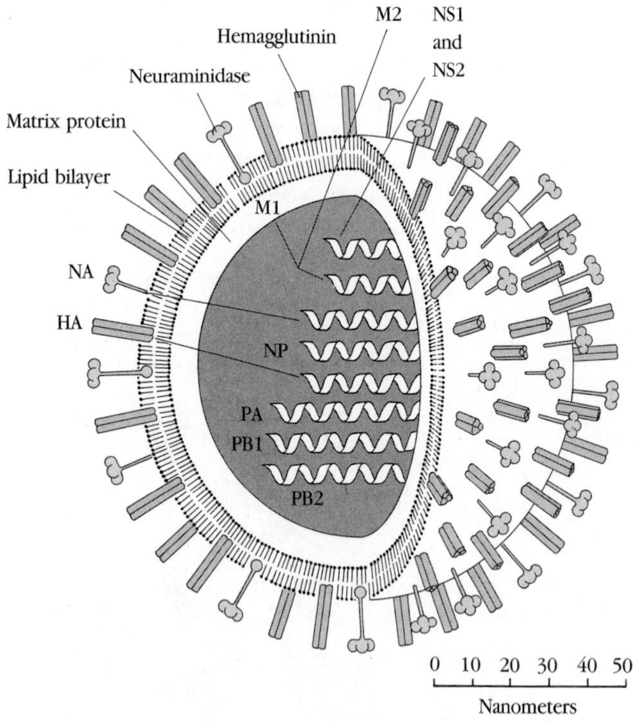

Figure 19-2 Representative structure of influenza. The envelope is covered with neuraminidase and hemagglutinin spikes. Inside is an inner layer of matrix protein surrounding the nucleocapsid, which consists of eight ssRNA strands associated with nucleoprotein. The eight RNA strands encode ten proteins: PB1, PB2, PA, HA (hemagglutinin), NP (nucleoprotein), NA (neuraminadase), M1, M2, NS1, and NS2.

to the nomenclature of the World Health Organization, each virus strain is defined by its animal host of origin (specified, if other than human), geographical origin, strain number, year of isolation, and antigenic description of HA and NA (Table 19-2). For example, A/SW/Iowa/15/30 (H1N1) designates a strain isolate 15 that arose in swine in Iowa in 1930, and A/Hong Kong/1/68 (H3N2) denotes a strain isolate 1 that arose in humans in Hong Kong in 1968; the H and N spikes are antigenically distinct in these two strains.

The distinguishing feature of influenza virus is its variability. The virus can change its surface antigens so completely that the immune response to one viral epidemic gives little or no protection against a subsequent epidemic. The antigenic variation results primarily from changes in the hemagglutinin and neuraminidase spikes protruding from the viral envelope (Figure 19-3). Two different mechanisms generate antigenic variation in HA and NA: *antigenic drift* and *antigenic shift*. Antigenic drift involves a series of spontaneous point mutations that occur gradually, resulting in minor changes in HA and NA. Antigenic shift results in the sudden emergence of a new subtype of influenza bearing an HA and possibly NA dramatically different from that of the preceding virus.

The first human influenza virus was isolated in 1934 and was given the subtype designation H0N1. This subtype persisted until 1947 when a major antigenic shift generated a new subtype, H1N1. This subtype supplanted the previous subtype and became prevalent worldwide until 1957 when H2N2 emerged. The H2N2 subtype prevailed for the next decade and was replaced in 1968 by H3N2. The last antigenic shift in 1977 saw the re-emergence of H1N1. With each antigenic shift, hemagglutinin and neuraminidase undergo major sequence changes, resulting in major antigenic variations for which the immune system displays an absence of memory. Thus each antigenic shift finds the population immunologically unprepared, resulting in a major pandemic of influenza.

Between pandemics the influenza virus undergoes antigenic drift, generating minor antigenic variations, which account for strain differences. The immune response contributes to the emergence of these different influenza strains. As an individual infected with a given influenza strain mounts an effective immune response, the strain is eliminated. However, the accumulation of point mutations alters the antigenicity of some variants sufficiently so that they are able to escape immune elimination. These variants become a new strain of influenza, causing another local epidemic cycle. The role of antibody in such immunologic selection can be demonstrated in the laboratory by mixing an influenza strain with monoclonal antibody specific for that strain and then culturing the virus in cells. The antibody will neutralize all unaltered viral particles and only those viral particles with mutations resulting in altered antigenicity will escape. Within a short period in culture, a new influenza strain can be shown to emerge.

Antigenic shift is thought to occur through genetic reassortment between influenza virions from humans and from various animals, including horses, pigs, and ducks. The fact that influenza contains eight separate strands of ssRNA makes possible the reassortment of the RNA strands of human and animal virions if a single cell is coinfected with both viruses. Evidence for in vivo genetic reassortment between influenza A viruses from human and domestic pigs was obtained by R. G. Webster and C. H. Campbell in 1971. After infecting a pig simultaneously with human Hong Kong influenza (H3N2) and with swine influenza (H1N1), they were able to recover virions expressing H3N1. In some cases, an apparent antigenic shift may represent the re-emergence of a previous strain that has remained hidden for several decades. For example, in May of 1977 a strain of influenza, A/USSR/77 (H1N1), appeared that proved to be identical to a strain that had caused an epidemic 27

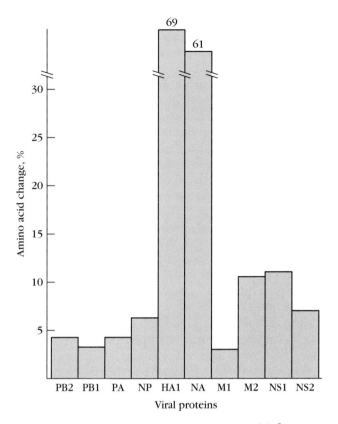

Figure 19-3 Amino acid sequence variation in 10 influenza viral proteins from two H3N2 strains and one H1N1 strain. The surface glycoproteins hemagglutinin (HA) and neuraminidase (NA) showed significant sequence variation; in contrast, the sequences of internal viral proteins, such as matrix proteins (M1 and M2) and nucleoprotein (NP), were largely conserved. [From G. G. Brownlee, 1986, in *Options for the Control of Influenza*, Alan R. Liss.]

years earlier. The virus could have been preserved over the years in a frozen state or in an animal reservoir. When such a re-emergence occurs, the HA and NA antigens expressed are not really new; however, they will be seen by the immune system as if they were new because no memory cells specific for these antigenic subtypes will exist in the population. Thus from an immunologic point of view, the re-emergence of a previous influenza A strain can have the same effect as an antigenic shift that generates a new subtype.

Host Response to Influenza Infection

Humoral antibody specific for the HA molecule is produced during an influenza infection. This antibody protects against influenza infection, but its specificity is strain-specific and is readily bypassed by antigenic drift in the HA and NA glycoproteins. Antigenic drift in the HA molecule results in amino acid substitutions in several antigenic domains at the molecule's distal end (Figure 19-4). Two of these domains are on either side of the conserved sialic acid–binding cleft, which is necessary for binding of virions to target cells. Serum antibodies to these regions, which are important in blocking initial viral infectivity, peak within a few days of infection and then decrease over the next 6 months; the titers then plateau and remain relatively stable for the next several years. This antibody does not appear to be required for recovery from influenza, as patients with agammaglobulinemia recover from the disease. Instead the serum antibody appears to play a significant role in resistance to reinfection by the same strain. When serum antibody levels are high for a particular HA molecule, both mice and humans are resistant to infection by virions expressing that particular HA molecule. If mice are infected with influenza virus and antibody production is experimentally suppressed, the mice recover from the infection only to become reinfected with the same viral strain.

Cell-mediated immunity involving CTLs specific for influenza-infected host cells develops 3–4 days after infection, reaches a peak by day 8 and then disappears by about day 20. In mice, transfer of influenza-specific T_C clones has been shown to confer immunity to a lethal dose of influenza virus on syngeneic adoptive-transfer recipients. Unlike the humoral response, which is specific for each influenza subtype, CTL activity can be cross-reactive; that is, CTLs sometimes recognize and kill syngeneic cells infected with any type A influenza subtype (Table 19-3). This cross-reactivity is important for the development of a better vaccine for influenza, since current vaccines—which are designed to induce antibodies to HA and NA—yield poor protection owing to the continual changes in these glycoproteins. If a vaccine could induce CTL memory that is cross-reactive for all three human pandemic viral subtypes (H1N1, H2N2, and H3N2), then the vaccine might be more protective. It is therefore important to determine which influenza antigens induce cross-reactive CTLs and to characterize the cross-reactive epitopes on these antigens. As discussed in Chapter 18, a vaccine intended to maximize CTL activity must be infectious and capable of replicating within host cells to some extent. Thus, inactivated influenza preparations, which cannot replicate in host cells, are relatively ineffective at inducing CTL activity.

One of the cross-reactive influenza antigens, an internal viral protein called *nucleoprotein*, is recognized by a subset of CTLs that are indeed cross-reactive for all three human pandemic influenza A subtypes. Different inbred strains of mice show individual variation in their ability to respond to influenza nucleoprotein. In some mice 40% of the cross-reactive CTL clones respond to influenza nucleoprotein, but in other strains none of

the cross-reactive CTL clones respond to the nucleoprotein. Among strains that respond to nucleoprotein, however, there are differences in the ability to recognize various peptides derived from nucleoprotein. Experiments described in Chapter 18 indicate that these differences are related to the MHC haplotype of the mouse strains. Furthermore, generation of CTL activity in response to a particular nucleoprotein peptide depends on expression of a particular class I MHC molecule on the target cells (see Table 18-6).

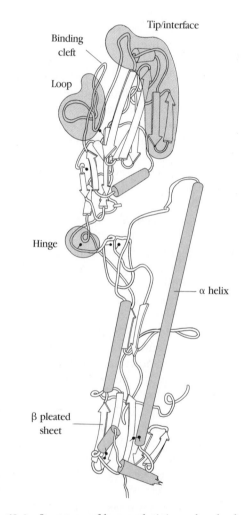

Figure 19-4   Structure of hemagglutinin molecule showing cleft that binds to sialic acid on host cells and regions where antigenic drift is prevalent (circled areas). Antibodies to two of these regions—designated the loop and tip/interface—are important in blocking viral infections. Continual changes in amino acid residues in these regions allow the influenza virus to evade the antibody response. Small black dots represent residues that exhibit a high degree of variation among virus strains. [From D. C. Wiley et al., 1981, *Nature* **289**:373.]

Table 19-3 Cross-reactivity of CTL response to influenza type A virus[*]

Subtype used to challenge primed lymphocytes in vitro	[^{51}Cr] release from infected target cells, %				
	H2N1	H2N2	H3N2	H0N1	Control (uninfected)
H2N1	48	50	52	35	1
H2N2	45	53	53	40	2
H3N2	46	52	52	37	3
H0N1	34	52	45	42	1

[*] Mice were primed with an H2N1 subtype of influenza. The mouse splenic lymphocytes were isolated and challenged in vitro with macrophages infected with the influenza subtypes indicated. The CTL activity generated was then measured by monitoring [^{51}Cr] release from syngeneic [^{51}Cr] labeled target cells infected with the indicated influenza subtypes.

SOURCE: Adapted from H. J. Zweerink, B. A. Askonas, D. Millican et al. 1977. *Eur. J. Immunol.* 7:630.

These results with influenza nucleoprotein peptides highlight the important role of the MHC in determining the immunodominant T-cell epitodes. In the design of a vaccine for influenza, the results from these mouse studies must be considered. A vaccine consisting only of nucleoprotein might not be immunogenic in all individuals, because (as suggested by the mouse data) some MHC haplotypes appear unable to respond to nucleoprotein. And if a synthetic peptide vaccine is chosen, it should consist of a "cocktail" of several peptides, because the mouse data reveal differences among class I MHC molecules in their ability to present different influenza nucleoprotein peptides.

Bacterial Infections

Immunity to bacterial infections is achieved by means of antibody unless the bacterium is capable of intracellular growth, in which case delayed-type hypersensitivity has an important role. Bacteria enter the body either through a number of natural entry routes (e.g., the respiratory tract, the gastrointestinal tract, and the genitourinary tract) or through unnatural routes opened up by breaks in mucous membranes or skin. Depending on the number of organisms entering and the virulence of the organism, different levels of host defense are enlisted. If the inoculum size and the virulence are both low, then localized tissue phagocytes may be able to mount a nonspecific defense and eliminate the bacteria. Larger inoculums or organisms with increased virulence tend to induce an immune response.

Immune Response to Extracellular and Intracellular Bacteria

Infection by extracellular bacteria induces production of humoral antibodies, which are ordinarily secreted by plasma cells in regional lymph nodes and the submucosa of the respiratory and gastrointestinal tracts. The antibodies act at several levels to bring about destruction of the invading organisms (Figure 19-5). Antibody that binds to accessible antigens on the surface of a bacterium can, together with the C3b component of complement, act as an opsonin that increases phagocytosis and thus clearance of the bacterium (see Figure 15-11). Antibody-mediated activation of the complement system can also induce localized production of immune effector molecules that help to develop an amplified and more effective inflammatory response. For example, the complement split products C3a, C4a, and C5a act as anaphylatoxins, inducing local mast-cell degranulation and thus vasodilation and the extravasation of lymphocytes and neutrophils from the blood into tissue space. Other complement split products serve as chemotactic factors for neutrophils, thereby contributing to the buildup of phagocytic cells at the site of infection. In the case of some bacteria—notably the gram-negative organisms—complement activation can lead to lysis of the organism. If the bacterium secretes an exotoxin or endotoxin, antibody may bind to the toxin and neutralize it. The antibody-toxin complexes are then cleared by phagocytic cells in the same manner as any antigen-antibody complex.

Infections caused by bacteria that are capable of intracellular growth within phagocytic cells tend to induce

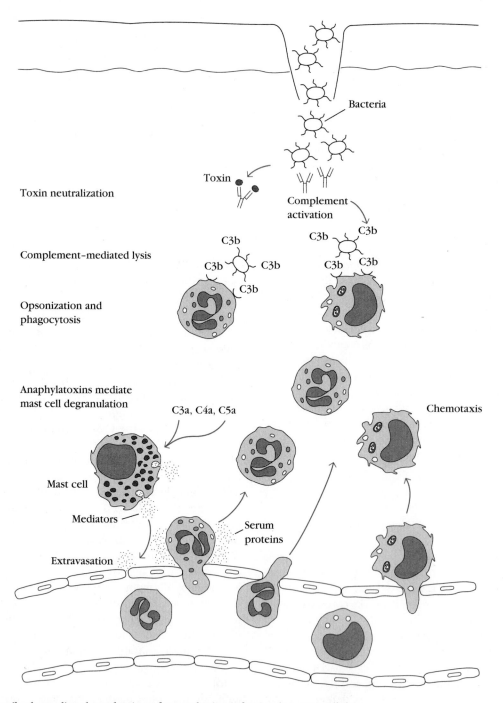

Toxin neutralization

Complement–mediated lysis

Opsonization and phagocytosis

Anaphylatoxins mediate mast cell degranulation

Mast cell

Mediators

Extravasation

Figure 19-5 Antibody-mediated mechanisms for combating infection by extracellular bacteria. (1) Antibody and the complement split product C3b bind to bacteria, serving as opsonins to increase phagocytosis. (2) Antibody neutralizes bacterial toxins. (3) Antibody induces complement-mediated lysis of bacteria. (4) C3a and C5a generated by antibody activation of the complement system induce local mast-cell degranulation, releasing substances that mediate vasodilation and extravasation of lymphocytes and neutrophils.

Table 19-4   Host immune responses to bacterial infection and bacterial evasion mechanisms

Infection process	Host defense	Bacterial evasion mechanisms
Attachment to host cells	Blockage of attachment by secretory IgA antibodies	Secretion of proteases that cleave secretory IgA dimers Antigenic variation in attachment structures
Proliferation	Phagocytosis (Ab- and C3b-mediated opsonization)	Production of surface structures (polysaccharide capsule, M protein, fibrin coat) that inhibits phagocytic cells Intracellular mechanisms for surviving within phagocytic cells
	Complement-mediated lysis and localized inflammatory response	Generalized resistance to complement-mediated lysis by gram-positive bacteria Insertion of membrane-attack complex prevented by long side chain in cell-wall LPS (some gram-negative bacteria) Secretion of elastase that inactivates C3a and C5a (*Pseudomonas*)
Invasion of host tissues	Ab-mediated agglutination	Secretion of hyaluronidase, which enhances bacterial invasiveness
Toxin-induced damage to host cells	Neutralization of toxin by antibody	

a cell-mediated immune response, specifically, delayed-type hypersensitivity. In this response cytokines secreted by T_{DTH} cells are important—notably IFN-γ, which activates macrophages to achieve more effective killing of intracellular pathogens (see Figure 13-13).

Bacterial Evasion of Host-Defense Mechanisms

Bacteria have evolved various mechanisms for enhancing their ability to colonize host mucous membranes and for circumventing host immune responses (Table 19-4). A number of gram-negative bacteria have pili (long hair-like projections), which enable them to attach to the membrane of the intestinal or genitourinary tracts, the first step in infection (Figure 19-6). Other bacteria, such as *Bordetella pertussis*, secrete adhesion molecules that attach to both the bacterium and the ciliated epithelial cells of the upper respiratory tract. Secretory IgA antibodies can block bacterial attachment to mucosal epithelial cells. However, some bacteria (e.g., *Neisseria*

gonorrhoeae, *Hemophilus influenzae*, and *Neisseria meningitidis*) secrete proteases that cleave secretory IgA at the hinge region; the resulting Fab and Fc fragments have a shortened half-life in mucous secretions and are not able to agglutinate microorganisms.

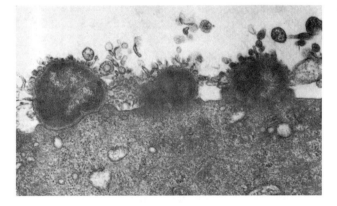

Figure 19-6   Electron micrograph of *Neisseria gonorrhoeae* attaching to urethral epithelial cells. Pili (P) extend from the gonococcal surface and mediate the attachment. [From M. E. Ward and P. J. Watt, 1972, *J. Inf. Dis.* **126**:601.]

Another way that bacteria evade the IgA response of the host and increase their ability to attach to epithelial cells is by changing their surface antigens. An example of this is provided by *N. gonorrhoeae*, which attaches to epithelial cells of the urethra or cervix by means of pili. In this organism, pilin, the protein component of the pili, has been shown to consist of constant, variable, and hypervariable amino acids. Variation in the pilin amino acid sequence is generated by gene rearrangements of the coding sequences. The pilin locus consists of one or two expression genes and 10–20 silent genes. Each gene is arranged into six regions called "minicassettes." Pilin variation is generated by a process of gene conversion in which one or more minicassettes from the silent genes replace a minicassette of the expression gene (Figure 19-7). This process generates enormous antigenic diversity of the pilin proteins, similar to that achieved by immunoglobulin-gene rearrangements. The continual changes in pilin protein structure may contribute to the pathogenicity of *N. gonorrhoeae*, by increasing the likelihood of expression of pili that bind more firmly to epithelial cells. In addition, the continual changes in the pilin sequence allows the organism to evade neutralization by humoral antibody.

Numerous bacteria have developed ways to resist phagocytosis or to counteract various complement-mediated immune responses. A number of bacteria, for example, possess surface structures that serve to inhibit phagocytosis. A classic example is *Streptococcus pneumoniae*, whose polysaccharide capsule is very effective in preventing phagocytosis. On other bacteria, such as *Streptococcus pyogenes*, a surface protein projection, called the M protein, inhibits phagocytosis. And some pathogenic *Staphylococci* secrete a coagulase enzyme that produces a fibrin coat around the organism, shielding it from phagocytic cells. Some bacteria are able to interfere with the complement system. In some gram-negative bacteria, for example, long side chains on the lipid A moiety of the cell-wall core polysaccharide help to resist complement-mediated lysis. *Pseudomonas* secretes an enzyme, elastase, that inactivates both the C3a and C5a anaphylatoxins, thereby diminishing the localized inflammatory reaction.

A number of bacteria escape host-defense mechanisms by their ability to survive intracellularly within phagocytic cells. Some, such as *Mycobacterium tuberculosis* and *Mycobacterium leprae*, do this by escaping the phagolysosome and growing within the more favorable environment of the cytoplasm. Other bacteria, such as *Mycobacterium avium* and *Chlamydia*, block lysosomal fusion with the phagolysosome; still others are resistant to the oxidative attack that takes place within the phagolysosome.

Contribution of the Immune Response to Bacterial Pathogenesis

In some cases disease is caused not by the bacterial pathogen but by the immune response to the pathogen. In some gram-negative bacterial infections, endotoxins (e.g., LPS) activate macrophages, resulting in the release of high levels of IL-1 and TNF-α. The activities of these

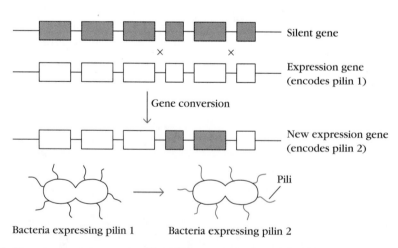

Figure 19-7 Variation of pilin sequences is generated by DNA rearrangements. The pilin locus consists of one or two expression genes and a series of 10–20 silent genes. Each gene contains a series of "minicassettes." One or more minicassettes of the expression gene can be replaced by a minicassette of one of the silent genes. [Modified from T. F. Meyer, 1990, *Annu. Rev. Microbiol.* **44**:460.]

cytokines can lead to fatal bacterial septic shock (see Chapter 11).

High levels of cytokines have also been shown to contribute to symptoms in staphylococcal food poisoning and toxic shock syndrome. Food poisoning by *Staphylococcal aureus* is caused by staphylococcal enterotoxins (SEs), which can be classified into five serologically distinct groups (A, B, C, D, and E). These enterotoxins act as potent mitogens, activating all T cells expressing a particular T-cell receptor V$_\beta$ gene family; for this reason, these enterotoxins are called "superantigens." Cytokines released by the large numbers of T$_H$ cells activated by these superantigens are responsible for many of the symptoms seen in staphylococcal food poisoning, including fever, diarrhea, and sometimes cardiovascular shock (see Chapter 11). A similar sequence of events appears to occur in toxic shock syndrome, an often fatal disease associated with tampon use. In this case a staphylococcal exotoxin called toxic shock syndrome toxin-1 (TSST-1) acts as a superantigen, inducing large scale-production of TNF by activated T$_H$ cells and macrophages.

The ability of some bacteria to survive intracellularly within phagocytic cells can result in chronic antigenic activation of T$_{DTH}$ cells, leading to tissue destruction by a DTH reaction. Cytokines secreted by these activated T cells can lead to extensive macrophage accumulation and activation (called a granuloma). The localized concentrations of lysosomal enzymes in these granulomas can cause extensive tissue necrosis. Much of the tissue damage seen with *Mycobacterium tuberculosis* is due to this delayed-type hypersensitivity response. (see Chapter 13).

Diphtheria (*Corynebacterium diphtheriae*)

Diphtheria is the prototype of a bacterial disease caused by a secreted exotoxin for which immunity can be induced by immunization with a toxoid. The causative agent, a gram-positive, rodlike organism called *Corynebacterium diphtheriae*, was first described by Klebs in 1883 and was shown a year later by Loeffler to cause diphtheria in guinea pigs and rabbits. Autopsies on the infected animals revealed that while bacterial growth was limited to the site of inoculation, there was widespread damage to a variety of organs including the heart, liver, and kidneys. This led Loeffler to speculate that the neurologic and cardiologic manifestations of the disease were caused by a toxic substance elaborated by the organisms. Loeffler's hypothesis was validated in 1888 when Roux and Yersin produced the disease in animals by injection of a sterile filtrate from a culture of *C. diphtheriae*. Two years later, von Behring showed that an antiserum to the toxin was able to prevent death in

infected animals. He prepared a toxoid by treating the toxin with iodine trichloride and demonstrated that the toxoid could induce protective antibodies in animals. However the toxoid was still quite toxic and therefore unsuitable for use in humans. In 1923 Ramon found that exposure of the toxin to heat and formalin rendered it nontoxic but did not destroy its antigenicity. Clinical trials with the formalin-treated toxoid revealed that it was able to confer a high level of protection to diphtheria upon recipients. As widespread use of the toxoid increased, the number of cases of diphtheria decreased dramatically. In the 1920s there were approximately 200 cases of diphtheria per 100,000 population in the United States. In 1989 the Centers for Disease Control reported only three cases of diphtheria in the United States.

Natural infection with *C. diphtheriae* occurs only in humans. The disease is spread from one individual to another by airborne respiratory droplets. The organism colonizes the nasopharyngeal tract, remaining in the superficial layers of the respiratory mucosa. Growth of the organism itself causes little tissue damage, and only a mild inflammatory reaction develops. The virulence of the organism is completely dependent on its potent exotoxin. The toxin causes destruction of the underlying tissue resulting in the formation of a tough fibrinous membrane ("pseudomembrane") composed of fibrin, white blood cells, and dead respiratory epithelial cells. The membrane itself can lead to suffocation. The exotoxin also is responsible for widespread systemic manifestations. Often there is pronounced myocardial damage (often leading to congestive heart failure) and neurologic damage (ranging from mild weakness to complete paralysis).

The toxin that causes diphtheria symptoms is encoded by the *tox* gene carried by phage β. Only strains of *C. diphtheriae* that carry phage β in a state of lysogeny (in which the β-prophage DNA persists within the bacterial cell) are able to produce the exotoxin. The exotoxin, which is synthesized as a single polypeptide precursor, can be dissociated into two fragments (A and B) by mild trypsin digestion. Fragment B binds to ganglioside receptors on susceptible cells, facilitating the transport of fragment A across the plasma membrane. Toxicity results from the inhibitory effect of fragment A on protein synthesis. This fragment catalyzes the covalent modification of elongation factor 2 (EF-2), which is present in mammalian cells but not in bacteria. Loss of EF-2 inhibits interaction of mRNA and tRNA on ribosomes, thus preventing further addition of amino acids to a growing polypeptide chain. Fragment A is extremely potent; a single molecule has been shown to kill a cell. Removal of fragment B from the exotoxin prevents fragment A from entering the cell, thus rendering the exotoxin nontoxic. As discussed in Chapter 7, an immunotoxin can be prepared by replacing fragment B with a monoclonal antibody specific for a tumor-cell surface antigen; in this way the toxin A fragment can be targeted to tumor cells (see Figure 7-10).

Today, diphtheria toxoid is prepared by treating diphtheria toxin with formaldehyde. The reaction with formaldehyde cross-links the toxin, resulting in an irreversible loss in its toxicity while enhancing its antigenicity. The toxoid is administered together with tetanus toxoid and inactivated *Bordetella pertussis* in a combined vaccine that is given to children beginning at 6–8 weeks of age (Table 18-2). Immunization with the toxoid induces the production of antibodies (antitoxin), which can bind to the toxin and neutralize its activity. Because antitoxin levels decline slowly over time, booster doses are recommended at 10-year intervals to maintain antitoxin levels within the protective range. Interestingly, antibodies specific for epitopes on fragment B of the diphtheria toxin are critical for toxin neutralization because these antibodies block binding of the toxin to cellular receptors and the subsequent translocation of fragment A into cells.

Lyme Disease (*Borrelia burgdorferi*)

In 1975 about 60 cases of a new and mysterious disease were reported in Lyme, Connecticut. The disease symptoms included unexplained "bull's-eye" rashes, headaches, and arthritis; in some cases severe neurologic complications developed, including excruciating headaches, meningitis, loss of memory, and mood swings. An epidemiologic study was initiated in hope of identifying the causative agent. The disease was shown to have a higher incidence in individuals living in heavily wooded areas, and a close geographic clustering of infected individuals was found. In addition, the disease was shown to be contracted during the summer months between June and September. Finally in 1977, nine patients with the disease remembered having been bitten by a tick at the site of the characteristic rash. Fortuitously, the tick had been saved by one patient and was examined by a noted authority on tickborne diseases, Willy Burgdorfer. He found the tick (an *Ixodes* species) to be teaming with a new species of gram-negative spirochete, which was subsequently named *Borrelia burgdorferi* after its discoverer.

As an infected tick takes a blood meal, *B. burgdorferi* enters the bloodstream. Experiments with fluorescent antibodies to *B. burgdorferi* have revealed the presence of low numbers of the spirochete at the site of the bite and in various organs including kidney, spleen, liver, cerebrospinal fluid, and brain tissue. The clinical symptoms of Lyme disease generally begin with a characteristic rash, beginning as a red papule and spreading to form what appears as a bull's eye 10–50 cm in diameter. Following the rash, arthritic symptoms and neurologic symptoms often develop. Roughly 80% of individuals with Lyme disease develop some degree of arthritic symptoms ranging from joint pain to chronic joint destruction. Neurologic symptoms develop in about 60% of Lyme patients. Most report headaches, but about 15% develop meningitis and encephalitis. The disease can be successfully treated with broad-spectrum antibiotics such as penicillin and tetracycline. Interestingly, though, soon after the antibiotic is administered, there is a temporary exacerbation of symptoms (called the Jarish-Herxheimer reaction).

Antibodies to a protein associated with the flagella of *B. burgdorferi* can often be detected after infection. However, these antibodies do not appear to confer protection against the spirochete and may even contribute to the pathogenesis of Lyme disease. Immune complexes, consisting of spirochete antigens and antibody, are thought to result in a type III hypersensitive reaction. Deposition of complexes near the original bite results in the characteristic rash; deposition of complexes in the joints is thought to induce an inflammatory response resulting in arthritic symptoms; deposition of the complexes in the vasculature and along the meninges leads to neurologic symptoms. As was discussed in Chapter 15, antigen-antibody complexes activate the complement system. Complement activation can result in direct lytic damage to the joint or vasculature. Alternatively, complement split products, such as C3a and C5a, will induce neutrophil chemotaxis and activation. Some of the tissue damage may then result from lysosomal enzymes released by the activated neutrophils.

Gail Habicht, Gregory Beck, and Jorge Benach have suggested that interleukin 1 (IL-1) is involved in the pathogenesis of Lyme disease. Like other gram-negative bacteria, *Borrelia* has a cell wall containing lipopolysaccharide (LPS). These researchers observed that when macrophages are cultured together with *B. burgdorferi*, the macrophages secrete high levels of IL-1. They suggested that high levels of IL-1 released by macrophages in Lyme disease may be responsible for many of the symptoms of the disease. For example, when IL-1 is injected into rabbit skin, a characteristic rash appears. Furthermore, when IL-1 is added to cultured synovial cells, the cells begin to secrete collagenase and prostaglandins. The release of collagenase in the joint could lead to the degradation of collagen and destruction of the joint. They have suggested that the exacerbation of symptoms seen with antibiotic treatment may result from massive killing of *B. burgdorferi*, releasing large quantities of LPS from the gram-negative cell wall. The LPS in turn is hypothesized to induce high-level IL-1 release, resulting in increased severity of symptoms, until the LPS levels subside.

In order to understand the role of the immune response in Lyme disease, some researchers have studied the infection in mice, which are a major reservoir of *B. burgdorferi*. Ticks acquire the spirochetes from infected mice and transmit them to humans. Unlike humans, however, normal mice infected with *B. burgdorferi* do not develop Lyme disease, although mutant *scid* mice, which lack functional T and B cells, are susceptible to the disease. This finding has led to the speculation that the immune response in normal mice protects the animals from the disease. Comparison of the immune response to *B. burgdorferi* in normal mice and humans has shown that mice produce high levels of antibodies to two envelope outer-surface proteins, whereas humans fail to do so; instead, most infected humans produce antibodies to a flagellar antigen. The ability of these antibodies to protect against Lyme disease was studied using *scid* mice. Monoclonal antibodies to the outer-surface proteins protected *scid* mice from disease, whereas monoclonal antibodies to the flagellar antigen did not. These results offer the possibility that a vaccine for Lyme disease consisting of the outer-surface proteins might induce protective antibodies in humans.

Protozoan Diseases

Protozoans are unicellular eukaryotic organisms. They are responsible for several serious diseases in humans, including amebiasis, Chagas' disease, African sleeping sickness, malaria, leishmaniasis, and toxoplasmosis. The type of immune response that develops and the effectiveness of the response depends in part on the location of the parasite within the host. Many protozoans have stages in which they are free within the bloodstream, and it is during these stages that humoral antibody is most effective. Many of these same pathogens are also capable of intracellular growth, and during these stages cell-mediated immune reactions are effective in host defense. In the development of vaccines for protozoan diseases, the branch of the immune system that is most likely to confer protection must be carefully considered.

Malaria (*Plasmodium* species)

Malaria, one of the most important diseases in the world today, is estimated to infect 600 million people worldwide. The disease may cause 1–2 million deaths every year. Malaria is caused by various species of the genus *Plasmodium*, of which *P. falciparum* is the most virulent and prevalent. The alarming development of mul-

tiple drug resistance in *Plasmodium* and the increased resistance of its vector, the *Anopheles* mosquito, to DDT underscore the importance of developing new strategies to hinder the spread of malaria.

Plasmodium *Life Cycle and Pathogenesis of Malaria*

The life cycle of *Plasmodium* is extremely complex, progressing through a remarkable series of developmental and maturational stages (Figure 19-8). The female *Anopheles* mosquito serves as the vector for *Plasmodium* transmission, and part of the parasite's life cycle takes place within the mosquito. While male *Anopheles* mosquitos feed on plant juices, the females feed on blood meals and thus acquire *Plasmodium gametocytes* from an infected individual. The male and female gametocytes fuse to form a zygote within the mosquito's gut. The zygotes multiply and differentiate into *sporozoites* within the salivary gland of the infected female mosquito. The sporozoite is a long, slender cell that is covered by 45-kD protein called the circumsporozoite (CS) antigen.

Human infection begins when *Plasmodium* sporozoites are introduced into an individual's bloodstream as an infected mosquito takes a blood meal. Within 30 min the sporozoites disappear from the blood as they migrate to the liver, where they infect liver hepatocytes. Sporozoites have been shown to adhere to hepatocytes in vitro, and the circumsporozoite antigen is thought to take part in the adhesion. The liver phase is characterized by extensive sporozoite multiplication and a complex series of transformations that culminate in about a week in the *merozoite* stage. It has been estimated that a liver hepatocyte infected with a single sporozoite can release 5,000–10,000 merozoites. The released merozoites infect red blood cells, initiating the symptoms and pathology of malaria. Within a red blood cell, merozoites replicate and undergo successive differentiations; eventually the cell ruptures and releases new merozoites, which go on to infect more red blood cells. Eventually some of the merozoites differentiate into male and female *gametocytes*. The gametocytes are ingested by an *Anopheles* mosquito, and the cycle repeats itself.

The symptoms of malaria are recurrent chills, fever, and sweating. The symptoms peak roughly every 48 h, when successive generations of merozoites are released from infected red blood cells. An infected individual eventually becomes weak and anemic and shows splenomegaly. The large numbers of merozoites formed can block capillaries, causing intense headaches, renal failure, heart failure, or cerebral damage—often with fatal consequences. There is speculation that some of the symptoms of malaria may be caused not by *Plasmodium* itself but instead by lymphokine production. This hypothesis stemmed from the observation that cancer patients treated in clinical trials with recombinant tumor necrosis factor (TNF) developed symptoms that mimicked malaria. The relation between TNF and malaria symptoms was studied by infecting mice with a mouse-specific strain of *Plasmodium*, which causes rapid death by cerebral malaria. Injection of these mice with antibodies to TNF was shown to prevent the rapid death.

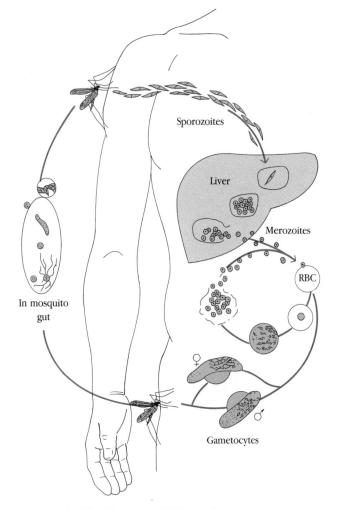

Figure 19-8 The life cycle of *Plasmodium*. Sporozoites enter the bloodstream when an infected mosquito takes a blood meal. The sporozoites migrate to the liver where they multiply, transforming liver hepatocytes into giant multinucleate schizonts, which release thousands of merozoites into the bloodstream. The merozoites infect red blood cells, which eventually rupture, releasing more merozoites. Eventually some of the merozoites differentiate into male and female gametocytes, which are ingested by a mosquito and differentiate into the sporozoite stage within the salivary gland of the mosquito.

Host Response to Plasmodium *Infection*

In endemic regions the immune response to malaria is poor. Children less than 14 years old mount the lowest immune response and consequently are most susceptible to infection. In some regions the childhood mortality rate for malaria reaches 50%, and worldwide the disease kills about a million children a year. The low immune response to malaria among children can be demonstrated by measuring serum antibody levels to the sporozoite stage. Only 22% of the children living in endemic areas have detectable antibodies to the sporozoite stage, whereas 84% of the adults have such antibodies. Even in adults the degree of immunity is far from complete, however, and most people living in endemic regions have lifelong low-level *Plasmodium* infections.

A number of factors may contribute to the low levels of immune responsiveness to *Plasmodium*. The maturational changes from sporozoite to merozoite to gametocyte allow the organism to keep changing its surface molecules, resulting in continual changes in the antigens seen by the immune system. The intracellular phases of the life cycle in liver cells and erythrocytes also reduce the degree of immune activation generated by the pathogen and allow the organism to multiply while it is shielded from the attacking immune system. Furthermore, the most accessible stage, the sporozoite, circulates in the blood for only about 30 min before it infects liver hepatocytes; it is unlikely that much immune activation can occur in such a short period of time. And even when an antibody response does develop to sporozoites, *Plasmodium* has evolved a way of overcoming that response by sloughing off the surface CS-antigen coat, thus rendering the antibodies ineffective.

Design of Malaria Vaccines

Clearly an effective vaccine for malaria should be designed to maximize the most effective immune defense mechanisms. Unfortunately, little is known of the roles that humoral and cell-mediated responses play in the development of protective immunity to this disease. Current approaches to design of malaria vaccines largely focus on the sporozoite stage. One experimental vaccine, for example, consists of *Plasmodium* sporozoites attenuated by x-irradiation. Mice, monkeys, and human volunteers have been shown to develop increased levels of both humoral and cell-mediated immunity to these x-irradiated sporozoites; mice immunized with x-irradiated sporozoites, for example, were protected when challenged with a mouse-specific strain of *Plasmodium*. As encouraging as these results are, an x-irradiated-sporozoite vaccine is not a feasible approach for immunizing the millions of people living in endemic regions. It has been estimated that it would take an enormous insectory to breed mosquitos in which to prepare enough x-irradiated sporozoites to vaccinate one small village in an endemic area.

Another vaccine approach has focused on identification of immunodominant B- and T-cell epitopes on the various *Plasmodium* stages. Once these epitopes are identified, synthetic peptide vaccines containing these epitopes could be prepared or monoclonal antibodies could be developed that are specific for these epitopes. Both of these approaches are currently being explored. The target antigen recognized by humoral antibodies in the x-irradiated-sporozoite vaccine is the circumsporozoite (CS) antigen. The CS antigen of *P. falciparum* contains 412 amino acids with a central region consisting of approximately 40 repeats of an Asn-Ala-Asn-Pro (NANP) sequence (Figure 19-9). This repeat was shown to constitute the immunodominant B-cell epitope of the x-irradiated-sporozoite vaccine. In addition, monoclonal antibodies specific for these repeats on the CS antigen were found to protect mice against a challenge of live plasmodia, suggesting that synthetic peptide vaccines based on the repeat might induce protective antibody. To design such a synthetic peptide vaccine, it was first necessary to determine the number of repeats that function as the immunodominant B-cell epitope. Experiments with synthetic peptides incorporating from one to five repeats of NANP demonstrated

that $(NANP)_3$ represented the entire epitope; that is, it could completely block antibody binding to sporozoites.

In one trial the $(NANP)_3$ synthetic peptide was conjugated to tetanus toxoid in alum and administered intramuscularly to 35 healthy male volunteers. Of these volunteers, 71% developed antibody to a 160-μg dose of the vaccine. Three of the volunteers with high serum antibody levels were subsequently infected with live *P. falciparum* by infected *Anopheles* mosquitos; four unimmunized volunteers were also infected. All four unimmunized volunteers developed merozoites in an average of 8.5 days. In contrast, one recipient of the vaccine appeared to be immune and never developed merozoites or any symptoms of malaria; the other two recipients developed merozoites, but they did not appear until day 11, considerably later than usual. Similar degrees of protection have been reported by other researchers. Such results show promise, but a success rate of one in three is not what one would hope for.

The $(NANP)_3$–tetanus toxoid trials illustrate one common problem with vaccines in which a synthetic peptide representing only the immunodominant B-cell epitope is coupled to an unrelated carrier protein. Although a humoral antibody response is generated to $(NANP)_3$, the T-cell response induced by this vaccine is directed to the tetanus toxoid carrier; therefore, the vaccine fails to generate a T-memory response specific for *Plasmodium*. What is needed is a vaccine incorporating both

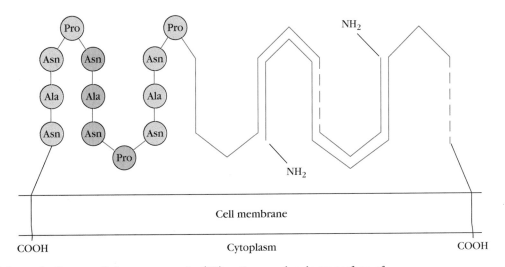

Figure 19-9 Schematic diagram of circumsporozoite (CS) antigen molecule on surface of *P. falciparum*. The central region consists of approximately 40 repeats of the tetrapeptide Asn-Ala-Asn-Pro (NANP). Three repeats—that is, $(NANP)_3$—serves as the immunodominant B-cell epitope on CS antigen. The polypeptide chain bends sharply at each Pro, and hydrogen bonds to itself or to an adjacent molecule. The entire molecule contains 412 amino acids; the central-repeat region (red), which is not to scale in the diagram, contains about 160 amino acids.

B- and T-cell immunodominant epitopes. In an attempt to identify T-cell epitopes on CS antigen, different inbred mouse strains were immunized with a recombinant vaccina virus expressing the CS antigen. Of the different mice strains tested, only mice possessing IA^b or IA^k class II MHC alleles were able to produce a high antibody response to the CS antigen. This would suggest that only IA^b and IA^k class II molecules can present peptides from the CS antigen to T_H cells and thereby achieve B-cell activation.

In order to identify the T-cell epitope on CS antigen that is recognized by IA^k-bearing mice, linear peptide sequences of the CS protein were analyzed by a computer program to identify peptides having significant amphipathic α helices. Such peptides present both hydrophobic and hydrophilic surfaces and are thought to bind effectively to MHC molecules and the T-cell receptor. The peptide sequence, designated Th2R had the highest amphipathic index (Figure 19-10). When IA^k-bearing mice were immunized with a synthetic peptide containing the B-cell epitope NANP conjugated to the Th2R peptide, the mice responded with a high level of antibody production. By analyzing peptide sequences for those properties known to be important for T-cell

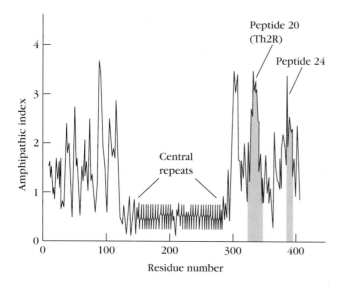

Figure 19-10 Identification of amphipathic peptides in circumsporozoite (CS) antigen of *P. falciparum*. Overlapping blocks of 11 residues were analyzed by computer and assigned an amphipathic index, which was plotted at the center position of each block. The area under each peak corresponds to the amphipathic score. The peaks with the highest amphipathic scores correspond to peptides 20 (Th2R) and 24. Th2R is the major T-cell eptiope on CS antigen recognized by IA^k-bearing mice. In humans, both Th2R and peptide 24 function as T-cell epitopes. [Adapted from M. F. Good et al., 1987, *Science* **235**:1059.]

epitopes (such as amphipathic helices), then, it was possible to design a successful synthetic vaccine for the IA^k-bearing mice. By continuing this process it is hoped that other T-cell epitopes can be identified that can be presented by other MHC alleles. Presumably an effective vaccine would include a mixture of these peptides.

CS antigen also appears to be poorly immunogenic for T cells in humans. For example, when peripheral blood lymphocytes from individuals living in malarial endemic areas were incubated with overlapping synthetic peptides spanning the entire length of CS antigen, the cells from 40% of the individuals did not proliferate (were not activated) in response to any of the peptides. Interestingly, among the 60% of cell samples that did respond to the synthetic peptides, the two peptides that were most recognized, peptides 20 (Th2R) and 24, were also the peptides having the highest amphipathic indices. Comparison of the sequence variation of CS peptides from one plasmodium to the next revealed that these two peptides (Th2R and 24) exhibited more variation than other peptide sequences. This variability might contribute to the ability of *Plasmodium* to escape the immune response. Some researchers speculate that the immune response may actually select for such variants, which would be more likely to escape an effective cell-mediated response. Because of this possibility, it might be fruitful to screen other sporozoite proteins for amphipathic sequences showing less variation.

The variation in the major T-cell epitopes of CS antigen may place a fundamental limit on the effectiveness of the cell-mediated immune response to *Plasmodium*. Yet a number of findings have suggested that cell-mediated immunity—acting in concert with humoral antibody or acting independently—is important in malaria. For example, when mice are immunized with x-irradiated sporozoites, they are immune to a subsequent challenge with live sporozoites, as mentioned above. However, if immunized mice are treated with anti-CD8 to deplete their $CD8^+$ T cells, that immunity is abolished (Table 19-5). In addition, T cells from mice rendered immune with x-irradiated-sporozoite vaccine are able to confer immunity on adoptive-transfer recipients. T cells could contribute to immunity to malaria either through a delayed-type hypersensitive response or by cell-mediated lysis by CTLs. $CD4^+$ cells may recognize sporozoite antigens associated with class II MHC molecules on liver Kupffer cells (a type of macrophage). The target for $CD8^+$ CTLs is thought to be sporozoite antigens presented by class I MHC molecules on infected liver hepatocytes. The ability of sporozoites to escape an effective cell-mediated immune response may allow such large numbers of merozoites to become established that successful elimination of *Plasmodium* by the immune system is reduced.

Table 19-5 Effect of removal of CD4$^+$ or CD8$^+$ T cells on immunity to *Plasmodium* infection in mice immunized with x-irradiated-sporozoite vaccine

Immunization (control)	In vivo treatment	Infected/Total mice	Median days to detectable parasitemia
No	None	15/15	5
Yes	None	0/10	Not detected
Yes	Anti-CD8	9/9	5
Yes	Anti-CD4	0/5	Not detected

* After immunization and in vivo treatment as indicated, mice were challenged with a mouse-specific strain of *Plasmodium*. The number that became infected and the development of parasitemia were monitored.

SOURCE: Data from W. R. Weiss, 1988, *Proc. Nat'l Acad. Sci. USA* **85**:573; cited in M. F. Good et al., 1988, *Annu. Rev. Immunol.* **6**:663.

African Sleeping Sickness (*Trypanosoma* Species)

Two species of African trypanosomes, which are flagellated protozoans, can cause sleeping sickness, a chronic, debilitating disease transmitted to humans and cattle by the bite of the tsetse fly. In the bloodstream a trypanosome differentiates into a long, slender form that continues to divide every 4–6 h. The disease progresses through several stages, beginning with an early (systemic) stage in which trypanosomes multiply in the blood and progressing to a neurologic stage in which the parasite infects the central nervous system, causing meningoencephalitis and eventually the loss of consciousness.

Following infection, the number of trypanosomes within the bloodstream increases and decreases rapidly in successive waves of parasitemia, which continue indefinitely. As parasite numbers increase, an effective humoral antibody response to trypanosomal surface antigens develops; these antibodies eliminate most of the parasites from the bloodstream, both by complement-mediated lysis and by opsonization and subsequent phagocytosis. Although most of the trypanosomes are successfully eliminated from the blood, about 1% of the organisms, which now bear an antigenically different surface glycoprotein, escape the initial antibody response. These surviving organisms now begin to proliferate in the bloodstream, and a new wave of parasitemia is observed. The successive waves of parasitemia reflect a unique mechanism of *antigenic variation* by which

the trypanosomes can evade the immune response to their glycoprotein antigens. This antigenic variation is so effective that each new variant that arises in the course of a single infection is able to escape the humoral antibodies generated in response to the preceding variant (Figure 19-11).

A trypanosome is covered by a glycoprotein coat, called *variant surface glycoprotein* (VSG), and it is the antigenic shift of this surface glycoprotein that enables the organism to escape immunologic clearance and so generate successive waves of parasitemia. Several unusual genetic processes generate the extensive variation in the VSG. An individual trypanosome carries a large repertoire of VSG genes, each encoding a different VSG primary sequence. *Trypanosoma brucei*, for example, contains more than 1000 VSG genes in its genome, clustered at multiple chromosomal sites. A trypanosome expresses only a single VSG gene at a single time. Activation of a VSG gene results in duplication of the gene and its transposition to a transcriptionally active expression site (ES) at the telomeric end of specific chromosomes. Activation of a new VSG gene displaces the previous gene from the telomeric expression site. A number of chromosomes in the trypanosome have transcriptionally active expression sites at the telomeric ends, so that a number of VSG genes can potentially be expressed, but unknown control mechanisms limit expression to a single VSG expression site at a time.

One interesting observation is that there appears to be some order to the VSG variation during infection. Each new variant arises not by clonal outgrowth from a single variant cell but instead from the growth of mul-

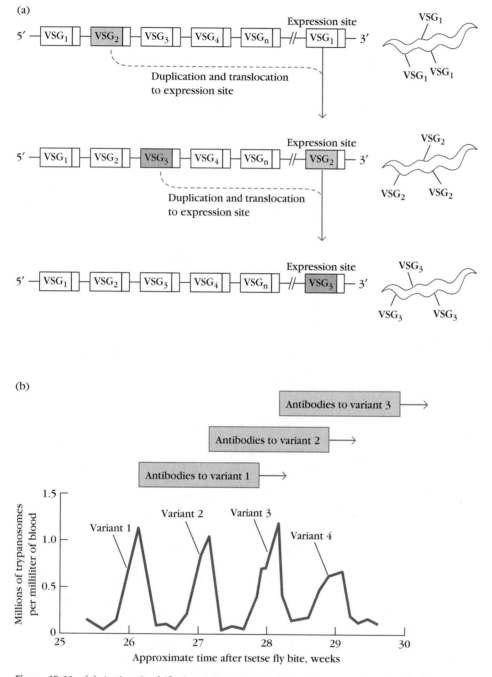

Figure 19-11 (a) Antigenic shifts in trypanosomes occur as gene segments encoding the variable surface glycoprotein (VSG) are duplicated and translocated to an expression site located close to the telomere. (b) Repeated antigenic shifts of VSGs in trypanosomes allows the organism to evade the humoral antibody response, resulting in successive waves of parasitemia. [Part (b) adapted from John Donelson, 1988, *The Biology of Parasitism*, Alan R. Liss.]

tiple cells that have activated the same VSG gene in the current wave of parasite growth. It is not known how this process is regulated among individual trypanosomes. Clearly the continual shifts in epitopes displayed by the VSG makes the development of a vaccine for African sleeping sickness extremely difficult.

Diseases Caused by Parasitic Worms (Helminths)

Unlike protozoans, which are unicellular and often grow within human cells, helminths are large multicellular organisms that do not ordinarily multiply within humans and are not intracellular pathogens. Although helminths are more accessible to the immune system than protozoans, most infected individuals carry relatively few of these parasites; for this reason the immune system is not strongly engaged and the level of immunity generated to helminths is often very poor. Parasitic worms are responsible for a wide variety of diseases in both humans and animals. More than a billion people are infected with *Ascaris*, a parasitic roundworm that infects the small intestine, and more than 300 million people are infected with *Schistosoma*, a trematode worm that causes a chronic debilitating infection. Several helminths are important pathogens of domestic animals and invade humans who ingest contaminated food. These helminths include *Taenia*, a tapeworm of cattle and pigs, and *Trichinella*, the roundworm of pigs that causes trichinosis.

Schistosomiasis (*Schistosoma* Species)

Several species of schistosomes are responsible for the chronic, debilitating, and sometimes fatal disease schistosomiasis (formerly known as bilharzia). Three species, *S. mansoni*, *S. japonicum*, and *S. haematobium*, are the major pathogens in humans, infecting individuals in Africa, the Middle East, South America, the Caribbean, China, Southeast Asia, and the Philippines. A rise in schistosomiasis infections in recent years has paralleled the increasing worldwide use of irrigation, which has expanded the habitat of the fresh water snail that serves as the intermediate host for schistosomes.

Infection occurs through contact with free-swimming infectious larvae, called cercariae, which are released from an infected snail at the rate of 300–3000 per day. When cercariae contact human skin, they secrete digestive enzymes that help them to bore into the skin, where they shed their tail and are transformed into schistosomules. The schistosomules enter the capillaries and migrate to the lungs, then to the liver, and finally to the primary site of infection, which varies with the species. *S. mansoni* and *S. japonicum* infect the intestinal mesenteric veins; *S. haematobium* infects the veins of the urinary bladder. Once established in their final tissue site, schistosomules mature into male and female adult worms. The worms mate and the females produce at least 300 spiny eggs a day. Unlike protozoan parasites, schistosomes and other helminths do not multiply within their hosts. The eggs produced by the female worm do not mature into adult worms in humans; instead, some of them pass into the feces or urine and are excreted to infect more snails. The number of worms in an infected individual increases only through repeated exposure to the free-swimming cercariae, and so most infected individuals carry rather low numbers of worms.

Most of the symptoms of schistosomiasis are initiated by the egg stage. Not all the eggs are eliminated through the feces or urine; as many as half of them remain in the host, where they invade the intestinal wall, liver, or bladder and cause hemorrhage. A chronic state can then develop lasting for 20 years or more in which the adult worms persist and the unexcreted eggs induce cell-mediated delayed-type hypersensitive reactions, resulting in large granulomas that are gradually walled off by fibrous tissue. Although the eggs are contained by the formation of the granuloma, often the granuloma itself obstructs the venous blood flow to the liver or bladder.

Although an immune response does develop to the schistosomes, it is not sufficient to eliminate the adult worms in most individuals, even though the intravascular sites of schistosome infestation should make the worm an easy target for immune elimination. Instead the worms survive for up to 20 years. The schistosomules would appear to be the forms most susceptible to immune attack, but because they are motile, they can evade the localized cellular buildup of immune and inflammatory cells. Adult schistosome worms also possess several unique protective mechanisms that help them to escape the immune defenses. The adult worm has been shown to decrease the expression of antigens on its outer membrane and also to enclose itself in a glycolipid and glycoprotein coat derived from the host, masking the presence of its own antigens. Among the antigens observed on the adult worm are the host's own ABO blood-group antigens and histocompatibility antigens! The immune response is of course diminished by this covering of the host's self-antigens, which probably contributes to the lifelong persistence of these organisms.

The role of humoral and cell-mediated responses in protective immunity to schistosomiasis is controversial. Following infection with *S. mansoni*, a humoral response develops that is characterized by large elevations in IgE antibody production, localized increases in mast cells and their subsequent degranulation, and increased numbers of eosinophils (Figure 19-12). The mediators

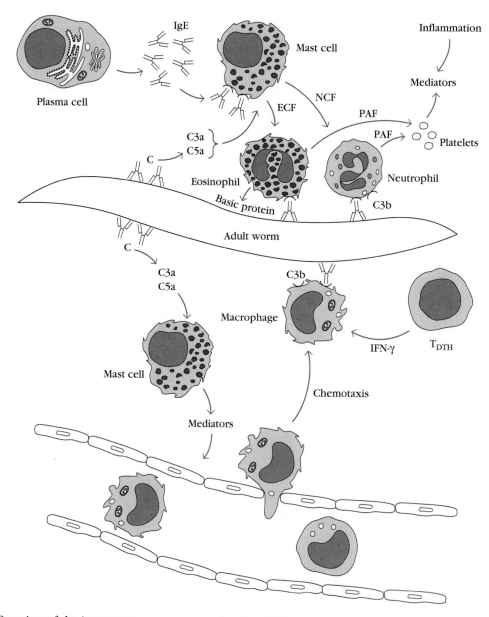

Figure 19-12 Overview of the immune response generated against *Schistosoma mansoni*. The response includes both humoral and cell-mediated components. C = complement; ECF = eosinophil chemotactic factor; NCF = neutrophil chemotactic factor; PAF = platelet-activating factor.

released from mast cells increase the infiltration of such inflammatory cells as macrophages and eosinophils. The eosinophils express Fcε and Fcγ receptors and bind to the antibody-coated parasite. Once bound to the parasite the eosinophil can participate in antibody-dependent cell-mediated cytotoxicity (ADCC), releasing mediators from its granules that damage the parasite. One eosinophil mediator, called basic protein, has been shown to be particularly toxic to helminths. The humoral manifestations suggest that cytokines derived from a T$_H$2-like CD4$^+$ T cell play an important role in the response.

IL-4 induces B cells to class-switch to IgE production, IL-5 induces bone marrow precursors to differentiate into eosinophils, and IL-3 (together with IL-4) induce localized mast cell increases.

Not all evidence points to the humoral IgE response as protective. When mice are immunized with *S. mansoni* vaccines, the protective immune response that develops is not an IgE response but rather is a cell-mediated T$_{DTH}$ response characterized by IFN-γ production and macrophage accumulation (Figure 19-12). Furthermore, inbred strains of mice with deficiencies in mast cells or

IgE develop protective immunity to the vaccine, whereas inbred strains with deficiencies in cell-mediated T_{DTH} responses fail to develop protective immunity to the vaccine. These studies suggest that the T_{DTH} response may be important in immunity to schistosomiasis. This had led Alan Sher and his colleagues to speculate that schistosomes may have evolved a cleaver defense mechanism by their ability to induce an ineffective T_H2-like response. This would ensure that sufficient levels of IL-10 are produced to inhibit the effective response generated by the T_H1-like subset.

Antigens present on the membrane of cercariae and young schistosomules look promising as possible vaccine components because these stages appear to be most susceptible to immune attack. Some monoclonal antibodies to cercariae and young schistosomules have been shown to passively transfer resistance to mice and rats that had been challenged with live cercariae. These protective monoclonal antibodies were then used to identify surface antigens on cercariae and schistosomules as possible candidates for vaccine development. With monoclonal-antibody affinity columns the schistosome membrane antigens were purified from crude membrane extracts. When mice were immunized and boosted with these purified antigens, they exhibited increased resistance to a later challenge with live cercariae. Schistosome cDNA libraries were then established and screened with the monoclonal antibodies to identify those encoding the surface antigens. Experiments using cloned cercariae or schistosomule antigens are presently under way to assess their ability to induce protective immunity in animal models. In developing an effective vaccine for schistosomiasis, however, a fine line separates a beneficial immune response, which at best limits the parasite load, from a detrimental response, which in itself becomes pathologic.

Summary

1.   The immune response to viral infections involves both humoral and cell-mediated components. Antibody to the viral receptor can block viral infections of host cells. However, a number of viruses, including influenza, are able to mutate their receptor molecules and thus evade the humoral antibody response. Once a viral infection has been established cell-mediated immunity appears to be more important. The cell-mediated response may develop in response to such internal viral proteins as the nucleoprotein of the viral core. These internal proteins are expressed together with class I MHC molecules on the membrane of infected host cells and serve to activate CTL activity.

2.   Immunity to bacterial infections is generally mediated by antibody unless the bacterium is capable of intracellular growth, in which case delayed-type hypersensitivity is important for host defense. Antibody can induce localized production of immune effector molecules of the complement system, thus facilitating development of an inflammatory response. Antibody can also activate complement-mediated lysis of the bacterium, neutralize toxins, and serve as an opsonin to increase phagocytosis. Bacteria can evade the humoral antibody response by several mechanisms. Some bacteria secrete protease enzymes that cleave IgA dimers, thus reducing the effectiveness of IgA in the mucous secretions. Other bacteria escape phagocytosis by producing surface capsules or protein that inhibit adherence to phagocytes, by secreting toxins that kill phagocytes, or through their ability to survive within phagocytes.

3.   Both humoral and cell-mediated immune responses have been implicated in immunity to protozoan infections. The effectiveness of the response depends in part on the site of the parasite. In general, humoral antibody is effective against blood borne stages, but once protozoans infect host cells, cell-mediated immunity is necessary. Protozoans escape the immune response through several mechanisms. Some—notably *Trypanosoma brucei*—are covered by a glycoprotein coat that is constantly changed by a genetic-switch mechanism. Others (including *Plasmodium*) slough off their glycoprotein coat after antibody has bound. In addition, the glycoprotein coat of *Plasmodium* contains few T-cell epitopes, and those that are present are in regions of the glycoprotein exhibiting the most variation among organisms.

4.   Because of their size, the helminths are extracellular parasites and are generally attacked by antibody-mediated defenses. Because relatively few of these organisms are carried in an affected individual and because they do not multiply within the host, immune system exposure to helminths is limited and consequently only a low level of immunity is induced.

References

BODMER, H. C., R. M. PEMBERTON, J. ROTHBARD, and B. A. ASKONAS. 1988. Enhanced recognition of a modified antigen by cytotoxic T cells specific for influenza nucleoprotein. *Cell* **52**:253.

BORST, P. 1991. Molecular genetics of antigenic variation. *Immunoparasit. Today* (March):A29.

BRAUN, R. 1988. Molecular and cellular biology of malaria. 1988. *Bioessays.* **8**:194.

GOOD, M. F., J. A. BERZOFSKY, and L. H. MILLER. 1988. The T cell response to the malaria circumsporozoite protein: An immunological approach to vaccine design. *Annu. Rev. Immunol.* 6:663.

GREVE, J. M., G. DAVIS, A. M. MEYER et al. 1989. The major human rhinovirus receptor is ICAM-1. *Cell* 56:839.

HABICHT, G. S., G. BECK, and J. L. BENACH. 1987. Lyme disease. *Sci. Am.* (July):

HALL, B. F., and K. A. JOINER. 1991. Strategies of obligate intracellular parasites for evading host defences. *Immunoparasit. Today* (March):A22.

LOCKSLEY, R. M., and P. SCOTT. 1991. Helper T-cell subsets in mouse leishmaniasis: induction, expansion, and effector. *Immunoparasit. Today* (March):A58.

MAHMOUD, A. A. F. 1989. Parasitic protozoa and helminths: biological and immunological challenges. *Science* 246:1015.

MCCONKEY, G. A., et al. 1990. The generation of genetic diversity in malarial parasites. *Annu. Rev. Microbiol.* 44:479.

MEYER, T. F., C. P. GIBBS, and R. HASS. 1990. Variation and control of protein expression in Neisseria. *Annu. Rev. Microbiol.* 44:451.

MIMS, C. A. 1987. *Pathogenesis of Infectious Disease.* Academic Press.

MITCHELL, G. F. 1987. Cellular and molecular aspects of host-parasite relationships. In *Progress in Immunology VI.* B. Cinander and R. G. Miller, eds. Academic Press.

PALA, P., and B. A. ASKONAS. 1986. Low responder MHC alleles for Tc recognition of influenza nucleoprotein. *Immunogenetics* 23:379.

PLAYFAIR, H. L., J. TAVERNE, C. A. W. BATE, and J. B. DE SOUZA. 1990. The malaria vaccine: anti-parasite or anti-disease? *Immunol. Today* 11:25.

ROTH, J. A. (ed.). 1988. *Virulence Mechanisms of Bacterial Pathogens.* American Society for Microbiology.

SIMON, M. M., U. E. SCHAIBLE, R. WALLICH, and M. D. KRAMER. 1991. A mouse model for *Borrelia burgdorferi* infection: approach to a vaccine against Lyme disease. *Immunol. Today* 12:11.

STAUNTON, D. E., V. J. MERLUZZI, R. ROTHLEIN et al. 1989. A cell adhesion molecule, ICAM-1, is the major surface receptor for rhinoviruses. *Cell* 56:849.

TAYLOR, P. M., J. DAVEY, K. HOWLAND et al. 1987. Class I MHC molecules rather than other mouse genes dictate influenza epitope recognition by cytotoxic T cells. *Immunogenetics* 26:267.

TOWNSEND, A. R. M., et al. 1986. The epitopes of influenza nucleoprotein recognized by cytotoxic T lymphocytes can be defined with short synthetic peptides. *Cell* 44:959.

VIGNALI, D. A. A. et al. 1989. Immunity to *Schistosoma mansoni* in vivo: contradiction or clarification? *Immunol. Today* 10:410.

Study Questions

1. The effect of the MHC on the immune response to peptides of the influenza virus nucleoprotein was studied in H-2^b mice that had been previously immunized with live influenza virions. The CTL activity of primed lymphocytes was determined by in vitro CML assays using H-2^k fibroblasts as target cells. The target cells had been transfected with different H-2^b class I MHC genes and were infected either with live influenza or incubated

For use with Question 1.

Target cell (H-2^k fibroblast)	Test antigen	CTL activity of influenza-primed H-2^b lymphocytes (% lysis)
(a) Untransfected	Live influenza	0
(b) Transfected class I D^b	Live influenza	60
(c) Transfected class I D^b	Nucleoprotein peptide 365–380	50
(d) Transfected class I D^b	Nucleoprotein peptide 50–63	2
(e) Transfected class I K^b	Nucleoprotein peptide 365–380	0.5
(f) Transfected class I K^b	Nucleoprotein peptide 50–63	1

with nucleoprotein synthetic peptides. The results of these assays are shown in the table on the previous page:

a. Why was there no killing of the target cells in system (a) even though the target cells were infected with live influenza?

b. Why was a CTL response generated to the nucleoprotein even though it is an internal viral protein?

c. Why was there a good CTL response in system (c) to peptide 365–380, whereas there was no response in system (d) to peptide 50–63?

d. If you were going to develop a synthetic peptide vaccine for influenza in humans, how would these results obtained in mice influence your design of a vaccine?

2. a. Describe the nonspecific defenses that operate when a disease-producing microorganism enters the body.

b. What additional defense mechanisms does the immune system contribute?

3. Discuss the role of humoral and the cell-mediated responses in immunity to influenza.

4. The humoral response to influenza is subtype-specific, whereas the cell-mediated response has been shown to cross-react with all influenza A subtypes.

a. Discuss the significance of this observation in terms of potential vaccine development for influenza.

b. Why might an internal viral protein, such as nucleoprotein, serve as a potential vaccine?

5. M. F. Good and co-workers analyzed the effect of MHC haplotype on the antibody response to a malarial circumsporozoite (CS) peptide antigen in several recombinant congenic mouse strains. Their results are shown in the table below:

a. Based on the results of this study, which MHC molecule(s) serve(s) as restriction element(s) for this peptide antigen?

b. Since antigen recognition by B cells is not MHC restricted, why is the humoral antibody response influenced by the MHC haplotype?

6. African trypanosomes, plasmodium, and influenza each have unique mechanisms allowing them to escape the immune response. Discuss each of these mechanisms.

For use with Question 5.

| Strain | H-2 alleles | | | | | Antibody response to CS peptide |
	K	IA	IE	S	D	
B10.BR	k	k	k	k	k	<1
B10.A (4R)	k	k	b	b	b	<1
B10.HTT	s	s	k	k	d	<1
B10.A (5R)	b	b	k	d	d	67
B10	b	b	b	b	b	73
B10.MBR	b	k	k	k	a	<1

SOURCE: Adapted from M. F. Good et al., 1988, *Annu. Rev. Immunol.* 6:633.

Immuno-deficiency Diseases

The immunodeficiency diseases include a diverse spectrum of illnesses that stem from various abnormalities of the immune system. The basic clinical manifestations are frequent, severe infections of long duration, which often are caused by organisms of normally low pathogenicity. An immunodeficiency disease may result from a primary congenital defect or may be acquired from a secondary cause, such as a viral or bacterial infection or a drug treatment. Acquired immune deficiency syndrome (AIDS) is the most significant immunodeficiency arising from secondary causes, in this case the retrovirus

HIV. Because of the worldwide impact of AIDS as well as its scientific importance, AIDS is covered separately in the next chapter. This chapter focuses on selected primary immunodeficiency diseases affecting the various branches of the immune system.

Classification of Immunodeficiencies

Immunodeficiency diseases can result from congenital or acquired defects in hematopoietic stem cells, T cells, B cells, phagocytic cells, and the complement system. The diseases discussed in this chapter are summarized in Table 20-1, classified according to the branch of the immune system that is primarily involved. Figure 20-1 shows the stages in hematopoiesis and development of leukocytes at which congenital defects result in various immunodeficiency diseases. The prevalence of several of these diseases is given in Table 20-2.

Phagocytic Deficiencies

Defects in phagocytic defense can result either from a reduction in the numbers of phagocytic cells or from a reduction in their function. In either case the hallmarks are recurrent bacterial or fungal infections. The clinical manifestations, which are generally related to the mag-

Table 20-1   Some immunodeficiency diseases

Disease	Characteristic immune-system deficiency	Possible mechanism
Phagocytic deficiencies		
Congenital agranulocytosis	Decreased neutrophil count	Decreased production of G-CSF
Leukocyte-adhesion deficiency (LAD)	Failure of neutrophils and monocytes to extravasate Defective CTL killing Defective T-cell help in B-cell activation	Defective synthesis of β chain of integrin family of adhesion molecules
Lazy-leukocyte syndrome	Decreased neutrophil chemotaxis	Not known
Chronic granulomatous disease (CGD)	Defective killing by neutrophils of phagocytosed bacteria	Decreased H_2O_2 production due to defective NADPH oxidase (cytochrome *b*)
Humoral deficiencies		
X-linked (Bruton's) hypogammaglobulinemia	Reduction in B-cell count Absence of immunoglobulins	Block in B-cell maturation due to defective V-D-J gene rearrangement
Common variable hypogammaglobulinemia	Decreased plasma-cell levels but usually normal B-cell levels Variable reduction in secreted Ig of all isotypes	Defective differentiation of B cells to plasma cells due to defective processing of Ig transcripts, lack of cytokine receptors on B cells, or abnormal T-cell response
Selective immunoglobulin deficiencies	Decreased levels of one or more Ig isotypes	Defect in maturation of plasma cells or necessary T-cell–derived cytokines
Cell-mediated deficiencies		
DiGeorge syndrome	Decreased T-cell counts	Lack of T-cell maturation due to absence of thymus
Nude mice	Decreased T-cell counts	Lack of T-cell maturation due to absence of thymus

nitude of the defect, range from mild skin infections to life-threatening systemic infections. The most common infectious organisms include *Staphylococcus aureus*, *Streptococcus pneumoniae*, *Escherichia coli*, various species of *Pseudomonas*, *Candida*, and *Aspergillis*.

Reduction in Neutrophil Count (Neutropenia)

Quantitative deficiencies in neutrophils can range from an almost complete absence of cells, called *agranulocytosis*, to a reduction in peripheral blood neutrophils below 1500/mm^3, called *granulocytopenia* or *neutro-*

Table 20-2 Prevalence of selected immunodeficiency diseases

Disease	Worldwide prevalence
IgA immunodeficiency	1:700
Heriditary angioedema (deficiency in C1 inhibitor)*	1:1000
Common variable hypogammaglobulinemia	1:70,000
Severe combined immunodeficiency disease (SCID)—all forms	1:100,000
X-linked (Bruton's) hypogammaglobulinemia	1:200,000

* Complement deficiences are discussed in Chapter 15.

Table 20-1 Some immunodeficiency diseases (*continued*)

Disease	Characteristic immune-system deficiency	Possible mechanism
Combined immunodeficiencies		
Reticular dysgenesis	Decreased numbers of all cells of lymphoid and myeloid lineages	Defective maturation of hematopoietic stem cells
Bare-lymphocyte syndrome	Some reduction in CD4$^+$ T-cell counts Reduced B-cell and T_C-cell activation Decreased T_{DTH}-cell activity	Failure to express class I or II MHC molecules on cells
Severe combined immuno-deficiency disease (SCID)	Marked reduction in T- and B-cell counts in all forms	Various mechanisms
X-linked SCID		Defective T- and B-cell maturation
Autosomal recessive SCID		Defective T- and B-cell maturation
ADA-deficiency SCID		Selective killing of lymphocytes by metabolites that accumulate in absence of adenosine deaminase (ADA)
PNP-deficiency SCID		Selective killing of lymphocytes by metabolites that accumulate in the absence of purine nucleoside phosphorylase (PNP)
CB-17 *scid* mouse		Aberrant D-J joining of Ig heavy-chain and TCR β- and δ-chain gene segments
Complement deficiencies		

See Table 15-7

446   CHAPTER 20   IMMUNODEFICIENCY DISEASES

penia. These quantitative deficiencies may be caused by congenital defects or may be acquired through extrinsic factors. Congenital neutropenias often involve a genetic defect affecting the myeloid progenitor stem cell that results in reduced production of neutrophils during hematopoiesis (see Figure 20-1). In *congenital agranulocytosis* myeloid stem cells are present in the bone marrow but rarely differentiate beyond the promyelocyte stage. As a result, children born with this condition show severe neutropenia with counts of less than 200 cells/mm³. These children frequently manifest bacterial infections as early as the first month of life. Experimental evidence suggests that this genetic defect results in decreased production of granulocyte colony-

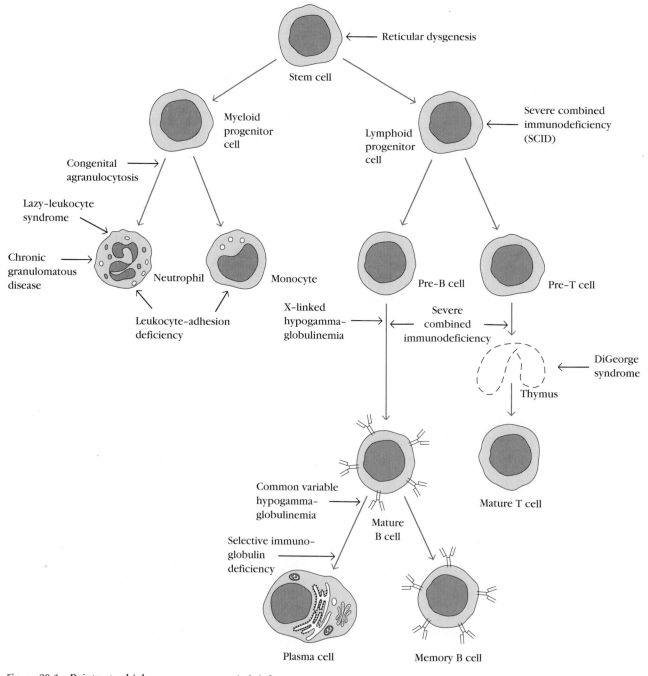

Figure 20-1   Points at which common congenital defects may result in various immunodeficiency diseases.

stimulating factor (G-CSF) and thus in a failure of the myeloid stem cell to differentiate along the granulocytic lineage (see Figure 3-2).

Most neutropenias are acquired through extrinsic factors rather than by congenital means. Because neutrophils have a short lifespan, the precursors divide rapidly in the bone marrow to maintain homeostatic levels of neutrophils. Radiation and certain drugs, including chemotherapeutic ones, cause neutropenia because of their increased effect on rapidly dividing cells. Occasionally neutropenia can develop in such autoimmune diseases as Sjögren's syndrome or systemic lupus erythematosus; in these conditions, autoantibodies cause neutrophil destruction. Transient neutropenia often develops after certain bacterial or viral infections. It is not uncommon for children to manifest neutropenia after certain viral infections, but this neutropenia is transient, and neutrophil counts return to normal as the infection is cleared.

Defective Phagocytic Function

An effective phagocytic defense system involves a series of processes that interact in sequence to ingest and kill microorganisms. These processes include the adherence of phagocytes to vascular endothelial cells, emigration across the vascular endothelium, chemotaxis through subendothelial connective tissue to the site of immune reaction, attachment to the microorganism, phagocytosis, and subsequent killing and digestion. A dysfunction in any one of these processes may severely limit the effectiveness of the phagocytic defense system (see Table 20-1).

Adherence Defect

The development of an effective inflammatory response involves the adherence of neutrophils and monocytes to capillary endothelial cells near the site of the immune reaction. These adherent neutrophils and monocytes migrate through the capillary wall into extravascular sites, where an effective inflammatory response develops. A recently described autosomal recessive defect, called *leukocyte-adhesion deficiency (LAD)*, involves an impairment of a variety of functions involving leukocyte adhesion. Included among the deficiencies is the inability of neutrophils, monocytes, and lymphocytes to adhere to vascular endothelial cells, thus preventing extravasation of these cells into the extravascular tissue spaces. Also impaired is the ability of CTLs and NK cells to adhere to their target cells. Individuals with this defect manifest recurrent bacterial infections and impaired wound healing.

The molecular basis of LAD has been shown to be defective biosynthesis of the β chain component (CD18)

of one subfamily of integrin adhesion molecules. The integrin molecules affected by this defect include the type 3 and type 4 complement receptors (CR3 and CR4), which bind the complement degradation product C3bi, and LFA-1, which binds the intercellular adhesion molecule, ICAM-1. CR3, CR4, and LFA-1 are all heterodimeric glycoproteins in which a unique α chain is noncovalently associated in the cell membrane with a common β chain. The β-chain defect in LAD results in a loss of all three membrane glycoproteins (Table 20-3).

Each of the three integrin receptors has its own role in leukocyte adhesion (Table 20-4). Monoclonal antibody to the β chain strongly inhibits adhesion of phagocytes to endothelial cells, random locomotion, and chemotaxis, suggesting that the β chain takes part in all these processes. Phagocytes from individuals with LAD show diminished in vitro adherence to cultured human endothelial cells. Activation of normal neutrophils with agents such as phorbol myristate acetate produces an increase in adherence from a baseline of from 5–10% to 50–80% after activation; unactivated neutrophils from individuals with LAD exhibit 2–5% adherence, and there is no appreciable increase in adherence after activation.

Chemotactic Defect

A large number of clinical disorders reflect defects in neutrophil chemotaxis. These disorders may be caused by an intrinsic defect in the neutrophil itself or by an extrinsic defect such as a complement deficiency and a corresponding reduction in the chemotactic factors of the complement cascade (C3a, C5a, C5b67). One syndrome, called *lazy-leukocyte syndrome*, involves a congenital defect in which neutrophil migration is severely impaired.

Killing Defect

Chronic granulomatous disease (CGD) is the most prevalent defect associated with defective intracellular killing of ingested bacteria. The disease is inherited as an X-linked recessive disorder that is manifested in boys during the first two years of life. (A milder autosomal recessive form of this disease has been observed; this form can also occur in girls and often is not recognized until young adulthood.) Clinically, CGD is characterized by disseminated granulomatous lesions in various organs. Children with this disease often die of septicemia by 7 years of age.

The deficiency in CGD is in the bactericidal activity of neutrophils. The neutrophils from affected individuals can phagocytose bacteria but are unable to kill bacteria that contain the enzyme catalase. (Catalase-negative bacteria are not a problem because bacteria form H_2O_2 dur-

Table 20-3   Percentage of granulocytes bearing CR3, CR4, and LFA-1 in patients with leukocyte-adhesion deficiency (LAD) and in normal controls*

	Percentage of cells bearing				
LAD status	CR3 M α chain	LFA-1 L α chain	CR4 X α chain	Common β chain	Unrelated molecule (CR1)
Severe:					
Patient 1	0.1	0.15	0.1	0.15	94
Patient 2	0.0	0.0	0.3	0.1	100
Moderate:					
Patient 3	6.0	11.0	7.0	4.4	92
Patient 4	4.0	31	3.5	2.5	99
Patient 5	4.0	26	4.0	6.0	87
Patient 6	3.0	24	2.0	4.0	109
Normal control	57.0	66.5	42.1	54.5	101

* Granulocytes were incubated with fluorochrome-labeled monoclonal antibody specific for the indicated receptor chains and then analyzed with a fluorescence-activated cell sorter (FACS) to determine the percentage of cells binding antibody (see Figure 6-16).

SOURCE: D. C. Anderson et al., 1986, *J. Infect. Dis.* **152**:668.

Table 20-4   Properties of integrin receptor molecules that are absent in leukocyte-adhesion deficiency (LAD)

		Receptor molecule*	
Property	LFA-1	CR3	CR4
CD designation	CD11aCD18	CD11bCD18	CD11cCD18
Subunit composition	αLβ2	αMβ2	αXβ2
Subunit molecular mass M_r (kD)			
α chain	175,000	165,000	150,000
β chain	95,000	95,000	95,000
Cellular expression	Lymphocytes Monocytes Macrophages Granulocytes Natural killer cells	Monocytes Macrophages Granulocytes Natural killer cells	Monocytes Macrophages Granulocytes
Ligand	ICAM-1 ICAM-2	C3bi	C3bi
Functions inhibited with monoclonal antibody	Extravasation CTL killing T-B conjugate formation ADCC	Opsonization Granulocyte adherence, aggregation, and chemotaxis ADCC	Granulocyte adherence and aggregation

* CR3 = type 3 complement receptor, also known as Mac-l; CR4 = type 4 complement receptor, also known as p 150,90. LFA-1, CR3, and CR4 have the same β chain but different α chains designated L, M, and X, respectively.

ing their own metabolism, and in the absence of catalase these bacteria cannot detoxify their own H_2O_2 and are unable to survive even in the defective phagocytes.) During normal phagocytosis there is a burst of respiratory oxidative activity, increased oxygen consumption, and a shift of glucose metabolism to the hexose monophosphate shunt. As glucose is metabolized, reduced pyridine nucleotides (NADH and NADPH) accumulate and convert O_2 into the bactericidal H_2O_2 and potent superoxides. The levels of H_2O_2 and superoxides are normally high enough to kill even catalase-positive bacteria. Neutrophils from CGD patients, however, show no increase in O_2 consumption, no increase in utilization of the hexose monophosphate shunt, and no H_2O_2 production during phagocytosis. The underlying defect appears to be in one of the genes encoding a subunit of cytochrome b, which is necessary for NADP recycling. The resulting decrease in the levels of reduced pyridine nucleotides leads to decreased H_2O_2 production; in this environment ingested catalase-positive bacteria can survive in neutrophils. The bacteria are carried by the cells into various organs, where they give rise to the characteristic disseminated granulomatous lesions.

Humoral Deficiencies

B-cell immunodeficiency disorders include a diverse spectrum of diseases ranging from the complete absence of mature recirculating B cells, plasma cells, and immunoglobulin to the selective absence of only certain classes of immunoglobulins (see Table 20-1). Patients with these disorders usually are subject to recurrent bacterial infections but display normal immunity to most viral and fungal infections because the T-cell branch of the immune system is largely unaffected. The most common infections in patients with humoral immunodeficiencies involve such encapsulated bacteria as staphylococci, streptococci, and pneumococci because antibody is critical for the opsonization and clearance of these organisms. The severity of the disorder parallels the degree of antibody deficiency.

X-Linked Infantile (Bruton's) Hypogammaglobulinemia

A severe *X-linked hypogammaglobulinemia*, described by Bruton in 1952, was the first immunodeficiency disorder to be recognized. Male infants with this disorder begin to manifest severe recurrent bacterial infections, especially of pneumococci, streptococci, staphylococci, and *Hemophilus influenzae*, at about 6 months as the level of passively acquired maternal antibody declines and they are left unprotected.

The defect causing this disorder involves the maturation of pre-B cells to mature B cells in the bone marrow (see Figure 8-17). Patients have normal numbers of pre-B cells in their bone marrow but lack (or have severely reduced levels of) mature B cells and plasma cells. Fluorescent-antibody staining to detect B cells reveals a complete absence of recirculating B cells and a lack of cells in the B-cell–dependent areas of the peripheral lymphoid tissues. The lymph nodes, for example, lack germinal centers and have diminished cell numbers in the cortex. Closer analysis of pre-B cells from affected individuals reveals cytoplasmic μ heavy chains but no κ or λ light chains. The cytoplasmic μ heavy chains are unusual in that they lack the V_H sequence and therefore are shorter than normal. The defect is in the V-D-J rearrangement process, which occurs during B-cell maturation, and appears to result in defective heavy-chain production in affected individuals.

X-linked hypogammaglobulinemia can be diagnosed relatively easily by serum immunoelectrophoresis, which reveals an absence (or severe reduction) of the serum γ-globulin fraction, usually with loss of all five immunoglobulin classes. Treatment of patients with this disorder requires periodic γ-globulin injections to passively protect them against common bacterial infections. Sinopulmonary infections are still common, however, because secretory IgA is not transferred by γ-globulin injections.

Common Variable Hypogammaglobulinemia

Common variable hypogammaglobulinemia (*CVH*) refers to a heterogeneous group of disorders that cause late-onset hypogammaglobulinemia. There appears to be no definitive genetic basis, although familial inheritance patterns have been reported. Patients with this disorder typically develop recurrent bacterial infections beginning between 15 and 35 years of age because their serum immunoglobulin levels are severely reduced.

A variety of immune deficiencies have been observed in affected individuals. In some cases, the number of mature B cells is reduced; usually, however, B-cell levels are normal and the intrinsic defect appears to be in the differentiation of mature B cells into plasma cells. In some cases a defect may render plasma cells unable to synthesize the secreted form of the antibody molecule. A variety of defects could block immunoglobulin secretion. One possible defect may be at the level of RNA processing of the primary transcript. A defect in polyadenylation of the primary Ig transcript might prevent the loss of the M1 and M2 exons, which is necessary for the expression of the secreted form of the antibody (see Figure 8-14). In other cases defective heavy-chain glycosylation may prevent immunoglobulin secretion by plasma cells. It has also been suggested that B cells may lack receptors for lymphokines that are necessary to trigger their activation and differentiation into antibody-secreting cells (see Figure 12-13); alternatively, the defect may reflect the T-cell role in the humoral response. Some CVH patients, for example, have been shown to have defective T_H cells, whereas others have an excess of T cells, which may act as suppressors and prevent plasma cells from secreting immunoglobulin.

Selective Immunoglobulin Deficiencies

Some immunodeficiency disorders involve a deficiency in a single immunoglobulin class or subclass. Most common is a selective IgA deficiency, which occurs in 1 in 600–800 people. Although some individuals are completely asymptomatic, many develop recurrent respiratory infections and gastrointestinal symptoms of malabsorption and infection. This is not surprising in view of the important role of secretory IgA in the mucous secretions of the respiratory and gastrointestinal tracts. Affected individuals also have an increased incidence of severe allergic reactions, presumably due to increased penetration of allergens through mucosal surfaces and subsequent stimulation of IgE production. The B cells of patients with IgA deficiency generally bear membrane IgA; the defect appears to be in the maturation of these cells to become plasma cells secreting IgA. It is not known whether the defect is in the B cell itself or whether the defect is at the level of T-cell help. It has been suggested that there may be a decrease in IL-5 or TGF-β, which are known to mediate a class switch to IgA. In some cases the defect has been shown in vitro to be caused by T-cell-mediated suppression of IgA production by B cells.

Cell-Mediated Deficiences

Because of the central role of T cells in the immune system, a T-cell deficiency can affect both the humoral and the cell-mediated responses. The impact on the cell-mediated system can be severe, with a reduction in both delayed-type hypersensitive responses and cell-mediated cytotoxicity. Whereas defects in the humoral system are associated primarily with infections by encapsulated bacteria, defects in the cell-mediated system are associated with increased susceptibility to viral, protozoan, and fungal infections. Intracellular pathogens such as *Candida albicans* (Figure 20-2), *Pneumocystis carinii*, and *Mycobacteria* are often implicated, reflect-

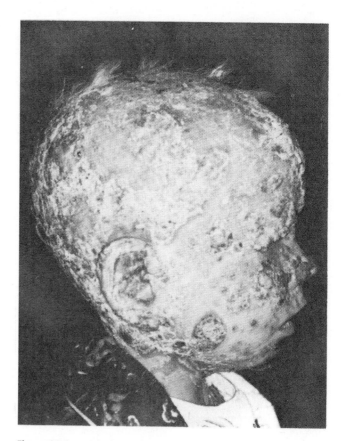

Figure 20-2   Chronic cutaneous candidiasis in a boy with defective cell-mediated immunity. [From R. J. Schlegel et al., 1970 *Pediatrics* **45**:926–936.]

ing the importance of T cells in eliminating intracellular pathogens. Infections with viruses that are rarely pathogenic for the normal individual (such as cytomegalo virus or even an attenuated measles vaccine) can become life-threatening. T-cell defects generally affect the humoral system, too, because of the requirement for T_H cells in B-cell activation. Generally there is some decrease in antibody levels, particularly in the production of specific antibody following immunization.

DiGeorge Syndrome (Congenital Thymic Aplasia)

In 1965 DiGeorge first described a syndrome characterized by the absence of a thymus: hypoparathyroidism, cardiovascular anomalies, characteristic facial features (Figure 20-3), and increased incidence of infections. The syndrome reflects a failure of the third and fourth pharyngeal pouches to develop between 10 and 12 weeks of gestation, a time when several organs, including the aortic arch of the heart, are developing. Children born with this syndrome are often diagnosed not because of infection but because of seizures on the first day of life due to low calcium in the blood, a result of the hypo-

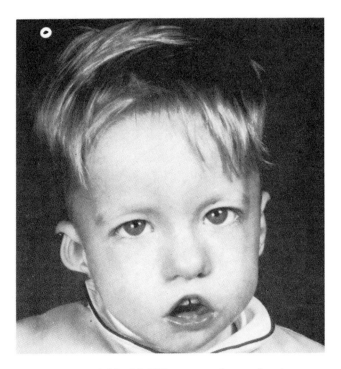

Figure 20-3 A child with DiGeorge syndrome showing characteristic dysplasia of ears and mouth and abnormally long distance between the eyes. [From F. S. Rosen, in R. Kretschmer et al., 1968 *N. Engl. J. Med.* **279**:1295.]

parathyroid condition. Cardiac defects are the most common cause of death. If the child survives the neonatal period, increased susceptibility to various opportunistic infections is observed. Generally these children have effective humoral immunity against common bacterial infections but are extremely susceptible to viral, pro-

tozoan, and fungal infections; even the common attenuated measles vaccine may be life-threatening to affected children.

Evaluation of children with complete DiGeorge syndrome reveals a severe decrease in the total number of T cells, which can be demonstrated by T-cell rosetting techniques or flow cytometry. Functionally, there is an absence of skin-test reactivity to common antigens, a decreased response to T-cell mitogens such as PHA, and decreased responsiveness to allogeneic cells in the mixed-lymphocyte reaction (MLR). In partial DiGeorge syndromes, the thymus is abnormally situated or is extremely small. In these cases there can be intermediate levels of T-cell numbers and responsiveness to T-cell mitogens or antigens.

Treatment for DiGeorge syndrome involves the grafting of fetal thymus tissue. The age of the thymus tissue is important: fetal thymuses older than 14 weeks of gestation should not be used because they have T cells that can cause graft-versus-host disease in the immune-suppressed recipient. The grafted thymic tissue provides a source of thymic hormones and a cellular environment in which T-cell stem cells can mature and differentiate. Once mature T cells are formed, unfortunately, the grafted thymus can sometimes be rejected by the very cells it helped to mature.

Nude Mice

An autosomal recessive thymic defect in mice resembles DiGeorge syndrome. Among the many defects exhibited by these mice is an absence of hair follicles, and they are called *nude* mice because of their strange hairless state (Figure 20-4). What makes these mice interesting

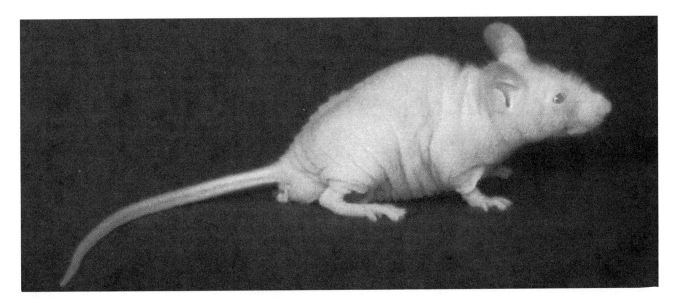

Figure 20-4 A nude mouse (*nu/nu*) [*Courtesy of Jackson Laboratory.*]

from an immunologic perspective is that they lack a thymus or have a vestigial thymus and show varying degrees of cell-mediated immunodeficiency. The defect is inherited and controlled by a recessive gene on chromosome 11; *nu/nu* homozygotes are hairless and lack a thymus, whereas *nu/+* heterozygotes are normal. This homozygous recessive gene has been bred into several inbred mouse strains, and these animals have served as important model systems. Because these mice lack a thymus, the pre-T cells fail to mature and there is a marked absence of cell-mediated immunity. This lack of a functioning cell-mediated response is best demonstrated in these mice by their ability to accept foreign skin grafts. Even xenogeneic grafts of human skin or chicken skin, feathers and all, are accepted by nude mice (Figure 20-5).

Combined Humoral and Cell-Mediated Deficiencies

As one might expect, combined deficiencies of the humoral and cell-mediated branches are the most serious of the immunodeficiency disorders (see Table 20-1). The onset of infections begins early in infancy and the prognosis for these infants is early death unless some therapeutic intervention reconstitutes the defective immune system. Considerable success has been achieved with bone marrow transplantation from HLA-matched donors.

Reticular Dysgenesis

Reticular dysgenesis is a rare, fatal congenital disease in which the lymphoid and myeloid stem cells fail to differentiate during hematopoiesis. Children born with this defect lack phagocytic cells of the monocyte and granulocyte series and also T and B lymphocytes. The developmental failure must therefore be at a very early developmental stage in hematopoiesis, before the stem cell differentiates into separate lymphoid and myeloid lineages (see Figure 20-1). Children born with this disorder die shortly after birth.

Bare-Lymphocyte Syndromes

Bare-lymphocyte syndromes are a group of severe combined immunodeficiency diseases caused by a deficiency in class I or class II MHC expression. The syndromes are categorized into three types: in the type I syndrome the class I MHC expression is defective; in the type II syn-

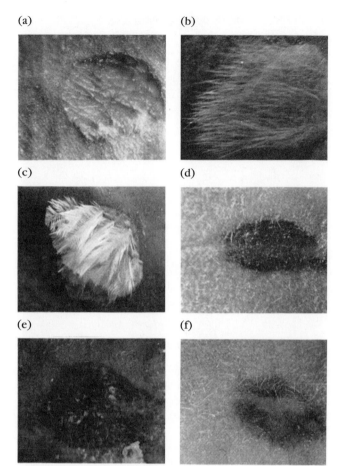

Figure 20-5   Grafts from other species (xenogeneic grafts) accepted by nude mice. The figure shows mice with the following grafts: (a) human skin after 60 days; (b) cat skin after 51 days; (c) chicken skin with feathers at 32 days; (d) chameleon skin at 41 days; (e) lizard skin at 28 days; and (f) tree frog skin at 40 days. [From D. D. Manning et al., 1973 *J. Exp. Med.* **138**:488.]

drome the class II MHC expression is defective; and in the type III syndrome both class I and class II MHC expression are defective. Patients with these syndromes lack the requisite MHC molecules necessary for antigen presentation to class I or class II restricted T cells. Consequently, individuals born with these deficiencies suffer recurrent bacterial and viral infections and often die by 5 years of age.

In patients with the type II syndrome the defect has begun to be unraveled at the molecular level. Patients with the type II defect do not express either class II MHC molecules or their mRNA in cells where class II MHC molecules are normally expressed such as B cells, macrophages, or dendritic cells. Even IFN-γ which normally induces increased class II MHC expression is unable to induce class II expression in patients with the type II syndrome. The fact that each of the class II MHC molecules (DP, DQ, and DR) are not expressed, suggests that these genes must be coordinately regulated. Because the promoter region of each class II MHC gene contains several conserved motifs, it has been speculated that coordinate expression of the class II MHC genes may be achieved by DNA-binding factors that bind to these conserved promoter motifs, activating each of the class II MHC genes. One hypothesis is that these DNA-binding factors may not be able to bind to the conserved promoter motif in bare lymphocyte syndrome, thus accounting for the coordinate loss of each of the class II MHC gene products. In a 1991 report in *Science*, Catherine Kara and Laurie Glimcher showed that type II bare lymphocyte syndrome was in some cases caused by a defect in the class II MHC promoter region, causing the chromatin structure to be less accessible to DNA-binding proteins. They speculated that the loss of a common DNA-binding factor in bare-lymphocyte syndrome may render the DNA less accessible to other transcriptional activating factors.

Severe Combined Immunodeficiency Disease (SCID)

Severe combined immunodeficiency disease (SCID)—a group of diseases resulting from defects in both humoral and cell-mediated immunity—is associated with increased susceptibility to viral, bacterial, fungal, and protozoan diseases; a failure to thrive and reduced weight gain are also usually observed. The degree of immune compromise is so severe that organisms that are nonpathogenic for the normal individual can cause serious or even life-threatening infections in the SCID patient. The disease received national attention in the 1970s when the plight of a boy named David, who lived his life inside a sterile plastic bubble, was much publicized.

SCID occurs in several forms and may be inherited as an X-linked recessive or autosomal recessive trait (see Table 20-1). The basic defect in most forms of human SCID has not been established. Possible causes include a defect in stem-cell differentiation or a defect in thymic and bone marrow processing. Bone marrow transplantation from HLA-identical siblings has met with some success in reconstituting the immune system in SCID children. Because 60% of SCID patients do not have HLA-identical siblings, marrow from haploidentical parental donors is often administered. The problem with HLA-mismatched bone marrow is that fatal graft-versus-host disease can develop. The fatal graft-versus-host disease can be avoided by treating the donor bone marrow with monoclonal anti-T-cell antibody + complement to deplete T cells prior to transplantation.

ADA Deficiency and PNP Deficiency

The defects causing two autosomal recessive forms of SCID have been established. In both cases the disease results from an inherited deficiency of an enzyme—either adenosine deaminase (ADA) or purine nucleoside phosphorylase (PNP). A deficiency of either enzyme results in accumulation of metabolites that are selectively toxic to dividing B and T cells. Thus individuals with either ADA or PNP deficiency have markedly reduced numbers of mature T and B cells.

Patients with ADA deficiency have been treated successfully with infusions of the purified enzyme. The gene encoding adenosine deaminase has been cloned, and in 1990 the first attempt at gene therapy in humans was performed on a young girl suffering from ADA-deficiency SCID. The gene therapy was accomplished with a retrovirus in which key retroviral genes had been replaced with the ADA gene. The patient's bone marrow cells were removed and infected in vitro with the engineered retrovirus; the genetically altered bone marrow cells then were reinfused back into the little girl. The results of this gene therapy are still being monitored.

SCID Mice and SCID-Human Mice

An autosomal recessive mutation resulting in severe combined immunodeficiency disease developed spontaneously in CB-17 mice. Like their human counterpart, CB-17 *scid* mice fail to develop mature T and B cells; these mice can be kept alive by housing them in a sterile environment. The absence of functional T and B cells enables the mice to accept allogeneic skin grafts. Apart from their lack of functional T and B cells, the mice appear to be normal in all respects. When normal mouse bone marrow cells are injected into *scid* mice, normal T and B cells develop and the mice are cured of the immunodeficiency. This finding has made these mice a valuable model system for study of immunodeficiency and the process of differentiation of bone marrow stem cells into mature T or B cells.

The CB-17 *scid* mice have a defect in the recombinase enzyme machinery, which normally catalyzes functional rearrangements of variable-region gene segments in immunoglobulin DNA and in T-cell receptor DNA. In the absence of a functional recombinase, these mice do not achieve the functional gene rearrangements required for B-cell and T-cell maturation. To demonstrate the *scid* defect, homogeneous B- and T-cell lines from affected mice were needed. These were obtained by taking bone marrow cells from *scid* mice and transforming them with Abelson murine leukemia virus to produce B-cell lines. The DNA gene rearrangements in these B-cell clones were then compared to those in normal CB-17 clones. Southern-blot analysis (with labeled J gene segments as probes) revealed aberrant DNA rearrangement in B-cell clones and also in T-cell thymomas from the *scid* mice. The defect, which appears to lie in the recombinase machinery, leads to aberrant joining of D and J gene segments in Ig heavy-chain DNA (see Figure 8-5) and in TCR β-chain and δ-chain DNA (see Figure 10-4). The finding of a similar defect in both B- and T-cell lineages suggests that the recombinase machinery is generally the same in both B and T cells. The defective recom-

binase enzyme in *scid* mice appears to recognize the D and J recognition signals and to excise the intervening DNA correctly. However, the enzyme does not join the D and J segments properly; instead, joining occurs at some distance from the functional D and J segments, resulting in deletion of one or both of the exons (Figure 20-6).

Interest in *scid* mice has mushroomed recently with the development of a new way to utilize these mice to study the human immune system. Implantation in *scid* mice of portions of human fetal liver, thymus, and lymph nodes causes the mice to become populated with mature human T and B lymphocytes (Figure 20-7). Because the mice lack mature T and B cells of their own, they do not reject the transplanted human tissue. The fetal liver provides a source of human stem cells, which mature into human B and T lymphocytes within the human thymus and lymph node implants. Because the human T cells are exposed to mouse major histocompatibility antigens while they are still immature within the human thymus implant, they later recognize mouse cells as self and do not mount an immunologic response against the mouse host. The beauty of this system is that it enables

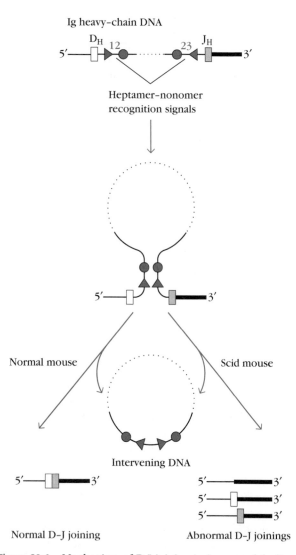

Figure 20-6 Mechanism of D-J joining in immunoglobulin heavy-chain DNA in normal mice and in *scid* mice. In *scid* mice, appropriate D_H and J_H recognition occurs and the intervening DNA is excised as a circular product, as in normal mice. However, the *scid* recombinase enzyme system does not properly join the D_H and J_H gene segments, so that either one or both segments are deleted during joining. The *scid* defect similarly affects joining of D and J gene segments in TCR β-chain and δ-chain DNA. [Adapted from G. D. Yancopoulos and F. W. Alt, 1988, *Science* **241**:1581.]

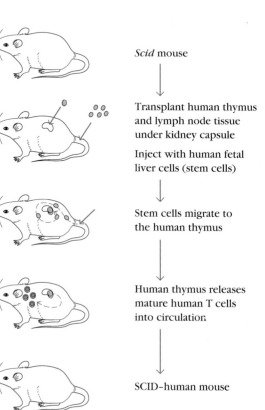

Figure 20-7 Production of SCID-human mouse.

one to study human lymphocytes within an animal model. The value of this model will become clear in the next chapter, because the SCID-human mouse is rapidly becoming an important animal model for the study of immune depletion in AIDS. There are, however, important ethical considerations that must be addressed concerning the use of human fetal tissue in research.

Complement Deficiencies

Immunodeficiency diseases resulting from deficiencies in the complement system were discussed in Chapter 15 and are mentioned only briefly here. Many of these deficiencies are associated with increased susceptibility to bacterial infections and/or with immune-complex diseases (see Table 15-7).

Summary

1. Immunodeficiency diseases can affect any component of the immune system. Disorders have been reported involving the phagocytic system, the complement system, the humoral system, and the cell-mediated system.

2. Phagocytic disorders can result from quantitative deficiencies (agranulocytosis or neutropenia) or from a functional defect in one of the steps of phagocytosis (leukocyte adhesion, chemotaxis, phagocytosis, or killing). Examples include congenital agranulocytosis, leukocyte-adhesion deficiency, lazy-leukocyte syndrome, and chronic granulomatous disease.

3. Humoral deficiencies can result from defects in B-cell maturation, intrinsic defects of mature B cells, ineffective T_H-cell activation, or inappropriate suppression by T cells. Examples of humoral deficiencies include X-linked infantile hypogammaglobulinemia, common variable immunodeficiency, and selective IgA deficiency.

4. Cell-mediated deficiencies can result from defective T-cell maturation due to thymic aplasia. DiGeorge syndrome is an example of a cell-mediated immune defect.

5. Combined humoral and cell-mediated deficiencies can result from stem-cell differentiation defects, defects in thymic or bursal processing, enzyme deficiencies that result in selective killing of T and B cells, or failure to express class II MHC molecules. Examples of these combined disorders include reticular dysgenesis, bare-lymphocyte syndrome, and the various forms of severe combined immunodeficiency disease (SCID).

References

ANDERSON, D. C., and T. A. SPRINGER. 1987. Leukocyte adhesion deficiency: an inherited defect in the Mac-1, LFA-1 and p150,95 glycoproteins. *Annu. Rev. Med.* **38**:175.

BOSMA, M. J., and A. M. CARROLL. 1991. The scid mouse mutant: definition, characterization, and potential uses. *Annu. Rev. Immunol.* **9**:323.

HOLZMANN, B., and I. L. WEISSMAN. 1989. Integrin molecules involved in lymphocyte homing to Pyer's patches. *Immunol. Rev.* **108**:45.

KANTOFF, P W., S. M. FREEMAN, and W. F. ANDERSON. 1988. Prospects for gene therapy for immunodeficiency diseases. *Annu. Rev. Immunol.* **6**:581

KARA, C. J., and L. H. GLIMCHER. 1991. In vivo footprinting of MHC class II genes: bare promoters in the bare lymphocyte syndrome. *Science* **252**:709.

MALYNN, B. A., et al. 1988. The *scid* defect affects the final step of the immunoglobulin VDJ recombinase mechanism. *Cell* **54**:453.

McCUNE, J. M., et al. 1988. The SCID-Hu mouse: murine model for the analysis of human hematolymphoid differentiation and function. *Science* **241**:1632.

ROSEN, F. S., M. D. COOPER, and R. J. WEDGWOOD. 1984. The primary immunodeficiencies. *New Eng. J. Med.* **311**:235 and 300.

SPICKETT, G. P., and J. FARRANT. 1989. The role of lymphokines in common variable hypogammaglobulinemia. *Immunol. Today* **10**(6):192.

VERMA, I. M. 1990. Gene therapy. *Sci. Am.* (**263**) 5:68.

YANCOPOULOS, G. D., and F. W. ALT. 1988. Reconstruction of an immune system. *Science* **241**:1581.

YEDNOCK, T. A., and S. R. ROSEN. 1989. Lymphocyte homing. *Adv. Immunol.* **44**:313.

Study Questions

1. Indicate whether each of the following statements is true or false. If you think a statement is false, explain why.

    a. DiGeorge syndrome is a congenital birth defect resulting in absence of the thymus.

    b. Bruton's agammaglobulinemia is a combined B-cell and T-cell immunodeficiency disease.

    c. The hallmark of a phagocytic deficiency is increased susceptibility to viral infections.

    d. In chronic granulomatous disease, H_2O_2 produced by catalase-negative bacteria results in bacterial killing in the defective granulocytes.

    e. Gamma-globulin injections are given to treat individuals with X-linked agammaglobulinemia.

f. $D_H J_H$ joining is defective in CB-17 *scid* mice.

g. Mice with the *scid* defect lack functional B and T lymphocytes.

h. A thymic transplant can restore the immune defect in CB-17 *scid* mice.

i. Children born with DiGeorge syndrome often manifest increased infections of encapsulated bacteria.

j. Failure to express class II MHC molecules in bare-lymphocyte syndrome affects cell-mediated immunity only.

2. a. How do rearranged Ig heavy-chain genes in *scid* mice differ from those in normal mice.

b. In *scid* mice, rearrangement of κ light-chain DNA is not attempted. Explain why.

c. If you introduced a functional μ heavy-chain gene into *scid* progenitor B cells by a gene-transfer method, would the κ light-chain DNA undergo a normal rearrangement? Explain your answer.

d. If you compared gene rearrangements in TCR α- and β-chain DNA in T-cell thymomas derived from *scid* mice and normal CB-17 mice, what differences would you detect?

3. a. Describe the procedure for preparing SCID-human mice.

b. Why are human fetal liver cells used in this procedure?

c. Why are the human cells not rejected by the recipient mouse?

d. Why does graft-versus-host disease not develop in the recipient mouse?

4. Granulocytes from patients with leukocyte-adhesion deficiency (LAD) express greatly reduced amounts of three integrin-type receptors: CR3, CR4, and LFA-1.

a. What is the nature of the defect that results in decreased or in no expression of these receptors in LAD patients?

b. What is the normal function of these integrin-type receptor molecules?

c. Would you expect LAD patients to exhibit normal levels of specific antibody following antigenic challenge? Explain your answer.

CHAPTER 21

The Immune System in AIDS

Since the early 1980s, the spread of the disease now known as acquired immunodeficiency syndrome (AIDS) has been dramatic. Many predict that AIDS eventually will cause millions of deaths and sorely stress health care systems worldwide in the next decade or two. AIDS—the epitome of an acquired immunodeficiency disease—renders its victims susceptible to various opportunistic infections and rare forms of cancer, which are the immediate cause of death. As the number of reported AIDS cases escalated, the acquisition of scientific information about AIDS exhibited a comparable surge, with reports in the scientific literature increasing logarithmically from 1982 to the present. Never has so much been learned about a disease and its causative agent in such a short time. This explosion of information about AIDS has expanded our understanding about the immune system to such an extent that this entire chapter is devoted to AIDS and the immunodeficiences associated with it.

Discovery and Incidence of AIDS

In the summer of 1981, five cases of *Pneumocystis carinii* pneumonia, all in young homosexual men from the same area of Los Angeles, were reported to the Centers for Disease Control (CDC), the agency of the U.S. Public Health Service responsible for monitoring infectious diseases in the United States. Soon after, the CDC began to get reports of *Pneumocystis carinii* pneumonia, Kaposi's sarcoma, and various opportunistic infections clustered in young homosexual men living in New York City, San Francisco, and Los Angeles. *Pneumocystis carinii* was known as a widespread and generally harmless protozoan rarely associated with pneumonia; Kaposi's sarcoma was a rare tumor of blood-vessel tissue associated with aging. What caught the attention of the CDC was that these diseases had previously been limited to individuals with impaired cell-mediated immunity. One might expect to see these diseases in individuals born with immune deficiencies, in transplant recipients receiving immunosuppressive drugs, or in cancer patients receiving chemotherapy, but to see them in young and previously healthy men with no obvious condition that would impair immunity was alarming. In December 1981, reports in the *New England Journal of Medicine* confirmed the linkage to immune system compromise by demonstrating that the original victims of the still-unnamed disorder had decreased counts of CD4$^+$ T cells. In early 1982 the CDC suggested that this distinct new disorder be called *acquired immunodeficiency syndrome*, now commonly known as AIDS. The syndrome appeared to be a collection of symptoms associated with an immune-system deficiency that was not inborn or imposed but somehow acquired.

Although AIDS was first identified in homosexual men in the United States, it soon began to be reported in other groups, including users of intravenous (IV) drugs, hemophiliacs, recipients of blood transfusions, sexual partners of AIDS patients, and eventually in infants of mothers with the disease. Such findings suggested that AIDS was transmissible; in order to monitor the disease, the CDC asked in 1982 that all AIDS cases be reported. Since that time the spectrum of clinical disease has broadened as the number of reported cases has increased exponentially. What began as five cases reported in a CDC newsletter in 1981 mushroomed to staggering proportions within a few years. Between 1980 and 1985

there were an estimated 70,000 cases of AIDS worldwide; by 1986 to 1988 the number of AIDS cases had risen to 300,000; and by 1989 to 1991 there were an estimated 700,000 cases. Projected estimates forecast 500,000 cases in the United States by 1992, and estimates by the CDC suggest that 1–2 million Americans have already been infected by the virus that causes AIDS. On a global scale a conservative estimate by the World Health Organization puts the number of people infected at 10 million: 6 million in Africa, 2 million in the Americas, 500,000 in Europe, 500,000 in Asia, and 30,000 in Oceania (Figure 21-1). The high rate of infection estimated by the World Health Organization among men and women (Table 21-1) and children portends economic and social disaster should an effective intervention not be forthcoming.

The Causative Agent and Infection Process

Initial attempts to identify the cause of AIDS in homosexual men focused on a number of hypotheses. Sperm was known to be immunosuppressive, and some investigators suggested that the entry of sperm antigens into the blood through rectal tearing might account for the immunosuppression seen in AIDS. Others thought that antigen overload might in itself suppress the immune system. In addition, amyl nitrite, a sexual stimulant used by some homosexuals, was known to have immunosuppressive capabilities. However, the development of AIDS in hemophiliacs who had received injections of factor VIII from pooled and concentrated human plasma began to point to a viral agent. Several known viruses such as Epstein-Barr virus and cytomegalovirus were considered. It was not long, however, before a new retrovirus was identified as being associated with AIDS by several independent groups.

Table 21-1   Estimated proportion of men and women infected with HIV*

	Men	Women
North America	1 in 75	1 in 700
South America	1 in 125	1 in 500
Western Europe	1 in 200	1 in 1400
Sub-Saharan Africa	1 in 40	1 in 40

* Incidence by sex is for adults aged 15 to 49.

SOURCE: WHO Communicable Disease Scotland Weekly Report 25/8/90 and *Science*, 1991, **25**:372.

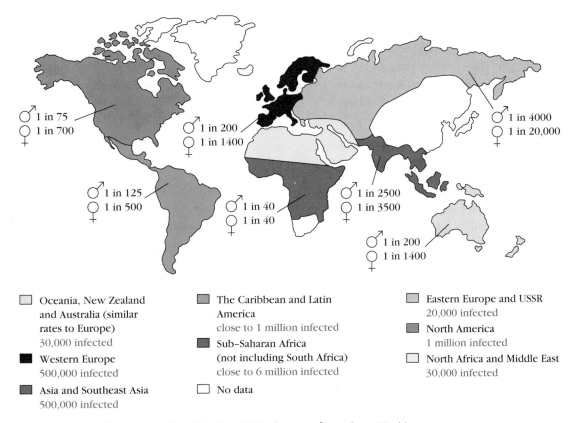

Figure 21-1 Amount and distribution of worldwide AIDS infections. [Data from World Health Organization. Adapted from *Science* **252**:372.]

Luc Montagnier's group at the Pasteur Institute isolated a retrovirus from a patient manifesting persistent generalized lymphadenopathy in 1983 and called it *LAV* for lymphadenopathy-associated virus. Soon after that Robert Gallo's group at the National Cancer Institute identified a retrovirus in 1984 and called it *HTLV-III* for human T-lymphotrophic virus type III. The virus was also independently identified by Jay Levy's group at the University of California at San Francisco and called *ARV* (AIDS-related virus). Subsequent studies revealed that the three viral isolates were the same virus. For a while all three names were used in the literature, leading to some confusion. Then, in 1986, an international committee renamed the virus *human immunodeficiency virus*, or *HIV*. Following the discovery of an antigenic variant in 1986, the original virus was designated HIV-1 and the variant HIV-2. Several related simian viruses have also been discovered in monkeys: SIV_{AGM} from the African green monkey, SIV_{MND} from mandrills, SIV_{MAC} from captive macaque (rhesus) monkeys, SIV_{SMM} from captive sooty mangabeys, and SIV_{CPZ} from wild chimpanzees.

Origins and Evolutionary Relationships of HIV

The retroviruses can be divided into two groups: transforming and cytopathic. The *transforming retroviruses* induce changes in cell growth that lead to cancer. These viruses often carry genes, called *oncogenes*, that influence cellular growth. Included in this group are bovine leukemia virus, equine infectious anemia virus, feline leukemia virus, avian type C virus, mammalian type C virus, and human T-cell lymphotrophic virus type I and II (HTLV-I and HTLV-II). The best studied of this group are HTLV-I and HTLV-II, which cause T-cell leukemia. Infection of T lymphocytes with HTLV-I or HTLV-II causes the cells to begin to express a receptor for IL-2, so that as a cell secretes IL-2, it autostimulates its own division in an unregulated way, causing T-cell leukemia (see Chapter 11).

The *cytopathic retroviruses* are members of the Lentivirus family. One branch of this group includes visna virus, caprine arthritis encephalitis virus, equine infectious anemia virus, and feline immunodeficiency virus. The other branch of this group includes human immunodeficiency virus (HIV-1 and HIV-2) and simian immunodeficiency virus (SIV). HIV-1, which is epidemic in Central Africa, the Americas, Europe, Asia, and Haiti, infects both humans and chimpanzees but causes immune suppression only in humans. HIV-2 was originally isolated from Senegal in West Africa and small numbers of cases have been reported outside Africa, in Europe, and the Americas. Most HIV-2 strains appear to spread more slowly than HIV-1 and to be less pathogenic; HIV-2 infects humans, chimpanzees, macaques monkeys, and baboons and thus has a broader host range than HIV-1. The infection of macaque monkeys with some strains of HIV-2 results in symptoms of immune suppression and holds promise as an animal model for AIDS. SIV$_{AGM}$ is endemic in African green monkeys, with an estimated 40% of the green monkey population in parts of Africa infected. SIV$_{AGM}$ infection of the African green monkey does not cause immune suppression, but injection of SIV$_{AGM}$ into macaques does lead to a fatal AIDS-like disease (simian AIDS, or SAIDS) and to death within 3–36 months.

Comparisons of the DNA sequences of various HIV-1, HIV-2, and SIV isolates have revealed that HIV-1 and HIV-2 exhibit only 40–50% sequence homology. The HIV-2 sequence appears to be more closely related to SIV$_{MAC}$, SIV$_{SMM}$, and SIV$_{AGM}$, showing 75% homology with some strains of these simian viruses. It is thought that SIV arose first as a nonpathogenic lentivirus in African nonhuman primates and that transmission of SIV to humans gave rise to HIV-2. HIV-1 and SIV$_{CPZ}$ genomes suggest an evolutionary relationship, although it is not known if SIV$_{CPZ}$ is the precursor to HIV-1 or if it arose from some other animal lentivirus.

HIV Morphology

HIV-1, HIV-2, and SIV share structural and molecular similarity with all members of the lentivirus family of retroviruses (Figure 21-2). The virus has an RNA viral genome with two associated molecules of an enzyme called *reverse transcriptase*. The retroviruses are named for the fact they have an RNA genome that is "reverse-transcribed" into DNA by reverse transcriptase. Surrounding the genome are two layers of protein forming a cylindrical protein core. The proteins composing the core are designated p17 and p24. Outside the core is a lipid bilayer envelope the virus acquires from an infected host cell by a process called *budding*. The host-cell membrane is modified by the insertion of two viral glycoproteins, gp120 and gp41. The gp41 glycoprotein spans the membrane; gp120 is noncovalently associated with gp41 but extends beyond the membrane.

(a)

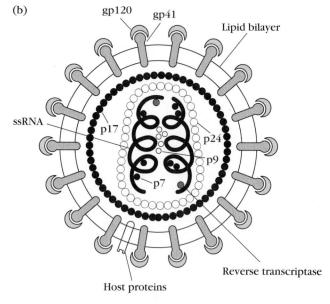

(b)

Figure 21-2   (a) Electron micrograph of HIV virions magnified 200,000 times. The glycoprotein projections are faintly visible as "knobs" extending from the periphery of each virion. (b) Cross-sectional diagram of HIV virion. Each virion expresses 72 glycoprotein projections composed of gp120 (light red) and gp41 (gray). Gp 41 is a transmembrane molecule that crosses the lipid bilayer of the envelope. Gp120 is noncovalently associated with gp41 and serves as the viral receptor for CD4 on host cells. The viral envelope also contains some host-cell membrane proteins such as class I and class II MHC molecules. Within the envelope is the viral core, or nucleocapsid, which includes a layer of a protein called p17 and an inner layer of a protein called p24. The HIV genome consists of two copies of ssRNA, which are associated with two molecules of reverse transcriptase (dark red) and nucleoid proteins p7 and p9. [Part (a) from micrograph by Hans Geldenblom of the Robert Koch, Institute in Berlin, in R. C. Gallo and L. Montagnier, 1988, The AIDS epidemic, *Sci. Am.* **259**:40; part (b) adapted from B. M. Peterlin and P. A. Luciw, 1988, *AIDS* **2**:S29.]

HIV Infection of Target Cells

Entry of HIV into target cells involves two steps: binding of virions to receptors on target cells followed by fusion of the viral envelope with the plasma membrane of the target cells. The two glycoproteins—gp120 and gp41— that make up the surface projections on HIV play vital roles in these initial steps in HIV infection. Once inside a target cell, the viral genome is integrated into the host-cell genome, forming a *provirus*, which may remain in a latent state or be activated and transcribed into viral proteins.

HIV Binding to Cells

The first step in HIV infection is binding of viral gp120 to receptors on target cells. Because the CD4 membrane molecule on the surface of T_H cells is the principal cellular receptor for HIV, the virus is said to be *lymphotrophic*. Other cells (e.g., macrophages, monocytes, dendritic cells, Langerhans' cells, hematopoietic stem cells, certain rectal-lining cells, and microglial cells) also express low levels of CD4 and thus exhibit some binding of HIV. HIV-1 has a 25-fold higher affinity for CD4 than HIV-2. The lower binding ability of HIV-2 may account, in part, for its lower pathogenicity compared to HIV-1. The importance of CD4 in HIV binding has been demonstrated by transferring the gene encoding CD4 into cells in culture (e.g., HeLa cells) that lack CD4; such cells, formerly resistant to HIV, become susceptible to HIV infection after transfection.

The CD4-binding sequence on gp120 was determined by researchers at Genetech, who transfected Chinese Hamster Ovary (CHO) cells with the CD4 gene. They found that soluble, cloned [^{125}I] labeled gp120 could bind to these transfected cells but not to untransfected controls. They then cleaved the gp120 molecule into peptide fragments, produced monoclonal antibody to each fragment, and tested the ability of each monoclonal antibody to inhibit binding of the radiolabeled gp120 to the CD4-transfected CHO cells. By using this procedure, they identified a largely conserved region of amino acids (397–439) near the carboxy terminus of gp120 that appeared to be involved in CD4 binding. Further evidence for the role of this sequence in CD4 binding was obtained by synthesizing a peptide with this sequence and showing that it could also block binding of soluble radiolabeled gp120 to the CD4-transfected CHO cells. When regions within the 397–439 sequence were deleted, a substantial reduction in binding to CD4 occurred.

Although the CD4 molecule is the high-affinity receptor for HIV, studies have shown that expression of CD4 by a cell is not always sufficient or necessary for HIV infection. For example, when the gene for CD4 is transfected into mouse cells, these transfected cells still cannot be infected with HIV even though they express CD4. This finding led to the suggestion that some other membrane molecule or intracellular event must be necessary for viral entry into cells. On the other hand, some cells that lack detectable CD4 can be infected with HIV, although it is not known how the virus enters these cells. For instance, HIV has been shown to infect some brain-derived cell lines that lack CD4, and to do so even in the presence of excess soluble CD4. These findings led some researchers at the VI International AIDS Conference in 1990 to propose that a membrane molecule other than CD4 may serve as a universal receptor for HIV, allowing the virus to bind to cells lacking CD4. These various results suggest that in some cases HIV can enter cells by some mechanism other than binding of gp120 to CD4.

Fusion of HIV with Cells

After binding of HIV to its receptor (principally CD4), the viral envelope fuses with the target-cell plasma membrane. The fusion event appears to be induced by a hydrophobic region near the amino terminus of gp41; this region is called the *fusogenic domain*. Following fusion, the HIV nucleocapsid is internalized, and the viral RNA is uncoated, establishing a productive infection (Figure 21-3a, steps 1–4).

HIV Replicative Cycle

Once the HIV RNA has been introduced into a target cell and uncoated, it is transcribed into DNA by the viral reverse transcriptase enzyme. The viral DNA is integrated into the host-cell genome, forming a provirus, which can remain in a latent state and be passed on to daughter cells. Activation of the provirus initiates transcription of the structural genes into mRNA, which is translated into viral proteins. The host plasma membrane is modified by insertion of gp41 and associated gp120; the viral RNA and capsid protein then assemble beneath the modified membrane, acquiring the modified host plasma membrane as its envelope in a process called *budding*. In some cases the process of budding goes on at a low level, allowing the infected cell to survive; in other cases the assembly of viral particles and budding is so massive that the host cell is lysed (see Figure 21-3b–d). The infection of macrophages and monocytes generally does not lead to cell death, and there is some speculation that HIV-bearing macrophages may serve as a major reservoir of HIV, carrying it to various organs and even across the blood-brain barrier.

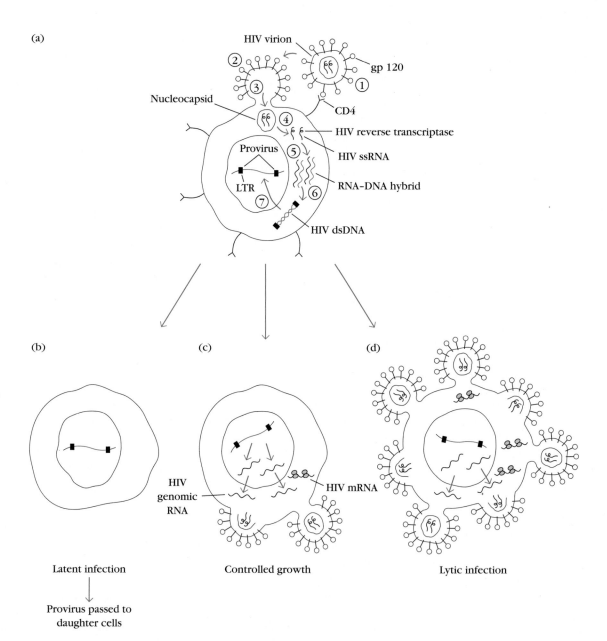

Figure 21-3 (a) HIV infection of susceptible cells begins with the binding of gp120 to CD4 membrane molecules (1). The viral envelope fuses with the plasma membrane of the cell (2) allowing entry of the HIV nucleocapsid containing the viral genome (3). The outer core proteins p17 and p24 are removed (4), releasing ssRNA and reverse transcriptase, which copies the ssRNA into RNA-DNA hybrids (5). Second-strand DNA synthesis proceeds (6) after the action of ribonuclease H, which partially degrades the original RNA template. The viral DNA duplex is then translocated to the nucleus and integrated into the host chromosomal DNA by the viral integrase enzyme (7). At this point the integrated HIV is referred to as a provirus. (b) The provirus can remain in a latent state for months to years. During this time cell division passes the proviral DNA on to progeny cells. (c) Activation of the provirus results in transcription of the proviral DNA and translation into viral structural protein. The virus leaves the infected host cell by budding out of the plasma membrane. In some cells this process goes on at low levels, referred to as controlled growth, allowing the host cell to survive. (d) In other cells activation of the provirus results in rapid viral assembly leading to massive membrane damage upon viral budding, so that the host cell is lysed by the process.

Viral Transmission: Role of HIV-Infected Cells

As mentioned in the previous section, HIV has been shown to infect numerous types of cells other than $CD4^+$ T cells (Table 21-2). Although the virus can exist as a provirus and replicate in any of these cells, the T cell is the major cell type to be depleted as a result of HIV infection. What this means is that other cells, notably macrophages and dendritic cells can harbor the virus, protecting it from the immune system and serving as a reservoir from which the virus can be transmitted throughout the body or from one individual to another. The ability of HIV to infect such macrophage-like cells as microglia cells in the brain may lead to some of the neurologic manifestations in AIDS. In addition, when lymph nodes from AIDS patients are examined, most of the viral particles are in or near the follicular dendritic cells rather than in $CD4^+$ cells, suggesting that dendritic cells also may be a major site of HIV replication.

A number of studies have suggested that HIV-infected cells are the primary means by which the virus is transmitted. Normally the level of free HIV is quite low in serum and vaginal fluid, and it is even lower in other body fluids such as urine, saliva, breast milk, and tears. The major transmission routes are by sexual intercourse, transfusions of blood or blood products, IV drug use involving shared needles, and transplacental transfer from an infected mother to the fetus; each of these routes are likely to involve cell-associated virus. It has been suggested that macrophages, dendritic cells, and lymphocytes carrying HIV may be the most important mode of transmission from one infected individual to another.

HIV Genome

The HIV genome appears to be more complicated than that of other known retroviruses. The organization of the HIV-1 genome is diagrammed in Figure 21-4, and the functions of the corresponding proteins are summarized in Table 21-3.

Most retroviruses (including HIV) carry three genes—designated *gag*, *env*, and *pol*—that, respectively, encode the viral core proteins, the envelope glycoproteins, and the nonstructural proteins required for replication. Each of these genes encodes a large polyprotein precursor, which is then cleaved to render the final gene products. The *pol* polyprotein is cleaved to generate three enzymes: reverse transcriptase, protease, and integrase. The *gag* gene encodes a precursor polyprotein that is cleaved by the *pol* protease to yield p24, p7, p9, and p17; p17 and p24 make up the protein core of the viral particle. The *env* gene encodes a glycosylated precursor polyprotein (gp160), which is cleaved to yield gp120 and gp41.

In addition to *gag*, *env*, and *pol*, the HIV genome includes at least six additional genes: virion infectivity factor (*vif*), viral protein R (*vpr*), transactivator (*tat*), regulator of expression of virion proteins (*rev*), negative factor (*nef*), and either viral protein U (*vpu*) in HIV-1 or viral protein X (*vpx*) in HIV-2. Two of these genes, *tat* and *rev*, are split genes, which are read in different reading frames on the polyribosome to yield the *tat* gene product or the *rev* gene product. The *tat*, *rev*, and *nef* genes encode regulatory proteins that control the expression of the structural genes *gag*, *pol*, and *env*. The protein encoded by *tat* upregulates transcription, and

Table 21-2 Cell types that can be infected by HIV

Hematopoietic/immune cells	Brain/glial cells	Others
T lymphocytes	Astrocytes and oligodendrocytes	Fibroblasts
B lymphocytes	Microglia	Sperm
Primary monocytes/macrophages	Glial cell lines	Liver sinusoid epithelium
Kuppfer cells (liver macrophages)	Fetal neural cells	Bowel epithelium
Monocyte cell lines	Brain capillary endothelium	Colon carcinoma cells
Bone marrow precursor cells		Osteosarcoma cells
Dendritic cells		Rhabdomyosarcoma cells
Langerhans' cells		Fetal chorionic villi
		Rabbit macrophages

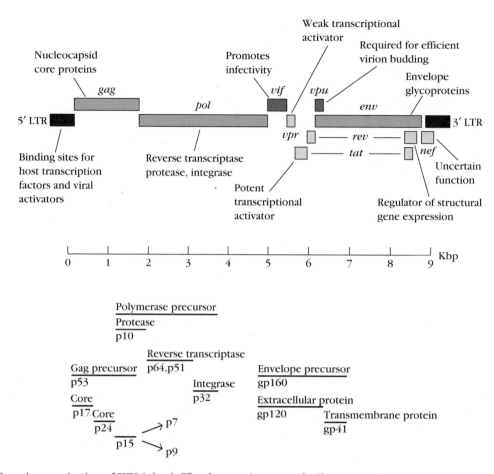

Figure 21-4 Genetic organization of HIV-1 (*top*). The three major genes (red)—*gag, pol,* and *env*—encode polyproteins, which are cleaved to yield the nucleocapsid core proteins, enzymes required for replication, and envelope core proteins (*bottom*). Of the remaining six genes, three (light gray) encode regulatory proteins that play a major role in controlling expression; two (dark gray) encode proteins required for virion maturation; and one (light red) encodes a weak transcriptional activator. As indicated, the coding sequences of several genes overlap. Differential RNA processing of the single primary transcript and translation of the resulting mRNAs in different reading frames yields the various gene products. Both *tat* and *rev* are split genes; the exons are spliced together during RNA processing, and depending on the reading frame during translation, either Tat or Rev is synthesized. The 5' long terminal repeat (LTR) contains sequences to which various regulatory proteins bind. The organization of the HIV-2 genome is very similar, except the *vpu* gene is replaced by *vpx* in HIV-2. See Table 21-3 for a summary of the functions of the viral proteins.

that encoded by *nef* may have the opposite effect; the protein encoded by *rev* promotes transcription of the viral structural proteins that are necessary for viral assembly in the lytic state. The *vif, vpu,* and *vpx* genes encode proteins required for virion maturation. The remaining HIV gene (*vpr*) encodes a regulatory protein that is a weak transcriptional activator. The proviral genes are flanked by repetitive sequences called *long terminal repeats* (*LTRs*), which contain essential regulatory sequences controlling viral expression and integration. The function of these sequences is discussed in the next section.

Activation of the HIV Provirus

As noted earlier, after the HIV genome is integrated into a host-cell genome, the resulting provirus may enter a latent state, during which viral replication and maturation proceeds at very low levels or not at all. During latency, the provirus in infected cells is passed on to daughter cells as the host genome is replicated during mitosis; however, because the viral structural genes are not expressed, new viral particles are not produced. This latency period—a characteristic feature of HIV infec-

Table 21-3 Proteins encoded by HIV-1 genes and their functions

Gene	Protein products	Functions of final products
gag	53-kD precursor (p53) ↓ p17, p24, p9, & p7	Nucleocapsid core proteins: p17: is associated with inner surface of envelope p24: forms inner protein layer of nucleocapsid p9: is a component of nucleoid core p7: binds directly to genomic RNA
env	160-kD precursor (gp160) ↓ gp120 & gp41	Envelope glycoproteins: gp120: protrudes from envelope and binds CD4 gp41: transmembrane protein, contains an external domian required for fusion with target cells
pol	Precursor ↓ p64, p51, p10, & p32	Enzymes: p64, p51: has reverse transcriptase activity; p64 also has RNase activity p10: has protease activity p32: has integrase activity
vif	p23	Promotes infectivity of cell-free virions
vpr	p15	Activates transcription weakly
tat	p14	Activates transcription strongly
rev	p19	Controls proportions of mRNAs for structural and regulatory proteins
nef	p27	Has uncertain regulatory functions*
vpu	p16	Is required for efficient viral assembly and budding from host cells

* Early studies suggested that the protein encoded by this gene inhibited HIV transcription; hence the gene was named *nef* for "negative factor." More recent studies, however, have called this function into question.

tion—may last for more than 10 years, during which time an HIV-infected individual is largely asymptomatic. When HIV progresses from latent infection to lytic infection, viral replication and maturation increase dramatically, the number of CD4$^+$ T cells begins to plummet, and the typical symptoms of AIDS begin to appear. A major research focus has been to try to understand the events that trigger lytic viral replication in the hope that it might be possible to inhibit the progression from latency to the lytic state, thus prolonging the asymptomatic latency period in HIV-infected individuals.

Considerable evidence indicates that an HIV-infected cell must be activated before the provirus can replicate. Stimulation of HIV-infected T cells with various antigens or T-cell mitogens, for example, has been shown to induce viral replication. As mentioned in the previous section, the proviral genes are flanked by sequences called LTRs, which play a role in regulating viral gene expression. Because these LTRs exhibit some sequence homology with cellular genes involved in T-cell activation,

R. C. Gallo has speculated that the signals that activate T cells may also activate the HIV provirus. A number of findings support Gallo's hypothesis. For example, activation of the provirus is induced by several nuclear-binding proteins that are synthesized in activated T cells. Two of these proteins, NFAT-1 and NF-κB, normally take part in the activation of several T-cell genes required for T-cell proliferation, including the genes encoding IL-2 and the high-affinity IL-2 receptor (see Chapter 11). These nuclear-binding proteins, however, also appear to regulate HIV proviral activation, thereby linking the state of HIV activation to the state of T-cell activation.

As illustrated in Figure 21-5, NF-κB has been shown to bind to the enhancer in the 5′ proviral LTR, initiating transcription of the provirus. Early in HIV expression, the predominant proteins expressed are the regulatory proteins Tat, Rev, and Nef. At this stage there is little expression of the structural proteins. In time, however, expression shifts from the regulatory proteins to the structural and enzymatic proteins encoded by *gag, env,* and *pol.* This shift in expression appears to depend on

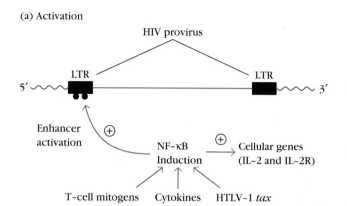

(a) Activation

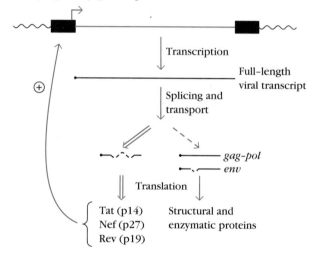

(b) Early regulatory–gene expression

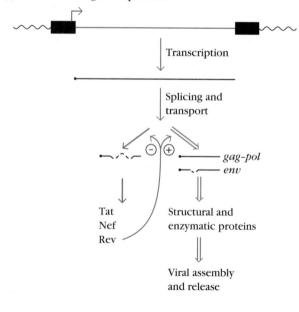

(c) Late structural–gene expression

the Rev protein (p19), which apparently can increase the transport and translation of mRNAs encoding the structural and enzymatic proteins necessary for viral assembly.

The finding that NF-κB increases in activated T cells suggests that increased antigenic stimulation of an HIV-infected individual would similarly increase the risk of viral activation. In the case of intravenous drug users, the high antigen exposure associated with IV drug use may induce early activation of the HIV provirus. In addition, many HIV-infected individuals are known to carry viruses (e.g., cytomegalovirus and Epstein-Barr virus) that activate lymphocytes, and these secondary infections may contribute to HIV activation and progression from the latent to the lytic state. Another way in which a latent HIV infection may progress to a lytic infection is by entry of allogeneic lymphocytes from semen into the bloodstream via anal intercourse. In this situation, a graft-versus-host reaction may develop in which the allogeneic lymphocytes attack host cells. This reaction could serve as an effective T-cell activating signal, initiating the expression of the proviral genome and replication of HIV virions in latently infected T cells.

Genetic Variation in HIV

HIV is capable of tremendous genetic variation, with mutations in the viral genome occurring at rates millions of times faster than what is observed in human DNA. In fact, sequencing studies reveal that no two AIDS patients carry the identical virus; furthermore, viral isolates taken from the same individual at different times also can differ substantially. The DNA sequence diversity seen in HIV is generated by its reverse transcriptase enzyme, which has been shown to be extremely error-prone and thus gives rise to numerous base substitutions, additions, and

Figure 21-5 Stages in the expression of HIV proviral DNA. (a) T-cell activation by mitogens, cytokines, or other viral gene products such as the HTLV-1 *tax* gene induces formation of various nuclear-binding factors including NF-κB. The NF-κB binds to the enhancer sequence in the proviral 5′ LTR, initiating transcription of the provirus. (b) Early in HIV expression the predominant products formed are the various regulatory proteins of HIV including Tat, Rev, and Nef. Tat and Nef act on the 5′ LTR to regulate HIV transcription. (c) Late in HIV expression there is a shift from production of regulatory proteins to production of the structural and enzymatic proteins encoded by *gag, env*, and *pol*. This shift appears to depend upon the levels of Rev, which can increase the transport and translation of the mRNAs encoding the structural and enzymatic proteins necessary for viral assembly. [Adapted from W. C. Greene, 1991, *New Engl. J. Med.* **324**:308.]

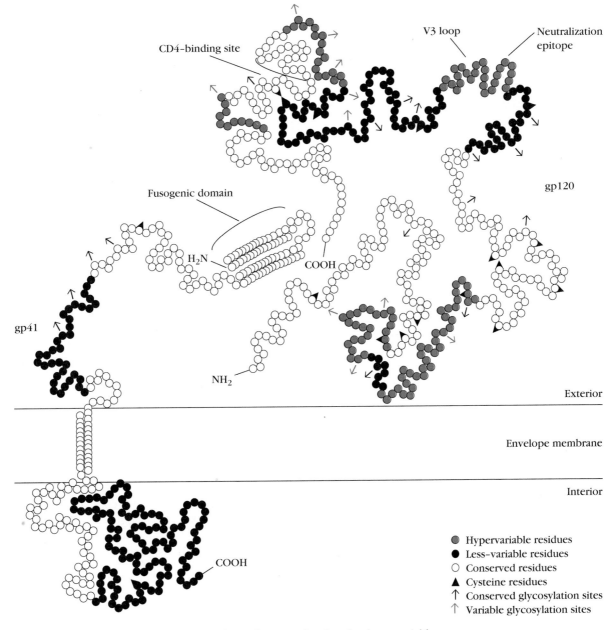

Figure 21-6 Schematic diagram of HIV-1 envelope glycoproteins showing hypervariable amino acid residues (red), less variable residues (black), and conserved residues (white). Neutralizing antibodies are produced predominantly to an epitope that overlaps with one of the hypervariable regions in gp120, designated the V3 loop. For this reason, neutralizing antibodies to HIV generally are strain-specific. Note that the CD4-binding site on gp120 and the fusogenic domain in gp41, both of which mediate essential viral functions, have conserved amino acid sequences. [Adapted from R. C. Gallo, 1988, *J. Acquired Immune Deficiency Syndromes* **1**:521.]

deletions. It has been estimated that between 5 and 10 errors are introduced into the HIV genome during each round of replication! As discussed in a later section, these changes make development of an HIV vaccine extremely difficult because antibodies or cell-mediated immunity directed against one isolate may not recognize another isolate.

Role of Immune System in Selecting HIV Variants

In one study HIV was isolated from peripheral blood lymphocytes from an infected individual on two different occasions separated by 16 months. The viral isolates recovered at these different times showed an average of 13% variation in their DNA sequences. This variation was enough to change the viral isolates' biological activity, as evidenced by differences in their ability to grow in T cells and in macrophages. The emergence of distinct HIV isolates in infected individuals results partly from immune-system selection of HIV variants.

After an individual is infected with HIV, specific neutralizing antibodies are made to viral protein and glycoprotein components. These antibodies bind to HIV and have been shown to block its ability to infect T cells in vitro. Furthermore, when HIV is grown in T-cell lines in the presence of human serum containing neutralizing antibody, a viral population resistant to the neutralizing antibody emerges after 4–5 weeks in culture. What this means is that although an individual may initially produce antibody that can inactivate HIV, the high mutation rate, coupled with the high rate of viral replication, enables some viral progeny to become resistant to the effects of the antibody. These resistant viruses survive and continue to infect additional cells and replicate, so that eventually there emerges a population of resistant viral particles.

Variation in the Envelope Glycoproteins

The external presentation of gp120 and gp41 on the envelope of HIV makes these two glycoproteins potential targets for antibody neutralization of viral infectivity. For this reason considerable research has focused on the structure and antigenicity of these two envelope glycoproteins. Gp120 and gp41, are synthesized from a glycosylated precursor protein (gp160) in the rough endoplasmic reticulum of infected cells. The precursor is cleaved, generating a small carboxyl-terminal fragment (gp41), which spans the membrane, and a larger amino-terminal fragment (gp120), which remains noncovalently associated with the gp41 on the membrane (see Figure 21-2b).

Of all the HIV proteins gp120 shows the most sequence variation, with gp41 ranking second. When the gp120 and gp41 sequences of different isolates are compared, some regions are constant from one isolate to another and other regions are hypervariable (Figure 21-6). The constant regions are thought to be conserved for some necessary viral function. For example, both the CD4-binding site in gp120 and the fusogenic domain in gp41 are conserved regions.

A number of laboratories have focused their research on producing neutralizing antibodies to accessible conserved regions of gp120 or gp41. Antibodies to the conserved region of gp120 that is the putative CD4-binding site have been shown to block binding of soluble gp120 to CD4. Unfortunately, these antibodies are not effective at blocking HIV infection, perhaps because there are so many gp120-CD4 interactions at the interface of the virus and cell that they act cooperatively, increasing the likelihood of HIV binding to the target cell and rendering the neutralizing antibody ineffective. Antibodies to this conserved region on gp120 are present in HIV-infected individuals, but the titer is low.

The V3 hypervariable region of gp120, which spans residues 307 to 330, extends as a loop formed by two disulfide-linked cysteine residues at position 303 and 337. The two cysteines are highly conserved and are present in all HIV-1 isolates studied to date. There is speculation that when gp120 binds to CD4, the V3 loop may interact with gp41, inducing a conformational change that exposes the fusogenic domain. The fusogenic domain may then mediate fusion of the viral envelope with the target-cell membrane (Figure 21-7).

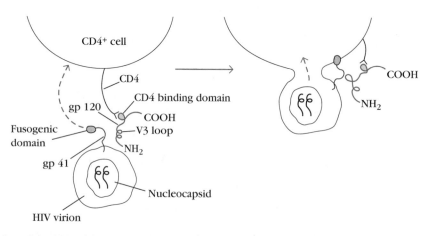

Figure 21-7 Proposed model of HIV fusion with a target cell. After viral gp120 (red) binds to CD4 on a target cell, the V3 loop is thought to interact with gp41, inducing a conformational change that exposes the fusogenic domain (gray) in gp41. This domain then mediates fusion between the viral envelope and target-cell plasma membrane, enabling the viral nucleocapsid to enter the cell.

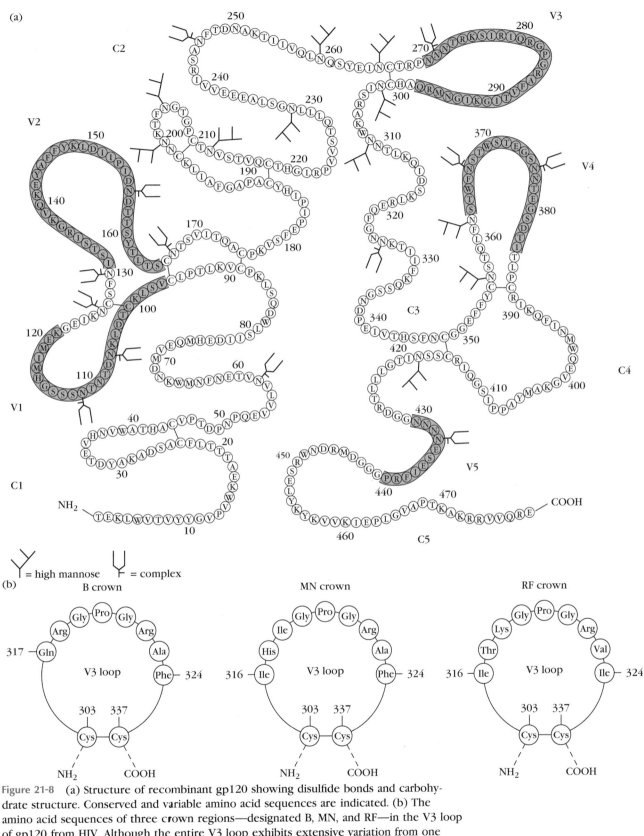

(a)

= high mannose   = complex

Figure 21-8 (a) Structure of recombinant gp120 showing disulfide bonds and carbohydrate structure. Conserved and variable amino acid sequences are indicated. (b) The amino acid sequences of three crown regions—designated B, MN, and RF—in the V3 loop of gp120 from HIV. Although the entire V3 loop exhibits extensive variation from one viral isolate to another, a significant percentage of isolates have a common crown sequence. Thus HIV isolates can be grouped into a small number of classes based on their crown sequence. Small numbers refer to residue positions in the overall gp120 sequence. [Part (a) from D. J. Capon and R. H. R. Ward. 1991. *Annu Rev. Immunol.* **9**:649.]

Antibodies to the V3 loop have been shown to be quite effective at neutralizing viral infectivity. Unfortunately, since the V3 loop is the most variable region of gp120 (and can differ by as much as 50% between HIV-1 isolates), the neutralizing antibody is strain-specific.

A small subregion within the V3 loop of gp120, however, is largely conserved. This subregion, which was identified by sequencing the V3 loop of over 200 HIV isolates, is located at the crown of the loop. HIV isolates can be grouped into a small number of classes based on the crown sequence. For example, 30% of HIV isolates in North America have a common crown sequence designated MN (Figure 21-8). Antibodies to the MN crown sequence of the V3 loop have been shown to block infectivity of all MN viral isolates. There is a great deal of interest in producing antibodies to the different crown sequences of the V3 loop as a possible vaccine approach. This approach is discussed in the section on vaccines.

Clinical Diagnosis of AIDS

The different stages of HIV infection have been classified by the Centers for Disease Control (Table 21-4). Initial HIV infection sometimes causes an acute mononucleosis-like illness, which is generally followed by an asymptomatic latency period. Often, however, individuals manifest no apparent symptoms at all upon initial HIV infection and pass without any indications into the asymptomatic latency period. Finally, a significant number of individuals infected with HIV have a persistent generalized lymphadenopathy, characterized by enlargement of multiple lymph nodes, but no concurrent illness. In all three cases, the individual is infected with HIV, and is antibody-positive in an ELISA or Western-blot test but is not yet diagnosed as having AIDS.

The disease manifestations initially recognized by the CDC as being indicative of AIDS were limited to a few opportunistic infections or Kaposi's sarcoma. It soon became apparent, however, that a much broader range of indicator diseases should be included in the diagnosis of AIDS. In an effort to reflect the diversity of disease symptoms in AIDS, the CDC classified the indicator diseases into five major categories: constitutional disease, neurologic disease, opportunistic disease, and secondary cancers, and a fifth miscellaneous category for all remaining types of indicator diseases. A positive AIDS diagnosis may be made if an individual tests positive for exposure to HIV and exhibits combinations of symptoms from one or more of these categories.

AIDS patients often have symptoms of constitutional disease, including persistent fever, involuntary weight loss greater than 10% of baseline, chronic diarrhea, and pronounced weakness. Many of these symptoms used to be classified in a non-AIDS diagnostic category called *AIDS-related complex* (*ARC*). It was soon noted, however, that patients with this diagnosis were dying without ever progressing to other indicator-disease symptoms, making it clear that many of the so-called ARC symptoms were in themselves sufficient to warrant a positive AIDS diagnosis. The term *AIDS wasting syndrome* is sometimes used to refer to the weight loss, chronic diarrhea, and weakness seen in this group of AIDS patients.

The neurologic diseases associated with AIDS includes dementia, myelopathy, and peripheral neuropathy. Neurologic symptoms are quite common, occurring in over 60% of AIDS patients. AIDS dementia complex is an insidious neurologic dysfunction that includes various cognitive, behavioral, and motor dysfunctions.

The opportunistic diseases commonly found in AIDS patients reflect their cell-mediated immune defect. They include *pneumocystis carinii* pneumonia (PCP), disseminated mycobacterial disease, cerebral toxoplasmosis, candidiasis (often infecting the oesophagus), extrapulmonary cryptococcosis, cytomegalovirus retinitis, disseminated coccidioidomycosis, disseminated histoplasmosis, tuberculosis (ofter involving extrapulmonary sites), and Herpes simplex virus mucocutaneous ulcers. *Pneumocystis carinii* pneumonia is diagnosed in about 57% of AIDS patients.

Finally, certain cancers are known to be associated with HIV infection, again indicating a cell-mediated defect. Kaposi's sarcoma stands out in this category, appearing in approximately 48% of AIDS patients, but other cancers are also observed, including various non-Hodgkins lymphomas, Burkitt's lymphoma, and immunoblastic sarcoma.

Effect of HIV Infection on T-Cell Counts

One of the early observations of immune-system impairment in HIV infection was a reduction in the number of $CD4^+$ T cells. Normally, the ratio of CD4 to CD8 T cells in the peripheral blood is about 2.0, but in AIDS patients the ratio is reversed, becoming less than 1.0 and sometimes reaching levels as low as 0.2. When lymphocytes are stained with fluorescent anti-CD4 monoclonal antibody and passed through a fluorescence-activated cell sorter, the $CD4^+$ T cells appear as a distinct peak; in AIDS patients this peak is markedly reduced. Furthermore, quantitation of the number of peripheral blood lymphocytes bearing the CD4 marker reveals a difference among clinical subgroups of AIDS patients (Figure 21-9). Although there was considerable variation in the counts among individuals in each group, the av-

Table 21-4   CDC classification of stages of HIV disease

I.   Acute infection: glandular fever-like illness lasting a few weeks

II. Asymptomatic: no symptoms at the time of infection

III. Persistant generalized lymphadenopathy (PGL): lymph node enlargement persisting for 3 or more months with no evidence of infection

IV. AIDS

    A. Constitutional disease, including one or more of the following:
       (i) Fever persisting for more than 14 days without infectious cause
       (ii) Weight loss greater than 10% of body weight with no apparent cause
       (iii) Diarrhoea persisting for more than 30 days without definable cause

    B. Neurological disease, including one or more of the following:
       (i) dementia
       (ii) myelopathy
       (iii) peripheral neuropathy

    C. Opportunistic infections, including one or more of the following:
       Pneumocystis carinii pneumonia
       Disseminated atypical mycobacterial disease
       Cerebral toxoplasmosis
       Oesophageal candidiasis
       Cryptosporidiosis
       Extrapulmonary cryptococcosis
       Cytomegalovirus retinitis
       Disseminated coccidioidomycosis
       Disseminated histoplasmosis
       Tuberculosis involving at least one extrapulmonary site
       Recurrent non-typhoid septicemia
       Extraintestinal strongyloidosis
       Progressive multifocal leucoencephalopathy

    D. Neoplasms
       Kaposi's sarcoma
       Primary lymphoma of the brain
       Non-Hodgkins lymphoma

    E. Other: clinical findings or diseases not classified above but which are attributed to HIV infection.

SOURCE: Adapted from Centers for Disease Control, 1986. *MMWR* **35**:335.

erage count for the control group differed significantly from those of all the HIV-infected groups exhibiting symptoms. Once the CD4$^+$ T cell count falls to 200/mm^3 and below, the individual is quite susceptible to opportunistic infections and neoplams. About 40% of the patients manifesting opportunistic infections had no detectable CD4$^+$ T cells at all. The very low number or complete absence of CD4$^+$ T cells in these patients probably explains their susceptibility to opportunistic infections, and also the finding that such patients have the shortest life expectancy of all AIDS patients.

The average CD8$^+$ T-cell count is actually higher in some subgroups of AIDS patients than in uninfected controls. Early in the disease, CTL activity against HIV-infected cells can be detected, but as the disease progresses, the CTL activity appears to decline. There is some evidence that at least some of the CD8$^+$ T cells in HIV-infected individuals may act to suppress the immune response.

Depletion of HIV-Infected CD4$^+$ T Cells

As explained previously, as long as the HIV provirus in an infected CD4$^+$ T cell remains in the latent state, no damage to the cell is evident. However, once the provirus is activated and new HIV virions begin to assemble and bud from the infected cell (Figure 21-10a), extensive damage to the cell membrane can occur, leading to death of the cell. In addition, the humoral or cell-mediated response generated against HIV may lead to destruction of HIV-infected CD4$^+$ T cells. Those infected CD4$^+$ T cells expressing gp120 and gp41 on their membrane can be killed by antibody + complement; those which express viral proteins associated with class I MHC molecules can be killed by a CTL response against the altered self-cells. Both processes represent a normal immune response against a virus, a process that should serve to eliminate virus-infected cells and thus prevent further spread of the virus. The irony in the case of HIV is that the immune response to eliminate the virus kills off the central cells of the immune system itself.

Depletion of Uninfected CD4$^+$ T Cells

Experiments have demonstrated that only one CD4$^+$ T cell out of 10^5-10^6 is actually infected with HIV in AIDS patients. Given that the infected cells represent less than 0.001% of the CD4$^+$ T-cell population, some mechanism(s) other than direct virus-mediated cell damage must lead to the dramatic depletion of CD4$^+$ T cells observed in AIDS patients. Some of the hypotheses that have been put forth to account for this depletion of uninfected T cells are described in this section.

In vitro experiments reveal that an HIV-infected CD4$^+$ T cell can form a giant multinucleated cell, called a syncytium, by fusing with as many as 50 uninfected CD4$^+$ T cells (Figure 21-10b). These giant multinucleated cells undergo lysis and death within 48 h after their formation. Some evidence suggests that soluble gp120 alone may interact with CD4 membrane molecules to induce cell fusion leading to syncytia formation. In one study a recombinant vaccinia virus containing the gp120 gene was able to cause syncytia formation

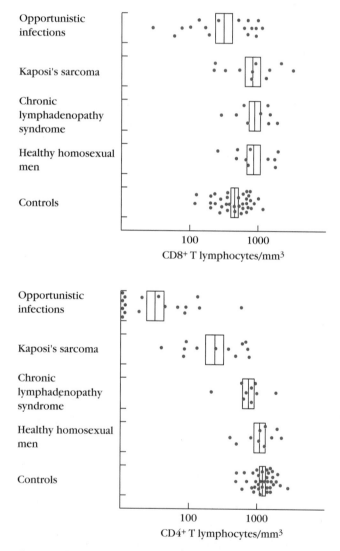

Figure 21-9 Quantitation of CD4 and CD8 T lymphocytes in normal controls and in clinical subpopulations of AIDS patients. [From H. C. Lane and A. S. Fauci. 1985. *Ann. Rev. Immunol.* **3**:477.]

(a)

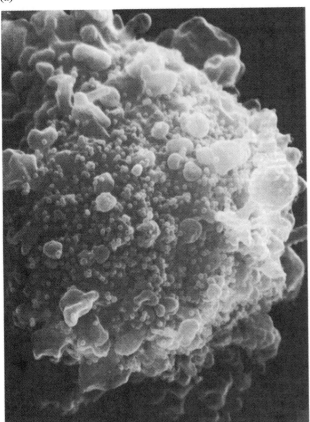

(b)

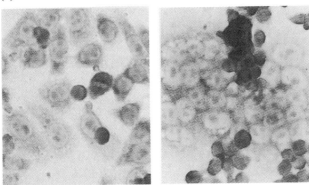

Figure 21-10 (a) Destruction of HIV-infected T cells can occur as HIV buds from the infected T cell. (b) Destruction of uninfected T cells can occur through syncytia formation caused by HIV. On the left HeLa cells lacking CD4 are exposed to HIV in culture. These cells cannot be infected and do not show syncytia formation. At right, CD4-transfected HeLa cells expressing CD4 are infected by HIV. Giant multinucleated syncytia are formed following HIV infection. [Part(a) photo courtesy of R. C. Gallo, 1988, *J. Acquired Immune Deficiency Syndromes* **1**:521–535; part(b) from J. N. Weber and R. A. Weiss, 1988, *Sci. Am.* (October):101.]

and subsequent cell death in a CD4$^+$ T-cell line in vitro. Taken together, these findings suggest that the fusion of activated HIV-infected CD4$^+$ T cells expressing gp120 with other, uninfected CD4$^+$ T cells may lead to the progressive depletion of CD4$^+$ T cells that is seen in AIDS patients. These findings also raise some concern about using gp120 (or a recombinant vaccinia virus carrying the gp120 gene) as a vaccine because the vaccine itself might induce syncytia formation. Not all researchers, however, think that syncytia formation is a primary cause of CD4$^+$ T-cell depletion in AIDS. Although syncytia formation has indeed been observed in the brain of some AIDS patients, the inability to detect widespread formation of syncytia in vivo has led some to suggest that the growth and lysis of these giant cells may be an in vitro phenomenon and bear little relevance to the disease process.

Several other hypotheses to account for depletion of uninfected CD4$^+$ T cells have focused on the large quantities of soluble gp120 in the blood and lymph of AIDS patients (Figure 21-11). The noncovalent interaction of gp120 and gp41 is unstable, allowing large quantities of free gp120 to be shed into the surrounding fluid. Because gp120 has a high affinity for CD4, it can bind to CD4 molecules on normal, uninfected CD4$^+$ T cells. Such binding might prevent antigen-mediated activation of T cells since CD4 plays a role both in stabilizing the interaction with an antigen-presenting cell and in transducing the activation signal (see Figure 10-9). Another possibility is that binding of soluble gp120 to CD4 membrane molecules may induce destruction of uninfected T cells by antibody + complement lysis or by antibody-dependent cell-mediated cytotoxicity. The density of CD4 molecules is considerably higher on CD4$^+$ T cells than on macrophages or other CD4-bearing cells. This difference may explain why the depletion of CD4$^+$ T cells can be extensive, while depletion of other CD4-bearing cells is much less, on which the density of CD4 is too low to induce antibody-mediated complement activation or antibody-dependent cell-mediated cytotoxicity.

The depletion of uninfected CD4$^+$ T cells seen in AIDS normally would stimulate T-cell maturation within the thymus to restore the peripheral CD4$^+$ T-cell numbers. It has been suggested that free gp120 interferes with T-cell maturation within the thymus by binding to CD4 on thymocytes, thus interfering with positive selection of class II MHC–restricted cells. In the experiments outlined in Figure 10-16a, antibody to class II MHC molecules selectively interfered with maturation of CD4$^+$ T cells. It is therefore possible that the binding of soluble gp120 to CD4 might interfere with the maturation process. Destruction of mature CD4$^+$ T cells in the periphery, coupled with a lack of replacement by developing

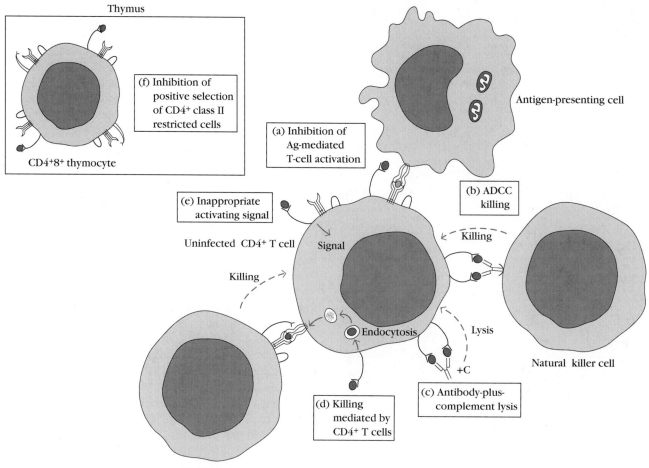

Figure 21-11 Possible mechanisms by which soluble gp120 may induce depletion of uninfected CD4$^+$ T cells. See text for discussion. C = complement.

thymocytes, could explain the progressive CD4$^+$ T-cell depletion seen in AIDS (Figure 21-11f).

Although CD8$^+$ T cells generally function as cytotoxic cells and CD4$^+$ T cells generally function as helper cells, the dichotomy is not absolute. As discussed in previous chapters, some CD8$^+$ T cells secrete lymphokines and appear to function in a helper capacity and some CD4$^+$ T cells have been shown to have cytotoxic activity. A recent experiment has suggested that in AIDS patients a CD4$^+$ T-cell subpopulation with cytotoxic activity may play a role in the destruction of uninfected CD4$^+$ T cells. In this study monocytes from a normal uninfected individual were cultured together with gp120, allowing the monocytes to endocytose, process, and present

gp120 peptides together with class II MHC molecules on their membrane. Normal lymphocytes from these same uninfected individuals were then added to the monocyte culture. A small number of T cells specific for the gp120 peptides presented by the monocytes were activated in the cell culture. These activated T cells were then isolated and cloned by a soft-agar technique. When one of these T-cell clones, which expressed CD4, was added to normal CD4$^+$ T cells in the presence of soluble gp120, the T-cell clone began to kill the normal uninfected T cells. Note that unlike most cytotoxic T cells, which are class I MHC restricted, this cytotoxic T cell bore the CD4 membrane molecule and was class II MHC restricted. Because antigen-activated human T cells express class II MHC molecules, some workers have speculated that binding of soluble gp120 to the CD4 molecule on activated uninfected T cells might result in receptor-mediated endocytosis of the gp120. The internalized gp120 might then be processed and presented together with class II MHC molecules on the cell membrane of uninfected CD4$^+$ T cells. Cytotoxic CD4$^+$ T cells specific for gp120 associated with class II MHC molecules could then selectively deplete these uninfected CD4$^+$ T cells (see Figure 21-11d).

M. S. Ascher and H. W. Sheppard have proposed another mechanism to account for depletion of uninfected CD4$^+$ T cells in AIDS patients. They suggest that binding of gp120 to CD4 may result in an inappropriate transmembrane activating signal, transduced by a particular tyrosine kinase known to be associated with the cytoplasmic tail of CD4 (see Figure 21-11e). According to this hypothesis, such inappropriate T-cell activation may prevent memory-cell formation, leading to eventual exhaustion of T memory cells and a gradual decrease of CD4$^+$ T cells. This hypothesis can account for some of the unusual findings seen in AIDS patients, such as the generalized level of nonspecific immune activation and the ensuing polyclonal B-cell activation, the spontaneous lymphocyte proliferation, and the increased autoimmune manifestations. In addition this model can account for the observed differences in the latency period in different individuals. A short latency would be expected in individuals having high antigen exposure because continual immune activation would be expected to hasten immune-cell depletion.

Immunologic Abnormalities in AIDS

The total collapse of the immune system in AIDS reflects the central role of CD4$^+$ T$_H$ cells in both humoral and cell-mediated responses and in the regulation of both responses. Some of the immunologic abnormalities seen in AIDS patients are listed in Table 21-5. One of the abnormalities that can be easily demonstrated is the reduced ability of T lymphocytes to proliferate in vitro in response to mitogens or soluble antigens. This is illustrated by the data in Table 21-6, which compares the in vitro proliferative response to pokeweed mitogen and tetanus toxoid of T lymphocytes from AIDS patients and normal controls. The researchers in this study wanted to know if the decrease observed with unfractionated T cells from AIDS patients reflected reduced numbers of T cells compared with controls or some inherent defect in the T cells. They therefore separated CD4$^+$ and CD8$^+$ T cells with an FACS, adjusted cell numbers so that comparable numbers of cells were present in the AIDS and control samples, and repeated

Table 21-5 Immunologic abnormalities associated with AIDS

Antibody production
Early: Enhanced IgG and IgA antibody-forming capacity but reduced IgM synthesis
Late: Immunoglobulin levels may still remain elevated but clonal proliferation of antigen-specific B cells does not occur

Delayed-type hypersensitivity
Early: Highly significant reduction in proliferative capacity. Reduction in DTH
Late: Elimination of proliferative capacity against soluble antigens and of DTH

Cytotoxic T cells
Early: Comparatively normal reactivity
Late: Reduction in activity but even at AIDS stage quite significant activity

the proliferation assays. The results with these adjusted samples showed that CD4$^+$ T cells from AIDS patients responded at near-normal levels to pokeweed mitogen; the low response to mitogen with the unfractionated cell sample thus reflected the smaller number of T cells in this sample compared with that of controls. On the other hand, the CD4$^+$ cells from AIDS patients, even when cell numbers were equalized, remained unable to respond to tetanus toxoid antigen.

This study demonstrates one of the earliest abnormalities seen in AIDS patients: the inability of T cells to proliferate in response to a specific antigen. The diminished T$_H$-cell response to antigen may result partly from the binding of gp120 to CD4 on T$_H$ cells. As discussed in Chapter 10, CD4 is essential for T$_H$-cell recognition of antigen, presumably because it stabilizes the TCR-antigen–MHC II complex. Given that monoclonal antibodies to CD4 can inhibit the T$_H$-cell response to antigen, it is not surprising that gp120 binding may have a similar inhibitory effect if it blocks the CD4 membrane molecule.

The pronounced decline in CD4$^+$ T cells in AIDS would be expected to impact significantly on the balance of lymphokines. Several findings suggest that an imbalance in expression of lymphokines or lymphokine receptors may contribute to the pathogenesis of AIDS. Elevated levels of IL-6, GM-CSF, and TNF-α have been reported in both serum and cerebrospinal fluid of AIDS

Table 21-6   Comparison of in vitro proliferative response of peripheral blood lymphocytes from AIDS patients and normal controls*

| | [³H] thymidine incorporated (cpm) | | | |
| | Pokeweed mitogen | | Tetanus toxoid | |
Cell sample†	AIDS	Control	AIDS	Control
Unfractionated	1,400 ± 800	10,800 ± 1,900	< 100	20,300 ± 6,400
CD4⁺ T cells	17,800 ± 2,600	19,600 ± 2,200	< 100	16,900 ± 1,200
CD8⁺ T cells	3,100 ± 515	4,400 ± 680	< 100	4,300 ± 600

* Lymphocytes were cultured in the presence of [³H] thymidine and either pokeweed mitogen or tetanus toxoid. At the end of a 5-day culture period, the amount of radioactivity (cpm) incorporated into cells was determined.

† Cell numbers in the unfractionated sample were not equalized and represent the cell counts in peripheral blood. After separation of CD4⁺ and CD8⁺ T cells, cell numbers in the AIDS and control samples were equalized.

SOURCE: Data from H. C. Lane and A. S. Fauci, 1985, *Annu. Rev. Immunol.* **3**:477.

patients, and HIV-infected macrophages and CD4⁺ T cells have been shown to express high levels of the receptor for TNF-α. In addition, in vitro studies suggest that certain lymphokines may contribute to the progression from latency to lytic infection. These studies have shown, for example, that TNF-α induces HIV expression in infected T cells and that TNF-α, IL-6, and GM-CSF induce HIV expression in infected monocytes (Table 21-7). TNF-α appears to induce production of nuclear-binding factors that bind to the viral LTR inducing transcription of HIV (see Figure 21-5). Abnormalities in the expression of IL-2 and the IL-2 receptor also occur in AIDS. As CD4⁺ T-cell numbers decline, there is a corresponding decline in the level of IL-2. In addition, HIV-infected T cells exhibit decreased expression of the high-affinity IL-2 receptor when stimulated in vitro with PHA compared with uninfected control cells. This decreased expression of the IL-2 receptor makes HIV-infected T cells less reactive to IL-2.

AIDS patients also show significant reductions in skin-test reactivity compared with uninfected controls, reflecting a decrease in T$_{DTH}$-cell function (Table 21-8). As discussed in Chapter 13, the delayed-type hypersensitive response is an important host-defense mechanism against intracellular pathogens such as *Pneumocystis carinii*, *Mycobacterium tuberculosis*, *Mycobacterium avium*, *Candida albicans*, *Histoplasma*, and *Cryptococcus*. Given the limited ability of AIDS patients to mount a DTH response, it is not surprising that they exhibit increased susceptibility to intracellular pathogens.

Table 21-7   Cytokine induction of HIV reverse transcriptase in HIV-infected monocytes

Cytokine	Reverse transcriptase activity (cpm/μl)
M-CSF	200
GM-CSF	950
IFN-γ	300
TGF-β	200
TNF-α	1200
IL-6	1250
IL-4	200
IL-3	200
IL-2	200
IL-1	200
Unstimulated	200

SOURCE: Data from A. S. Fauci, 1989, Cytokine induction of HIV expression, *Colloque Des Cent Gardes*, Marnes La Coquette, Paris, France.

Although the level of CD8$^+$ T$_C$ cells is near normal in AIDS patients, the ability to generate CTLs from T$_C$ cells, which requires IL-2 (see Figure 13-1), is impaired because of the reduced levels of IL-2. Therefore, despite the presence of adequate numbers of T$_C$ cells, AIDS patients have limited abilities to eliminate virus-infected cells and tumor cells. In one study, the cytolytic activity of CD8$^+$ T cells from AIDS patients infected with cytomegalovirus (CMV) and from CMV-infected controls was compared. In CML assays (see Figure 9-5b) with CMV-infected target cells, the T cells from the AIDS patients showed lower ability to kill CMV-infected target cells than did T cells from the controls. Moreover, because HIV antigens are not expressed on latently infected host cells, these cells are safe from CTL-mediated killing until activation of the provirus initiates expression of the viral antigens. IL-2 also stimulates the activation and proliferation of natural killer (NK) cells, which are important in nonspecific killing of tumor cells. Because of their reduced IL-2 levels, AIDS patients have diminished NK-cell activity; not surprisingly they commonly develop various types of tumors.

Many HIV-infected individuals can produce antibodies to various HIV gene products, including both envelope glycoproteins (gp160, gp41, and gp120) and core proteins (p55, p17, and p24). Unfortunately the presence of high titers of circulating antibody to HIV proteins in no way indicates protective immunity. One reason the antibody has so little effect seems to be frequent antigenic drift in HIV. Furthermore, the decline of CD4$^+$ T$_H$ cells in AIDS patients eventually affects the functioning of B cells in the humoral response. As AIDS progresses, patients are increasingly unable, for lack of T$_H$ cells, to mount a humoral antibody response to new antigens. The decline in antibody levels as AIDS progresses can be so pronounced that some patients screen as antibody-negative in the HIV ELISA test during advanced stages of the disease. Some studies have indicated that anti-HIV antibody may actually be detrimental because binding of antibody-HIV immune complexes to Fc receptors on macrophages and subsequent receptor-mediated endocytosis may lead to increased HIV infection of macrophages.

Several observations indicate that immune regulation is disturbed in AIDS patients, although the mechanisms underlying these disturbances are not entirely clear. For example, many AIDS patients exhibit various autoimmune manifestations including the presence of autoantibodies and immune complexes, a disease similar to systemic lupus erythematosus, glomerulonephritis, autoimmune thrombocytopenia purpura, and various skin disorders. These autoimmune symptoms may reflect a decline in T-cell–mediated immune suppression (see Chapter 17). In addition, a generalized loss of regulation in the humoral branch results in a nonspecific increase

Table 21-8 Skin-test reactivity to various test antigens in AIDS patients and normal controls

Antigen	No. responding/no. tested (%)	
	AIDS patients ($n = 20$)	Controls ($n = 10$)
Control	0	0
Tetanus	10	90
Diphtheria	5	80
Streptococcus	15	70
Tuberculosis	0	60
Candida	10	90
Trichophyton	0	80
Proteus	40	50

SOURCE: Data from H. C. Lane and A. S. Fauci, 1985, *Annu. Rev. Immunol.* **3**:477.

in immunoglobulins of the IgG and IgA classes, presumably because B cells are being activated in a nonspecific, unregulated way; the loss of specific T-cell–mediated suppression may be partly responsible. It is also possible that the presence of cytomegalovirus and Epstein-Barr virus in AIDS patients may be partly responsible, since these viruses are known to activate B cells nonspecifically.

Serological Profile of HIV Infection

Following HIV infection a sequence of serological events occur that can be used to diagnose HIV infection and to predict the progression from latency to lytic infection, culminating in an AIDS diagnosis (Figure 21-12). Following infection the virus appears to replicate actively and the viral core protein p24 can be detected in the serum by ELISA or RIA. The p24 antigen is detectable in the serum for only a few weeks following infection and then disappears as the antibody response (*seroconversion*) develops. In most cases the time between infection and seroconversion is 6 weeks, but in some individuals the lag period has lasted for more than 3 years.

At seroconversion IgM antibody to HIV antigens can be detected. Within a few weeks of seroconversion, antibody of the IgG class appears that is specific for many of the viral structural proteins including gp160, gp120, gp41, p24, and p17. The appearance of antibody to the

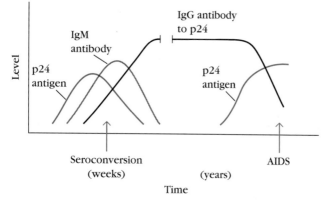

Figure 21-12   Serological profile of HIV infection.

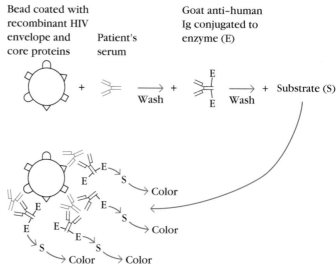

Figure 21-13   The ELISA test for HIV infection indicates the presence of serum anti-HIV antibodies.

p24 core protein is particulary useful as its presence correlates with viral latency. As the antibody to p24 begins to decline, there is a corresponding increase in the appearance of p24 antigen in the serum. The decline in antibody to p24 and increase in p24 antigen are associated with the progression from latency into lytic infection and have been used to clinically predict the onset of overt disease.

Screening Tests for HIV Infection

The standard screening test for HIV infection is an ELISA for serum antibody to HIV in which viral antigens are absorbed onto a solid phase (Figure 21-13). The patient's serum is added, unbound antibody is washed away, and then an enzyme-conjugated goat antihuman immunoglobulin reagent is added. After excess reagent is washed away, the substrate for the enzyme is added. A colored reaction product indicates that the patient has antibody to the HIV antigens and must therefore have been exposed to the virus. There is a lag period between the time of HIV infection and the appearance of enough antibody to be detected in the ELISA assay. Because of the lag period, potentially infectious individuals may screen negative for HIV infection. The importance of the lag period between HIV infection and seroconversion was demonstrated in 1991 by a news report of the transmission of HIV from an infected organ donor to a number of transplant recipients. In this case, the organ donor had been infected with HIV but had not yet seroconverted. Thus when an ELISA test was performed prior to organ transplantation, the donor screened as negative for HIV infection. The lag period is often referred to as a "window of opportunity" and is a time

when a HIV infected individual will screen as negative using an ELISA test for HIV-specific antibody. Also, as mentioned previously, AIDS patients often test negative for antibody in the late stages of the disease, when serum antibody levels drop as a result of depleted levels of T_H cells.

More sensitive and expensive tests, such as the Western blot and the polymerase chain reaction (PCR), are used to confirm HIV infection or to detect low-level infection. In a Western-blot assay, HIV proteins and glycoproteins are separated by electrophoresis and then transferred to a nitrocellulose membrane. The patient's serum is added to the nitrocellulose and allowed to react, and then a radiolabeled goat antihuman immunoglobulin reagent is added (see Figure 6-14). The presence of radioactive bands corresponding to the molecular weight of HIV antigens indicates the presence in the patient of antibody to HIV. In 1987 the CDC recommended that a positive HIV ELISA test should be confirmed by another ELISA and then by a positive Western blot. The polymerase chain reaction can be used to amplify a small number of proviral DNA copies isolated from a large amount of cellular DNA (see Figure 2-8). The PCR technique has made it possible to demonstrate HIV infection in a number of individuals who had tested negative by the ELISA and Western-blot assays.

Development of an AIDS Vaccine

The development of a vaccine requires knowledge of the infectious agent, characterization of the immune response to the agent, and determination of what type of immune response is protective. There are no shortcuts, and the development of most vaccines has been a long and arduous process. For example, the development and testing of the most recent hepatitis B vaccine took 17 years. Human clinical trials of a vaccine must be conducted according to guidelines set by the Food and Drug Administration (FDA). A vaccine is first tested in appropriate animals to determine whether it is safe. Three phases of human clinical trials are then conducted. Phase I and phase II human trials are intended to evaluate the safety, dosage, and immunogenicity of a vaccine preparation. Phase III trials are designed to determine the effectiveness of a vaccine.

The first human phase I clinical trial of an AIDS vaccine began in September 1987 when 81 volunteers were immunized with genetically engineered gp160. Phase II trials, with larger numbers of volunteers, attempt to extend the phase I findings on safety, dosage, and immunogenicity. Phase III trials require much larger numbers of volunteers so that the degree of vaccine protection afforded by the vaccine can be assessed by statistical measures. Because of the high mortality of HIV infection, the FDA has tried to shorten some aspects of the review process. All AIDS-related drug and vaccine treatments, for instance, have been given a special designation, 1-AA, that automatically moves them ahead in the review process.

Factors Hindering Vaccine Development

Despite the extensive efforts to develop an AIDS vaccine and the actions of the FDA to hasten testing and review, several properties of HIV itself hamper vaccine development. As discussed earlier, HIV is constantly mutating and changing its surface glycoproteins, allowing it to evade the immune response. Such antigenic shift, which occurs in several other viruses, including influenza, has hampered the development of an effective vaccine for influenza. In HIV the mutation rate is 65 times higher than it is in influenza. Clearly this property poses serious problems in developing a vaccine that is effective against myriad antigenically diverse strains. In addition, the HIV genome can integrate into the genome of host cells and lie dormant as a provirus for years. Throughout this latent stage, the virus presents no antigenic targets at all, either to induce an immune response or to be attacked by immune mechanisms induced by a vaccine.

A major problem in developing an AIDS vaccine has been the lack of a suitable animal model. The chimpanzee is the only natural animal model for HIV-1 infection; however, although HIV can produce a persistent infection in the chimpanzee, the infection does not lead to an immune deficiency (Table 21-9). Testing of a potential vaccine in chimpanzees must therefore focus on inhibition of viral replication rather than on the immunodeficiency manifestations. Moreover, use of chimpanzees for AIDS-vaccine testing poses an increasing

threat to the already dwindling chimpanzee population. The pharmaceutical industry has been pushing vigorously for the World Health Organization to relax restrictions on the importation of chimpanzees from Africa. The contention is that a shortage of captive chimpanzees (fewer than 600 in the United States) is impeding the development of vaccines for AIDS. Yet a 1988 paper in *Nature* from scientists in the United States, the Netherlands, Germany, and France highlights the threat of extinction to wild chimpanzees. The authors maintain that many chimpanzees of breeding age will be killed as attempts are made to capture infants for export; they estimate that 10 chimpanzees die for every infant that eventually reaches its overseas destination. Certainly these issues point to the need for proper management, sharing of research information among competing groups, and attention to priorities as vaccine trials go forward in chimpanzees in research laboratories around the world.

A more satisfactory animal model is available for HIV-2 infection: the macaque monkey. Not only can these monkeys be infected with HIV-2, but infected animals also develop symptoms of immunosuppression somewhat similar to AIDS. Macaque monkeys also are easier to work with and to breed than chimpanzees; however, concerns about species preservation also apply to them.

Development of SCID-human mice has given AIDS researchers some optimism in their search for a practical animal model. There are two distinct approaches to developing the SCID/hu mouse that have each proved useful. The approach developed by M. McCune, previously described in Figure 20-7, reconstitutes the immune sys-

Table 21-9 Infectivity and pathogenicity of HIV-1, HIV-2, and SIV_{AGM} in various animals

Virus	Animal	Infection	AIDS
HIV-1	Human	+	+
	Chimpanzee	+	−
	SCID-human mouse	+	?
HIV-2	Human	+	+
	Chimpanzee	+	−
	Macaque (rhesus) monkey	+	+
	Baboon	+	−
SIV_{AGM}	African green monkey	+	−
	Macaque (rhesus) monkey	+	+ (SAIDS)

tem of the SCID mouse with human fetal liver, mesenteric lymph node, and thymus. The other approach developed by D. Mosier reconstitutes the SCID mice with human peripheral blood mononuclear cells. In both systems the mice become populated with human T and B lymphocytes and with other white blood cells. When these SCID-human mice are challenged with HIV the human CD4$^+$ T cells and myeloid cells have been shown to become infected. Mosier has recently reported a significant depletion in the CD4$^+$ T cells of SCID-human mice within 8 weeks of HIV infection (Figure 21-14). Additionally, these mice have already proved to be valuable by allowing researchers to evaluate the efficacy of antiviral agents and vaccines in vivo. McCune reported with his system that azido-3'-deoxythymidine (AZT), the first therapeutic drug approved for AIDS patients, inhibits HIV infection in these mice. McCune's research group is presently using these mice to define therapeutic levels of AZT and dideoxyinosine (ddI) for use in humans. And a recent report by Mosier has shown that when SCID mice were reconstituted with peripheral blood cells from human volunteers that had been immunized with a recombinant vaccinia virus vaccine expressing gp160, the mice were protected from a later challenge with live HIV. Certainly the SCID-human mice provide a ray of hope for developing a workable animal model to study the mode of immune suppression in AIDS and for evaluating potential drug or vaccine therapies.

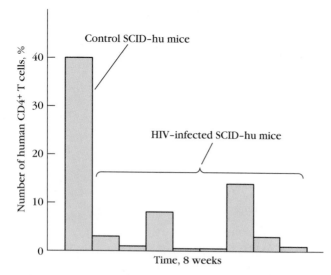

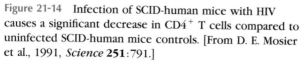

Figure 21-14   Infection of SCID-human mice with HIV causes a significant decrease in CD4$^+$ T cells compared to uninfected SCID-human mice controls. [From D. E. Mosier et al., 1991, *Science* **251**:791.]

Experimental AIDS Vaccines

Ever since HIV was identified as the causative agent of AIDS, tremendous effort has been directed toward the development of a safe and effective vaccine. Several types of vaccines have been designed, including whole inactivated virus, live recombinant viruses, recombinant DNA products, synthetic peptides, and anti-idiotype antibodies. At the VII International Conference on AIDS in Florence, Italy in the summer of 1991, it was reported that 13 vaccine trials in humans are currently underway.

Inactivated Whole Viruses

Inactivated preparations of HIV-1 have been produced by irradiating the virus and treating it with formaldehyde. This procedure, similar to that used to develop the Salk polio vaccine, inactivates the HIV genome and releases much of the gp120 from the envelope. SIV$_{AGM}$ has also been chemically inactivated with formaldehyde. The results of trials with these vaccines are summarized in Table 21-10.

In the two trials of inactivated SIV, macaque monkeys were immunized with the vaccine and then challenged with doses of live SIV considerably higher than the established minimum infectious dose. All the unvaccinated controls became infected and all developed SAIDS, whereas none of the vaccinated monkeys developed SAIDS during the trial period, although some of them became infected.

Inactivated HIV-1 has been tested in chimpanzees that were subsequently challenged with live HIV and in HIV-infected humans. In one trial, the vaccine was given to three chimpanzees, two of which were already infected with HIV. Following two booster injections with the vaccine, all three chimpanzees were given a large injection of live HIV. All three vaccinated chimps were shown to clear the HIV, and all three have remained free of virus. Although these animal trials with inactivated SIV and HIV are hopeful, it is important to keep in mind that the animals were vaccinated and subsequently challenged with the same strain of SIV or HIV. In light of the incredible mutation rate of HIV, it can not be inferred that this procedure will protect against an unrelated strain of the virus.

The inactivated-HIV vaccine was tested in 1988–1989 in clinical phase I trials on 19 HIV-infected humans who manifested early symptoms of AIDS; the objective was to boost their immune response to viral antigens. Of these 19 individuals, 7 showed an increase in their CD4$^+$ T-cell count following vaccination, and 6 of these 7 also showed an increase in cell-mediated immunity, demonstrated by skin testing. However, in 4 of the 19 vaccine recipients the level of CD4$^+$ T cells decreased following vaccination, as did the skin-test response. It is not known

Table 21-10 Trials with inactivated SIV$_{AGM}$ and HIV-1 vaccines

Date	Recipient (no.)	Inactivated vaccine	Challenge	Observations
June 1989	Macaques (6)	SIV	Live SIV	2/6 no detectable SIV 4/6 detectable SIV 6/6 no SAIDS/no deaths
	Macaques (4)—controls	None	Live SIV	4/4 SAIDS 3/4 died
Dec. 1989	Macaques (9)	SIV	Live SIV	8/9 no detectable SIV 8/9 no SAIDS
	Macaques (7)—controls	None	Live SIV	7/7 detectable SIV 7/7 SAIDS
June 1989	Chimpanzee (3)	HIV	Live HIV	3/3 no detectable HIV
1988–1989	HIV-infected humans (19)	HIV	None	7/19 increased CD4$^+$ T cells; of these, 6/7 increased skin-test response 4/19 decreased CD4$^+$ T cells; of these, 4/4 decreased skin-test response

why some individuals responded positively to the vaccine and others did not. In any case, the inactivated-vaccine approach is not without potential risks, as work with feline leukemia virus (FeLV), a retrovirus that causes leukemia in cats, has demonstrated. When cats were vaccinated with an irradiated and formaldehyde-treated preparation of FeLV, some of them actually developed enhanced susceptibility to infection compared with unvaccinated controls.

Cloned Envelope Glycoproteins

Several groups have applied gene-engineering techniques to clone the gp120 gene or the entire gp160 gene in order to produce large quantities of gp120 or gp160 for immunization. The first of the cloned gp160 vaccines, which was produced by MicroGeneSys Inc., was administered in September 1987 to 140 healthy seronegative volunteers. The vaccine induced humoral antibodies and activated T$_H$ cells. The humoral antibodies elicited in the volunteers were shown to inhibit viral replication in vitro, but the inhibition was always strain-specific—a result of the antigenic variation of gp160. A June 1990 report in *Nature* by P. Berman and colleagues of Genentech suggests that recombinant gp120 may prove to be an effective vaccine. They immunized two chimpanzees with recombinant gp160 and immunized two chimpanzees with recombinant gp120 and then challenged both groups of chimpanzees with live HIV-1. A control unimmunized group and the two animals immunized with gp160 became infected with

HIV-1 within 7 weeks of challenge. However, the two chimpanzees that were immunized with the recombinant gp120 were reported to show no signs of HIV infection, even by the very sensitive PCR technique, for more than 6 months. Vaccine trials in HIV-infected individuals using recombinant gp120 or gp160 are currently under way in several cities. One limitation with vaccines of this sort is that they are soluble proteins and therefore are processed as an exogenous antigen; thus, they are not very likely to induce a significant CD8$^+$ CTL response.

In order to induce CD8$^+$ CTLs specific for gp120 or gp160, it is necessary to introduce the antigen by a route that will favor antigen processing and presentation together with class I MHC molecules. Two types of vaccines discussed in Chapter 18 are being developed to accomplish this end (see Figure 18-5b). Gjp120-containing liposomes have been constructed which would fuse with cells, enabling the gp120 to be processed by an endogenous pathway. Gp120 also has been incorporated into immunostimulating complexes (ISCOMs), which are particles with a mean diameter of 35 nm that hold protein antigens in an adjuvant-containing micelle. ISCOMs can penetrate the plasma membrane and deliver the antigen to the cytoplasm where it would likely be processed as an endogenous antigen together with class I MHC molecules. One recent report described the sucessful induction of CD8$^+$ CTLs specific for gp120 using gp120-containing ISCOMs.

Presently there are several concerns about vaccines employing gp120 or gp160. One concern, mentioned already, is that gp120 itself might induce syncytia formation and thus increase T-cell depletion. Another concern is that a strong humoral-antibody response might increase the cellular spread of HIV infection through binding of antibody-HIV complexes to Fc receptors on macrophages. A third concern stems from the observation that gp160 shares amino acid sequences in common with certain class II MHC molecules. It is not known whether individuals possessing these class II MHC molecules might be at risk for developing some type of autoimmune reaction when immunized with gp160. Finally, the tremendous genetic variation in gp120 and gp160 among different HIV strains makes it unlikely that any one vaccine would provide protection against an unrelated HIV strain.

Recombinant Viruses Carrying HIV Genes

Recombinant vector vaccines are another approach that may prove useful in the search for an effective AIDS vaccine. Vaccinia virus and the Sabin polio virus are both live attenuated viruses that have proved to be safe and successful vaccines for smallpox and polio, respectively. Both of these viruses can be engineered to carry genes from HIV-1, and the recombinant virus can then be used as an HIV vaccine. Because the recombinant virus is attenuated (not inactivated), it is able to infect host cells and would therefore be expected to induce CTL activity. As with any attenuated vaccine, the prolonged exposure to the viral antigens tends to induce a very good immune response without the need of additional boosters.

Vaccinia virus, which is a large virus, can be engineered to carry several dozen foreign genes without impairing its capacity to infect host cells and to replicate in them. A genetically engineered vaccinia virus can be administered simply by dermal scratching; the virus causes a limited localized infection in host cells (see Figure 18-4). The foreign genes are expressed by the vaccinia, and if the foreign gene product is a viral envelope protein, it is inserted into the membrane of the infected host cell and there stimulates the development of T-cell–mediated immunity. Vaccinia virus carrying gp160 has been shown to infect host cells at the site of scarification; the gp160 is glycosylated, cleaved into gp120 and gp41, and inserted into the plasma membrane of the infected host cells. A number of HIV genes have been engineered into vaccinia virus, including *env, tat, pol,* and *gag.*

In experiments conducted by researchers at the Oncogen Corporation, chimpanzees were immunized with vaccinia virus carrying the gp120 gene. The vaccine induced production of protective antibodies to gp120 and sensitization of T_C cells. When the sensitized T_C cells from the immunized chimpanzees were tested in an in vitro CML reaction, they killed target cells infected with the recombinant vaccinia virus. These initial findings appeared hopeful, but unfortunately later clinical trials revealed that the immunized chimpanzees were not protected from infection with live HIV-1.

Trials of this same type of vaccine were being conducted by Daniel Zagury and co-workers of the Pasteur Institute. Healthy human volunteers (including Zagury himself) were immunized by scarification with recombinant vaccinia virus expressing the gp160 envelope glycoprotein. The primary response was weak, and the volunteers were subsequently boosted intramuscularly with their own cells, which had first been infected in vitro with the recombinant vaccinia virus. These individuals showed enhanced in vitro cell-mediated immunity to HIV following each booster immunization. Such an approach to large-scale clinical trials is limited logistically by the difficulty of immunization with autologous cells infected in vitro with recombinant vaccinia virus. Zagury's vaccinia-based HIV vaccine trials have been controversial. Among the issues raised was the degree of informed consent in the test trials on human subjects in Zaire without the prior approval of a Zairian or French human subjects ethics committee. Consequently, the French minister of health, Bruno Durieux, recently imposed a ban on these vaccine trials. In addition, the National Institutes of Health in the U.S. recently rescinded permission for Robert Gallo at the National Cancer Institute to collaborate with Zagury in these trials. Adding to the controversy was the finding that three recipients of the vaccine died from disseminated vaccinia infection. Although, vaccinia is a safe vaccine in healthy individuals, the attenuated virus can cause disseminated lesions in individuals with immune-system compromise. At the VII International Conference on AIDS in Florence, Zagury announced that he would discontinue the vaccinia vaccine trials. This case demonstrates the importance of ethical awareness in scientific research, particularly where the welfare of human subjects is involved.

Synthetic Crown-Sequence Peptides

The principal neutralizing epitope of HIV overlaps with the V3 loop of gp120 (see Figure 21-6), and antibodies to the V3 loop have been shown to protect chimpanzees from HIV infection. Because of the high level of variation in the V3 loop, antibody neutralization is always strain-specific. However, the so-called crown sequence in the V3 loop is conserved to a considerable degree (see Figure 21-8). Approximately 30% of North American HIV isolates have the crown sequence designated MN. Synthetic peptides of different HIV crown sequences, including the MN sequence, have been prepared and

483

tested for their ability to activate T-cell proliferation and cytotoxicity in vitro. These synthetic peptides appear to activate a population of T_H cells and to induce some cytotoxic activity; however, because these peptides are processed as exogenous antigens, the cytotoxic T cells induced were all $CD4^+$, class II restricted. These studies suggest that cocktails of synthetic peptides, representing the crown sequences of the predominant HIV isolates, might induce protective antibody or $CD4^+$ cytotoxic T cells.

Cloned CD4

A number of laboratories have cloned CD4 and used it as a vaccine in an effort to block HIV infection. Because gp120 binds to CD4 with such high affinity, the hope is that soluble CD4 may bind effectively to gp120 on HIV

and thus block viral binding to host cells (Figure 21-15a). In vitro studies have revealed that soluble cloned CD4 can indeed inhibit HIV binding and infection of T cells and can also inhibit syncytia formation. In a recent study four SIV-infected macaques were given daily intramuscular injections of 2 mg of soluble cloned CD4 for 50 days. Before the CD4 treatment, SIV could be isolated from peripheral-blood cultures or bone marrow cultures from all the infected monkeys. Within 2 weeks of the first CD4 injection, the virus could not be recovered from either peripheral-blood or bone-marrow cultures in three of the four monkeys. Cell cultures from these three monkeys remained free of SIV for 18–43 days after the CD4 injections were stopped. The one monkey that failed to show this effect had already shown severe T-cell depletion at the beginning of the study and died 3 days after the end of treatment; autopsy suggested

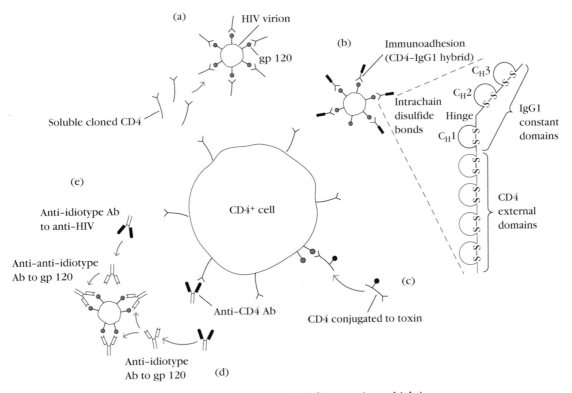

Figure 21-15 Various approaches for interfering with the gp120-CD4 interaction, which is necessary for HIV to infect $CD4^+$ target cells. (a) Injection of soluble cloned CD4, which can bind to gp120 on HIV virions. (b) Injection of an immunoadhesin formed from the constant region of IgG1 and the external domains of CD4. Like soluble CD4, this immunoadhesin binds to gp120, but its half-life in the blood is considerably longer than that of CD4. (c) Injection of soluble CD4 linked to a toxin. Binding of this reagent to viral gp120 on HIV-infected target cells leads to death of the cell. (d, e) Injection of anti-CD4 antibody (d) or of anti-idiotype antibody specific for the paratope on anti-HIV antibody (e) induces production of antibodies that bind to gp120 without exposing the individual to HIV or to HIV components.

that death was due to simian AIDS rather than to the CD4 treatment. Results with soluble cloned CD4 look hopeful, and phase 1 clinical trials in AIDS patients are now under way.

One of the problems with a soluble CD4 vaccine in humans is that CD4 has a half-life of only 30–120 min in serum, which necessitates frequent injections. D. J. Capon and colleagues reported overcoming this limitation in an ingenious way by linking the CD4 gene to the constant-region gene of human IgG1. The CD4-immunoglobulin hybrid encoded by this recombinant gene, called an *immunoadhesin*, exhibits the high-affinity binding of gp120 characteristic of CD4 but has the longer serum half-life characteristic of IgG1 (see Figure 21-15b). Initial animal studies with this immunoadhesin revealed that its half-life is 200-fold longer than that of soluble CD4; in humans the half-life of this immunoadhesin is expected to approach 21 days. It is also possible to engineer immunoadhesions with different immunoglobulin Fc regions to induce different effector functions such as opsonization or complement activation.

Another approach utilizing soluble CD4 that has been tried is to conjugate a toxin chemically to CD4. Any HIV-infected cell expressing gp120 on its membrane should bind the soluble CD4 toxin and be killed (see Figure 21-14c). It is hoped that alternating administration of soluble CD4, to bind the free virus and inhibit infection of additional T cells, followed by CD4-toxin, to kill HIV-infected cells, might prove effective.

Anti-Idiotype Antibodies

Anti-idiotype antibody specific for the antigen-binding site (the paratope) on anti-HIV antibody is an attractive vaccine approach, especially when undesirable or uncontrollable side effects might be induced with an attenuated or killed whole-pathogen vaccine. When anti-idiotype antibody specific for the paratope is administered, an animal makes antibody to the binding site on the anti-idiotype antibody, and this antibody (called anti-anti-idiotype antibody) will also bind to the original antigen (see Figure 14-5). In this way an animal can become immune to an antigen without having to see the antigen; it is exposed instead to anti-idiotype antibody. Kaprowski has produced anti-idiotype antibody to HIV antigens and then injected it into animals to produce anti-anti-idiotype antibody, which also binds to HIV antigens. The beauty of this scheme is that it avoids immunizing with the virus or viral components. Following the same principle, researchers have immunized animals with anti-CD4 monoclonals to generate an anti-idiotype response to the antibody. This induced anti-idiotype antibody blocks the CD4-binding site on HIV (see Figure 21-15d, e).

Summary

1.　HIV—an enveloped retrovirus containing ssRNA as its genome—is the causative agent for AIDS. The virus infects host cells when its envelope glycoprotein gp120 binds to CD4 molecules on cell membranes. Upon entry into a cell, the virus copies its RNA into DNA with a viral reverse transcriptase. The DNA can then integrate into the host chromosomal DNA forming a provirus, which can remain in a latent state for varying periods of time.

2.　Activation of an HIV-infected $CD4^+$ T cell also triggers activation of the provirus, resulting in transcription of the viral structural proteins and assembly of viral particles at the host cell's plasma membrane. Viral particles are released from the host cell by a process called budding, in which portions of the host-cell plasma membrane modified with viral glycoproteins become the viral envelope. Destruction of the host-cell plasma membrane in this process can lead to cell death.

3.　Destruction of $CD4^+$ T_H cells following HIV infection leads to severe immune-system depression, reflecting the necessary role of T_H cells in activation of B cells and T_C cells, delayed-type hypersensitivity, and IL-2–mediated activation of NK cells.

4.　Since less than 0.001% of the $CD4^+$ T cells in an HIV-infected individual are actually infected with the virus, the extensive depletion of T_H cells that is observed means that uninfected $CD4^+$ T_H cells also are destroyed. Several mechanisms have been proposed to account for destruction of uninfected T_H cells. One theory is that binding of soluble gp120 to CD4 on uninfected cells may lead to their destruction by antibody + complement lysis or antibody-dependent cell-mediated cytotoxicity. Another hypothesis speculates that soluble gp120 may induce an unusual population of $CD4^+$ T_C cells specific for gp120 peptides presented by class II MHC molecules on activated T_H cells. Still other hypotheses suggest that soluble gp120 may either block or enhance T_H-cell activation by binding to CD4 membrane molecules.

5.　Several approaches are being tried in the extensive effort to develop an effective AIDS vaccine. Experimental vaccines that have been developed and tested to some extent include the following: inactivated HIV, cloned envelope glycoproteins, recombinant vaccinia virus carrying HIV envelope-protein genes, synthetic peptides of the gp120 crown sequence, soluble CD4 and CD4-IgG1 hybrids (immunoadhesins), and anti-idiotype antibody specific for gp120 epitopes or the CD4-binding site on gp120. Development of an effective AIDS vaccine has been hampered by the extensive antigenic variation exhibited by HIV; the ability of HIV to exist as a provirus in host cells, where it is unaccessible to the immune system; and the lack of a good animal model for AIDS.

References

ASCHER, M. S.,and H. W. SHEPPARD. 1990. AIDS as immune system activation. *J. Acquired Immune Deficiency Syndromes* 3:177.

BOLOGNESI, D. P. 1990. Progress in vaccine development against SIV and HIV. *J. Acquired Immune Deficiency Syndromes* 3:390.

CAPON, D. J., S. M. CHAMOW, J. MORDENTI et al. 1989. Designing CD4 immunoadhesins for AIDS therapy. *Nature* 337:525.

CAPON, D. J., and R. H. R. WARD. 1991. The CD4-gp120 interaction and AIDS pathogenesis. *Annu. Rev. Immunol.* 9:649.

CENTERS FOR DISEASE CONTROL. 1990. HIV/AIDS surveillance report. April:1.

FAUCI, A. S. 1988. The human immunodeficiency virus: infectivity and mechanisms of pathogenesis. *Science* 239:617.

GALLO, R. C. 1990. Mechanism of disease induction by HIV. *J. Acquired Immune Deficiency Syndromes* 3:380.

GERMAINE, R. N. 1988. Antigen processing and CD4$^+$ T cell depletion in AIDS. *Cell* 54:441.

GREENE, W. C. 1991. The molecular biology of human immunodeficiency virus type I infection. *N Engl. J. Med.* 324:308.

KARON, J. M., T. J. DONDERO, and J. W. CURRAN. 1988. The projected incidence of AIDS and estimated prevalence of HIV infection in the United States. *J. Acquired Immune Deficiency Syndromes* 1:542.

LAURENCE, J. 1988. Vaccines and immunology overview. *AIDS* 2 (Suppl. 1):91.

McCUNE, J. M., et al. 1990. Suppression of HIV infection in AZT-treated SCID-hu mice. *Science* 247:564.

McCUNE, J. M., H. KANESHIMA, J. KROWKA et al. 1991. The SCID-hu mouse: A small animal model for HIV infection and pathogenesis. *Annu. Rev. Immunol.* 9:399.

MOSIER, D. E., R. J. GULIZIA, S. M. BAIRD et al. 1991. Human immunodeficiency virus infection of human-PBL-SCID mice. *Science* 251:791.

MURPHEY-CORB, M., et al. 1989. A formalin inactivated whole SIV vaccine confers protection in macaques. *Science* 246:1293.

NAMIKAWA, R., et al. 1988. Infection of the SCID-hu mouse by HIV-1. *Science* 242:1684.

PETERLIN, B. M., and P. A. LUCIW. 1988. Molecular biology of HIV. *AIDS 1988* 2:29–40 (supplement 1).

ROSENBERG, Z. F., and A. S. FAUCI. 1990. Immunopathogenic mechanisms of HIV infection: cytokine induction of HIV expression. *Immunol. Today* 11:176.

TILL, M. A., V. GHETIE, T. GREGORY et al. 1990. Immunoconjugates containing ricin A chain and either human anti-gp41

or CD4 kill H9 cells infected with different isolates of HIV but do not inhibit normal T or B cell function. *J. Acquired Immune Deficiency Syndromes* 3:609.

WEISS, R. A., P. R. CLAPHAM, M. O. MCCLURE et al. 1988. Human immunodeficiency viruses: neutralization and receptors. *J. Acquired Immune Deficiency Syndromes* 1:536.

WIGZELL, H. 1988. Immunopathogenesis of HIV infection. *J. Acquired Immune Deficiency Syndromes* 1:559.

Study Questions

1. Indicate whether each of the following statements is true or false. If you think a statement is false, explain why.

    a. HIV-1 and HIV-2 are more closely related to each other than to SIV.

    b. HIV-1 causes immune suppression in both humans and chimpanzees.

    c. SIV is endemic in the African green monkey.

    d. The *nef* gene of HIV appears to increase proviral transcription.

    e. T-cell activation increases transcription of the HIV proviral genome.

    f. HIV can only infect cells expressing CD4.

    g. Patients with advanced stages of AIDS always have detectable antibody to HIV.

    h. The polymerase chain reaction is a sensitive test that can be used to detect antibodies to HIV.

    i. Production of antibody to HIV sometimes increases the likelihood of HIV infection.

2. Soluble CD4 is currently being administered to AIDS patients. What is the rationale of this approach? What is a major limitation of this approach and what experimental procedures are being developed to overcome this limitation?

3. Would you expect to see much p17 and p24 in the blood of HIV-infected individuals in the asymptomatic latency period?

4. If p24 levels begin to increase dramatically in the blood of an HIV-infected individual, what would this indicate about HIV infection?

5. Why do clinicians monitor the level of skin-test reactivity in HIV-infected individuals? What change might you expect to see in skin-test reactivity with progression into AIDS?

6. What type of immune response would probably be induced by immunization with a recombinant vaccinia virus carrying the HIV gene encoding gp120?

Transplantation Immunology

Transplantation, as the term is used in immunology, refers to the act of transferring cells, tissues, or organs from one site to another. The surgical procedures for many kinds of transplantation were developed by the turn of the century. With the surgical technology in place, scientists began to ask whether organs or tissues might be transplanted from one individual to another. In the early 1900s a Viennese surgeon observed that he could surgically remove a kidney from an animal and then transplant it back into the same animal and restore kidney function. When the kidney was transplanted to a different animal, however, it soon ceased to function. Experimental transplantation between animals continued through the 1920s and 1930s;

however, every attempt was a dismal failure. Autopsies revealed massive infiltrations of white blood cells into the donated organ or tissue.

In the 1940s P. B. Medawar made several observations that convinced him that graft rejection was due to an immunologic response. While working with burn patients during World War II, he had noticed that grafts of skin from one site to another on the same patient were readily accepted, whereas grafts from relatives were rejected. In one patient a skin graft from a brother had been rejected; when a second graft from the same donor was attempted, the rejection occurred much faster and with much greater intensity. This observation led Medawar to experiment with animals and to discover that prior sensitization with donor cells led to heightened rejection of a subsequent graft. In 1945 he published a paper suggesting that graft rejection resulted from an immunologic response to the donor organ.

Medawar's suggestion proved to be correct. No matter how skilled the surgeon is, a surgically successful transplant can be thwarted by an immunologic attack. The very system that had evolved to recognize and destroy altered self-cells was simply performing its function by recognizing and destroying the foreign cells of the graft. The subdiscipline of transplantation immunology sought to understand the immunologic basis of graft rejection. Active experimentation sought to diminish immune-system activation and thus promote graft acceptance. Various immunosuppressive agents were developed to diminish the immunologic attack. Within just 10 years of Medawar's 1945 paper, the first kidney transplantation in humans was successfully performed. Today transplantations that once were widely publicized have become commonplace events. Transplantations of kidney, heart, lung, liver, bone marrow, and cornea are performed with ever-increasing frequency and success. This chapter describes the mechanisms underlying graft rejection and various procedures that are used to prolong graft survival.

The Immunologic Basis of Graft Rejection

The degree of immune response to a graft varies with the type of graft. Various terms are used to denote different types of transplants. *Autograft* refers to self-tissue transferred from one body site to another in the same individual. These grafts are often performed on patients with burns by transferring healthy skin to the burned area. *Isografts* are grafts between genetically identical individuals. In inbred strains of mice an isograft can be performed from one mouse to another syngeneic mouse. In humans an isograft can be performed between genetically identical (monozygotic) twins. Neither auto-

grafts nor isografts are usually rejected, owing to the genetic identity between graft and host. *Allografts* are grafts between genetically different members of the same species. In mice an allograft is performed by transferring tissue or an organ from one inbred strain to another. In humans most organ grafts from one individual to another are allografts, unless an identical twin is available as a donor. Because an allograft is genetically dissimilar to the host, it is often recognized as foreign by the immune system and is rejected in an allograft reaction. *Xenografts* are grafts between different species such as the graft of a baboon heart to a human. Obviously, xenografts exhibit the greatest genetic disparity and therefore engender the most vigorous graft rejection.

Rejection Displays Specificity and Memory

The time sequence of allograft rejection varies according to the tissue involved. In general, skin grafts are rejected faster than more vascularized tissues such as kidney or heart. Despite these time differences, the immune response culminating in graft rejection, always displays the attributes of specificity and memory. If an inbred mouse of strain A is grafted with skin from strain B, primary graft rejection—known as *first-set rejection*—takes place (Figure 22-1). As the reaction develops, the vascularized transplant becomes infiltrated with lymphocytes, monocytes, and other inflammatory cells; there is decreased vascularization of the transplanted tissue by 6–9 days, visible necrosis by 10 days, and complete rejection by 14 days. Immunologic memory is demonstrated when another strain B graft is transferred to the original strain A mouse. A graft-rejection reaction develops more quickly than after the first graft with complete rejection occurring within 5–6 days; this secondary response is designated *second-set rejection*. The specificity of second-set rejection can be demonstrated by grafting an unrelated strain C graft at the same time as the second strain B graft. Rejection of the strain C graft proceeds according to first-set rejection kinetics, whereas the strain B graft is rejected in an accelerated second-set fashion.

Role of Cell-Mediated Immunity

In the early 1950s A. Mitchison showed in adoptive-transfer experiments that lymphocytes, but not serum antibody, could transfer allograft immunity. Later studies began to implicate T cells in allograft rejection. For example, nude mice, which lack a thymus and conse-

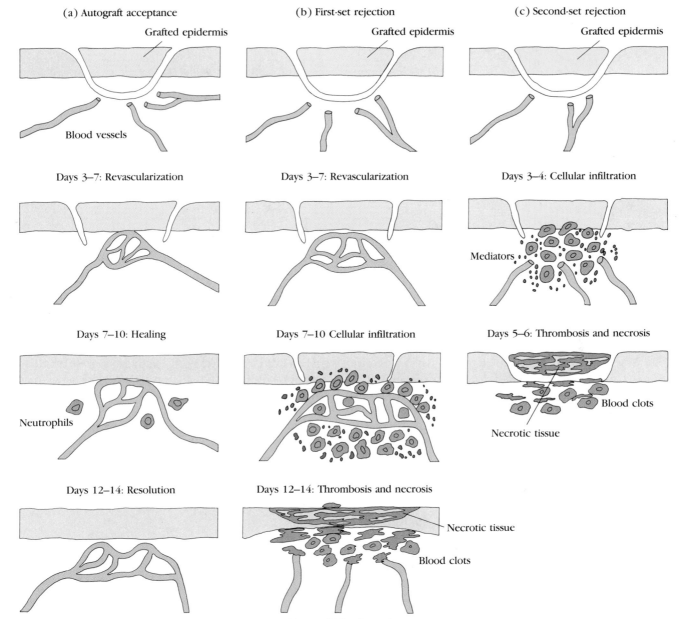

Figure 22-1 Schematic diagrams of the process of graft acceptance and rejection. (a) Acceptance of autograft is completed within 12–14 days. (b) First-set rejection of an allograft begins 7–10 days after grafting, with full rejection occurring by 12–14 days. (c) Second-set rejection of an allograft begins within 3–4 days, with full rejection by 5–6 days. The cellular infiltrate that invades an allograft contains lymphocytes, phagocytes, and other inflammatory cells.

quently lack functional T cells, were found to be incapable of allograft rejection; indeed these mice even accept xenografts (see Figure 20-6). In other studies, T cells derived from an allograft-primed mouse were shown to transfer second-set graft rejection to unprimed syngeneic recipients, as long as that recipient was grafted with the same allogeneic tissue (Figure 22-2).

Analysis of the T-cell subpopulations involved in allograft rejection has implicated both CD4+ and CD8+ populations. In one study the role of CD4+ and CD8+ T-cell subpopulations in rejection of skin allografts was analyzed by injecting the recipient mice with monoclonal antibodies to deplete one or both types of T cells and then measuring the rate of graft rejection. As shown

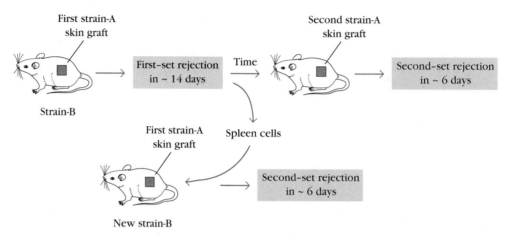

Figure 22-2   T cells derived from an allograft-primed mouse mediate second-set rejection of an allograft (from the same allogeneic strain) in an unprimed mouse.

in Figure 22-3, removal of the CD8$^+$ population alone had no effect on graft survival, and the graft was rejected at the same rate as in control mice (15 days). Removal of the CD4$^+$ T-cell population alone prolonged graft survival from 15 days to 30 days. However, removal of both the CD4$^+$ and the CD8$^+$ T cells resulted in long-term survival (up to 60 days) of the allografts. This study indicates that both CD4$^+$ and CD8$^+$ T-cell subpopulations participate in rejection and that the collaboration of both subsets results in more pronounced graft rejection.

Transplantation Antigens

Tissues that are antigenically similar are said to be *histocompatible*; such tissues do not induce an immunologic response that leads to tissue rejection. Tissues displaying significant antigenic differences are *histoincompatible*; such tissues induce an immune response leading to tissue rejection. The various antigens that determine histocompatibility are encoded by more than 40 different loci, but the loci responsible for the most vigorous allograft-rejection reactions are located within the major histocompatibility complex (MHC). The organization of the MHC—called the H-2 complex in mice and the HLA complex in humans—was described in Chapter 9 (see Figure 9-1). Because the MHC loci are closely linked, they are usually inherited as a complete set, called the haplotype, from each parent. Within an inbred strain of mice, all animals are homozygous at each MHC locus. When mice from two different inbred strains are mated, all the F$_1$ progeny inherit one haplotype from each parent (see Figure 9-2b); these F$_1$ offspring can accept grafts from either parent. MHC inheritance in

outbred populations is very different because the high polymorphism exhibited at each MHC locus gives a high probability of heterozygosity at most loci. In matings between outbred mice, there is only a 25% chance that any two offspring will inherit identical MHC haplotypes (see Figure 9-2c), unless the parents share one or more haplotypes in common. Therefore, for purposes of organ or bone marrow grafts, there is a 25% chance of identity within the MHC between siblings. With parent-to-child grafts, the donor and host will always have one haplotype in common but will be mismatched for the other haplotype.

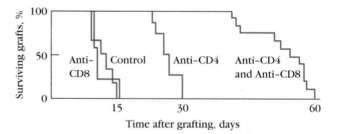

Figure 22-3   Experimental demonstration of the role of CD4$^+$ and CD8$^+$ T cells in allograft rejection in mice. Animals were treated with either anti-CD4 or anti-CD8 monoclonal antibody and then grafted with allogeneic skin; the rate of graft rejection was monitored and compared with that in untreated grafted controls. Removal of CD8$^+$ T cells alone had no effect on graft survival, whereas removal of CD4$^+$ T cells prolonged graft survival by about 15 days. However, removal of both T-cell populations resulted in much longer graft survival. [Adapted from S. P. Cobbold, G. Martin, and H. Waldmann, 1986, *Nature* **323**:165.]

Tissue identity at the MHC is not the sole factor determining tissue acceptance. When tissue is transplanted between genetically different individuals, even if their MHC antigens are identical, the transplanted tissue is likely to be rejected because of differences at various minor histocompatibility loci. Unlike the major histocompatibility antigens, which are recognized directly by T_H and T_C cells (see Chapter 10), minor histocompatibility antigens are recognized only when they are presented in the context of self-MHC molecules. In addition, the tissue rejection induced by minor histocompatibility differences is usually less vigorous than that induced by major histocompatibility differences. Still, reaction to these minor tissue differences often results in graft rejection. For this reason, transplantation even between HLA-identical individuals requires some degree of immune suppression.

Mechanisms Involved in Graft Rejection

Graft rejection is caused principally by a cell-mediated immune response to alloantigens (primarily MHC molecules) expressed on cells of the graft. Both delayed-type hypersensitive and cell-mediated cytotoxicity reactions have been implicated. The process of graft rejection can be divided into two stages: (1) a sensitization phase in which antigen-reactive lymphocytes of the recipient proliferate in response to alloantigens on the graft and (2) an effector stage in which immune destruction of the graft takes place.

Sensitization Stage

During the sensitization phase, $CD4^+$ and $CD8^+$ T cells recognize alloantigens expressed on cells of the foreign graft and proliferate in response. Both major and minor histocompatibility alloantigens can be recognized. In general the response to the minor histocompatibility antigens is weak, although the combined response to several minor differences can sometimes be quite vigorous. Foreign class I and class II MHC molecules are recognized directly by host $CD4^+$ or $CD8^+$ cells, presumably because they resemble self-MHC associated with antigen. Antigen-presenting cells that enter the graft can also endocytose the foreign alloantigens (both major and minor histocompatibility molecules) and present them as processed peptides together with self-MHC molecules.

Immunologic involvement varies with different types of transplants. When skin is grafted, for example, the graft at first does not contain functional blood vessels. Host lymphocytes, carried to the tissue by capillaries or lymphatics, encounter the foreign antigens of the skin graft and are carried by the afferent lymphatics to regional lymph nodes. Effector lymphocytes are generated in the regional nodes and are carried by the lymphatics back to the graft to mount an immunologic attack. In kidney or heart transplants the blood vasculature is immediately restored by suturing major blood vessels of the graft together with those of the host. Blood-borne lymphocytes encounter the alloantigens of the graft and are carried by blood vessels to the spleen or by the lymphatics to regional lymph nodes. Here, within the spleen or lymph nodes effector cells are generated and are then transported back to the graft by blood or lymph vessels.

A number of cell types, which vary depending upon the type of graft, have been shown to play an important role in presenting alloantigens to the host lymphocytes. In some organ and tissue grafts (e.g., grafts of kidney, thymus, and pancreatic islets), a population of donor cells called *passenger leukocytes* has been shown to migrate from the graft to the regional lymph nodes. Because passenger leukocytes express the allogeneic MHC antigens of the donor graft, they are recognized as foreign and therefore stimulate immune activation of T lymphocytes in the lymph node (Figure 22-4). These passenger leukocytes have been shown to be dendritic cells, which express high levels of class II MHC molecules (together with normal levels of class I MHC molecules) and are widespread in most mammalian tissues with the exception of the brain. In organ transplantations in which passenger leukocytes play a role in presenting alloantigens to the host immune system, depletion of these cells from the organ before grafting has been shown to prolong survival of the graft in an allogeneic host. One way of depleting the passenger leukocytes in a graft is to first transplant the graft into an immune-suppressed allogeneic animal and then later transplant it into a normal allogeneic recipient. While the graft is in the immune-suppressed animal, the passenger leukocytes migrate out of the graft. Now when the graft is placed in the normal allogeneic animal, the depleted passenger-leukocyte population will be less able to induce a rejection reaction. Another method of removing passenger leukocytes is to culture a graft in vitro prior to transplantation. In one study, removal of passenger leukocytes from rat pancreatic islet tissue by prior in vitro culture even enabled xenogeneic tissue to be accepted by some recipient mice!

Passenger leukocytes are not the only cells in a graft that can present alloantigens to the immune system. In fact, in skin grafts and some other grafts, passenger leukocytes do not seem to play any role at all. Other cell types that have been implicated in alloantigen presentation to the immune system include Langerhans, cells and endothelial cells lining the blood vessels. Both of these cell types express class I and class II MHC antigens.

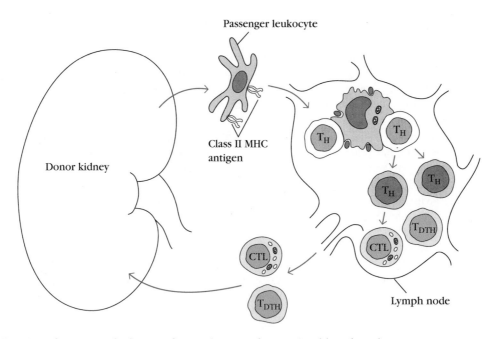

Figure 22-4   Migration of passenger leukocytes from a donor graft to regional lymph nodes of the recipient results in the activation of T_H cells in response to any different class II MHC antigens expressed by the passenger leukocytes. These activated T_H cells (gray) then induce generation of T_{DTH} cells and/or CTLs (red), both of which mediate graft rejection.

Recognition of the foreign alloantigens expressed on the cells of a graft induces vigorous T-cell proliferation in the host. This proliferation can be demonstrated in vitro in a mixed-lymphocyte reaction. Both dendritic cells and vascular endothelial cells from an allogeneic graft induce vigorous proliferation of host T cells in an MLR. The major proliferating cell is the CD4$^+$ T cell, which recognizes class II alloantigens directly or alloantigen peptides presented by host antigen-presenting cells (see Table 13-1). This amplified population of activated T_H cells is thought to play a central role in inducing the various effector mechanisms of allograft rejection.

Effector Stage

A variety of effector mechanisms participate in allograft rejection. The most common are cell-mediated reactions involving delayed-typed hypersensitivity and CTL-mediated cytotoxicity; less common mechanisms are antibody+complement lysis and destruction by antibody-dependent cell-mediated cytotoxicity (ADCC). The hallmark of graft rejection involving cell-mediated reactions is an influx of T lymphocytes and macrophages into the graft. Histologically, the infiltration in many cases resembles that seen during a delayed-type hypersensitive response in which lymphokines produced by T_{DTH} cells promote macrophage infiltration (see Figure

13-12). Recognition of foreign class I alloantigens on the graft by host T_C cells can lead to CTL-mediated killing (see Figure 13-5). In some cases graft rejection is mediated by CD4$^+$ T cells that function as class II MHC–restricted cytotoxic cells.

In each of these effector mechanisms, cytokines secreted by T_H cells play a central role (Figure 22-5). For example, IL-2, IFN-γ, and TNF-β have each been shown to be important mediators of graft rejection. IL-2 promotes T-cell proliferation and is necessary for the generation of effector CTLs (see Figure 13-4). IFN-γ is central to the development of a DTH response, promoting the influx of macrophages into the graft and their subsequent activation into more destructive cells. TNF-β has been shown to have direct cytotoxic activity on the cells of a graft. A number of cytokines promote graft rejection by inducing expression of class I or class II MHC molecules on graft cells. The interferons (α, β, and γ), TNF-β, and TNF-α all increase class I MHC expression, and IFN-γ increases class II MHC expression as well. During a graft rejection episode, these cytokines will increase, inducing a variety of cell types within the graft to express class I or class II MHC molecules. In rat cardiac allografts, for example, dendritic cells are initially the only cells that express class II MHC molecules, but as an allograft reaction begins, localized production of IFN-γ in the graft induces vascular endothelial cells and myocytes to begin to express class II MHC molecules as well.

Clinical Mainfestations of Graft Rejection

Graft rejection reactions have various time courses depending upon the type of tissue or organ grafted and the immune response involved. *Hyperacute* rejection reactions occur within the first 24 h after transplantation; *acute* rejection reactions usually begin in the first few weeks after transplantation; and *chronic* rejection reactions can occur from months to years after transplantation.

Hyperacute Rejection

In rare instances a transplant is rejected almost immediately—so quickly in fact that the grafted tissue never becomes vascularized. These hyperacute reactions are caused by pre-existing host serum antibodies specific for antigens of the graft. The antigen-antibody com-

plexes that form activate the complement system, resulting in an intense infiltration of neutrophils into the grafted tissue. The ensuing inflammatory reaction causes massive blood clots within the capillaries, preventing vascularization of the graft (Figure 22-6).

Several mechanisms can account for the presence of pre-existing antibodies specific for allogeneic MHC antigens. Recipients of repeated blood transfusions sometimes develop significant levels of antibodies to MHC antigens expressed on white blood cells present in the transfused blood. If some of these MHC antigens are the same as those on a subsequent graft, then the antibodies can react with the graft, inducing a hyperacute rejection reaction. With repeated pregnancies women are exposed to the paternal alloantigens of the fetus and may develop antibodies to these antigens. If a woman receives a graft expressing any of these same MHC antigens, again it is subject to a hyperacute rejection

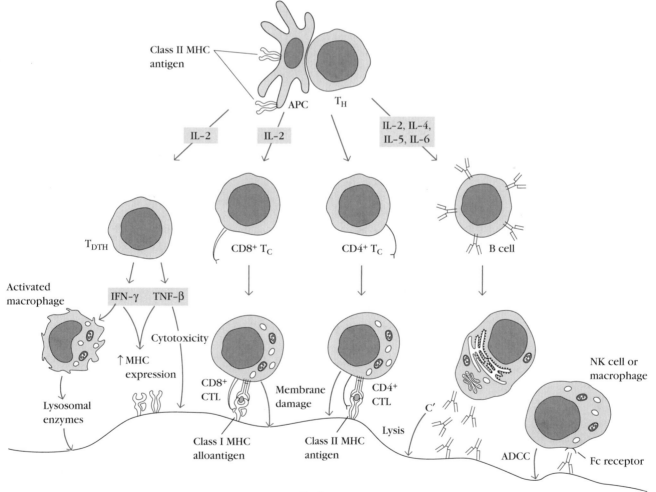

Figure 22-5 Effector mechanisms involved in allograft rejection. The generation or activity of the various effector cells (red) depends directly or indirectly on activated T_H cells (gray).

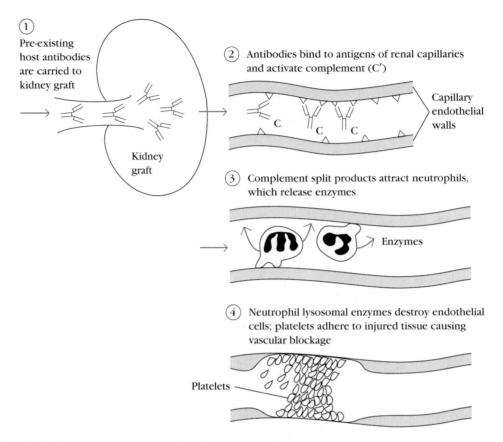

Figure 22-6   Steps in the hyperacute rejection of a kidney graft. In this type of rejection
reaction, the graft never becomes vascularized.

reaction. Finally, individuals who have had previous
grafts sometimes have high levels of antibodies to the
allogeneic MHC antigens of this graft; these antibodies
will mediate hyperacute rejection of any subsequent
graft that expresses some of the same allogeneic antigens. In some cases the pre-existing antibodies participating in hyperacute graft rejection may be specific for
blood-group antigens in the graft. If tissue typing and
ABO blood-group typing are performed prior to transplantation, these pre-existing antibodies can be detected
and grafts that would result in hyperacute rejection can
be avoided.

Acute Rejection

Allograft rejection that is cell-mediated manifests as an
acute rejection of the graft beginning about 10 days after
transplantation (see Figure 22-2). Histopathologic examination reveals a massive infiltration of macrophages
and lymphocytes at the site of tissue destruction, sugges-
tive of T_H-cell activation and proliferation. Acute graft
rejection is effected by the mechanisms described previously (see Figure 22-5).

Chronic Rejection

Chronic rejection reactions develop months or years
after the acute rejection reactions have subsided. The
mechanisms of chronic rejection include both humoral and cell-mediated responses. Chronic rejection
reactions are often difficult to manage with immunosuppressive drugs and may necessitate another
transplantation.

Tissue Typing

Since differences in blood-group and major histocompatibility antigens are responsible for the most intense
graft rejection reactions, various tissue-typing procedures have been developed to screen potential donor
and recipient cells and assess the likelihood of tissue
compatibility. Initially, donor and recipient are screened
for ABO blood-group compatibility by typing their RBC
antigens (see Figure 16-12). The A, B, and O antigens
are expressed on donor RBCs, epithelial cells, and endothelial cells. Antibodies produced in the recipient to
any of these antigens that are present on transplanted

tissue will induce antibody+complement lysis of the incompatible cells.

HLA typing of potential donors and a recipient can be accomplished with a microcytotoxicity test (Figure 22-7). In this test white blood cells from the potential donors and recipient are distributed into a separate series of wells on a microtiter plate, and then monoclonal antibodies specific for various class I and class II MHC alleles are added to different wells. After incubation, complement is added to the wells, and cytotoxicity is assessed by the uptake or exclusion of various dyes (e.g., trypan blue or eosin Y) by the cells. If the white blood cells express the MHC allele for which a particular monoclonal antibody is specific, then the cells will be lysed on addition of complement, and these dead cells will take up a dye such as trypan blue. HLA typing based on antibody-mediated microcytotoxicity can indicate the presence or absence of various MHC alleles. The results of such typing of a hypothetical family are shown in Table 22-1. In this example, only siblings 1 and 4 are fully HLA compatible.

Even when a fully HLA-compatible donor is not available, transplantation may be successful. For example, in Table 22-1, sibling 1 shares some HLA antigens with sibling 2 and with the father. In this situation, a one-way MLR can be used to assess quantitatively the degree of class II MHC compatibility between potential donors and a recipient (see Figure 9-6). Lymphocytes from a potential donor that have been treated with mitomycin C or x-irradiated serve as the stimulator cells, and lymphocytes from the recipient serve as responder cells. Proliferation is indicated by the uptake of [³H] thymidine. The greater the class II MHC differences between the donor and recipient cells, the more [³H] thymidine uptake will be observed in an MLR assay. Intense proliferation of the donor lymphocytes indicates a poor prognosis for graft survival. The advantage of the MLR over microcytotoxicity typing is that it gives a better indication of the degree of T_H-cell activation generated in response to the class II MHC antigens of the potential graft. The disadvantage of the MLR is that it takes about 6 days to run the assay. If the potential donor is a cadaver, for example, it is not possible to wait 6 days for the results of the MLR, and in that case the microcytotoxicity test must be relied on.

General Immunosuppressive Therapy

Allogeneic transplantation requires some degree of immunosuppression if the transplant is to survive. Most of the immunosuppressive treatments that have been developed have the disadvantage of being nonspecific; that is, they result in generalized immunosuppression, which places the recipient at increased risk for infection. In addition, many immunosuppressive measures are aimed at slowing the proliferation of activated lymphocytes. However, because any rapidly dividing nonimmune cells (e.g., epithelial cells of the gut or bone marrow hematopoietic stem cells) are also affected, serious or even life-threatening complications can occur.

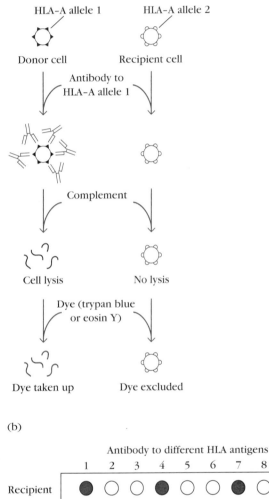

Figure 22-7 Microcytotoxicity HLA typing. (a) White blood cells from potential donors and the recipient are added to separate wells of a microtiter plate. The example depicts only one HLA antigen on donor and recipient cells and shows the reaction sequence on addition of antibody to one of these antigens. (b) Because cells express numerous HLA antigens, they are separately tested with a battery of monoclonal antibodies specific for various HLA antigens. Here, donor 1 shares antigens 1, 4, and 7 with the recipient, whereas donor 2 has no antigens in common with the recipient.

Table 22-1   HLA tissue typing of a hypothetical family based on microcytotoxicity testing with monoclonal antibodies to various HLA-A, -B, -C, and -DR allelic antigens

Family member	Allelic antigens at each locus														
	A				*B*				*C*			*DR*			
	1	2	3	9	5	7	8	12	1	2	4	1	2	3	7
Father	+	−	+	−	−	+	+	−	+	−	−	−	+	+	−
Mother	−	+	−	+	+	−	−	+	−	+	+	+	−	−	+
Sib 1	+	−	−	+	−	−	+	+	+	−	+	−	−	+	+
Sib 2	+	+	−	−	+	−	+	−	+	+	−	+	−	+	−
Sib 3	−	+	+	−	+	+	−	−	−	+	−	+	+	−	−
Sib 4	+	−	−	+	−	−	+	+	+	−	+	−	−	+	+

Family member	Inferred genotype								Haplotype designation
	A,	B,	C,	DR	A,	B,	C,	DR	
Father	A1,	B8,	C1,	D3	A3,	B7,	—,	D2	a/b
Mother	A2,	B5,	C2,	D1	A9,	B12,	C4,	D7	c/d
Sib 1	A1,	B8,	C1,	D3	A9,	B12,	C4,	D7	a/d
Sib 2	A1,	B8,	C1,	D3	A2,	B5,	C2,	D1	a/c
Sib 3	A3,	B7,	—,	D2	A2,	B5,	C2,	D1	b/c
Sib 4	A1,	B8,	C1,	D3	A9,	B12,	C4,	D7	a/d

SOURCE: Adapted from A. Svejgaard et al., 1979, *The HLA System. An Introductory Survey*, S. Karger, Basel, cited in W. E. Paul, 1984, *Fundamental Immunology*. Raven, Press.

Mitotic Inhibitors

Azathioprine (Imuran), a potent mitotic inhibitor, is often given just before and after transplantation to diminish T-cell proliferation in response to the alloantigens of the graft. Azathioprine acts on cells in the S phase of the cell cycle to block synthesis of inosinic acid, which is a precursor of the purines adenylic and guanylic acid. Both B-cell and T-cell proliferation is diminished in the presence of azathioprine. Functional immune assays such as the MLR, CML, and T$_{DTH}$reactions show a significant decline following azathioprine treatment, indicating an overall decrease in T-cell numbers.

Two other mitotic inhibitors that are sometimes used in conjunction with other immunosuppressive agents are cyclophosphamide and methotrexate. Cyclophosphamide is an alkylating agent that inserts into the DNA helix and becomes cross-linked, leading to disruption of the DNA chain. It is especially effective against rapidly dividing cells and therefore is sometimes given at the time of grafting to block proliferating T cells. Methotrexate acts as a folic acid antagonist to block purine biosynthesis.

Corticosteroids

The corticosteroids, which are cholesterol derivatives, include prednisone, prednisolone, and methylprednisolone. The lipophilic nature of these hormones enables them to cross the plasma membrane and bind to receptors in the cytosol; the receptor-corticosteroid complexes are subsequently transported to the nucleus where they bind to specific regulatory DNA sequences, either up-regulating or down-regulating transcription.

The corticosteroids are potent anti-inflammatory agents that exert their effects at many levels of the immune response. Corticosteroid treatment results in marked depletion of circulating lymphocytes due either to steroid-induced lymphocyte lysis (lympholysis) or to alterations in lymphocyte-circulation patterns resulting in a decrease in circulating lymphocytes. Some species, including the hamster, mouse, rat, and rabbit, are particularly sensitive to corticosteroid-induced lympholysis. In these animals corticosteroid treatment at dosages as low as $10^{-7} M$ causes such widespread lympholysis that the weight of the thymus is reduced by 90%; the spleen and lymph nodes also shrink visibly. Immature thymocytes in these species appear to be particularly sensitive to corticosteroid-mediated killing. It has been suggested that the corticosteroid-receptor complex may activate an endonuclease enzyme that induces DNA degradation. Mature thymocytes may lack this endonuclease enzyme and therefore may escape corticosteroid-induced lympholysis. In humans, guinea pigs, and monkeys, the corticosteroids do not induce lympholysis but rather affect lymphocyte-circulation patterns, causing a decrease in thymic weight and a marked decrease in the number of circulating lymphocytes.

Corticosteroids also reduce both the phagocytic and killing ability of macrophages and neutrophils, and this effect may contribute to their anti-inflammatory action. In addition, chemotaxis is reduced, so that fewer inflammatory cells are attracted to the site of T_H-cell activation. In the presence of corticosteroids class II MHC expression and IL-1 production by macrophages is dramatically reduced; such reductions would be expected to lead to corresponding reductions in T_H-cell activation. Corticosteroids also stabilize the lysosomal membrane, so that decreased levels of lysosomal enzymes are released at the site of inflammation.

Cyclosporin

Cyclosporin is a fungal metabolite that specifically suppresses antigen-activated T lymphocytes. Because cyclosporin has a somewhat selective mode of action, the drug has become a mainstay for immunosuppressive therapy in heart, liver, kidney, and bone marrow transplantation. Cyclosporin has been shown to block transcriptional activation of the T_H-cell genes encoding several lymphokines, including IL-2, IL-4, and IFN-γ. In addition, there is some evidence that it suppresses IL-2 receptor expression at various times in the cell cycle. Although the mechanism of cyclosporin action remains unknown, recent evidence suggests that cyclosporin may inhibit signal transduction from the T-cell receptor to the nucleus, thus preventing transcription of various lymphokine genes. T-cell activation involves several nuclear-binding proteins that bind to sequences in the lymphokine promoter regions. One of these proteins, called the nuclear factor of activated T cells (NFAT) binds to the IL-2 enhancer region and thereby promotes IL-2 transcription (see Chapter 10). In the presence of cyclosporin, transcriptional activation induced by NFAT binding to the IL-2 enhancer region is blocked. Reduced production of lymphokines, especially IL-2, diminishes T_H-cell proliferation and the activation of various effector populations involved in graft rejection, including T_{DTH} cells, CTLs, activated macrophages, and NK cells.

Cyclosporin prolongs graft survival in kidney, liver, heart, and heart-lung transplants. In one study of 209 kidney transplants from cadaver donors, the 1-year survival rate was 64% among recipients receiving other immunosuppressive treatments and 80% among those receiving cyclosporin. In liver transplantation, 6-month survival rates in one series climbed from 33% without cyclosporin to 76% with cyclosporin (Figure 22-8). Despite these impressive results, cyclosporin does have some negative side effects, the most notable of which is its toxicity to the kidneys. Acute nephrotoxicity is quite common, in some cases progressing to chronic nephrotoxicity and drug-induced kidney failure.

Total Lymphoid Irradiation

Because lymphocytes are extremely sensitive to x-rays, x-irradiation can be used to eliminate recipient lymphocytes before grafting. In total lymphoid x-irradiation the recipient receives multiple x-ray exposures to the thymus, spleen, and lymph nodes and then receives the

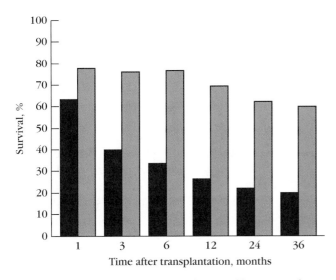

Figure 22-8 Comparison of survival rates of liver transplants in 84 patients who were immunosuppressed with azathioprine and corticosteroids (black) and in 55 patients who were immunosuppressed with cyclosporin and corticosteroids (red). [Adapted from S. M. Sabesin and J. W. Williams, 1987, *Hosp. Pract.* July 15, p. 75.]

transplant. The typical protocol involves daily x-irradiation treatments of about 200 rads per day for several weeks until a total of 3400 rads has been administered. The recipient is grafted in this immune-suppressed state. Because the bone marrow is not x-irradiated, lymphoid stem cells proliferate and renew the population of recirculating lymphocytes. These newly formed lymphocytes appear to be more tolerant to the antigens of the graft.

Antilymphocyte Serum

Antilymphocyte serum can be prepared by immunizing an animal with allogeneic or xenogeneic thymocytes, spleen cells, lymph-node cells, or thoracic-duct lymphocytes. For transplantation in humans, antilymphocyte serum is often prepared by immunizing a horse or a rabbit with human lymphocytes. The injection of antilymphocyte serum at the time of grafting results in decreased levels of circulating lymphocytes (lymphocytopenia) and in decreased cell-mediated immunity; it has variable effects on humoral immunity. The lymphocyte depletion does not appear to be caused by antibody-+-complement lysis; it may be that antibody coats the lymphocytes and acts as an opsonin, promoting phagocytosis of antibody-coated cells mediated by Fc receptors on phagocytes (see Figure 15-11a).

In experimental animals antilymphocyte serum has been shown to prolong kidney, liver, and cardiac allografts. In human transplantation the serum is always given along with other immunosuppressive drugs, and so it has been difficult to determine its individual effectiveness. Further, it is difficult to predict the effectiveness of a particular serum batch, perhaps because of variation in the concentrations of antibodies specific for one or another lymphocyte membrane molecule or variation in the major antibody isotypes. Some antilymphocyte sera may be quite effective at lymphocyte depletion, and others may be quite poor. Finally, a major drawback to the use of horse or rabbit antilymphocyte serum in humans is that it may induce a potent antibody response in the recipient to the antigenic determinants of the foreign antiserum that can result in serum sickness or anaphylactic shock.

Monoclonal Antibody Therapy

The major limitation with each of the immunosuppressive treatments discussed thus far is that they lack specificity and therefore result in more-or-less generalized immunosuppression and increase the recipient's risk for infection. Ideally what is needed is an antigen-specific immunosuppressant that will reduce the immune response to the alloantigens of the graft while preserving the response to unrelated antigens. Monoclonal antibodies have the potential of serving as such specific immunosuppressive agents, although the needed techniques are still in their infancy. So far, monoclonal antibodies have been successfully used to suppress T-cell activity in general or the activity of broad subpopulations of T cells. The technology has not yet advanced to the point of using monoclonal antibodies to suppress only alloantigen-activated T cells, but animal models suggest that monoclonal antibodies are the immune suppressors of the future.

Monoclonal antibody to the CD3 molecule of the T-cell-receptor complex has been shown in some cases to block T-cell activation. Injection of such monoclonal antibodies results in a rapid depletion of T cells from the circulation. This depletion appears to be caused by binding of antibody-coated T cells to Fc receptors on phagocytic cells, which then phagocytose and clear the T cells from the circulation. The success of anti-CD3 monoclonal antibody in reversing rejection episodes in animal models has led to its approval by the Food and Drug Administration for clinical trials where it has been shown, in some cases, to reverse acute rejection.

Monoclonal antibodies specific for the IL-2 receptor (anti-TAC) have been used successfully to increase graft survival. Since the IL-2 receptor is expressed only by activated T cells, exposure to the anti-TAC monoclonal antibody following grafting should specifically block proliferation of T cells activated in response to the alloantigens of the graft. In one experiment, treatment of mice and rats with an anti-TAC monoclonal antibody markedly increased the acceptance of cardiac and kidney transplants from allogeneic donors (Table 22-2).

Both CD3 and IL-2 receptor are expressed on all activated T cells. Monoclonal antibodies specific for membrane molecules that are present only on particular T-cell subpopulations also have been developed. For example, monoclonal antibody to CD4 has been shown to prolong graft survival. In one study, monkeys were given a single large dose of anti-CD4 just before they received a kidney transplant. Graft survival in the anti-CD4–treated animals was markedly increased compared with that in untreated control animals. Interestingly, the anti-CD4 did not reduce the CD4$^+$ T-cell count but instead appeared to induce the T cells to enter an immunosuppressed state.

Monoclonal antibody therapy, which usually is employed to deplete or inactivate T cells in graft recipients, also has been used to treat bone marrow before it is transplanted. Such treatment is designed to deplete the immunocompetent T cells in the bone marrow transplant, which can cause graft-versus-host disease, as discussed in the next section. The effectiveness of an anti-T-cell monoclonal antibody in reducing T-cell populations can be maximized by selecting monoclonal

Table 22-2 Effect of treatment with anti-TAC monoclonal antibody* on survival of cardiac allografts in rats

Anti-TAC dose (μg/kg/day)	Treatment period (days after grafting)	Mean graft survival in days (range)
—	—	8 (4–9)
25	0–9	13 (12–14)
100	0–9	14 (13–16)
300	0–9	20 (20–21)
300	5–9	17 (15–26)
300	5–9/15–19	27 (26–28)

* Anti-TAC binds to the IL-2 receptor.

SOURCE: Data from J. W. Kupiec-Weglinski et al., 1986, *Proc. Nat'l, Acad. Sci. USA.*

antibody isotypes that are good activators of the complement system.

One difficulty with monoclonal antibody intervention in the prolonging of graft survival is that the antibodies are generally of mouse origin. The recipient often develops an antibody response to the mouse monoclonal antibody, rapidly clearing it from the body. To avoid this limitation, human monoclonal antibodies and mouse/human chimeric antibodies (see Chapter 7) are being evaluated in experimental trials.

Because cytokines appear to play an important role in allograft rejection, another strategy to prolong graft survival is to inject animals with monoclonal antibodies specific for the implicated cytokines, particularly TNF-α, IFN-γ, and IL-2. Monoclonal antibodies to TNF-α have been shown to prolong bone marrow transplants in mice and to reduce the incidence of graft-versus-host disease. Monoclonal antibodies to IFN-γ and to IL-2 are each reported in some cases to prolong cardiac transplants in rats. Anti-cytokine antibodies have not yet been used in human transplantations.

Clinical Transplantation

The clinical results of transplantation of various cells, tissues, and organs in humans have improved considerably in the past few years, largely because of the use of immunosuppressive agents such as cyclosporin. Nowadays, kidney and corneal transplantations are performed with high success rates; heart, lung, and liver

transplantations are accomplished with somewhat lower, but still promising, success rates. In contrast, transplantations of bone marrow and pancreas exhibit even lower rates of success and are performed as a last resort only after other treatment possibilities have been exhausted.

Bone Marrow Transplants

In the past decade bone marrow transplantation has been increasingly adopted as a therapy for a number of malignant and nonmalignant hematologic diseases, including leukemia, lymphoma, aplastic anemia, thalassemia major, and immunodeficiency diseases in general. In 1990, over 4000 allogenic bone marrow transplantations were performed. The bone marrow, which is obtained from a donor by multiple needle aspirations, consists of erythroid, myeloid, monocytoid, megakaryocytic, and lymphocytic lineages. The graft, which usually consists of about 10^9 cells per kilogram of host body weight, is injected intravenously into the recipient. The first successful bone marrow transplantations were performed between identical twins. However, development of the tissue-typing procedures described earlier now makes it possible to identify allogeneic donors with identical or near-identical HLA antigens as the recipients.

Graft-Versus-Host Disease

In the usual procedure, the recipient of a bone marrow transplant is immunologically suppressed before grafting. Leukemia patients, for example, are often treated with cyclophosphamide and total-body irradiation to kill all cancerous cells. The immune-suppressed state of the recipient makes graft rejection rare; however, because the donor bone marrow contains immunocompetent cells, the graft may reject the host, causing *graft-versus-host disease* (*GVHD*). This is quite common in bone marrow transplantation, affecting between 50 and 70% of transplant patients. Graft-versus-host disease develops as donor T cells recognize alloantigens on the host cells. The activation and proliferation of these T cells and the subsequent production of cytokines generate inflammatory reactions in the skin, gastrointestinal tract, and liver. If it is severe, GVHD can result in generalized erythroderma of the skin, gastrointestinal hemorrhage, and liver failure.

GVHD involves both an afferent phase and an efferent phase. In the afferent phase, T_H cells from the donor bone marrow recognize recipient peptide-MHC complexes displayed on antigen-presenting cells. Antigen presentation, together with IL-1 induces T_H activation, production of IL-2, and proliferation. Cytokines elaborated by the T_H cell induce the effector phase of GVHD by activating a variety of secondary effector cells including

NK cells, CTL, and macrophages. The CTL cell may act directly to cause tissue damage in GVHD. However, cytokines such as TNF may play an even more important role in the effector phase of GVHD. TNF is released by a variety of cells including T_H cells, CTL, NK cells and macrophages. TNF has been shown to mediate direct cytolytic damage to cells. The role that TNF plays in GVHD in mice can be demonstrated by the ability of monoclonal antibody to TNF to block the development of GVHD following bone marrow transplantation in mice.

Various treatments are administered to prevent GVHD in bone marrow transplantation. The transplant recipient is usually placed on a regimen of immunosuppressive drugs, which often include cyclosporin and methotrexate. Another approach has been to deplete T cells from the donor bone marrow before transplantation with anti-T-cell antisera or monoclonal antibodies specific for T cells. Complete T-cell depletion from donor bone marrow, however, makes it more likely that the marrow will be rejected, and so the usual procedure is now a partial T-cell depletion. Apparently a low level of donor T-cell activity, which results in a low-level GVHD, is actually beneficial because it prevents any residual host T cells from becoming sensitized to the graft. In leukemia patients low-level GVHD also seems to result in destruction of leukemic cells, thus making it less likely for the leukemia to recur.

Organ Transplants

The impact of basic scientific research on clinical medicine is highlighted by the success rates for organ transplantation. In the case of kidney transplants, the early survival rate in 1967 was 45%; it has now been improved to about 90%. Currently more than 10,000 kidney transplantations are performed every year in the United States. Heart, heart-lung, and liver transplantations are also being done with remarkable success (Table 22-3). A number of other experimental transplantations (e.g., of the pancreas and parts of the intestine) have been performed but have not yet attained a level of success that warrants widespread application.

Several factors have contributed to the increase in successful organ transplants, most notably HLA typing and immunosuppressive treatments. Comparisons of HLA antigen differences and graft survival have shown that matching of the class II D antigens is most important for success. The data in Figure 22-9, for example, reveal that survival of kidney grafts depends primarily on donor-recipient matching of the HLA-D antigens; matching or mismatching of the class I HLA-A and HLA-B antigens has little effect on graft survival unless there is mismatching of the D antigens. In heart transplants, due to a shortage of transplantable organs and insufficient time, it is not possible to match HLA antigens prior to grafting. In order to assess the effect that differences in HLA antigens have on heart-transplant success, a number of studies have compared HLA antigen differences to graft-recipient survival rates. In one study of heart-transplant recipients, the 1000-day survival rate of the recipients was 90% when there was a single mismatch in HLA-DR antigens between the donor and recipient; the survival rate dropped to 65% when two HLA-DR antigens were mismatched.

An important finding that has emerged from experimental transplant models is that the critical period for graft rejection is from 2 to 4 weeks after grafting. If immunosuppressive drugs or monoclonal antibody therapy can prevent graft rejection during this critical period when acute graft rejection would normally occur, then the prognosis for long-term graft survival improves dramatically. A number of reasons have been suggested for the decrease in immunogenicity shown by grafts that survive the critical period. One suggestion is that passenger leukocytes leave the graft, home to draining lymph nodes, and induce immune activation soon after grafting. If immune activation is decreased with immunosuppressive drugs or monoclonal antibodies until these allogeneic leukocytes die off, the potential for immune activation will dramatically decrease. There is also some speculation that, with time, continual alloantigen expression by the graft may induce a state of immunologic tolerance.

Transplantation of human pancreatic islet cells has been shown to reverse insulin-dependent diabetes mellitus, which is caused by degeneration of the insulin-producing islet cells of the pancreas. In the past, however, islet-cell allografts have often been rejected, even when the recipient is given potent immunosuppressive therapy. In an attempt to find a way to reduce rejection of islet-cell grafts, A. M. Posselt, A. Naji, and their col-

Table 22-3 Survival rates for organ allografts in humans

Organ allograft	1-Year survival rate (%)
Kidney (sibling)	90
Kidney (cadaver)	80
Heart	80
Heart-lung	74
Liver	70
Pancreas	40

SOURCE: J. R. Batchelor and Y. L. Chai, 1986, *Prog. Immunol.* 6:1002.

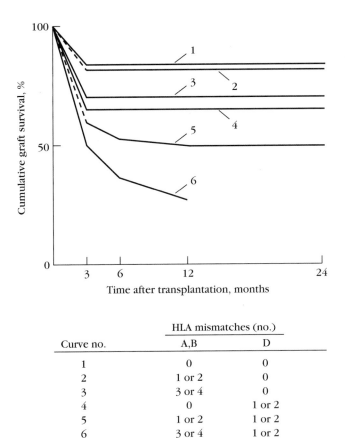

Figure 22-9 The effect of HLA-A, -B and -D antigen matching on survival of kidney grafts. Mismatching of HLA-A or HLA-B antigens has little effect on graft survival unless HLA-D is also mismatched. [Adapted from T. Moen, et al., 1980, *N. Eng. J. Med.* **303**:850.]

| | HLA mismatches (no.) | |
Curve no.	A,B	D
1	0	0
2	1 or 2	0
3	3 or 4	0
4	0	1 or 2
5	1 or 2	1 or 2
6	3 or 4	1 or 2

leagues injected rat pancreatic islet cells directly into the thymus of an allogeneic diabetic recipient rat. They found that the allogeneic islet cells survived indefinitely in the recipient, suggesting that the presence of alloantigens in the thymus induced the host's developing thymocytes to become tolerant to the alloantigens on the islet cells. This novel approach, reported in 1990, may well be applicable to other types of transplants and offers the promise of significantly improving graft survival rates without compromising the recipient's immune system.

Transplants to Immunologically Privileged Sites

There are certain sites in the body, called *immunologically privileged sites*, where an allograft can be placed without engendering a rejection reaction. These sites include the anterior chamber of the eye, the cornea, the cheek pouch of the Syrian hamster, the testes, and the brain. Each of these sites is characterized by an absence of lymphatic vessels and sometimes an absence of blood vessels as well. Consequently, the alloantigens of the graft are not generally able to sensitize the recipient's lymphocytes, and the graft shows an increased likelihood of acceptance, even when HLA antigens are not matched.

The privileged location of the cornea has allowed cornea transplants to be highly successful. The brain is another immunologically privileged site because the blood-brain barrier prevents the entry and exit of many molecules into or out of the brain. Transplantations of fetal brain-stem neurons into primates has been shown to reduce the symptoms of Parkinson's disease, and recently human fetal neurons have been transplanted into several patients with Parkinson's disease. The successful transplantation of allogeneic pancreatic islet cells into the thymus, discussed in the preceding section, has led to the speculation that the thymus may also be an immunologically privileged site.

Summary

1. Graft rejection is an immunologic response displaying the attributes of specificity, memory, and self/nonself recognition. The reaction generally involves the cell-mediated branch of the immune system with tissue damage mediated by T_{DTH} cells and/or CTLs.

2. The immune response is generated to differences in tissue antigens on the transplanted tissue. Although more than 40 different loci encode these antigen differences, the loci responsible for the most vigorous graft-rejection reactions are contained within the major histocompatibility complex (MHC), called the HLA complex in humans. Even when a donor and recipient have identical HLA antigens, differences in minor histocompatibility loci outside the MHC can also contribute to graft rejection.

3. The process of graft rejection can be divided into a sensitization stage and an effector stage. During the sensitization stage, passenger leukocytes, derived from the donor graft, migrate from the graft to the regional lymph nodes, where they are recognized as foreign by immune T cells, stimulating T-cell proliferation. Following T-cell proliferation, a population of effector cells is generated, which migrates to the graft and mediates graft rejection.

4. The degree to which a recipient and potential graft donors are matched for MHC antigens can be assessed by tissue typing. In the microcytotoxicity test, monoclonal antibodies are used to detect the presence of various class I and class II MHC antigens on donor and recipient cells. The more MHC antigens that a donor and recipient have in common, the more likely is a graft to survive. The mixed-lymphocyte reaction (MLR) can be used to quantitatively assess the class II MHC compatibility of a recipient and potential donors. In an MLR assay, donor and recipient lymphocytes are incubated together in the presence of [^{3}H] thymidine; the uptake of the labeled thymidine is directly related to T_H-cell proliferation. The closer the MHC match, the less proliferation occurs.

5. Graft rejection can be suppressed by specific and nonspecific immunosuppressive agents. Nonspecific agents include purine analogs, corticosteroids, cyclosporin A, total lymphoid x-irradiation, and antilymphocyte serum. Experimental approaches using monoclonal antibodies offer the possibility of specific immunosuppression. These approaches include blocking proliferation of antigen-activated T cells with monoclonal antibodies to the IL-2 receptor or depletion of T-cell populations with monoclonal antibodies to CD3 or CD4.

6. A major complication in bone marrow transplantation is a graft-versus-host reaction mediated by the lymphocytes contained within the donor marrow. T-cell depletion from the donor marrow with antibody specific for T-cell populations reduces the risk of graft-versus-host disease. Transplantations of a variety of organs are being performed with remarkable success. HLA typing together with immunosuppressive therapy have contributed to the high success rate for organ transplants.

References

AUCHINCLOSS, H., and H. J. WINN. 1989. Murine CD8$^+$ T cell helper function is particularly sensitive to cyclosporin suppression in vivo. *J. Immunol.* **143**:3940.

CERILLI, C. J. 1988. *Organ Transplantation and Replacement.* J. B. Lippincott Co.

COLVIN, R. B. 1990. Cellular and molecular mechanisms of allograft rejection. *Annu. Rev. Med.* **41**:361.

DIAMANTSTEIN, T., and H. OSAWA. 1986. The interleukin-2 receptor, its physiology and a new approach to selective immunosuppressive therapy by anti-interleukin-2 receptor monoclonal antibodies. *Immunol. Rev.* **92**:527.

EMMEL, E. A., et al. Cyclosporin A specifically inhibits function of nuclear proteins involved in T cell activation. In press.

FERRARA, J. L. M. and H. J. DEEG. 1991. Graft-versus-host disease. *N. Engl. J. Med.* **324**:667.

GREEN, C. J. 1986. Experimental transplantation. *Prog. Allergy* **38**:123.

MASON, D. W., and P. J. MORRIS. 1986. Effector mechanisms in allograft rejection. *Annu. Rev. Immunol.* **4**:119.

POSSELT, A. M., et al. 1990. Induction of donor-specific unresponsiveness by intrathymic islet transplantation. *Science* **249**:1293.

ROMOND, E. H., et al. 1989. Bone marrow transplantation. *Hosp. Prac.* (July 15):169.

SABESIN, S., and J. W. WILLIAMS. 1987. Current status of liver transplantation. *Hosp. Prac.* (July 15):75.

WALDMANN, H. 1989. Manipulation of T-cell responses with monoclonal antibodies. *Annu. Rev. Immunol.* **7**:407.

Study Questions

1. You are a pediatrician treating a child who needs a kidney transplant. The child does not have an identical twin, but both parents and several siblings will donate a kidney if the MHC match with the patient is good.
    a. What is the best possible MHC match that the pediatrician could achieve in this situation?
    b. In which relative(s) might he find it? Why?
    c. What test(s) would he perform in order to find the best-matched kidney?

2. Indicate in the Response column in the table on the facing page, whether a skin graft from each donor to each recipient listed would result in a rejection (R) or an acceptance (A) response. If you believe a rejection reaction would occur, then indicate in the right-hand column whether it would be a first-set rejection (FSR), occurring in 12–14 days, or a second-set rejection (SSR), occurring in 5–6 days. All the mouse strains listed in the table have different H-2 haplotypes.

3. a. Briefly outline the mechanisms involved in graft-versus-host disease (GVHD).
    b. Under what conditions is GVHD likely to occur?
    c. Some researchers have found that GVHD can be diminished by prior treatment of the graft with monoclonal antibody and complement or monoclonal antibody conjugated to toxins. List at least two cell-surface antigens to which monoclonal antibodies could be prepared and used for this purpose, and give the rationale for your choices.

4. a. A child who requires a kidney transplant has been offered a kidney from both parents and from five siblings. Cells from each of the potential donors are screened with monoclonal antibodies to the HLA-A, -B and -C antigens in a microcytotoxicity assay. In addition, ABO blood-group typing is performed. Based on the results in the table on the facing page, a kidney graft from which donor is the most likely to survive?

For use with Question 2.

Donor	Recipient	Response	Type of rejection
BALB/c	C3H		
BALB/c	Rat		
BALB/c	Nude mouse		
BALB/c	C3H, had previous BALB/c graft		
BALB/c	C3H, had previous C57Bl/6 graft		
BALB/c	BALB/c		
BALB/c	F_1 (BALB/c × C3H)		
BALB/c	F_1 (C3H × C57Bl/6)		
F_1 (BALB/c × C3H)	BALB/c		
F_1 (BALB/c × C3H)	BALB/c, had previous F_1 graft		

For use with Question 4a.

	ABO type	HLA-A type	HLA-B type	HLA-C type
Recipient	O	*A1/A2*	*B8/B12*	*Cw3*
Potential donors:				
Mother	A	*A1/A2*	*B8/B12*	*Cw1/Cw3*
Father	O	*A2*	*B12/B15*	*Cw3*
Sibling A	O	*A1/A2*	*B8/B15*	*Cw3*
Sibling B	O	*A2*	*B12*	*Cw1/Cw3*
Sibling C	O	*A1/A2*	*B8/B12*	*Cw3*
Sibling D	A	*A1/A2*	*B8/B12*	*Cw3*
Sibling E	O	*A1/A2*	*B8/B15*	*Cw3*

b.   Now a one-way MLR is performed using various combinations of mitomycin-treated lymphocytes. The results are expressed as counts per minute of [^{3}H] thymidine incorporated; the stimulation index is listed above in parentheses. Based on these results, a graft from which donor is the most likely to be accepted?

For use with Question 4b.

Responder cells	Mitomycin C–treated stimulator cells					
	Patient	Sib A	Sib B	Sib C	Sib D	Sib E
Patient	1,672 (1.0)	1,800 (1.1)	13,479 (8.1)	5,210 (3.1)	13,927 (8.3)	13,808 (8.3)
Sib A	1,495 (1.6)	933 (1.0)	11,606 (12.4)	8,443 (9.1)	11,708 (12.6)	13,430 (14.4)
Sib B	25,418 (9.9)	26,209 (10.2)	2,570 (1.0)	13,170 (5.1)	19,722 (7.7)	4,510 (1.8)
Sib C	10,722 (6.2)	10,714 (5.9)	13,032 (7.5)	1,731 (1.0)	1,740 (1.0)	14,365 (8.3)
Sib D	15,988 (5.1)	13,492 (4.2)	18,519 (5.9)	3,300 (1.1)	3,151 (1.0)	18,334 (5.9)
Sib E	5,777 (6.5)	8,053 (9.1)	2,024 (2.3)	6,895 (7.8)	10,720 (12.1)	888 (1.0)

CHAPTER
23

Cancer and the Immune System

As the death toll from infectious disease has declined in the Western world, cancer has become the second-ranking cause of death, led only by heart disease. Current estimates project that one person in three in the United States will develop cancer, and that one person in five will die from cancer. From an immunologic perspective, cancer cells can be viewed as altered self-cells that have escaped normal growth-regulating mechanisms. This chapter examines the unique properties of cancer cells, paying particular attention to those properties that can be recognized by the immune system. The immune responses that develop to cancer cells, as well as the methods by which cancers manage to evade those responses, are then described. Finally, current clinical and experimental tumor immunotherapies are discussed.

Cancer: Origin and Terminology

In a mature animal, a balance usually is maintained between cell renewal and cell death in most organs and tissues. The various types of mature cells in the body have a given lifespan; as these cells die, new cells are generated by the proliferation and differentiation of various types of stem cells. Under normal circumstances, the production of new cells is so regulated that the numbers of any particular type of cell remain constant. Occasionally, though, cells arise that are no longer responsive to normal growth-control mechanisms. These cells give rise to clones of cells that can expand to a considerable size, producing a *tumor*, or *neoplasm*. A tumor that is not capable of indefinite growth and does not invade the healthy surrounding tissue extensively is *benign*. A tumor that continues to grow and becomes progressively invasive is *malignant*; the term *cancer* refers specifically to a malignant tumor. In addition to uncontrolled growth, malignant tumors exhibit *metastasis*; in this process, small clusters of cancerous cells dislodge from a tumor, invade the blood or lymphatic vessels, and are carried to other tissues, where they continue to proliferate. In this way a primary tumor at one site can give rise to a secondary tumor at another site (Figure 23-1).

Malignant tumors are classified according to the embryonic origin of the tissue from which the tumor is derived. *Carcinomas* are tumors arising from endodermal or ectodermal tissues such as skin or the epithelial lining of internal organs and glands. *Sarcomas*, which arise less frequently, are derived from mesodermal connective tissues such as bone, fat, and cartilage. The *leukemias* and *lymphomas* are malignant tumors of hematopoietic cells of the bone marrow. Leukemias proliferate as single cells, whereas lymphomas tend to grow as tumor masses.

Figure 23-1 Tumor growth and metastasis. (a) A single cell develops altered growth properties at a tissue site. (b) The altered cell proliferates, forming a mass of localized tumor cells, or benign tumor. (c) The tumor cells become progressively more invasive, invading the underlying basal lamina. The tumor is now classified as malignant. (d) The malignant tumor metastasizes by generating small clusters of cancer cells that dislodge from the tumor and are carried by the blood or lymph to other sites in the body. [Adapted from J. Darnell, H. Lodish, and D. Baltimore, 1990, *Molecular Cell Biology*, 2d ed., Scientific American Books.]

(a)

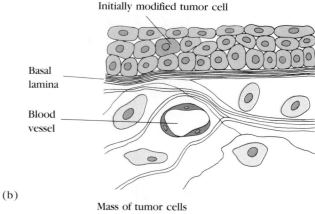

Initially modified tumor cell

Basal lamina

Blood vessel

(b)

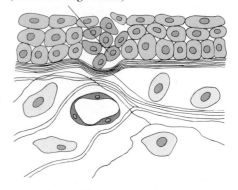

Mass of tumor cells (localized benign tumor)

(c)

Invasive tumor cells

(d)

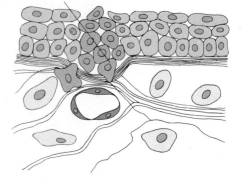

Tumor cells invade blood vessels, allowing metastasis to occur

Properties of Cancer Cells

A central thrust of cancer research has been to elucidate the differences between normal and cancer cells in the hope that an understanding of these differences might lead to some kind of cure for cancer. One might have hoped that all cancer cells might have some basic property in common that allows them to escape from normal growth controls, but no such universal property has been found to account for the cancerous state. Instead, a variety of properties distinguish a cancer cell from its normal cellular counterpart.

Cancer Cells Are Clonally Derived

Most cancers arise from a single neoplastic cell possessing a regulatory defect, which is inherited by the clonal progeny. This monoclonal origin of cancer cells has been proved for a variety of cancers. For example, in chronic myelogeneous leukemia the cancer cells have a translocation between chromosome 22 and chromosome 9. When DNA from these leukemic cells is cloned and sequenced, the exact site of the translocation is found to be the same for all leukemic cells from any one patient but to differ from patient to patient.

Cancer Cells Display Changes in In Vivo Growth Regulation

The most significant characteristic of cancer cells in the body of a person or experimental animal is their uncontrolled, invasive manner of growth. Normal cells are capable of rapid proliferation to meet the needs of the organism, but such proliferation is carefully regulated. If a portion of a rat's liver is surgically removed, for example, the liver quickly begins to regenerate. Initially the rate of cellular proliferation in the regenerating liver is faster than that in most malignant tumors. However, after 4 days the rate of cellular proliferation drops; by 7 days, when the liver has completely regained its normal size, cellular proliferation returns to the low levels characteristic of normal liver cells. Cancer cells, on the other hand, do not respond to normal regulatory constraints. For example, primary tumors of the liver, called *hepatomas*, proliferate much more slowly than a regenerating liver, but they continue to grow indefinitely, producing masses of tumor cells within the liver.

Cancer Cells Have Altered Tissue-Specific Affinities

Normal cells proliferate in certain microenvironments of organs or tissue, where they recognize other cells by unknown mechanisms. The tissue-specific affinity of normal cells can be observed in vitro if one dissociates liver and kidney cells from tissue by mild trypsinization. When the liver and kidney cells are then mixed together (in the absence of trypsin), the cells aggregate in a tissue-specific manner to form small fragments of liver or kidney tissue. Cancer cells have lost this tissue-specific affinity. When normal kidney cells are mixed with cancerous liver cells, the cells no longer aggregate separately but instead aggregate randomly, forming clumps of cancerous liver cells and kidney cells.

The loss of their tissue-specific affinity enables cancer cells to grow beyond the normal boundaries of tissues and to metastasize and grow in diverse tissue sites. Ironically, some tumors appear to acquire tissue-specific homing receptors that enable the cancer cells to extravasate to specific but "wrong" tissues in a manner that is analogous to the tissue-specific homing observed in lymphocytes. The acquisition of these homing receptors may account for the tendency of certain types of cancers to metastasize preferentially to particular tissues.

Biochemical Changes Occur in Cancer Cells

A number of biochemical changes that have been identified in cancer cells may contribute to their ability to invade and metastasize. One of the first biochemical changes observed in cancer cells, noted by Warburg in 1920, was an increase in glycolytic activity, which may allow tumors to grow to a large size with decreased oxygen requirements. Tumor invasion into an adjacent tissue begins with destruction of the limiting basement membrane, a principal constituent of which is type IV collagen. Invasive tumors have been shown to secrete a type IV collagenase, which destroys the basement-membrane barrier, facilitating tumor invasion into the underlying stroma or connective tissue. A number of other enzymes (e.g., cathepsins, hyaluronidases, proteoglycans, and type I, II, and III collagenases) weaken the extracellular matrix and contribute to further tumor invasion. As tumors enlarge in size beyond $1-2$ mm^3, the supply of oxygen and nutrients becomes limiting. A number of tumors have been shown to secrete tumor angiogenesis factors, which induce the formation of blood vessels within the tumor to supply the necessary oxygen and nutrients for sustained tumor growth.

Cancer Cells Have a Disorganized Cytoskeleton

The cytoskeleton of cancer cells displays striking changes compared to that of normal cells. Whereas normal cells possess an organized network of microtubules and microfilaments, the cytoskeleton of cancer cells is disorganized. One of the consequences of the cytoskeletal changes is an overall change in the morphology of cancer cells.

Cancer Cells Exhibit Various Chromosomal Abnormalities

Instead of the usual diploid complement of chromosomes, cancer cells generally exhibit *aneuploidy*, that is, an increase or decrease in the number of chromosomes. In addition, banding analysis of tumor cells reveals deletions, translocations, and gene duplications in a variety of tumors (Figure 23-2). One of the first cancer-associated chromosomal changes to be discovered was found in patients with chronic myelogenous leukemia. The leukemic cells of all patients with this disease contain an unusual chromosome, called the Philadelphia chromosome, which develops from a reciprocal translocation between chromosome 9 and chromosome 22. Burkitt's lymphoma is another cancer in which chromosomal translocations can be detected, in this case between chromosome 8 and chromosomes 2, 14, or 22. Trisomy, in which a particular chromosome occurs in triplicate, has been detected in several tumors. In other tumors entire chromosomes are missing or deletions of various chromosomal bands occur. For example, in retinoblastoma, an inherited childhood cancer, a chromosomal deletion is present in the long arm of chromosome 13. Because the deleted region appears to encode a product that suppresses cell growth, the deletion results in the loss of the growth-suppressing factor and thus in uncontrolled cancerous growth.

Cancer Cells Have Different In Vitro Growth Properties

Normal cells can be cultured in vitro at 37°C in the presence of increased CO_2 and a medium containing nutrients and serum. In most cell cultures derived from embryos or organs, a few cell types tend to grow best and become predominant. The major cell types that pre-

dominate in culture are the fibroblast, which is derived from embryonic mesoderm, and the epithelial cell, derived from ectodermal or endodermal embryonic cells. Normal fibroblast and epithelial cells have certain growth properties in culture in common. They secrete

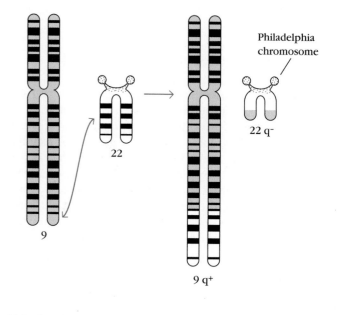

(a) Chronic myelogenous leukemia

(b) Burkitt's lymphoma

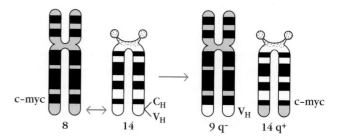

Figure 23-2 Chromosomal translocations in (a) chronic myelogenous leukemia (CML) and (b) Burkitt's lymphoma. Leukemic cells from all patients with CML contain the so-called Philadelphia chromosome, which results from a translocation between chromosomes 9 and 22. Cancer cells from some patients with Burkitt's lymphoma exhibit a translocation that moves part of chromosome 8 to chromosome 14. It is now known that this translocation involves c-*myc*, a cellular oncogene. Abnormalities such as these are detected by banding analysis of metaphase chromosomes. Normal chromosomes are shown on the left, and translocated chromosomes on the right.

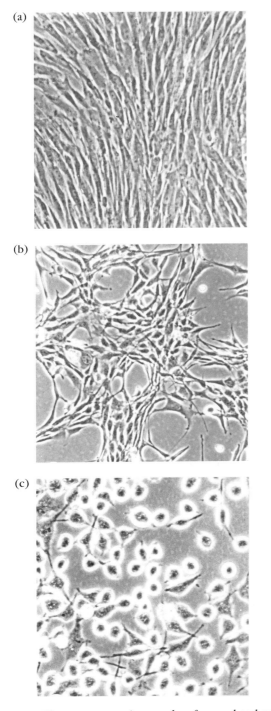

(a)

(b)

(c)

Figure 23-3 Phase-contrast micrographs of normal and cancerous rat embryo fibroblasts grown in culture. (a) Normal cells grow in an ordered fashion, forming a confluent layer of regularly arranged cells that adhere to surface. (b) Cells transformed with polyoma virus become neoplastic, showing a disorganized, criss-crossed pattern of growth. (c) Cells transformed with Abelson murine leukemia virus lose the ability to adhere to the surface and therefore appear almost round. [From J. Darnell, H. Lodish, and D. Baltimore, 1990, *Molecular Cell Biology*, 2d ed., Scientific American Books. *Courtesy of L.-B. Chen.*]

a matrix of extracellular glycoproteins, such as fibronectin and collagen, by which the cells adhere to the surface of the tissue-culture dish; such cells are referred to as "anchorage-dependent." The cells grow in an oriented fashion, generally until a confluent monolayer of cells is formed on the surface of the dish (Figure 23-3a). At this point the cells exhibit density-dependent inhibition of growth, and they stop growing. Both fibroblasts and epithelial cells can be subcultured. After a treatment with trypsin to disrupt the adherent protein matrix, an aliquot of the cells is transferred to fresh tissue-culture media to generate secondary cultures. This procedure of subculturing can be continued for a finite number of times. Finally the cells reach a point at which it takes longer and longer to form monolayers. For most normal human embryo fibroblasts, the ability to divide is limited to approximately 50 population doublings.

Tissue-culture studies comparing normal and neoplastic cells have provided valuable information on the changes associated with cancer. Cancer cells tend to require fewer growth factors for culture and often can grow without the addition even of serum. As cancer cells grow in culture they do not remain oriented but instead form random cellular patterns (Figure 23-3b, c). Often the cancerous cells are no longer anchorage-dependent and are able to proliferate into clones when suspended in liquid tissue-culture media. The cells no longer display density-dependent inhibition of growth but instead proliferate to much higher cell densities in culture, forming multiple layers with visible piles of cells. Perhaps the most notable change in such cancerous cells is their property of immortal growth. Whereas normal cells can be subcultured only a finite number of times, cancerous cells can be subcultured indefinitely.

Malignant Transformation of Cells

Treatment of normal cultured cells with chemical carcinogens, irradiation, and certain viruses can alter the morphology and growth properties of the cells. In some cases this process, referred to as *transformation*, makes the cells able to induce tumors when they are injected into animals; such cells are said to have undergone *malignant transformation*, and they often exhibit in vitro culture properties similar to those of cancer cells. They have decreased requirements for growth factors and serum, are no longer anchorage-dependent, grow in a density-independent fashion—and they are immortal. The process of malignant transformation has been studied extensively as a model of cancer induction.

Transformation Induced by Chemical or Physical Carcinogens

In the early 1900s two Japanese researchers applied coal tar to the ears of rabbits repeatedly over a period of a year and found that tumors appeared. Since this initial demonstration of chemically induced malignant transformation in animals, various chemical and physical agents have been shown to induce transformation by mutagenesis. Some chemical carcinogens, such as alkylating agents, are directly mutagenic; others are not mutagenic in vitro but are converted into potent mutagens in vivo, usually by enzymes of the liver. Physical carcinogens, such as ultraviolet light and ionizing radiation, are also potent mutagens. Ultraviolet light induces the formation of thymine dimers, and x-irradiation induces a range of mutations including chromosome breakage. The importance of these mutations in the induction of cancer is illustrated in certain diseases such as xeroderma pigmentosum. This rare disease in humans is caused by a defect in the gene encoding a DNA-repair enzyme called UV-specific endonuclease. Individuals with this disease are unable to repair UV-induced thymine dimers and consequently develop skin cancers.

Induction of malignant transformation with chemical or physical carcinogens appears to involve multiple steps and at least two distinct phases: *initiation* and *promotion*. Initiation involves changes in the genome but does not, in itself, lead to malignant transformation. Following initiation, promoters stimulate cell division and lead to malignant transformation.

Virus-Induced Transformation

The first evidence that a virus could induce malignant transformation came from the experiments of Peyton Rous in 1910. Rous prepared cell-free filtrates of chicken sarcomas and injected them into healthy chickens; he found that these filtrates alone could induce the formation of sarcomas. When Rous characterized the filtrate, he discovered that an RNA virus (which came to be called the Rous sarcoma virus) was the agent responsible for malignant transformation. In 1966, at the age of 85, Rous received a Nobel prize for this work. Since Rous' initial discovery, a number of DNA and RNA viruses have been shown to induce malignant transformation.

Two of the best-studied DNA viruses known to cause malignant transformation are SV40 and polyoma. In both cases the viral genomes, which integrate randomly into the host chromosomal DNA, include several genes that are expressed early in the course of viral replication. SV40 encodes two early proteins called T and t, and polyoma encodes three early proteins called T, mid-T,

and t. Each of these proteins plays a role in malignant transformation of virus-infected cells.

Most RNA viruses replicate in the cytoplasm and do not induce malignant transformation. The exceptions are retroviruses, which transcribe their RNA into DNA by means of a reverse transcriptase enzyme and then integrate the DNA transcript into the host's chromosomal DNA. This process is similar in the cytopathic retroviruses such as HIV-1 and HIV-2 (see Figure 21-3a) and in the transforming retroviruses, which induce changes in the host cell that lead to malignant transformation. In some cases, retroviral-induced transformation is related to the presence of *oncogenes*, or "cancer genes," carried by the retrovirus. One of the best-studied transforming retroviruses is the Rous sarcoma virus. This virus carries an oncogene called v-*src*, which encodes a 60-kD phosphoprotein (v-Src) that catalyzes the addition of phosphate to tyrosine residues on proteins. The first evidence that oncogenes alone could induce malignant transformation came from studies on the v-*src* oncogene from Rous sarcoma virus. When the v-*src* oncogene from Rous sarcoma virus was cloned and transfected into normal cells in culture, the cells underwent malignant transformation.

Oncogenes and Cancer Induction

In 1971 Howard Temin suggested that oncogenes might not be unique to transforming viruses but might also be found in normal cells; indeed, he proposed that oncogenes might be acquired by a virus from the genome of an infected cell. He called these cellular genes *proto-oncogenes* or *cellular oncogenes* (c-*onc*) to distinguish them from their viral counterpart (v-*onc*). In the mid-1970s J. M. Bishop and H. E. Varmus set out to determine whether these putative proto-oncogenes exist in normal cells. Using a radioactive v-*src* DNA probe, they identified a homologous DNA sequence in normal chicken cells, which was designated c-*src*. Since these early discoveries, numerous cellular oncogenes have been identified.

Sequence comparisons of viral and cellular oncogenes reveal that they are highly conserved in evolution. For example, sequences related to *src* have been detected in species as distant as humans, *Drosophila*, and even yeast, implying that the proteins encoded by these genes may have fundamental functions related to regulation of cellular growth or differentiation. Although most proto-oncogenes consist of a series of exons and introns, their viral counterparts consist of uninterrupted coding sequences, suggesting that the virus might have acquired the oncogene sequence via an intermediate RNA transcript from which the intron sequences were removed during RNA processing. The actual coding sequences of viral oncogenes and cellular proto-oncogenes exhibit a high degree of homology; in some cases a single point mutation is all that distinguishes a viral oncogene from the corresponding proto-oncogene. It is now believed that most, if not all, oncogenes (both viral and cellular) are derived from cellular genes that encode various growth-controlling proteins. In addition, the proteins encoded by a particular oncogene and its corresponding proto-oncogene appear to have very similar functions. As discussed below, the conversion of a proto-oncogene into an oncogene appears in many cases to involve a change in the level of expression of a normal growth-controlling protein.

Function of Oncogene and Proto-oncogene Products

In normal cells, proto-oncogenes generally are expressed at relatively low levels, and their expression is often limited to certain stages of the cell cycle and cellular differentiation. A number of proto-oncogenes are activated as cells enter the cell cycle, moving from G_0 into G_1 or from G_1 into the S phase of DNA synthesis. For example, as discussed in Chapter 11, within 45 min following T_H-cell activation, three proto-oncogene products—c-Fos, c-Myc, and c-Abl—can be detected (see Table 11-6). In this situation, these products serve a normal function in T_H-cell proliferation and/or differentiation.

Various oncogene products have been shown to act at different levels to regulate cellular growth (Table 23-1). A number of them function as growth factors or growth-factor receptors. The *sis* oncogene, for example, encodes a form of platelet-derived growth factor, and oncogenes such as *fms*, *erbB*, and *neu* encode growth-factor receptors. In normal cells the expression of these growth factors and receptors is carefully regulated. Usually one population of cells secretes a growth factor that acts on another population of cells carrying a growth-factor receptor, thus stimulating proliferation of the second population. Inappropriate expression of either a growth factor or its receptor can result in uncontrolled proliferation.

Another group of oncogene products acts to transmit signals from the membrane by regulating levels of second messengers, which in turn regulate gene activity or other cellular functions. The proteins encoded by the *src* and *abl* oncogenes, for example, function as protein kinases, and the Ras proteins have GTP-binding activity. Both protein kinases and GTP-binding proteins have been shown to activate second messengers. Still other oncogene products act at the nuclear level by binding to

DNA or DNA-associated proteins. The *jun* and *fos* oncogenes, for example, encode a transcription factor called AP1, which binds to a number of promoter and enhancer sequences including the IL-2 enhancer (see Chapter 11). The *myc*, *myb*, and *ski* oncogene products are nuclear proteins with DNA-binding activity, which may help to regulate transcription.

Conversion of Proto-oncogenes into Oncogenes

In 1972 Robert J. Huebner and George J. Todaro suggested that mutations or genetic rearrangements of proto-oncogenes by carcinogens or viruses might alter the normal, regulated function of these genes, converting them into potent cancer-causing oncogenes (Figure 23-4). Experimental evidence has been accumulating that supports Huebner and Todaro's hypothesis. For example, some malignantly transformed cells contain multiple copies of cellular oncogenes, resulting in increased

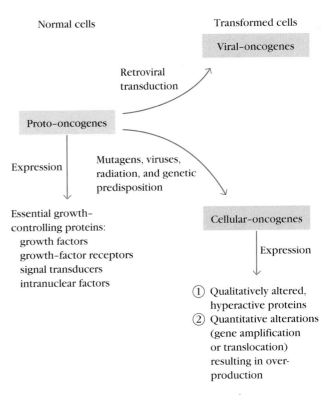

Figure 23-4 Conversion of proto-oncogenes into oncogenes can involve mutation, resulting in production of qualitatively different gene products, or DNA amplification or translocation, resulting in overproduction of gene products.

production of oncogene products (Table 23-2). Several groups have identified c-*myc* oncogenes in homogeneously staining regions (HSRs) of chromosomes from cancer cells; these HSRs represent long tandem arrays of amplified genes. The nerve-cell cancers, called neuro-

blastomas, have frequently been shown to have HSRs of amplified c-*myc* oncogenes (Figure 23-5). In some cases amplification of c-*myc* has been correlated with increased malignancy. For example, in small-cell carcinoma of the lung, the most malignant variants exhibit

Table 23-1   Selected oncogenes and their protein products

| Type/name | Oncogene found in: | | Protein product | |
	Retrovirus	Nonviral tumor	Subcellular location	Nature
Growth factors				
sis	Simian sarcoma		Secreted	A form of PDGF
Growth-factor receptors				
fms	McDonough feline sarcoma		Plasma membrane	CSF-1 receptor
erbB	Avian erythroblastosis		Plasma membrane	EGF receptor
neu (*erbB-2*)		Neuroblastoma	Plasma membrane	Related to EGF receptor
erbA	Avian erythroblastosis		Nucleus	Thyroid hormone receptor
Signal transducers				
src	Rous avian sarcoma		Cytoplasm	Tyrosine kinase
abl	Abelson murine leukemia		Cytoplasm	
Ha-*ras*	Harvey murine sarcoma	Bladder, mammary, and skin carcinomas	Plasma membrane	
N-*ras*		Neuroblastoma and leukemias	Plasma membrane	GTP-binding protein with GTPase activity
Ki-*ras*	Kirsten murine sarcoma	Lung and colon sarcomas	Plasma membrane	
Nuclear factors				
jun	Avian sarcoma virus 17		Nucleus	Transcription factor AP1
fos	FBJ osteosarcoma		Nucleus	
myc	Avian MC29 myelocytomatosis		Nuclear matrix	DNA-binding proteins possibly involved in regulating transcription
N-*myc*		Neuroblastoma	Nuclear matrix	
myb	Avian myeloblastosis		Nuclear matrix	

SOURCE: Adapted from J. Darnell, H. Lodish, and D. Baltimore, 1990, *Molecular Cell Biology*, 2d ed., Scientific American Books.

Table 23-2 Amplification of oncogenes in human tumors

Amplified gene	Tumor	Degree of amplification
c-*myc*	Promyelocytic leukemia cell line, HL60	20 ×
	Small-cell lung carcinoma cell lines	5–30 ×
N-*myc*	Primary neuroblastomas (stages III and IV) and neuroblastoma cell lines	5–1000 ×
	Retinoblastoma cell line and primary tumors	10–200 ×
	Small-cell lung carcinoma cell lines and tumors	50 ×
L-*myc*	Small-cell lung carcinoma cell lines and tumors	10–20 ×
c-*myb*	Acute myeloid leukemia	5–10 ×
	Colon carcinoma cell lines	10 ×
c-*erbB*	Epidermoid carcinoma cell line	30 ×
	Primary gliomas	*
c-K-*ras-2*	Primary carcinomas of lung, colon, bladder, and rectum	4–20 ×
N-*ras*	Mammary carcinoma cell line	5–10 ×

* No amplification given.

SOURCE: Modified from H. E. Varmus, 1984, *Annu. Rev. Genet.* **18**:553.

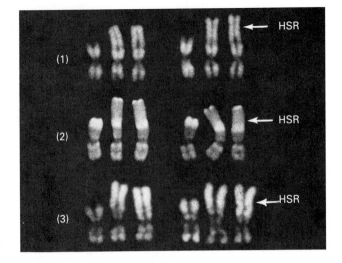

Figure 23-5 Homogeneously staining regions (HSRs), representing large tandem arrays of the c-*myc* oncogene, can be seen in chromosomes from neuroblastoma cells. Chromosomes are stained with quinicrine in preparation 1, with chromomycin A3 in preparation 2, and with Hoechst stain in preparation 3. In each set of three chromosomes, a normal chromosome is shown on the left and two HSR-containing chromosomes are shown on the right. [From S. Latt et al., 1985, *Biopolymers* **24**:77.]

the greatest amplification of c-*myc* compared with normal lung cells.

As noted earlier, some cancer cells exhibit chromosomal translocations. It turns out that these translocations usually involve movement of a proto-oncogene from one chromosome to another chromosomal site. In many cases of Burkitt's lymphoma, for example, c-*myc* is moved from its usual position on chromosome 8 to a position near the immunoglobulin heavy-chain enhancer on chromosome 14, a move that increases synthesis of the c-Myc protein.

Mutation in proto-oncogenes has also been associated with cellular transformation and may be a major mechanism by which chemical carcinogens or x-irradiation convert a proto-oncogene into a cancer-inducing oncogene. A single-point mutation in c-*ras* has been de-

tected in human lung carcinoma, prostate carcinoma, bladder carcinoma, and neuroblastoma. This single mutation appears to reduce the GTPase activity of the Ras protein and may alter its function in the regulation of cellular growth. Finally, viral integration into the host-cell genome may in itself serve to convert a proto-oncogene into a transforming oncogene. For example, avian leukosis virus (ALV) is a retrovirus that does not carry any viral oncogenes and yet is able to transform B cells into lymphomas. This particular retrovirus has been shown to integrate within the c-*myc* proto-oncogene between exon 1 and exons 2 and 3. Exon 1 of c-*myc* has an unknown function; exons 2 and 3 encode the Myc protein. Insertion of the virus at this position has been shown in some cases to allow the provirus promoter to increase transcription of exons 2 and 3, resulting in increased synthesis of c-Myc.

Elevation of Growth Factors and Their Receptors in Tumor Cells

A variety of tumors have been shown to express significantly increased levels of growth factors or growth-factor receptors. In adult T-cell leukemia, discussed in Chapter 11, T cells infected with the HTLV-I or HTLV-II retrovirus show constitutive expression of

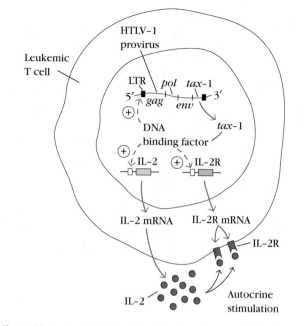

Figure 23-6 In adult T-cell leukemia, infection of T cells with HTLV-1 leads to constitutive expression of IL-2 and the IL-2 receptor (IL-2R), resulting in antigen-independent autostimulation of T-cell proliferation. Tax-1, encoded by the HTLV-1 genome, binds to the 5′ LTR, promoting transcription of the provirus. Tax-1 also stimulates expression of an unknown DNA-binding factor (or factors) that binds to the promoters (open boxes) of the IL-2 and IL-2R genes. As a result, IL-2 and IL-2R are expressed in the absence of antigen activation, leading to proliferation of infected T cells.

IL-2 and the IL-2 receptor, enabling the cells to autostimulate their own proliferation in the absence of antigen activation (Figure 23-6). Expression of the receptor for epidermal growth factor has also been shown to be amplified in many cancer cells. And in breast cancer, increased synthesis of the growth-factor receptor encoded by c-*neu* has been linked with a poor prognosis.

One of the best examples of the association between increased expression of growth factors and cancer induction involves transforming growth factor (TGF-α). TGF-α, which is secreted by a variety of transformed cells, is similar in both structure and function to epidermal growth factor (EGF), and like EGF it is also able to bind to the EGF receptor on cells. Increased expression of both TGF-α and the EGF receptor have been observed in many cancer cells and in cells that have been transformed with retroviruses, viral oncogenes, and carcinogens. TGF-α is thought to act as an autocrine activator of the EGF receptor. The effects of TGF-α overproduction have been studied by producing transgenic mice containing a TGF-α transgene linked to a metallothionine promoter. In these mice, the level of TGF-α expression could be controlled by adjusting their

zinc intake. Experiments with these mice revealed that when TGF-α expression was high, they developed carcinomas of the liver and breast and also exhibited enlargement of the pancreas; however, when TGF-α expression was low, none of these changes was observed. Thus overexpression of the gene encoding TGF-α enables it to function as an oncogene in this system.

Tumors of the Immune System

Tumors of the immune system are classified as lymphomas or leukemias. Lymphomas, which proliferate as solid tumors within a lymphoid tissue such as the bone marrow, lymph nodes, or thymus, include Hodgkin's and non-Hodgkin's lymphomas. Leukemias tend to proliferate as single cells and are detected by increased cell numbers in the blood or lymph. Leukemia can develop in lymphoid or myeloid lineages. Historically the leukemias were classified as acute or chronic according to the clinical progression of the disease. The acute leukemias appeared suddenly and progressed rapidly, whereas the chronic leukemias were much less aggressive and developed slowly as mild, barely symptomatic diseases. These clinical distinctions apply to untreated leukemias; with current treatments the acute leukemias often have a good prognosis, and permanent remission can often be achieved. Now the major distinction between acute and chronic leukemias is the maturity of the cell involved. Acute leukemias tend to arise in less mature cells, whereas chronic leukemias arise in mature cells. The acute leukemias include acute lymphocytic leukemia (ALL) and acute myelogenous leukemia (AML); these diseases can develop at any age and have a rapid onset. The chronic leukemias include chronic lymphocytic leukemia (CLL) and chronic myelogenous leukemia (CML); these diseases develop slowly and are seen in adults.

A number of B- and T-cell leukemias and lymphomas have been shown to involve chromosomal translocations in which a proto-oncogene is translocated into the immunoglobulin genes or T-cell-receptor genes. One of the best-characterized involves the translocation of c-*myc* in Burkitt's lymphoma and in mouse plasmacytomas. In 75% of Burkitt's lymphoma patients, c-*myc* is translocated from chromosome 8 to the Ig heavy-chain gene cluster on chromosome 14 (see Figure 23-6). In the remaining patients, c-*myc* remains on chromosome 8 and the κ or λ light-chain genes are translocated to a region 3′ of c-*myc*. Kappa-gene translocations from chromosome 2 to chromosome 8 occur 9% of the time, and λ-gene translocations from chromosome 22 to chromosome 8 occur 16% of the time.

Translocations of c-*myc* to the Ig heavy-chain gene cluster on chromosome 14 have been analyzed in some detail. In some cases the entire c-*myc* gene is translocated head-to-head to a region near the heavy-chain enhancer. In other cases exons 1, 2, and 3 or exons 2 and 3 of c-*myc* are translocated head-to-head to the S_μ or S_α switch site (Figure 23-7). In each case the translocation removes the *myc* coding exons from the regulatory mechanisms operating in chromosome 8 and places them in the immunoglobulin-gene region, which is a very active region that is expressed constitutively in these cells. Transgenic mice have proved to be an interesting experimental system in which to study the consequences of constitutive *myc* expression in lymphoid cells. In one study mice containing a transgene consisting of all three c-*myc* exons and the immunoglobulin heavy-chain enhancer were produced. Of 15 transgenic pups born, 13 developed lymphomas of the B-cell lineage within just a few months of birth.

Various hypotheses have been suggested to account for *myc*-related oncogenesis. Some researchers have suggested that the presence of the immunoglobulin enhancer may result in overproduction of the *myc* gene product. Another hypothesis, based on the unusual level of mutations observed in exon 1 of c-*myc* after translocation, is that somatic mutation within the immunoglobulin V-region genes may induce mutations in the oncogene that lead to faulty regulation through its exon 1 or to changes in the function of its protein product.

Tumor Antigens

The subdiscipline of tumor immunology involves the study of cell-membrane antigens on tumor cells and the immunologic response to these antigens. Two types of tumor antigens have been identified on tumor cells: *tumor-specific antigens* (*TSAs*) and *tumor-associated antigens* (*TAAs*). Tumor-specific antigens are unique to tumor cells and do not occur on other cells in the body. Tumor-associated antigens are not unique to the tumor cells and instead are also expressed on normal cells under conditions that fail to induce a state of immunologic tolerance to the antigen. The expression of the antigen on the tumor may occur under conditions that enable the immune system to respond to the antigen. Tumor-associated antigens may be antigens that are expressed on normal cells during fetal development when the immune system is immature and unable to respond or they may be antigens that are normally present at extremely low levels on normal cells but which are expressed at much higher levels on tumor cells.

Tumor antigens, whether tumor-specific or tumor-associated, must be capable of inducing either a humoral or cell-mediated immune response. Although a few tumor antigens have been shown to induce the production of humoral antibodies, most tumor antigens fail to induce humoral antibodies and instead induce a cell-mediated response. The presence of tumor antigens that elicit a cell-mediated response has been demonstrated by the

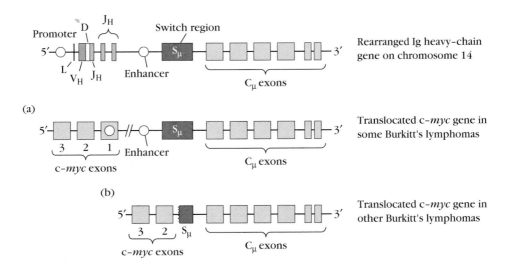

Figure 23-7 Analysis of the c-*myc* gene translocation to the immunoglobulin heavy-chain gene cluster on chromosome 14 in Burkitt's lymphoma has revealed several insertion sites. (a) Insertion of the entire c-*myc* gene near the heavy-chain enhancer. (b) Insertion of exons 2 and 3 of c-*myc* at the S_μ switch site. Only exons 2 and 3 of c-*myc* are coding exons.

rejection of tumors transplanted into syngeneic recipients; because of this phenomenon, these tumor antigens are referred to as *tumor-specific transplantation antigens (TSTAs)* or *tumor-associated transplantation antigens (TATAs)*. It has been difficult to characterize tumor transplantation antigens because they do not generally elicit an antibody response and therefore they cannot be isolated by immunoprecipitation. Many are peptides that are presented together with MHC molecules on the surface of tumor cells and have been characterized by their ability to induce antigen-specific CTLs.

Tumor-Specific Antigens

Tumor-specific antigens have been demonstrated on tumors induced with chemical or physical carcinogens and on some virally induced tumors. It has been much more difficult to demonstrate the presence of tumor-specific antigens on spontaneously occurring tumors. This may be because the immune response to such tumors has eliminated all of the tumor cells bearing recognizable antigens and in this way has selected for cells bearing lower levels of tumor-specific antigens.

Chemically- or Physically-Induced Tumor Antigens

A variety of chemical and physical carcinogens have been used to induce tumors in animals. Methylcholanthrene and ultraviolet light are two carcinogens that have been used extensively to generate tumorigenic cell lines. When syngeneic animals are injected with killed cells from a carcinogen-induced tumor-cell line, the animals develop a specific immunologic response that is unique for the specific tumor-cell line and does not recognize other tumor-cell lines induced in syngeneic animals by the same chemical or physical carcinogen (Table 23-3). Even when the same chemical carcinogen induces two separate tumors at different sites in the same animal, the tumor antigens are distinct and the immune response to one tumor does not protect against the other tumor.

The tumor-specific transplantation antigens of chemically-induced tumors have been difficult to characterize because they cannot be identified by induced antibodies but only by their T-cell–mediated rejection. One experimental approach that has allowed identification of genes encoding some TSTAs is outlined in Figure 23-8. When a mouse tumor-cell line is treated in vitro with a chemical mutagen, it is possible to convert the cell line from a tumorigenic line, designated tum^+, that forms progressive tumor growth to a mutant cell line that is no longer capable of inducing a tumor in syngeneic mice. These mutant tumor-cell lines are designated as tum^- variants. Most tum^- variants have been shown to express TSTAs that are not expressed by the original tum^+

tumor-cell line. When tum^- cells are injected into syngeneic mice, these unique TSTAs are recognized by specific CTLs, which destroy the tumor cells, thus preventing tumor growth.

To identify the genes encoding the TSTAs of a tum^- cell line, a cosmid DNA library is prepared from the tum^- cells. Genes from the tum^- cells then are transfected back into the original tum^+ cells, and the transfected tum^+ cells are tested for their ability to activate cloned CTLs specific for the tum^- TSTA. A number of diverse TSTAs have been identified by this method. The genes encoding these TSTAs have in some cases been shown to differ from normal cellular genes by a single-point mutation. In one case the mutated protein encoded by a particular tum^- gene was shown to be presented as a short peptide in association with a class I MHC molecule on the tum^- cells or on the transfected tum^+ cells. This experimental system has shown that at least some TSTAs may represent mutated forms of normal cellular proteins. In addition, these TSTAs are not always cell-membrane molecules of the tumor but sometimes are cytoplasmic proteins that are processed and presented as short peptides together with class I MHC molecules on the surface of the tumor cells where they can be recognized by CTLs as altered self-cells.

Table 23-3   Immune response of syngeneic animals to transplanted tumor cells induced with methylcholanthrene (MCA) or polyoma virus (PV)*

Transplanted killed tumor cells	Source of live tumor cells for challenge	Tumor growth
Chemically induced		
MCA-induced sarcoma A	MCA-induced sarcoma A	−
MCA-induced sarcoma A	MCA-induced sarcoma B	+
Virally induced		
PV-induced sarcoma A	PV-induced sarcoma A	−
PV-induced sarcoma A	PV-induced sarcoma B	−
PV-induced sarcoma A	SV40-induced sarcoma C	+

* Tumors were induced either with MCA or PV, and killed cells from the induced tumors were injected into syngeneic animals, which were then challenged with live cells from the indicated tumor-cell lines. The absence of tumor growth after live challenge indicates that the immune response induced by tumor antigens on the killed cells provided protection against the live cells.

Virally-Induced Tumor Antigens

In contrast to chemically-induced tumors, virally-induced tumors express tumor antigens shared by all tumors induced by the same virus. For example, when syngeneic mice are injected with killed cells from a particular polyoma-induced tumor, the recipients are protected against subsequent challenge with live cells from any polyoma-induced tumors (see Table 23-3). Likewise, when lymphocytes are transferred from mice with a virus-induced tumor into normal syngeneic recipients, the recipients reject subsequent transplants of all syngeneic tumors induced by the same virus.

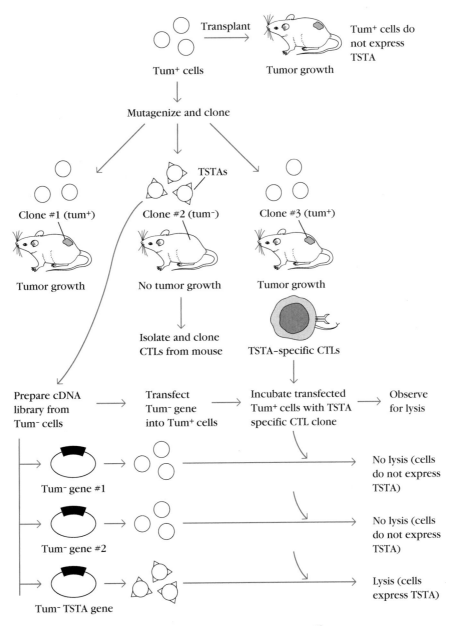

Figure 23-8   General procedure for identification of genes encoding tumor-specific transplantation antigens (TSTAs). Most TSTAs can be detected only by the cell-mediated rejection they elicit. In the first part of this procedure, a nontumorigenic (tum⁻) cell line is generated; this cell line expresses a TSTA that is recognized by syngeneic mice, which mount a cell-mediated response against it. To isolate the gene encoding the TSTA, a cosmid gene library is prepared from the tum⁻ cell line, the genes are transfected into tum⁺ cells, and the transfected cells are incubated with TSTA-specific CTLs.

In the case of both SV40 and polyoma-induced tumors, the presence of tumor antigens is related to the neoplastic state of the cell. Although viral antigens have not yet been established in human cancers, Burkitt's lymphoma cells have been shown to express a nuclear antigen of the Epstein-Barr virus that may indeed be a tumor-specific antigen for this type of tumor.

The nature of virally induced tumor antigens has been studied extensively in mice bearing polyoma- and SV40-induced tumors. In both cases the tumor antigens are encoded by viral genes shown to play a role in malignant transformation. For SV40 the early viral protein designated *large T* (where "T" stands for tumor) serves as a tumor-specific antigen. In the case of polyoma virus the tumor-specific antigen is the early viral protein called *middle T* (or mid-T). In both cases the tumor antigens are not part of the envelope proteins of the virion but instead are proteins expressed primarily in the nucleus of the tumor cell. At first the nuclear location of these tumor antigens was a surprise to researchers, but as data began to accumulate on antigen-processing pathways, it became clear that these nuclear proteins might be processed in tumor cells and presented with class I or class II MHC molecules on the tumor-cell membrane, thus serving to activate T_H and T_C cells.

The potential value of these virally induced tumor antigens can be seen in animal models. In one experiment mice immunized with a preparation of genetically

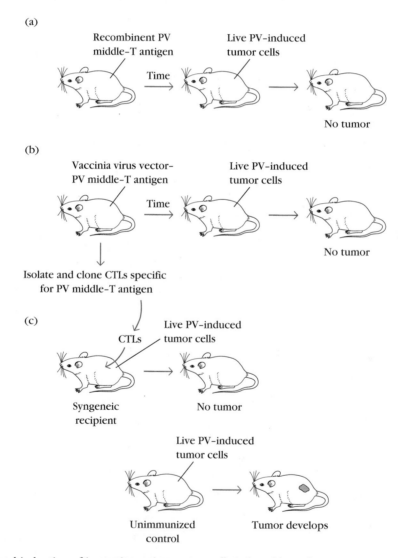

Figure 23-9 Experimental induction of immunity against tumor cells induced by polyoma virus (PV) has been achieved by immunizing mice with recombinant polyoma middle-T antigen (a), with a vaccinia vector vaccine containing the gene encoding middle-T antigen (b), or with CTLs specific for middle-T antigen (c). Unimmunized mice (*bottom*) develop tumors when injected with live polyoma-induced tumor cells, whereas the immunized mice do not.

engineered polyoma-virus tumor antigen were shown to be immune to subsequent injections of live polyoma-induced tumor cells. In another experiment mice were immunized with a vaccinia virus vaccine engineered with the gene encoding the polyoma middle-T antigen. These mice also developed immunity, rejecting later injections of live polyoma-induced tumor cells (Figure 23-9). Clearly if virally induced tumor antigens can be demonstrated on some human tumors, immunotherapeutic approaches to the treatment of these human tumors might be possible.

Tumor-Associated Antigens

The majority of tumor antigens are not unique to tumor cells but also are present on normal cells and are called tumor-associated antigens. These antigens may be expressed only on fetal cells but not on adult cells, or they may be antigens expressed at low levels on normal cells but at much higher levels by tumor cells. Several growth-factor receptors are expressed at significantly increased levels on tumor cells and can serve as tumor-associated antigens. Among these growth-factor receptors is the EGF receptor. A variety of tumor cells have been shown to express the EGF receptor at levels 100 times greater than that in normal cells. Another example of a tumor-associated antigen is a protein, designated p97, on melanoma cells. This protein functions as a transferrin growth factor by aiding in the transport of iron into cells. Whereas normal cells express less than 8,000 molecules of p97 per cell, melanoma cells express 50,000–500,000 molecules of p97 per cell. The gene encoding p97 has been cloned, and a recombinant vaccinia virus vaccine has been prepared carrying the cloned gene. When this vaccine was injected into mice, it induced both humoral and cell-mediated immune responses, which protected the mice against live melanoma cells expressing the p97 antigen. Results such as this highlight the importance of identifying tumor antigens as potential targets of tumor immunotherapy.

Oncofetal Tumor Antigens

Oncofetal antigens, as the name implies, are found not only on cancerous cells but also on normal fetal cells. These antigens appear early in embryonic development, before the immune system acquires immunocompetence; if these antigens later appear on cancer cells, they are recognized as nonself and induce an immunologic response. Two examples of oncofetal antigens are alpha-fetoprotein (AFP) and carcinoembryonic antigen (CEA). Although the serum concentration of AFP drops from milligram levels in fetal serum to nanogram levels in

normal adult serum, elevated AFP levels are found in a majority of patients with liver cancer (Table 23-4). CEA is a membrane glycoprotein found on gastrointestinal and liver cells of 2- to 6-month-old fetuses. Approximately 90% of patients with advanced colorectal cancer, and 50% of patients with early colorectal cancer have increased levels of CEA in their serum; some patients

Table 23-4 Elevation of alpha-fetoprotein (AFP) and carcinoembryonic antigen (CEA) in serum of patients with various diseases

Disease	No. of patients tested	% of patients with high AFP or CEA levels*
		AFP > 400 μg/ml
Alcoholic cirrhosis	NA	0
Hepatitis	NA	1
Hepatocellular carcinoma	NA	69
Other carcinoma	NA	0
		CEA > 10 ng/ml
Cancerous:		
Breast carcinoma	125	14
Colorectal carcinoma	544	35
Gastric carcinoma	79	19
Noncarcinoma malignancy	228	2
Pancreatic carcinoma	55	35
Pulmonary carcinoma	181	26
Noncancerous:		
Alcoholic cirrhosis	120	2
Cholecystitis	39	1
Nonmalignant disease	115	0
Pulmonary emphysema	49	4
Rectal polyps	90	1
Ulcerative colitis	146	5

* Although trace amounts of both AFP and CEA can be found in some healthy adults, none would have levels greater than those indicated in the table.

with other types of cancer also exhibit increased CEA levels. However, because AFP and CEA can be found in trace amounts in some normal adults and in some non-cancerous disease states, the presence of these oncofetal antigens is not diagnostic of tumors but rather serves to monitor tumor growth. If, for example, a patient has had surgery to remove a colorectal carcinoma, CEA levels are monitored following surgery. An increase in the CEA level is an indication of resumed tumor growth.

Oncogene Proteins as Tumor Antigens

A number of tumors have been shown to express tumor-associated antigens encoded by cellular oncogenes. These antigens are also present in normal cells encoded by the corresponding proto-oncogene. In many cases there is no qualitative difference between the oncogene and proto-oncogene products; instead, the increased levels of the oncogene product can be recognized by the immune system. For example, as noted earlier, human breast-cancer cells exhibit elevated expression of the *neu* oncogene, which encodes a growth-factor receptor, whereas normal adult cells express only trace amounts of the Neu protein. Because of this difference in the Neu level, anti-Neu monoclonal antibodies can recognize and selectively eliminate breast-cancer cells without damaging normal cells.

A few tumors have been shown to express a qualitative change in a proto-oncogene product. Single-point mutations in the *ras* proto-oncogene have been detected in a number of tumors including 17 out of 17 cases of malignant prostate cancer. If these qualitative changes can be recognized effectively by the immune system as tumor-specific antigens, they will lend themselves to various cancer immunotherapy approaches.

Immune Response to Tumors

In experimental animals tumor antigens can be shown to induce humoral and cell-mediated immune responses, which in some cases result in tumor elimination. Generally the tumor antigens on UV-induced tumors or tumors induced by oncogenic viruses tend to induce a strong immune response, the tumor antigens on chemically induced tumors tend to induce less immune reactivity, and tumors that arise spontaneously in animals tend to be poorly immunogenic. It is not known why spontaneous tumors lack tumor antigens capable of inducing strong immune reactivity. One theory is that the immune response eliminates any tumor cells bearing strong tumor antigens and that only weakly immunogenic tumor cells survive. The various humoral and cell-

mediated responses that have been shown to play a role in tumor immunity are discussed in this section.

Role of the T$_C$ Cells

Tumor-bearing mice generate T$_C$ cells with specificity for the tumor cells. The activity of these T$_C$ cells can be measured in an in vitro CML assay against [^{51}Cr] labeled tumor cells (see Figure 9-5). In this reaction the CTLs can be shown to recognize tumor antigens associated with class I MHC molecules, so that there is a direct membrane interaction between CTLs and the tumor cells. The mechanism of CTL-mediated killing, which was described in Chapter 13, involves movement of cytoplasmic granules in the CTL to the site of membrane interaction with the cancer cell, where the granules are exocytosed. A principal constituent of the granular contents is the 70-kD protein called perforin, which resembles the C9 complement component. Perforin molecules polymerize and insert into the cancer-cell membrane to form a 5- to 20-nm pore (see Figure 13-8). Another constituent of the perforin-containing granule is the soluble toxin TNF-β (lymphotoxin). It has been hypothesized that formation of the perforin pore on the membrane of the cancer cell may facilitate entry of TNF-β.

The protective effect of CTLs against tumor cells can be demonstrated in vivo with the Winn assay (Figure 23-10). In this assay lymphocytes are isolated from the spleens or lymph nodes of mice undergoing successful tumor regression. The lymphocytes are then mixed with live tumor cells from the same animals and injected into syngeneic recipients. As a control, lymphocytes isolated from normal mice are mixed with the live tumor cells and injected into syngeneic recipients. After an appropriate time, the tumors are removed from the recipients and weighed. One of the problems in extrapolating these results to real-life tumor immunity is that the ratio of the cytotoxic cells mixed with the tumor cells must be quite high to ensure direct contact between the two cell types. In reality such high ratios of CTLs to tumor cells may be achieved only at the periphery of a tumor, where CTLs can contact it. This has led some to question the actual role of CTLs in tumor immunity.

Role of Natural Killer Cells

Natural killer (NK) cells acquired their name from the observation that normal animals have high levels of lymphocytes capable of lysing a wide variety of tumor cells. Unlike B and T cells, these lymphocytes do not exhibit immunologic memory; that is, prior priming with a given tumor does not heighten NK-cell reactivity to a later challenge with the same tumor. NK cells are a heterogeneous group of large granular lymphocytes that constitute 0.6–2.4% of the total lymphocyte population. As noted in Chapter 13, NK cells do not express membrane-bound immunoglobulin, the T-cell receptor, or CD3. Although it is not known how NK cells recognize tumor cells, it is known that the recognition is not MHC-restricted. In some cases Fc receptors on NK cells can bind to antibody-coated tumor cells, bringing the NK cell into contact with the tumor and facilitating tumor-cell killing. In this type of killing, referred to as antibody-dependent cell-mediated cytotoxicity (ADCC), the antibody provides the antitumor specificity but the killing is done by the nonspecific NK cell (see Figure 13-10). NK cells are thought to exocytose granules containing perforin, which mediates pore formation in tumor cells (much like CTLs do). In addition, a soluble NK cytotoxic factor (NKCF) found to be secreted by NK cells appears to be cytotoxic only for tumor cells. The importance of NK cells in tumor immunity can be seen in a genetic defect in the mouse strain called beige and in Chédiak-Higashi syndrome in humans. In both cases there is marked impairment of NK cells and an increased incidence of certain types of cancer.

In addition to NK cells there are some T_C cells that express either the $\alpha\beta$ or $\gamma\delta$ T-cell receptor and CD3 but are not MHC-restricted and appear to resemble NK cells in their nonspecific tumor recognition and killing. This cell population is sometimes grouped among the NK cells, but they should actually be referred to as natural cytotoxic cells (NC cells) or as T_C cells with NK-like function rather than as NK cells. The cytotoxic activity of both NK and NC cells can be enhanced by in vitro treatment with IFN-γ or IL-2. This finding is being exploited in one type of experimental immunotherapy, which is described later in this chapter.

Role of Macrophages

Numerous observations indicate that macrophages play a significant role in the immune response to tumors. For example, macrophages are often observed to cluster around tumors, and their presence is often correlated with tumor regression. Also, macrophages isolated from tumor-bearing animals have been shown to inhibit tumor growth in vitro.

The antitumor activity of macrophages probably is mediated by several macrophage products. Activation of macrophages with IFN-γ and macrophage-activating factor (MAF) not only increases their secretion of various products but also increases their cytotoxicity to tumor cells. Activated macrophages secrete increased levels of lysosomal enzymes. These enzymes can reach high levels around a tumor, especially if antitumor antibodies bind to Fc receptors on macrophages and serve to bridge the macrophages to the tumor. Macrophages also secrete a cytokine called tumor necrosis factor α (TNF-α) that has potent antitumor activity. The gene for TNF-α has been isolated; when cloned TNF-α is injected into tumor-bearing animals, it has been found to induce hemorrhage and necrosis of the tumor.

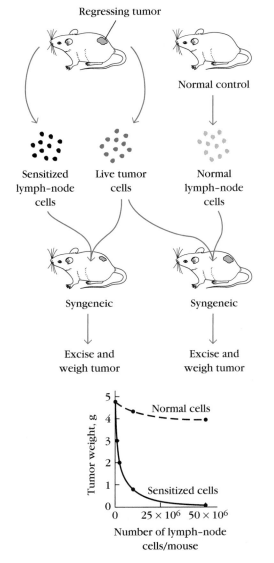

Figure 23-10 Winn assay for assessing CTL-mediated immunity to tumor cells in vivo. Constant numbers of live tumor cells are mixed with varying numbers of lymph-node cells from mice showing tumor regression or from normal control mice and then injected into syngeneic recipients. After 3 weeks, the resulting tumors are removed and weighed. Typical results are shown in the graph at the bottom.

Role of Humoral Antibody

Tumor-cell antigens often elicit the production of specific serum antibodies. These antibodies can play a protective role in eliminating the tumor through several mechanisms. In some cases the antibody can activate the complement system, leading to assembly of the membrane-attack complex (MAC), pore formation, and complement-mediated lysis. Some tumors, however, have been shown to endocytose the MAC pore and repair the membrane before the cell is lysed. In these cases complement split products such as C3a, C4a, C5a, and C5b67 can still play a significant role by inducing localized mast-cell degranulation and the release of mediators that facilitate the influx of inflammatory cells, especially neutrophils and macrophages. Antibodies bound to tumor cells may also facilitate antibody-dependent cell-mediated cytotoxicity (ADCC). Both macrophages and NK cells have receptors for the Fc region of certain antibody classes. The antibody thus serves to bring these nonspecific immune cells into contact with the tumor.

Paradoxically, in some cases antibodies have been shown to interfere with the immune response to a tumor. A number of experiments have demonstrated that tumor-specific antibody can block in vitro CML reactions to tumor cells, perhaps by binding to the tumor antigens and masking them from CTLs or NK cells. The role of antibody in enhancing tumor growth is discussed more fully later in this chapter.

Immune Surveillance Theory

The immune surveillance theory was first conceptualized in the early 1900s by Paul Ehrlich. He suggested that cancer cells frequently arise in the body but are recognized as foreign and eliminated by the immune system. Some 50 years later Lewis Thomas suggested that the cell-mediated branch of the immune system had evolved to patrol the body and eliminate cancer cells. According to these concepts, tumors arise only if cancer cells are able to escape immune surveillance, either by reducing their expression of tumor antigens or by an impairment in the immune response to these cells.

Among the early observations that seemed to support the immune surveillance theory was the increased incidence of cancer in transplantation patients on immunosuppressive drugs. Other findings, however, were difficult to reconcile with this theory. Nude mice, for example, lack a thymus and consequently lack functional T cells. According to the immune surveillance theory these mice should show an increase in cancer, but instead nude mice are no more susceptible to cancer than other mice. Furthermore, although individuals on immunosuppressive drugs do show an increased incidence of cancer, the cancers are largely restricted to cancers of the immune system. Contrary to what the immune surveillance theory would have predicted, other common cancers, such as lung, breast, and colon cancer are not increased in these individuals. One possible explanation for the selective increase in immune-system cancers is that the immunosuppressive agents themselves may exert a direct carcinogenic effect on immune cells.

Experimental data concerning the effect of tumor-cell dosage on the ability of the immune system to respond also are incompatible with the immune surveillance theory. For example, animals injected with very low or very high doses of tumor cells develop tumors, whereas those injected with intermediate doses do not. The mechanism by which a low dose of tumor cells "sneaks through" is difficult to reconcile with the immune surveillance theory. Finally, this theory assumes that cancer cells and normal cells exhibit qualitative antigen differences. In fact, as discussed in previous sections, many types of tumors do not express tumor-specific antigens, and any immune response that develops must be induced by quantitative differences in antigen expression by normal cells and tumor cells.

The basic concept of the immune surveillance theory—that malignant tumors arise only if the immune system is somehow impaired or if the tumor cells lose their immunogenicity, enabling them to escape immune surveillance—at this time remains unproven. Nevertheless, it is clear that an immune response can be generated to tumor cells and therapeutic approaches aimed at increasing that response may serve as a defense against malignant cells.

Tumor Evasion of the Immune System

Although the immune system clearly can respond to tumor cells, the fact that so many individuals die each year from cancer suggests that the immune response to tumor cells often is ineffective. This section describes several mechanisms by which tumor cells appear to evade the immune system.

Immunologic Enhancement of Tumor Growth

Following the discovery that antibodies could be produced to tumor-specific antigens, attempts were made to protect animals against tumor growth by active immunization with tumor antigens or by passive immunization with antitumor antibodies. Much to the surprise of the researchers, these immunizations did not protect against tumor growth; in many cases they actually enhanced the growth of the tumor. The tumor-enhancing ability of immune sera subsequently was studied in in vitro CML reactions. Serum taken from animals with progressive tumor growth was found to block the CML reaction, whereas serum taken from animals with regressing tumors had little or no blocking activity. K. E. and I. Hellstrom extended these findings by showing that children with progressive neuroblastoma had high levels of some kind of blocking factor in their sera and that children with regressive neuroblastoma did not have such factors. Since these first reports, blocking factors have been found to be associated with a number of human tumors.

In some cases, antitumor antibody itself acts as a blocking factor. Presumably the antibody binds to tumor-specific antigens and masks the antigens from cytotoxic T cells. In many cases the blocking factors are not antibodies alone but rather antibodies complexed to tumor antigens. These immune complexes have been shown to block the in vitro CML reaction to tumor cells and may inhibit T_C-cell activity either by blocking tumor antigens or by binding to Fc receptors on the T_C cells. The complexes also may inhibit ADCC by binding to Fc receptors on NK cells or macrophages and blocking their activity.

Antigenic Modulation

Certain tumor-specific antigens have been observed to disappear from the surface of tumor cells in the presence of serum antibody and then to reappear after the antibody is no longer present. This phenomenon, called *antigenic modulation*, is readily observed when leukemic T cells are injected into mice previously immunized with a leukemic T-cell antigen (TL antigen). These mice develop high titers of anti-TL antibody which binds

Table 23-5 Some tumors with altered MHC expression and the biological consequences of this alteration

Experimental tumor systems	Altered MHC expression	Biological consequences
AKR mouse leukemia	Absence of H-2K	Increased tumorigenicity
Murine D122 Lewis lung carcinoma	Reduced H-2K/H-2D ratio	Increased metastasis
Methylcholanthrene-induced murine T10 sarcoma	Absence of H-2K and increased H-2D	Increased metastasis
SV40-transformed mouse cells	Absence of H-2K	Increased tumorigenicity
Radiation leukemia virus (RadLV)– transformed mouse cells	Absence of class I	Lethal leukemogenesis
Herpes simplex virus type 2 (HSV-2)– infected cells	Reduced class I molecules	Resistant to lysis by CTLs
Human Burkitt's lymphoma	Absence of class I	Resistant to lysis by CTLs
Human urothelial cell line TGr III	Reduced class I	Increased tumorigenicity and invasiveness
Human small-cell lung cancer	Deficient class I	Increased tumorigenicity and early metastasis
Human neuroblastoma	Deficient class I	Increased N-*myc* oncogene expression
Human mucinous colorectal carcinoma	Reduced class I	Poor prognosis
Human melanomas	Reduced class I	Increased invasiveness and thicker primary form

SOURCE: From K. M. Hui, 1989, *BioEssays* **11**:23.

to the TL antigen on the leukemic cells and induces capping, endocytosis, and/or shedding of the antigen-antibody complex. As long as antibody is present, these leukemic T cells fail to display the TL antigen and thus cannot be eliminated.

Reduction in Class I MHC Molecules on Tumor Cells

Since CD8$^+$ CTLs recognize only antigen associated with class I MHC molecules, any alteration in the expression of class I MHC molecules on tumor cells may exert a profound effect on the CTL-mediated immune response. Malignant transformation of cells is often associated with

a reduction (or even a complete loss) of class I MHC molecules, and a number of tumors have been shown to express decreased levels of class I MHC molecules (Table 23-5). Class I MHC expression can be quantitated with radiolabeled monoclonal antibody to β_2-microglobulin, which is invariant and is always expressed together with class I molecules on the cell membrane. In many cases the decrease in class I MHC expression is accompanied by progressive tumor growth, and so the absence of MHC molecules on a tumor is generally an indication of a poor prognosis. For example, malignant porocarcinoma cells have been found to stain poorly with radiolabeled antibody to β_2-microglobulin, indicating weak class I MHC expression, whereas benign porocarcinoma cells stain well with the radiolabeled antibody, owing to their strong class I MHC expression.

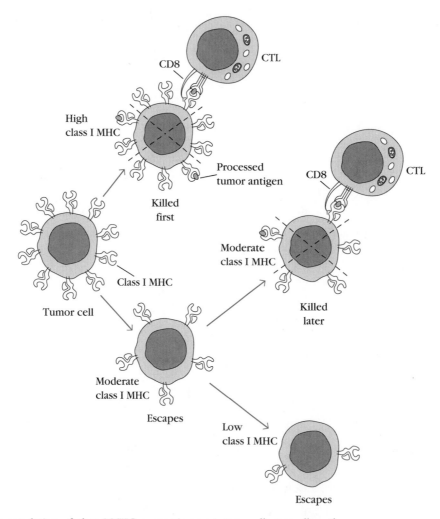

Figure 23-11   Down regulation of class I MHC expression on tumor cells may allow the tumor to escape CTL-mediated recognition. The immune response may play a role in selecting for tumor cells expressing lower levels of class I MHC molecules by preferentially eliminating those cells expressing high levels of class I molecules. With time, malignant tumor cells may express progressively fewer MHC molecules and thus escape CTL-mediated destruction.

The correlation between strong class I MHC expression and tumor progression has been studied extensively in AKR-strain mice, which have a high incidence of spontaneously occurring leukemias. Leukemic cells from these mice often have normal levels of class I H-2D molecules but significantly reduced levels of class I H-2K molecules. On the other hand, in vitro CML assays of lymphocytes from AKR mice, using leukemic cells as the target cells, reveal that only tumor antigens associated with H-2K molecules are recognized. The relationship between expression of H-2K molecules and tumor progression was studied in AKR mice by inoculating groups of mice with one of two leukemic cell lines: one with no detectable H-2K molecules and one with a high level of H-2K molecules. With the cell line lacking H-2K, only 3×10^3 cells were enough to produce a tumor, whereas with the line expressing high H-2K nearly a thousand-fold greater inoculum (2×10^6 cells) was required to induce a tumor. However, when a cloned gene encoding H-2K was transfected into the class I–deficient leukemic cell line, even substantial inoculum sizes failed to induce a tumor, presumably because class IK–restricted CTLs were able to kill the transfected leukemic cells. As illustrated in Figure 23-11, the immune response itself may play a role in selecting tumor cells with decreased class I MHC expression.

Cancer Immunotherapy

The discussion in this and previous chapters indicates that various immune mechanisms exist for responding to tumor cells, although the response frequently is not sufficient to prevent tumor growth. One approach to cancer treatment is to augment or supplement these natural defense mechanisms. Several types of cancer immunotherapy in current use or under development are described in this concluding section.

Immune Adjuvants

A number of immunotherapeutic approaches involve nonspecific activation of the immune system to boost the response to tumor cells. Several adjuvants previously shown to enhance immune responses to various microorganisms have also been shown to enhance antitumor responses. The most widely used adjuvant in tumor immunotherapy is the attenuated strain of *Mycobacterium bovis*, called bacillus Calmette-Guérin (BCG). This adjuvant activates macrophages and thus gives rise to increased production of IL-1, which stimulates T_H-cell activation, resulting in generalized increases in both humoral and cell-mediated responses. The effects of BCG as a tumor immunoagent are clearest when it is injected directly into a tumor, thereby stimulating localized immune activation within the tumor. A number of clinical studies have reported beneficial effects of BCG in slowing the growth of metastatic breast tumors, basal-cell tumors, and malignant melanoma. At first these reports were hailed as a "cancer cure," but continuing studies have shown that although the immune response to such tumors is definitely heightened by BCG treatment, the increase is not usually enough to eliminate the tumors. Other adjuvants that have been tried usually have shown less antitumor activity than BCG. These agents include *Corynebacterium parvum*, an antihelminth drug called levamisole, and azimezone and isoprinosine, which are mitogens that can activate lymphocytes in the absence of antigen.

Dinitrochlorobenezene (DNCB) is an allergen that induces delayed-type hypersensitive reactions when painted on the skin of test animals. Painting DNCB directly on skin cancers generates a localized DTH response that leads in some cases to complete regression of the cancers. DNCB has been shown to be particularly effective when painted on basal-cell carcinomas, causing complete regression in a third of the tumors and partial regression in another third of them.

Cytokine Therapy

Cloning of the various cytokine genes has facilitated their large-scale production. A variety of experimental and clinical approaches have been developed to use recombinant cytokines, either singly or in combination, to augment the immune response against cancer. A number of cytokines have been evaluated in cancer immunotherapy including: interferons α, β, and γ; IL-1, IL-2, IL-4, and IL-5; GM-CSF and TNF. There are scattered hopeful results from these trials but many obstacles remain. The most notable obstacle is the complexity of the cytokine network itself. This complexity makes it very difficult to know precisely how intervention with a given recombinant cytokine will affect the production of other cytokines. And since some cytokines act antagonistically, it is possible that intervention with a recombinant cytokine, designed to enhance a particular branch of the immune response, may actually lead to suppression. In addition, cytokine immunotherapy is plagued by difficulties with administering the cytokines in a localized fashion. In some cases systemic administration of high levels of a given cytokine has been shown to lead to serious and even life-threatening consequences. The results of several experimental and clinical trials with cytokine intervention in cancer will be presented. It is important to keep in mind that these trials are in their infancy.

Interferons

Interferons—a family of glycoproteins produced by a variety of cell types—either interfere with viral replication or play a role in the regulation of the immune response. The first to be characterized were interferon alpha (IFN-α), derived from leukocytes, and interferon beta (IFN-β), derived from fibroblasts. These glycoproteins are released from virus-infected cells and then confer antiviral protection on neighboring cells. Interferon gamma (IFN-γ) was discovered later and was shown to be a lymphokine secreted by activated T cells. Unlike IFN-α and IFN-β, which predominantly function to induce an antiviral state, IFN-γ acts by enhancing the function of various immune-system cells.

Large quantities of purified recombinant preparations of all three interferons are now available, each of which contains multiple molecules with differing biological activities. In clinical trials the recombinant interferons have shown some promise in the treatment of human cancer. To date, most of the clinical trials have involved INF-α. Daily injections of recombinant IFN-α have been shown to induce partial or complete tumor regression in some patients with hematologic malignancies such as leukemias, lymphomas, and myelomas and with solid tumors such as melanoma, Kaposi's sarcoma, renal cancer, and breast cancer. The effectiveness of IFN-α in inducing tumor regression depends in part on the degree of tumor malignancy. For example, when patients with relapsing non-Hodgkin's lymphoma were treated with daily injections of recombinant IFN-α, 15 out of 30 patients with low-level or intermediate-level malignancies exhibited complete or partial remission, whereas 6 of 7 patients with highly malignant lymphomas were completely unresponsive to the interferon treatment.

Interferon-mediated antitumor activity may involve several mechanisms. All three types of interferons have

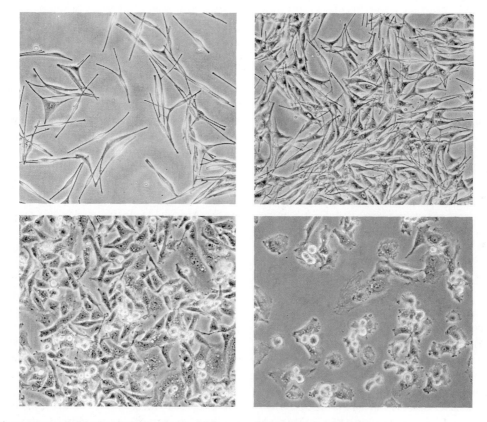

Figure 23-12 Photomicrographs of cultured normal melanocytes (*top*) and of cultured cancerous melanoma cells (*bottom*) in the presence and absence of tumor necrosis factor α (TNF-α). Note that in the presence of TNF-α, the cancer cells stop proliferating, whereas TNF-α has no inhibitory effect on proliferation of the normal cells. [From L. J. Old, 1988, *Scientific American* **258**:59.]

been shown to increase class I MHC expression on tumor cells; IFN-γ has also been shown to increase class II MHC expression on macrophages. Given the evidence for decreased expression of class I MHC molecules on malignant tumors, the interferons may act by restoring MHC expression, thereby increasing CTL activity against tumors. In addition, the interferons have been shown to inhibit cell division of both normal and malignantly transformed cells in vitro. It is possible that some of the antitumor effects of the interferons are related to this ability to directly inhibit tumor-cell proliferation. Finally, IFN-γ increases the activity of T_C cells, macrophages, and NK cells, all of which play a role in the immune response to tumor cells, as described in an earlier section.

Tumor Necrosis Factors: TNF-α and TNF-β

TNF-α and TNF-β are two chemically related polypeptides encoded by genes within the class III region of the major histocompatibility complex. TNF-α and TNF-β exhibit approximately 28% sequence homology and elicit similar biological effects involving myriad localized inflammatory reactions. TNF-α is secreted primarily by activated macrophages and NK cells, and TNF-β is secreted primarily by activated T_H cells. Both factors have been shown to exhibit direct antitumor activity, killing some tumor cells and reducing the rate of proliferation of others while sparing normal cells (Figure 23-12). In the presence of TNF-α or TNF-β a tumor undergoes visible hemorrhagic necrosis and tumor regression. TNF-α has also been shown to inhibit tumor-induced vascularization (angiogenesis) by damaging the vascular endothelial cells in the vicinity of a tumor, thereby decreasing the flow of blood and oxygen that is necessary for progressive tumor growth.

Progress in understanding the functional activity of TNF-α and TNF-β has been facilitated by the recent cloning of their genes and the production of large amounts of both factors by recombinant DNA technology. Phase I clinical trials of recombinant TNF-α in cancer patients appeared quite promising, and again early news stories hailed TNF-α as the "cure for cancer." Later reports showed that although TNF-α holds some promise, it is far from being an antitumor wonder drug. Some patients treated with TNF-α have had complete tumor regression, but only if TNF-α was injected directly into the tumor. For other patients direct tumor injection elicited some effects, but tumor regression was not complete. There are also some problems with TNF-α therapy including its extremely short half-life, which necessitates frequent injections, and several adverse side effects, such as fever, chills, blood-pressure changes, and decreased counts of white blood cells.

In October, 1991, Dr. Steven Rosenberg at the National Cancer Institute reported an attempt to vaccinate cancer patients with genetically engineered cancer cells. Melanoma cells from a patient with advanced malignant melanoma were surgically removed from the patient and genetically engineered with the gene for TNF. After genetically engineering the melanoma cells, the patient was injected in the thigh with 2 million of the engineered tumor cells. A few weeks after this procedure the lymphocytes will be harvested from the patients lymph nodes, clonally expanded in tissue culture, and returned to the patient. It is hoped that the engineered melanoma cells will act as a vaccine to activate tumor-specific lymphocytes which can then be further expanded in tissue culture.

In Vitro-Activated LAK and TIL Cells

Animal studies have shown that lymphocytes can be activated against tumor antigens in vitro by culturing the lymphocytes with x-irradiated tumor cells in the presence of IL-2. These activated lymphocytes mediate more effective tumor destruction than untreated lymphocytes when they are reinjected into the original tumor-bearing animal. It is difficult, however, to activate in vitro enough lymphocytes with antitumor specificity to be useful in cancer therapy. In 1980 Steven Rosenberg, who was sensitizing lymphocytes to tumor antigens by this method, found that in the presence of high concentrations of cloned IL-2 and without the addition of tumor antigens, large numbers of activated lymphoid cells were generated that could kill fresh tumor cells but not normal cells. He called these cells *lymphokine-activated killer (LAK)* cells. LAK cells appear to be a heterogeneous population of lymphoid cells that includes natural killer (NK) cells and natural cytotoxic (NC) cells; the relative numbers of the two cell types depend on the source of the lymphocytes and the conditions of IL-2 activation. Because large numbers of LAK cells can be readily generated in vitro and because these cells are active against a wide variety of tumors, their effectiveness in tumor immunotherapy has been evaluated.

In one study, infusion of LAK cells + recombinant IL-2 into tumor-bearing animals was found to mediate effective tumor-cell destruction (Figure 23-13). These results laid the foundation for clinical trials in which peripheral-blood lymphocytes were removed from patients with various advanced metastatic cancers and were activated in vitro to generate LAK cells. Patients were then infused with their autologous LAK cells together with IL-2. A trial with 25 patients in 1985 resulted in cancer regression in some patients. A more extensive trial on 222 patients in 1987 resulted in complete regression in 16 patients. However, a number of undesirable side effects are associated with the high levels of IL-2 required for LAK-cell activity. The most noteworthy is vascular leak syndrome, which involves emigration of lymphoid cells and plasma from the peripheral blood into the tissues, leading to shock.

Tumors contain lymphocytes that have infiltrated the tumor and presumably are taking part in an anti-tumor response. By taking small biopsy samples of tumors, one can obtain a population of these lymphocytes and expand it in vitro with IL-2. These activated *tumor-infiltrating lymphocytes* are called *TIL cells*. Many TIL cells have a wide range of antitumor activity and appear to be indistinguishable from LAK cells. However, some TIL cells have specific cytolytic activity against their autologous tumor. These tumor-specific TIL cells are of interest because they have increased antitumor activity and require 100-fold lower levels of IL-2 for their activity than do LAK cells. In one recent study TIL cells were expanded in vitro from biopsy samples taken from patients with malignant melanoma, renal-cell carcinoma, and small-cell lung cancer. The expanded TIL cells were reinjected into autologous patients together with continuous infusions of recombinant IL-2. Renal-cell carci-

nomas and malignant melanomas showed partial regression in 29% and 23% of the patients, respectively.

This approach has recently been extended by genetically engineering TIL cells from two patients with malignant melanomas to carry the gene encoding TNF-α. These engineered TIL cells were then infused into the autologous patients, who currently are being monitored. It is hoped that the TIL cells will attack the tumor, releasing high localized concentrations of TNF-α, which then will mediate tumor destruction.

Monoclonal Antibodies

Various monoclonal antibodies have been tested experimentally as immunotherapeutic agents for cancer. The preparation and potential uses of immunotoxins specific for tumor cells was discussed in Chapter 7. These agents consist of the inhibitor chain of a toxin (e.g., diphtheria toxin) linked to an antibody against a tumor-specific or tumor-associated antigen (see Figure 7-10). In vitro studies have demonstrated that these "magic bullets" can kill tumor cells without harming normal cells.

In another approach, monoclonal antibody to CD3, which is known to activate T cells in vitro, has been administered to mice in an effort to induce nonspecific T-cell activation in vivo. In one study, T cells from C3H-strain mice that had previously been activated by injections of anti-CD3 monoclonal antibody were isolated and analyzed. In comparison with control mice, the T cells from treated mice exhibited increased expression of IL-2 and increased functional activity in both MLR and CML assays. To determine whether such nonspecific T-cell activation might increase tumor immunity, C3H mice were injected with live fibrosarcoma cells with or without anti-CD3 and the tumor volume was measured over time. The fibrosarcoma tumor was chosen because it grows progressively in most C3H mice and kills the mice by developing into a large tumor mass. In one experiment, only 35% of mice injected with 4 μg of anti-CD3 had tumors 4 weeks after being injected with live fibrosarcoma cells, whereas 95% of the untreated mice had tumors. In the treated mice that did develop tumors, the tumor volume was significantly lower than in the untreated controls. When the treated mice were later given a secondary challenge with live fibrosarcoma cells, they were immune and did not develop tumors. Interestingly, the F(ab')₂ fragment of anti-CD3 was ineffective in reducing tumor development.

Although these findings with anti-CD3 are hopeful for tumor immunotherapy, the experiments also demonstrated the fine line between immune enhancement and immune suppression. The concentration of the anti-CD3 monoclonal was shown to be critical: a 4-μg dose enhanced tumor immunity but a 40-μg dose appeared

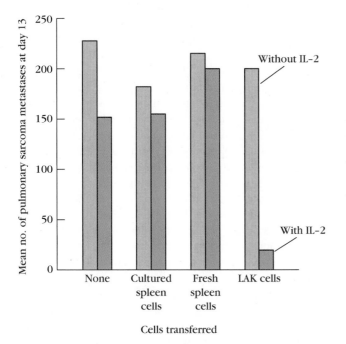

Figure 23-13 Experimental demonstration of tumor-destroying activity of LAK cells + IL-2. Spleen cells or LAK cells, in the presence or absence of recombinant IL-2, were infused into mice with pulmonary sarcoma. The animals were evaluated 13 days later for the number of pulmonary sarcoma metastases. The LAK cells were prepared by isolating lymphocytes from tumor-bearing animals and incubating them in vitro with high concentrations of IL-2. Note that tumor regression occurred only when LAK cells and IL-2 were infused. [Data from S. Rosenberg et al., 1988, *Annals of Internal Medicine*, **108**:853.]

to be immunosuppressive, causing enhanced tumor growth and earlier death (Figure 23-14). Until the steps leading to immune activation and immune suppression are more clearly understood, approaches such as this one are clearly too risky for clinical human trials.

Monoclonal antibodies can also be used to bridge activated T cells directly to a tumor. In this approach two different monoclonal antibodies are produced; one specific for a tumor-cell membrane molecule and one specific for the CD3 membrane molecule of the TCR complex. A hybrid monoclonal antibody, or heteroconjugate, is then prepared with specificity for the tumor antigen and for CD3 (see Chapter 7). In vitro experiments with these heteroconjugates have revealed that they are able to cross-link and activate T cells directly on the surface of the tumor cell.

The finding that a variety of tumors express significantly increased levels of growth-factor receptors suggests that treatment with monoclonal antibodies against these receptors might inhibit tumor-cell activity. Monoclonal antibodies to the EGF receptor, to the p97 (transferrin) receptor, and to the IL-2 receptor have each been produced. A phase 1 clinical trial at Memorial Sloan-Kettering Cancer Center is presently under way in which patients with squamous-cell lung carcinoma are being treated with monoclonal antibody to EGF receptor.

Tumor-Cell Vaccines

In a novel approach to developing tumor vaccines, a patient's own tumor cells are killed by x-irradiation, mixed with BCG, and reinjected into the patient. One woman treated in this way had been diagnosed in 1986 with advanced malignant melanoma with literally hundreds of tumors on her right leg. Within 7 weeks after receiving this experimental vaccine, the tumors in her leg had disappeared, and the woman was still alive more than 3 years after treatment. Recent reports indicate that about 25% of patients with malignant melanoma have shown complete or partial remission after treatment with killed autologous tumor cells + BCG.

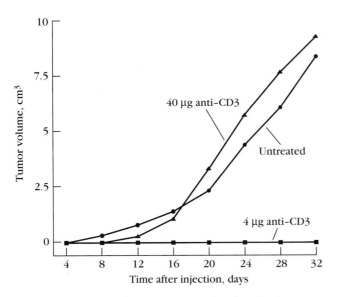

Figure 23-14 Effect of anti-CD3 monoclonal antibody on tumor growth in C3H mice. Animals were injected with live fibrosarcoma cells and simultaneously with 4 μg or 40 μg of anti-CD3 or with saline buffer; tumor volume was then determined at various times after the injections. The low dose of anti-CD3 inhibited tumor growth effectively, whereas the high dose did not do so and even appeared to enhance tumor growth somewhat in comparison with untreated controls. [Adapted from J. D. Ellenhorn, et al., 1988, *Science*, **242**:569.]

Summary

1. Tumor cells differ from normal cells in numerous ways. Among these differences are changes in growth regulation, various biochemical changes, cytoskeletal changes, chromosomal abnormalities, and the ability to grow indefinitely in in vitro culture.

2. Normal cells can be transformed by chemical and physical carcinogens and by transforming viruses. Transformed cells exhibit altered growth properties and are sometimes capable of inducing cancer when they are injected into animals. A study of transformed cells has revealed the important role of cellular and viral oncogenes in the transformation process.

3. In a number of B- and T-cell leukemias and lymphomas, proto-oncogenes have been translocated to the immunoglobulin or T-cell-receptor genes. In its new site the translocated gene may come under the influence of an enhancer and be transcribed at higher levels or may undergo an unusually high level of mutation owing to somatic mutation mechanisms at work in the B-cell immunoglobulin genes.

4. Tumor cells display a number of surface structures that can be recognized as antigenic by the immune system. Among these antigens are oncofetal antigens, virally encoded antigens, and increased levels of oncogene products. The immune response to tumors includes CTL-mediated lysis, NK-cell activity, macrophage-mediated tumor destruction, and destruction mediated by ADCC. Several cytotoxic factors, including TNF-α and TNF-β, help to mediate tumor-cell killing. Tumors may evade the immune response by modulating their tumor antigens, by reducing their expression of class I MHC molecules, and by antibody-mediated or immune-complex–mediated inhibition of CTL activity.

5. Experimental cancer immunotherapy has taken a variety of approaches. In some cases, injections of lymphokines such as IFN-α and TNF-α have been shown to have beneficial effects. In another approach lymphocytes are activated in vitro with high concentrations of IL-2, thereby inducing LAK cells or TIL cells with antitumor activity. Infusions of LAK cells + IL-2 have reduced tumor development in experimental animals. Monoclonal antibodies specific for tumor antigens have also been used to produce immunotoxins. Monoclonal antibodies to CD3 and to various growth-factor receptors are being evaluated. Finally, vaccines of killed autologous tumor cells mixed with BCG have shown some success in treatment of malignant melanomas.

References

CORY, S., and J. M. ADAMS. 1988. Transgenic mice and oncogenesis. *Annu. Rev. Immunol.* **6**:25.

HELLSTROM, K. E., and I. HELLSTROM. 1989. Oncogene-associated tumor antigens as targets for immunotherapy. *FASEB* **3**:1715.

HUBER, B. E. 1989. Therapeutic opportunities involving cellular oncogenes: novel approaches fostered by biotechnology. *FASEB* **3**:5.

HUI, K. M. 1989. Re-expression of major histocompatibility complex (MHC) class I molecules on malignant tumor cells and its effect on host-tumor interaction. *BioEssays* **11**:22.

JHAPPAN, C., et al. 1990. TGF-α overexpression in transgenic mice induces liver neoplasia and abnormal development of the mammary gland and pancreas. *Cell* **61**:1137.

KRADIN, R. L., et al. 1989. Tumor infiltrating lymphocytes and interleukin-2 treatment of advanced cancer. *Lancet* (March 18):577.

LANG, R. A., and A. W. BURGESS. 1990. Autocrine growth factors and tumourigenic transformation. *Immunol. Today* **11**:244

LURQUIN, C., A. V. PEL, B. MARIAME et al. 1989. Structure of the gene of Tum⁻ transplantation antigen P91A: the mutated exon encodes a peptide recognized with Lᵈ by cytolytic T cells. *Cell* **58**:293.

MARX, J. 1990. Oncogenes evoke new cancer therapies. *Science* **249**:1376.

RUSSEL, S. J. 1990. Lymphokine gene therapy for cancer. *Immunol. Today* **11**:196.

SANDGREN, E. P., N. C. LUETTEKE, R. D. PALMITER et al. 1990. Overexpression of TGF-α in transgenic mice: induction of epithelial hyperplasia, pancreatic metaplasia, and carcinoma of the breast. *Cell* **61**:1121.

SCHREIBER, H., P. L. WARD, D. A. ROWLEY, and H. J. STAUSS. 1988. Unique tumor-specific antigens. *Annu. Rev. Immunol.* **6**:465.

SHOWE, L. C., and C. M. CROCE. 1987. The role of chromosomal translocations in B and T cell neoplasia. *Annu. Rev. Immunol.* **5**:253.

TOPALIAN, S. L., D. SOLOMON, and S. A. ROSENBERG. 1989. Tumor-specific cytolysis by lymphocytes infiltrating human melanomas. *J. Immunol.* **142**:3714.

Study Questions

1. Indicate whether each of the following statements is true or false. If you think a statement is false, explain why.

   a. Cancer cells divide much more rapidly than normal cells.

   b. The c-*myc* gene is expressed in activated T_H cells.

   c. Multiple copies of cellular oncogenes are sometimes observed in cancer cells.

   d. Viral integration into the cellular genome may convert a proto-oncogene into a transforming oncogene.

   e. All oncogenic retroviruses carry viral oncogenes.

   f. The immune response against a virus-induced tumor protects against another tumor induced by the same virus.

   g. LAK cells are tumor-specific.

2. You are a clinical immunologist studying acute lymphoblastic leukemia (ALL). Leukemic cells from most patients with ALL have the morphology of lymphocytes but do not express cell-surface markers characteristic of mature B or T cells. You have isolated cells from ALL patients that do not express membrane Ig but do react with monoclonal antibody against a normal pre-B cell marker (B-200). You therefore suspect that these leukemic cells are pre-B cells. How would you confirm this commitment to the B-cell lineage by means of genetic analysis?

3. In a recent experiment melanoma cells were isolated from patients with early or advanced stages of malignant melanoma. At the same time T cells specific for tetanus toxoid antigen were isolated and cloned from each patient.

   a. When early-stage melanoma cells were cultured together with tetanus toxoid antigen and the tetanus toxoid–specific T-cell clones, the T-cell clones were observed to proliferate. This proliferation was blocked by addition of chloroquine or by addition of monoclonal antibody to HLA-DR. Proliferation was not blocked by addition of monoclonal antibody to HLA-A, -B, -DQ, or -DP. What might these findings indicate about the early-stage melanoma cell in this experimental system?

b. When the same experiment was repeated with advanced-stage melanoma cells, the tetanus toxoid T-cell clones failed to proliferate in response to the tetanus toxoid antigen. What might this indicate about advanced-stage melanoma cells?

c. When early and advanced malignant melanoma cells were fixed with paraformaldehyde and incubated with processed tetanus toxoid, only the early-phase melanoma cells could induce proliferation of the tetanus toxoid T-cell clones. What might this indicate about early-stage melanoma cells?

d. How might you confirm your hypothesis experimentally?

5. What is the rationale behind the use of anti-CD3 as an antitumor immunoagent? What is a critical consideration with this approach?

6. Various lymphokines have been evaluated for use in tumor immunotherapy. List four lymphokines that have been shown to enhance antitumor immunity and describe the mechanisms by which they are thought to do so.

Glossary

Acquired immunity an immune reaction involving lymphocytes that displays the features of specificity, diversity, memory, and self/nonself recognition.

Acute phase proteins hepatocyte-derived serum proteins that are produced during the early stages of an inflammatory response.

Acquired immunodeficiency syndrome (AIDS) a disease caused by a retrovirus, HIV, that causes significant depletion of $CD4^+$ T cells resulting in diminished immune responsiveness and increased susceptibility to a variety of infections and cancers.

Adoptive transfer transfer of an immune response by transferring lymphocytes from an antigen primed donor to an unprimed recipient.

Adherent cells cells of the monocyte/macrophage lineage that normally adhere to glass or plastic.

Adjuvant A substance which nonspecifically enhances or potentiates an immune response to an antigen.

Affinity a measure of the binding strength (association constant) between a receptor (e.g., one binding site on an antibody) and a ligand (e.g., antigenic determinant).

Affinity maturation the increase in average antibody affinity to an antigen produced during the secondary immune response.

Agretope the region of a processed peptide that binds to a MHC molecule.

Allele one of several alternate forms of a gene at a single locus that controls a particular characteristic.

Allelic exclusion the restriction of a lymphocyte to expression of only one of two possible allelic forms of a single gene.

Allergen nonparasitic antigens that induce an allergic reaction that is usually a type I hypersensitivity reaction.

Allergy an immune response induced by an environmental antigen that has deleterious effects resulting in significant tissue damage and inflammation.

Allogeneic genetic variation between members of the same species.

Alloantiserum antiserum produced by one member of a species specific for the allelic antigens of another individual of the same species.

Allograft a tissue transplant between allogeneic individuals.

Alternative complement pathway antibody independent complement activation involving C3 – C9 and factors B, D, H, I, and P.

Anaphylatoxins complement split products, C3a, C4a, and C5a, which are released following complement activation that induce mast cell degranulation resulting in histamine release and smooth muscle contraction.

Anaphylaxis an immediate type I hypersensitivity reaction, triggered by IgE mediated mast cell degranulation, releasing pharmacologically active mediators that produce vasodilation and smooth muscle contraction. The reaction leads to shock and is often fatal.

Antibody a protein (immunoglobulin) produced by B lymphocytes that recognizes a particular foreign antigenic determinant and facilitates clearance of that antigen.

Antibody-dependent cell-mediated cytotoxicity (ADCC) a type of cell-mediated cytotoxic reaction in which a target cell with bound antibody is recognized by an effector cell bearing Fc receptors and is subsequently lysed without involving complement.

Antigen a foreign substance that binds specifically to antibody or T-cell receptors and elicits an immune response.

Antigenic determinant the site on an antigenic molecule that is recognized and bound by antibody.

Antigen presenting cell (APC) macrophages, dendritic cells, B cells, and other cells that can process and present antigen peptides in association with class II MHC molecules. $CD4^+$ T cells recognize the antigen associated with the class II MHC molecule on the APC.

Atopy clinical manifestation of type I hypersensitivity (IgE mediated allergy) including allergic rhinitis (hayfever), eczema, asthma and various food allergies.

Autologous derived from the same individual.

Autograft tissue graft from one part of the body to another in the same individual.

Autosomal refers to all the chromosomes except the sex chromosomes.

Autoimmunity an abnormal immune response against self-antigens.

Avidity the functional binding strength between two molecules such as an antibody and an antigen. Avidity differs from affinity because it reflects the valency of the antigen-antibody interaction.

B lymphocytes lymphocytes that mature in the bone marrow and are precursors of antibody-secreting plasma cells.

β_2-Microglobulin an invariant protein that is associated on the membrane with the class I MHC molecule.

Bacillus Calmette-Guerin (BCG) an attenuated form of *Mycobacterium bovis* used as a specific vaccine and as an adjuvant component.

Bence-Jones protein monoclonal immunoglobulin light chains present (usually as dimers) in the urine of some patients with multiple myeloma.

Blast cell a cell stage distinguished by a higher cytoplasm-to-nucleus ratio than a resting cell, occuring in lymphocytes after activation and before cell division.

Bursa of Fabricus a primary lymphoid organ in birds found at the junction of the hind gut and cloaca which serves as a site for B cell maturation.

Carcinoembryonic antigen (CEA) antigen found in embryonic and malignant tissues, generally absent from normal adult tissues.

Carcinoma a cancer of epithelial origin.

Carrier an immunogenic molecule containing antigenic determinants recognized by T cells. The carrier is conjugated to a non-immunogenic hapten molecule, rendering the hapten immunogenic.

Carrier effect an experimental observation that a secondary immune response to a hapten-carrier conjugate requires prior priming for both hapten and carrier determinants.

CD antigens cell membrane molecules used to differentiate human leukocyte subpopulations. CD membrane molecules are identified by monoclonal antibodies. All monoclonal antibodies that identify the same membrane molecule are grouped into a common cluster of differentiation or CD.

CD2 a glycoprotein expressed on most thymocytes, all peripheral T cells, and on large granular lymphocytes. The molecule serves as a signal transducing molecule and as a cell-adhesion molecule. The ligand for CD2 is LFA-3.

CD3 a complex of polypeptides: γ, δ, and ϵ, complexed to either a homodimer of $\zeta\zeta$ chains or to a heterodimer of $\zeta\eta$. The complex is associated with the T-cell receptor and serves as a signal transducing membrane molecule.

CD4 a cell surface glycoprotein found on the subset of T cells (usually T_H) that recognizes antigenic peptides complexed to class II MHC.

CD8 a cell surface glycoprotein found on the subset of T cells (usually T_C) that recognizes antigenic peptides complexed to class I MHC.

Cell-mediated immunity (CMI) a branch of immune response mediated by the transfer of immune T cells that plays an important role in protection against intracellular bacteria, viruses, cancer, and in graft rejection.

Cell-mediated lympholysis (CML) generally refers to cytotoxic T-cell mediated destruction of another cell in an in vitro culture.

Chemotaxis increased directional movement of cells in response to the concentration gradient of some chemotactic factors.

Chimera an animal or tissue composed of elements derived from genetically distinct individuals.

Class I MHC major histocompatibility molecule composed of an integral membrane polypeptide noncovalently associated with β_2-microglobulin and found on all nucleated cells of the body. Class I MHC is encoded by H-2 K, D, and L in mice and by HLA-A, B, and C in humans.

Class II MHC major histocompatibility molecule consisting of two integral membrane polypeptides encoded by H-2 IA and IE in mice and HLA-DR, DQ, and DP in humans. These molecules are expressed on macrophages, B cells, dendritic cells, and other antigen-presenting cells.

Class III MHC gene products of a MHC region, distinct from class I and class II MHC molecules, that include some compo-

nents of the complement system, steroid 21-hydroxylase enzymes, and tumor necrosis factors α and β.

Classical complement pathway activation of a sequential enzymmatic cascade involving C1–C9 and ultimately leading to cell lysis.

Class switching the process by which a B cell undergoes gene rearrangement to express a new heavy chain isotype without altering the specificity of the antibody produced.

Clonal anergy a theory for immunological nonresponsiveness (tolerance) in which antigen-reactive lymphocytes are present but are functionally inactive.

Clonal deletion a theory for immunological unresponsiveness (tolerance) in which contact with self-antigen results in death of the self-reactive lymphocyte.

Clonal selection a central theory of immunology in which antigen binds to and stimulates a particular lymphocyte to undergo mitosis and develop into a clone of cells with the same antigenic specificity as the original parent cell.

Clone cells arising from a single progenitor cell.

Clonotype a unique marker or gene product expressed by members of a single clone.

Colony stimulating factors (CSFs) a group of factors that induce the proliferation and differentiation of hematopoietic cells and some additional cells.

Complement a group of serum proteins that participate in an enzymmatic cascade, ultimately resulting in a cytolytic membrane attack complex.

Complete Freund's adjuvant (CFA) a solution composed of mineral oil, an emulsifying agent, and heat-killed mycobacteria in which antigen is emulsified that serves to nonspecifically potentiate the immune response to the antigen.

Combined immunodeficiency deficiency in both humoral and cell-mediated branches of the immune response.

Congenic (coisogenic) individuals that differ genetically at a single genetic locus or region.

Con A (concanavalin A) a tetrameric protein extracted from jack beans which binds to sugars containing α-D-mannose or α-D-glucose. The molecule is able to crosslink glycoproteins on the surface of cells and is a potent mitogen of T cells in many species.

Conjugate a complex formed by covalent binding of two molecules: e.g., a toxin molecule bound to an antibody, an immunoglobulin bound to fluorescein. Also used to denote the close binding of two cells to each other.

Constant region (C region) the nearly invariant region of heavy and light immunoglobulin chains and the corresponding regions of the chains of the T-cell receptor.

Coomb's test a diagnostic test used to detect antibody bound to the membrane of a red blood cell by the addition of an anti-immunoglobulin antibody.

Cross-reactivity reaction of antibodies or T-cell receptors with more than one antigen due to shared epitopes.

Cyclosporin A an immunosuppressive drug commonly used to prevent graft rejections.

Cytokines a group of secreted low molecular weight proteins that regulate the intensity and duration of an immune response by stimulating or inhibiting the proliferation of various immune cells or their secretion of antibodies or other cytokines.

CTL cytotoxic T lymphocytes that are capable of mediating lysis of target cells following recognition of processed antigen presented by an MHC molecule on the target cell.

Cytotoxic having the property of cell killing.

Cortex the outer or peripheral layer of an organ.

Degranulation discharge of the content of cytoplasmic granules by basophils and mast cells.

Delayed type hypersensitivity (DTH) a type IV hypersensitive response mediated by sensitized T lymphocytes. The response is characterized by the release of growth and differentiation factors in response to antigen with the recruitment and activation of macrophages. The response generally occurs within 48–72 hrs and manifests as chronic inflammatory lesions, granuloma formation, tuberculin reactivity, and contact hypersensitivity.

Dendritic cell a type of antigen-presenting cell that has long membrane processes resembling dendrites of nerve cells found in the lymph nodes, spleen, thymus, skin and other tissues.

Desensitization tolerance to an allergen or loss of sensitization to an antigen.

Determinant the portion of an antigen molecule that is recognized by a complementary section of an antibody or T-cell receptor.

Diapedesis the passage of cells through unruptured vessel walls into surrounding tissue.

Differentiation antigen a cell surface molecule identified by the use of specific antibodies which is found only at a particular developmental stage or on cells of a particular lineage.

Dinitrophenol (DNP) a commonly used hapten.

DiGeorge syndrome a congenital immunodeficiency syndrome characterized by the absence of a thymus, hypoparathyroidism, and cardiovascular anomalies. The absence of a thymus results in the absence of mature functional T cells and consequently an absence of cell-mediated immunity.

Diversity segment that portion of an immunoglobulin heavy-chain gene or T-cell receptor gene, situated between the V and J gene segments, that encodes part of the hypervariable or complementarity determining regions and therefore is critical in determining specificity.

Domains the homologous structural units into which the immunoglobulin heavy and light chains are organized. Each unit consists of about 110 amino acids and an intrachain disulfide loop of about 60 amino acids that is folded into a three-dimensional structure known as the immunoglobulin fold.

E Rosette a human T lymphocyte surrounded by a cluster, or rosette, of red blood cells.

Edema an abnormal accumulation of fluid in intercellular spaces. Often results as a failure of the lymphatic system to drain off normal leakage in capillaries.

Effector cells cells capable of mediating an immune function, such as cell-mediated cytotoxicity.

Endogenous originating within the organism or cell.

ELISA enzyme-linked immunosorbent assay. An assay in which antibody or antigen can be quantitated by using an enzyme-linked antibody and a colored substrate to measure the activity of the bound enzyme.

Endocytosis a process by which cells ingest extracellular macromolecules by enclosing the macromolecule by a small portion of the plasma membrane which invaginates and then pinches off to form an intracellular vesicle containing the ingested material.

Endosome a series of compartments in which endocytosed macromolecules must pass on their way to lysosomes.

Endotoxins lipopolysaccharides found in the cell walls of gram-negative bacteria that are responsible for many of the pathogenic effects associated with these organisms.

Enhancement prolonged graft survival by pre-exposure to donor's tissues.

Eosinophil a granulocyte present at less than 5% of peripheral leukocytes, containing granules of cationic proteins which may modulate an inflammatory reaction.

Epitope the antigenic determinant or antigen site that interacts with an antibody or T-cell receptor.

Epstein-Barr virus (EBV) the causative agent of Burkitt's lymphoma and infectious mononucleosis; it can transform human B cells into stable cell lines.

Equilibrium dialysis measures the affinity of a monovalent antigen and its antibody.

Equivalence a measure of the proportion of antibody to antigen which yields the maximum precipitate in liquids and gels.

Erythema redness produced in localized inflammatory reactions caused by the movement of erythrocytes into tissue spaces when capillary dilation or rupture occurs.

Erythroblastosis fetalis a condition involving hemolysis due to the production of maternal antibodies against the Rh antigens on the erythrocytes of the fetus.

Erythropoiesis the generation of red blood cells.

Exon a continuous segment of DNA that encodes part of a gene product.

Exotoxins pathogenic proteins secreted by gram-positive and gram-negative bacteria.

Exudate fluid with a high content of protein, salts and cellular debris which accumulates extravascularly, usually as a result of inflammation.

Fab fragment a monovalent antigen-binding fragment of an immunoglobulin obtained by papain digestion that is composed of the light chain and part of the heavy chain.

F(ab')$_2$ fragment a bivalent antigen-binding fragment of an immunoglobulin obtained by pepsin digestion that contains both light chains and part of both heavy chains.

Fc fragment the crystallizable, non-antigen binding portion of an immunoglobulin molecule derived from digestion with papain. Contains the carboxy-terminal portion of heavy chains and the binding sites for Fc receptors on cells and the C1q component of complement.

Fc receptor Cellular membrane receptor specific for the Fc portion of certain classes of immunoglobulin. Found on some lymphocytes, mast cells, macrophage/monocytes and other accessory cells.

Flare a diffuse area of redness on the skin caused by local vasodilation.

Fibroblast a cell present in connective tissue that plays an important role in wound healing by producing collagen and other materials that lie between the cells of connective tissue.

Fluorescein isothiocyanate (FITC) a green fluorescent

dye or fluorochrome used to conjugate with antibodies and other proteins.

Fluorescent antibody an antibody conjugated to a fluorochrome.

Framework regions relatively conserved sequences of amino acids located on either side of the CDRs in heavy and light chain variable regions of immunoglobulin. It is the conserved sequence of the framework region that generates the basic β pleated sheet structure of the V_H and V_L domains.

GALT gut-associated lymphoid tissue, including palatine tonsils, Peyer's patches, the appendix, and lymphocytes in the submucosa.

Gamma globulins serum proteins (immunoglobulins) which show the greatest electrophoretic mobility towards the negative (cathode) electrode.

Genome the total genetic material contained in the haploid set of chromosomes.

Genotype the combined genetic material inherited from both parents: also, the alleles present at one or more specific loci.

Gene locus the specific location of a gene on a chromosome.

Germinal center a region within lymph nodes and the spleen populated mostly by proliferating B cells.

Germ line the unmodified genetic material that is transmitted from one generation to the next through the gametes.

Giant cells large, multinucleate cells often seen in granulomatous reactions that result from the fusion of macrophages.

Glomerulonephritis inflammation of the capillary loops in the renal glomeruli that often occurs as a result of immune complex deposition.

Graft versus host reaction a reaction that develops when a graft contains immunocompetent T cells that recognize and attack the host cells.

Granulocyte any of the myeloid cells (eosinophils, basophils, and neutrophils) characterized by the presence of cytoplasmic granules.

Granulopoiesis the formation of mature granulocytes from their precursors.

Granuloma a tumor-like mass or nodule of granulation tissue containing lymphocytes, multinucleate giant cells, activated macrophages (epithelioid cells), and fibroblasts that arises due to a chronic inflammatory response associated with an infectious disease or antigen persistence in tissues.

H-2 major histocompatibility complex of the mouse.

Haplotype a set of alleles present on one parental chromosome.

Hapten a compound of low molecular weight that is not immunogenic by itself but that, when coupled to a larger carrier molecule, can elicit antibodies directed against the hapten.

Heavy chain the larger polypeptide of an immunoglobulin molecule, composed of one variable region and three to four constant regions. The isotype of the antibody is determined by the constant regions.

Helper T cells a subclass of T lymphocytes that, when activated by antigen presenting cells, release growth and differentiation factors which enhance both cell-mediated and humoral immune responses.

Hemagglutinin a molecule capable of causing agglutination of red blood cells.

Hematopoiesis generation or development of red and white blood cells.

Heterologous (xenogeneic) originating from a different species.

HLA (human leukocyte antigen) the human major histocompatibility complex.

Hinge region a region of the immunoglobulin heavy chains between the Fc and Fab regions which gives flexibility to the molecule allowing the two binding sites to function independently.

Histamine an amine found in basophil and mast cell granules that causes a vasoactive effect in surrounding tissues when released following degranulation.

Histocompatible acceptance of grafts between individuals matching in major histocompatibility antigens.

High endothelial venule (HEV) an area of capillary venule comprised of specialized cells with a plump, cuboidal ("high") shape through which lymphocytes migrate to enter various lymphoid organs.

Humoral refers to extracellular fluid including the plasma and lymph. Humoral immunity refers to immunity that can be transferred by antibodies present in the plasma, lymph, and tissue fluids.

Homologous originating from the same source or species. Also refers to similarity in amino acid sequences between molecules.

HTLV (human t lymphotrophic virus) a retrovirus which infects human CD4$^+$ T cells and causes adult T cell leukemia.

HIV (human immunodeficiency virus) a retrovirus that infects human CD4$^+$ T cells and causes acquired immunodeficiency syndrome (AIDS).

Host the recipient of a graft, implant or transplant derived from another organism.

hnRNA (heterogeneous nuclear RNA) nuclear RNA which contains the primary transcripts of DNA prior to processing to form mRNA.

Humoral immunity immunity that can be transferred by antibodies present in the plasma, lymph, and tissue fluids.

Hybridoma a cell line derived by fusion of a lymphocyte and a tumor cell. In the production of monoclonal antibodies, B cells are fused with myeloma cells. The resulting hybridoma continues to secrete the antibody of the normal B cell but retains the immortal growth properties of the cancerous myeloma cell. T-cell hybridomas can also be produced by fusing normal T cells with cancerous T cells.

Hypersensitivity exaggerated immune response causing damage to the individual. Types I, II, and III are mediated by antibody, while Type IV is mediated by T cells.

Hypervariable regions amino acid sequences within the variable regions of heavy and light immunoglobulin chains and of the T cell receptor which show the most variability and contribute most to the antigen-binding site. Synonymous with complementarity determining regions (CDRs).

Idiotope a single antigenic determinant of the variable region of an antibody or T cell receptor.

Idiotype set of antigenic determinants (idiotopes) of the immunoglobulin or T cell receptor variable regions.

Immune complex a macromolecular complex of antibody bound to antigen, sometimes including components of the complement system. Precipitation of macromolecules may occur resulting in immune complex disease (Type III hypersensitivity).

Immunogen a substance capable of eliciting an immune response. All immunogens are antigens; however some antigens, such as haptens, are not immunogens.

Immunization the process of rendering a state of immunity. Active immunity may occur with inoculation of a specific antigen, while passive immunity may result from administration of specific antibodies from immune individuals.

Immunoadsorption removal of antibody or antigen from a sample by precipitation with a complementary antigen or antibody or by adsorption to a solid-phase system to which the antibody or antigen is bound.

Immunocompetent cell a cell capable of participating in an immune response.

Immunoglobulin (Ig) antibody.

Immunoglobulin fold the conserved homologous structure of the domains that consists of a sandwich of two β pleated sheets, each containing three or four antiparallel β strands of amino acids, stabilized by the intrachain 60 amino acids disulfide bond.

Immunoglobulin superfamily proteins containing domains that resemble an immunoglobulin domain including the T-cell receptor and MHC membrane molecules. The high degree of conservation in amino acid sequences among this family indicates a probable ancestral relation among these genes.

Inflammation a tissue response to injury or other trauma characterized by pain, heat, redness, and swelling. The response consists of altered patterns of blood flow, an influx of phagocytic and other immune cells, removal of the foreign antigen, and healing of the damaged tissue.

Innate immunity natural, nonspecific host defenses that exist prior to exposure to a specific antigen.

Intron noncoding gene segments which separate exons or coding regions. Introns are initially transcribed in the primary transcript but are removed by RNA splicing during formation of mRNA.

Interferons (IFN) a family of glycoproteins produced by a variety of cell types that induce an antiviral state in cells and help to regulate the immune response. Interferon alpha (IFN-α) is derived from various leukocytes, interferon beta (IFN-β) is derived from fibroblasts and interferon gamma (IFN-γ) is produced by T lymphocytes.

Interleukins (IL) a group of low molecular weight proteins (cytokines) secreted by leukocytes that function as growth and differentiation factors.

Insulin a hormone produced by the beta cells of the Islets of Langerhans of the pancreas, which regulates carbohydrate, lipid and amino acid metabolism.

Insulitis cellular infiltration of the pancreatic Islets of Langerhans resulting in inflammation seen in the early stages of insulin dependent diabetes mellitus.

In vitro refers to experiments involving living cells or cellular components performed outside the body.

In vivo refers to experiments carried out in a living organism.

Internal image a site on some anti-idiotypic antibodies (Ab-2) that binds to the paratope of the antibody (Ab-1) and mimics the original antigen. Since the internal image idiotope stimulates immune responses reactive to the antigen, it may be immunogenically substituted for the foreign antigen.

Ir gene immune response genes, which determine T-cell responsiveness to a particular antigen and map within the class II region of the MHC.

Isotype usually refers to antibody class (e.g., IgM, IgG, IgA, IgD, and IgE). Each isotype is encoded by a separate immunoglobulin constant region gene sequence that is carried by all members of a species.

Isotypic determinants antigenic determinants specific for an immunoglobulin class or subclass within a species.

Isotype switch genetic rearrangement of heavy chain constant region genes in antibody-producing B lymphocytes resulting in conversion of one antibody class (isotype) to another.

Isograft graft between genetically identical individuals.

J chain a polypeptide that joins or links subunits of polymeric IgA and IgM.

J gene joining gene segment encoding part of the variable region of the immunoglobulin light and heavy chains and the heterodimers of the T-cell receptor. J gene segments are recombined during differentiation of B cells and T cells.

Kappa κ chain one of two immunoglobulin light chain isotypes.

K (killer) cell a lymphoid cell bearing Fc receptors, but lacking B and T cell differentiating antigens, which destroys target cells by antibody-dependent cell-mediated cytotoxicity (ADCC).

Kaposi's sarcoma a neoplastic lesion common in individuals afflicted with AIDS, characterized by multiple bluish nodules in the skin and hemorrhages.

Karyotype the chromosomal constitution of a given cell.

Kuppfer cells fixed macrophages which line the blood sinuses of the liver and act as antigen presenting cells.

Kinins inflammatory peptides released during an inflammatory response which act as vasodilators inducing smooth muscle contraction and increased vascular permeability.

LAK cell lymphokine-activated killer cell.

Lambda chain one of two immunoglobulin light chain isotypes.

Langerhans cell a type of dendritic cell found in the skin, bearing Fc receptors and class II MHC antigens, that serves as an antigen-presenting cell.

Large granular lymphocytes (LGLs) lymphoid cells that are defined by morphological criteria, containing large cytoplasmic lysosomes, that may serve as natural killer (NK) or killer (K) cells.

Lectins a group of proteins, usually derived from plants, which specifically bind sugars and oligosaccharides present on the membrane glycoproteins of animal cells. Certain lectins, such as concanavalin A (Con A) and phytohemagglutinin (PHA), are also mitogenic.

Leukemia cancer originating in any class of hemopoietic cells that tends to proliferate as single cells within the lymph or blood.

Leukocyte "white cell," refers to any blood cell that is not an erythrocyte.

Leukocyte functional antigens (LFAs) a family of molecules (LFA-1, LFA-2, and LFA-3) that mediate intercellular adhesion.

Leukopenia reduction in the number of circulating white blood cells.

Leukotrienes mediators of type I hypersensitivity formed as the mast cell or blood basophil undergoes degranulation. The leukotrienes are metabolic products of arachidonic acid produced by the lipoxygenase pathway.

Ligand a molecule recognized by a receptor structure.

Light chain the smaller of the two polypeptides present in immunoglobulin molecules. Two light chains of the same isotype are found in each immunoglobulin, each possessing one variable and one constant region.

Linkage disequilibrium the situation in which two alleles occur together at a greater frequency than is expected from the product of their individual frequencies.

Lipopolysaccharides (LPS) gram negative bacterial endotoxins that have mitogenic and inflammatory effects.

Locus chromosomal location of a gene.

Ly markers a group of cell surface markers on murine lymphocytes. These are now more commonly referred to by their CD designation.

Lymph the intercellular tissue fluid which circulates through the lymphatic vessels.

Lymphadenopathy enlargement of the lymph nodes.

Lymph nodes small secondary lymphoid organs containing populations of lymphocytes, macrophages, and dendritic cells which serve as sites of filtration of foreign antigen and activation of lymphocytes.

Lymphoid pertaining to cells of the lymphoid series.

Lymphokines a generic term for cytokines produced by activated lymphocytes, especially T cells, that act as intercellular mediators of the immune response.

Lymphokine activated killer cells (LAK) killer and natural killer cells which, when activated by IL-2, exhibit more effective killing of their target cells.

Lymphoma a cancer of lymphoid cells that tends to proliferate as solid tumors.

Lymphopoiesis the differentiation of lymphocytes from hematopoietic stem cells.

Lymphotoxin (LT) tumor necrosis factor beta (TNF-β) produced by activated T cells.

Lysogeny process in which the phage genome is associated with the bacterial genome in a way that allows the virus to remain unexpressed or latent.

Lysosomes cytoplasmic granules found in many types of cells, containing hydrolytic enzymes, which play an important role in the digestion of phagocytosed materials.

Lysozyme a crystalline, basic enzyme found in tears, saliva, egg white, and nasal secretions which digests mucopeptides of bacterial cell walls and therefore acts as a nonspecific antibacterial agent.

Lytic pathway the complement pathway which leads to the formation of C5-C9, the membrane attack complex.

MHC (major histocompatibility complex) a complex of genes encoding cell-surface molecules that are responsible for rapid graft rejection and are required for antigen presentation to T cells.

Macrophage a large, myeloid cell derived from monocytes that can function as a phagocytic cell, antigen-presenting cell, and as a cytotoxic cell in ADCC.

Macrophage-activating factor (MAF) a lymphokine that augments the cytotoxic and phagocytic functions of macrophages.

Malignant tumors which have the capacity to invade and alter the normal tissue.

Marginal zone a B cell rich area in the periarteriolar lymphoid sheath of the spleen containing lymphoid follicles that can develop into germinal centers.

Margination adhesion of leukocytes to blood vessel endothelium; occurs normally and is more pronounced in the early stages of inflammation.

Mast cell a bone marrow derived cell found in tissues. It resembles peripheral blood basophils and bears Fc receptors for IgE. Upon antigen crosslinkage of the bound IgE, the mast cell degranulates, releasing histamines and other mediators.

Medulla the innermost or central region of an organ.

Megakaryocyte a white blood cell which produces platelets via cytoplasmic budding.

Membrane attack complex (MAC) complex of complement components C5–C9 formed by the lytic pathway creating a membrane pore in target cells.

Memory (immunologic) a characteristic of a specific immunological response in which secondary exposure to a given antigen produces a faster and greater response.

Memory cells clonally expanded progeny of T and B cells formed following a primary antigenic response. It is responsible for the speed and heightened levels of the secondary immunological response.

Metastasis in tumors refers to the tendency of cells to detach from the primary tumor and migrate to a secondary site.

MHC restriction the requirement that T cells recognize antigen only when antigenic peptides are displayed in association with self MHC molecules.

Migration-inhibition factor (MIF) a lymphokine which inhibits macrophage movement and is involved in delayed-type hypersensitivity.

Mitogen any substance that non-specifically induces DNA synthesis and cell division.

Mixed lymphocyte reaction (MLR) T cell proliferation induced in response to cells expressing allogeneic MHC molecules.

Minor histocompatibility antigens antigens encoded by genes outside of the MHC complex that contribute to graft rejection.

Monoclonal derived from a single cell.

Monoclonal antibody homogeneous antibody produced by a clone of hybridoma cells.

Monocyte a mononuclear, myeloid phagocytic cell which circulates briefly in the bloodstream before migrating to the tissues to become a macrophage.

Monokine cytokine secreted by activated monocytes or macrophages.

Mucosal-associated lymphoid tissue (MALT) lymphoid tissue found in the mucosa of the respiratory and gastrointestinal tracts.

Multiple myeloma a cancer of the immunoglobulin secreting plasma cell characterized by uncontrolled proliferation of plasma cells and high levels of immunoglobulin in serum and urine.

Myeloma protein the antibodies produced by myeloma cells.

Murine pertaining to mice.

NK (natural killer cell) a large, granular lymphocyte having cytotoxic ability. The cell lacks immunoglobulin or T-cell receptors but can recognize and destroy some tumor cells without MHC restriction.

Necrosis death of individual cells or groups of cells, leading to disruption and atropy of tissue.

Neoplasm new or abnormal growth, a benign or malignant tumor.

Neoplasia generation of a neoplasm, often refers to uncontrolled cell proliferation.

Network theory theory proposing that the immune system is regulated by a network of idiotype and anti-idiotype reactions involving antibodies and T-cell receptors.

Neutrophil a circulating, phagocytic granulocyte involved in early inflammatory responses. It possesses Fc receptors and can participate in antibody-dependent cell-mediated cytotoxicity (ADCC).

Nude mouse homozygous genetic defect *(nu/nu)* carried by an inbred mouse strain that results in an absence of a thymus and consequently a marked deficiency in T lymphocytes. The mice are also hairless, hence their name.

Null cells a small group of peripheral blood lymphocytes that fail to express the membrane molecules characteristic of T and B cells. Included in this group are the natural killer cells that participate in ADCC.

NZB/NZW related mouse strains displaying autoimmunity that serves as an animal model for systemic lupus erythematosus.

Oncogene genes whose products are capable of causing cellular transformation. Oncogenes derived from viruses are denoted v-onc, while their cellular counterparts, or protooncogenes, are denoted c-onc.

Oncofetal antigen an antigen that is present during fetal development but generally is absent in adult tissues. The antigen is also expressed by tumor cells.

Oncogenic causing cancer.

Opsonin a substance, such as an antibody or C3b, which binds to an antigen and enhances phagocytosis.

Opsonization deposition of opsonins on the antigen promoting a stable, adhesive contact with the appropriate phagocyte.

Ouchterlony technique immunoprecipitation technique involving the diffusion of antigen and antibody within a gel, forming a visible band of precipitation in the region of equivalence.

Papain proteolytic enzyme used to obtain Fab and Fc fragments in the hydrolysis of immunoglobulin.

PAF (platelet activating factor) A substance released by basophils and mast cells that causes aggregation and lysis of platelets.

Paratope an idiotope or antigenic site on an antibody or a T-cell receptor involved in binding to the epitope of an antigen.

Passive cutaneous anaphylaxis (PCA) In vivo technique to determine antigen-specific IgE responsible for immediate type I hypersensitivity reactions.

Passive immunity immune protection conferred by the transfer of immune products, such as antibody or sensitized T cells, produced by another individual.

PAGE polyacrylamide gel electrophoresis.

Patching cross-linkage and reorganization of membrane molecules into patches or clumps.

Pathogen a disease-causing organism.

PBL peripheral blood lymphocytes.

PFCs (plaque-forming cells) antibody-forming cells observed in vitro by their ability to lyse antigen-sensitized erythrocytes in the presence of complement, forming hemolytic plaques.

Pepsin proteolytic enzyme used to obtain $F(ab')_2$ and smaller peptide fragments of the Fc fragment in the hydrolysis of immunoglobulin.

Perforin cytolytic product of CTL cells which, in the presence of Ca^{2+}, polymerizes to form transmembrane pores in target cells.

Peyer's patches lymphoid nodules along the small intestine which function to trap antigens from the gastrointestinal tract and provide sites where mature, immunocompetent lymphocytes can interact with the antigen.

PHA (phytohemagglutinin) a plant lectin derived from kidney beans which is a potent T cell mitogen.

Phagocyte cells which engulf cellular and particulate matter, including monocytes/macrophages and neutrophils.

Phagosome intracellular vacuole containing ingested particulate materials; formed by invagination of the cell membrane during phagocytosis.

Phagolysosome product of the fusion of a lysosome and a phagosome. Ingested material in the phagosome is digested by degradative enzymes of the lysosome.

Phylogeny the evolutionary history of a species.

Pinocytosis a type of endocytosis in which a cell ingests extracellular fluid and soluble materials contained within that fluid.

Plasma the cell-free, fluid portion of the blood which contains all clotting factors.

Plasma cell differentiated antibody-producing cell derived from an activated B cell.

Plasmacytoma a plasma cell tumor.

Plasmapheresis a technique in which plasma is removed from a patient's blood by continuous-flow centrifugation. The red blood cells are then resuspended in a suitable medium and returned to the patient.

Platelet (thrombocyte) a small anuclear membrane bound cytoplasmic structure derived from megakaryocytes, containing vasoactive substances and clotting factors important in blood coagulation, inflammation, and allergic reactions.

Pokeweed mitogen (PWM) a lectin derived from pokeweeds that acts as a B cell mitogen.

Polyclonal the products of many different clones of lymphocytes.

Polymorphism presence of multiple alleles at a specific gene locus.

Primary immune response the initial cellular and humoral immune response to antigen exposure, comprised largely of IgM immunoglobulins and sensitized T cells.

Primary lymphoid organs organs in which lymphocytes mature to become antigenically committed, immunocompetent cells. In mammals the bone marrow and thymus are primary lymphoid organs, allowing maturation of B cells and T cells, respectively.

Private specificity antigenic specificity on an MHC molecule that is unique to a particular haplotype.

Properdin factor P.

Prophylaxis a vaccine or other preventive treatment.

Prostaglandins biologically active lipid derivatives of arachidonic acid which modulate the inflammatory response by inhibiting platelet aggregation, increasing vascular permeability, and inducing contraction of smooth muscles.

Protein A a protein derived from the Cowan strain of *Staphylococcus aureus* which binds to the Fc region of some IgG molecules. Protein A can be used to detect IgG.

Proto-oncogene the normal cellular counterparts of viral oncogenes.

Prozone effect the absence of immune precipitation or agglutination due to an excess of antibody compared to antigen.

Pseudogenes genes that are stable components of the genome but are incapable of being expressed. They are thought to have been derived by mutation of an ancestral active gene.

Public specificity antigenic determinant on an MHC molecule that is common to the many allelic forms of a particular MHC molecule.

Pyrogens fever-causing substances released by activated white blood cells.

Pyogenic pus producing.

Qa antigens class I MHC murine antigens encoded by a region within the Tla complex.

Reagin IgE antibody that mediate type I immediate hypersensitivity reactions.

Receptor cellular structure found on the cell membrane which has high affinity for particular proteins or peptides.

Recombinational diversity generation of diversity by the joining of DNA segments from different sets of genes.

Respiratory burst increase in oxidative metabolism of macrophages following phagocytosis.

Reticuloendothelial system (RES) a collective term for the diffuse system of phagocytic cells associated with the connective tissue throughout most of the body.

Retrovirus a type of RNA virus which uses a reverse transcriptase to produce a DNA copy of its genome.

Rheumatoid factor autoantibody found in the serum of individuals with rheumatoid arthritis and other connective tissue diseases.

RIA radioimmunoassay.

Ricin a potent toxin derived from castor bean seeds which can be conjugated to monoclonal antibodies to form an immunotoxin.

Sarcoma tumor of supporting or connective tissue.

Secondary response more rapid and heightened immune response that occurs following second exposure to an antigen.

Second-set graft rejection acute, rapid rejection of an allograft in an individual immunized by a previous graft.

Secretory IgA dimeric IgA linked to a secretory component that is found in mucous secretions.

Secretory component an epithelial cell derived protein derived from a poly Ig receptor that binds to dimeric IgA and pentameric IgM and transports the immunoglobulin across the mucous membrane. A part of the poly Ig receptor is released as the secretory component associated with the dimeric IgA or pentameric IgM in the mucous secretions.

Sensitized lymphocytes lymphocytes that, when exposed to antigen, respond and clonally expand, generating an immune response.

Serum fluid portion of the blood which is free of cells and clotting factors.

Serum sickness type III hypersensitivity reaction that develops when antigen is administered intravenously, resulting in large amounts of antigen-antibody complexes. The deposition of the immune complexes at various sites leads to vasculitis, glomerulonephritis, and rheumatoid arthritis. Serum sickness often develops when individuals are immunized with antiserum derived from another species.

sIg surface immunoglobulin.

SLE systemic lupus erythematosus.

Slow-reacting substance of anaphylaxis (SRS-A) leukotrienes derived from mast cells and basophils which are potent bronchoconstrictors, causing smooth muscle contraction.

Somatic hypermutation a mechanism by which B cells increase antibody diversity by introducing point mutations into rearranged immunoglobulin variable region genes.

Southern blot technique using electrophoretic separation of DNA fragments, transfer or blotting of ssDNA to a suitable filter, and hybridization of the separated ssDNA fragments with a complementary radioactive nucleic acid probe.

Specificity capacity for discrimination between antigenic determinants by antibody or lymphocyte receptor.

Stem cell cell from which differentiated cells derive.

Syngeneic genetically identical members of the same species.

T cell lymphocytes that are dependent upon the thymus for their differentiation and possess a rearranged T cell receptor.

T-cell receptor (TCR) surface antigen-recognition molecule of T lymphocytes, consisting of either an $\alpha\beta$ heterodimer or a $\gamma\delta$ heterodimer; associated with CD3 molecules on mature T cells.

T dependent antigen antigen dependent upon the presence of helper T cells in eliciting an immune response.

T independent antigen antigen which may be affected by, but is not dependent upon, the presence of T helper cells in eliciting an antibody response.

Thy-1 (Theta antigen) glycoprotein present on the surface of most thymocytes and peripheral T cells.

Thymocyte developing T cells that are present in the thymus.

Thymosin thymic hormone.

Thymus lymphoid organ in the thoracic cavity which is the site of T-cell maturation.

Titer a term used to denote the relative strength of an antiserum. The titer is the reciprocal of the last dilution of an antiserum capable of mediating some measurable effect such as precipitation or agglutination.

Tolerance state of induced immunological unresponsiveness.

Tolerogen substance which may induce a state of immunological tolerance.

Toxoid toxin that has been altered to eliminate its toxicity but retains its immunogenicity.

Transformation refers to the change in a normal cell as it becomes malignant.

Tuberculin crude protein fraction isolated from supernatants of *Mycobacterium tuberculosis* cultures.

Tumor-associated antigens cell-membrane antigens found on tumor cells also on normal cells.

Tumor necrosis factors (TNFα and TNFβ) two related cytokines produced by macrophages (TNFα) and some T cells (TNFβ). Both cytokines were named for the cytotoxic effect that they have on tumor cells but not on normal cells. In addition, both TNFs act on a variety of cells inducing a myriad of inflammatory effects.

Tumor-specific *antigens* cell membrane antigens found on tumor cells but not on normal cells.

V genes genes that in combination with J genes or DJ genes encode the variable regions of immunoglobulins and T cell receptors.

V region amino terminal amino acid sequence of an antibody or T-cell receptor that shows many sequence differences between antibodies or TCRs of different specificities; responsible for antigenic specificity of light and heavy chain immunoglobulin and T-cell receptors.

Vaccine preparation of antigenic material used to induce immunity against pathogenic agents.

Vaccination intentional introduction of a harmless or less harmful version of a pathogen to induce a specific immunological response that protects the individual against a later exposure to the pathogen.

Variola smallpox.

Vasculitis inflammation of the blood vessels.

Virulence a measure of the infectious ability of a pathogen.

Western blot detection of protein antigens that have been electrophoretically separated and transferred to a filter such as nitrocellulose by labeling the antigenic bands with radioactive or enzyme-conjugated antibodies.

Wheal and flare a reaction characteristic of type I immediate hypersensitivity in the skin, involving a sharply delineated swelling of the skin (wheal) with surrounding redness (flare).

White pulp periarteriolar sheaths containing myeloid cells and lymphocytes of the spleen.

Xenogeneic relationship between individuals of different species.

Xenograft graft or tissue transplanted from one species to another.

Answers to Study Questions

Chapter 1

1.

Statement	Humoral	Cell-mediated
a. Involves class I MHC molecules		x
b. Most likely responds to viral infection		x
c. Involves T helper cells	x	x
d. Involves processed antigen	x	x
e. Most likely responds to an organ transplant		x
f. Involves T cytotoxic cells		x
g. Involves B cells	x	
h. Involves CD8		x
i. Most likely responds to bacterial infection	x	
j. Involves secreted antibody	x	

2. The secondary immune response involves an amplified population of memory cells. The response is more rapid and achieves higher levels than the primary response.
3. Clonal selection accounts for the amplified number of antigen-reactive memory cells that characterize the secondary response.
4. Only antigen activated T_H cells express a membrane receptor for IL-2.
5. (a) Both antibody and the T-cell receptors display fine specificity for antigen, and subtle modifications in an antigen prohibit its binding to antibody or the T-cell's receptor. The MHC molecules do not possess such fine specificity, and a variety of unrelated peptide antigens can be bound by the same MHC molecule. (b) Antibody is expressed only on cells of the B-cell lineage; the T-cell receptor is expressed by cells of the T-cell lineage; the class I MHC molecule is expressed by virtually all nucleated cells; the class II MHC molecule is expressed only by specialized cells that function as antigen presenting cells (e.g., B cells, macrophages, and dendritic cells). (c) Antibody can bind to protein or polysaccharide antigens; the T cell receptors recognize only peptides associated with molecules of the MHC; the MHC molecules bind only processed peptides.

Chapter 2

1. (a) The genomic clone contains intervening sequences (introns) that are removed during processing of the primary transcript and therefore do not encode the protein product. (b) DNA must be microinjected into a fertilized egg so that the DNA (transgene) will be passed on to all daughter cells. (c) Primary lymphoid cultures have a finite life span and contain a heterogeneous population of cells.
2.

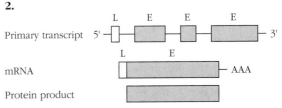

3. Because the transfected DNA integrates into a small percentage of cells, a selection marker needs to be included so that only cells in which the DNA has integrated will grow.
4. The mouse would become a mosaic in which the transgene would have incorporated into some of the somatic cells but not all.
5.

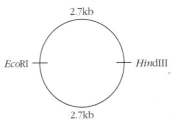

6. Isolate mRNA from activated T cells and transcribe into cDNA using reverse transcriptase. Insert cDNA into a suitable expression vector, such as plasmid DNA carrying an ampicillin selection gene. Transfer the recombinant plasmid DNA into *E. coli* and grow in the presence of ampicillin to select for bacteria containing the plasmid DNA. Test the bacterial culture supernatant for the presence of IL-2 by seeing if the monoclonal antibody to IL-2 reacts with the culture supernatent. Once a bacterial culture is identified that is secreting IL-2, the cDNA can be cloned.

Chapter 3

1. (a) Paracortical areas, follicles, and germinal centers; (b) Paracortical areas; (c) Since the T_H cell is needed for B-cell activation, there will be no areas of rapidly proliferating cells within the thymus; (d) Follicles and germinal centers.

2. They have receptors for M-CSF. If the cell also secreted M-CSF, it could autostimulate its own proliferation.

3. The primary lymphoid organs are the bone marrow in mammals (bursa of Fabricus in birds) and the thymus. These organs function as sites for B cell (bone marrow) or T-cell (thymus) maturation.

4. The secondary lymphoid organs are the spleen, lymph nodes, Peyer's patches, tonsils, adenoids, appendix. These organs function to trap antigen and provide sites for lymphocytes to interact with the antigen and undergo clonal selection.

5. These cells secrete thymic hormones that are necessary for thymocyte maturation into functional T cells within the thymus. These cells also display high levels of class I and class II MHC molecules which are recognized by the maturing thymocytes during positive and negative selection in the thymus.

6. Antigenic commitment is the random rearrangements of genes encoding the T-cell's receptor or B cell's immunoglobulin receptor. This process enables each mature B or T cell to express a single receptor specificity, and therefore the cell is committed to respond to a single antigenic specificity. Antigenic committment takes place in the primary lymphoid organs (bone marrow and thymus). Antigen is not involved in this process. The mature, antigenically committed T or B cells leave the primary lymphoid organs and are carried to secondary lymphoid organs, such as the spleen and lymph nodes. Here antigen interaction stimulates clonal selection into a population of memory cells and effector cells. The long lived memory cells are responsible for immunological memory.

7. The increased expression of ICAM's on vascular endothelial cells facilitates adherence of leukocytes to the blood vessel wall and thus increases the extravasation of leukocytes into the tissue spaces to sites of immune activation.

8. If the pluripotent stem cell was being successively enriched in the bone marrow, then progressively fewer bone marrow cells would be able to restore hematopoiesis in the lethally X-irradiated mice. If the mice lived, then it indicated that the pluripotent stem cell was present. If the mice died, it indicated that the pluripotent stem cell had been lost during the enrichment process and was no longer present.

9. In a neonatal mouse, thymectomy will eliminate T cell maturation causing the mouse to be immunodeficient and die. In an adult mouse, thymectomy will not have a profound effect because many of the recirculating T cells have a long life span.

10. Use fluorescein and rhodamine tagged monoclonal antibodies specific for cell membrane markers of B cells (i.e., surface immunoglobulin) and T cells (i.e., T-cell receptor or CD3).

11. (a) Mouse A might have a defect in the vascular addres-

sins of the cervical lymph nodes. Lymphocytes are capable of homing to control lymph nodes but not to mouse A nodes. (b) Mouse B lymphocytes could possibly lack a homing receptor, and therefore the cells fail to home even to control lymph nodes. (c) To determine if either hypothesis is correct, use various F1-monoclonal antibodies specific for homing receptors and vascular addressins, and compare the level of staining of mouse A and B to the control mouse.

Chapter 4

1. (a) True; (b) True; (c) False: a hapten cannot stimulate an immune response unless it is conjugated to a larger protein carrier. However, the hapten can combine with pre-formed antibody specific for the hapten. (d) True; (e) False: a T cell can only recognize peptides that have been processed and presented by MHC molecules. These epitopes tend to be amphipathic and, therefore, often represent internal peptides. (f) True; (g) True; (h) False: Each MHC molecule binds a number of different peptides. It is not yet known what features various different peptides share in common that enable them to bind to the same MHC molecule; (i) False: internal viral proteins can be processed and displayed by MHC molecules and activate T_H or T_C cells; (j) False: it is likely that the MHC differences between the two strains will bind different sets of peptides. Therefore, what is immunogenic for one strain may not be immunogenic for another strain.

2. (a) The UV-inactivated vaccine would be processed as an exogeneous antigen. Exogeneous antigens are internalized through phagocytosis or endocytosis and enter the endosomal processing pathway. These antigens are then presented by class II MHC molecules on the membrane of antigen-presenting cells. (b) The attenuated virus replicates within the host cells and is, therefore, seen as an endogenous antigen. Endogenous antigens are processed within the cytoplasm or endoplasmic reticulum and are presented by class I MHC molecules on the membrane of any nucleated cell. Since T_C cells are generally CD8$^+$, they are class I MHC restricted. Therefore, the attenuated virus would be more likely to activate a T_C cell.

3. Generally, more amphipathic peptides are more likely to bind to MHC molecules and are therefore more likely to induce a T cell response. Even if a peptide binds to the MHC within a given animal, it is still possible that there will not be a response to the peptide if the animal does not have T cells responsive to the particular peptide/MHC.

4. L cells are not antigen-presenting cells and, therefore, do not express their own class II MHC molecules. The class II MHC genes were transfected into the L cells so that the T-cell response to various peptide/MHC combinations could be assessed without the complication of additional class II MHC molecules. Had the genes been transfected into a macrophage, then other IA or IE MHC molecules would also be expressed by the cell, and these class II MHC molecules might also bind the peptides.

5. See Table 4-4.

Chapter 5

1. (a) True; (b) True; (c) False: both IgM and IgD have identical V_H and V_L domains and, therefore, have the same specificity for antigen; (d) True; (e) False: multiple isotypes can appear on the surface of a B cell. The mature B cell expresses both IgM and IgD. Memory B cells can express additional isotypes such as IgG, IgA or IgE; (f) True; (g) True; (h) False: both heavy and light chain variable regions are approximately 110 amino acid residues; (i) False; secreted IgM is a pentamer. Because of its larger size and valency, it is able to crosslink antigens more effectively than IgG.

2. (a) The molecule would have the following structural features: H_2L_2 basic unit: 2 identical heavy chains and 2 identical light chains; H—H, H—L joined by disulfide bonds; and each chain is organized into a series of domains of approximately 110 amino acids, stabilized by an intra-domain disulfide bridge of about 60 amino acid residues; single C domain on light chains; several (3–4) C domains on heavy chain. The amino terminal domain of the heavy and light chains should show sequence variation. (b) Both the antisera to the whole human IgG and the human κ chain should cross-react with the new immunoglobulin class. Both antisera have antibodies specific for the light chain. The new isotype would be expected to contain either kappa or lambda light chains. (c) Reduce the interchain disulfide bonds of the new isotype with mercaptoethanol and alkylation. Separate the heavy and light chains. Immunize a rabbit with the heavy chain. The rabbit antisera should only react with the new isotype but not with any other known isotypes.

3. Advantages of IgG compared to IgM are: (1) its ability to cross the placenta and protect the developing fetus; (2) the higher serum concentration of IgG allows larger numbers of antibodies to bind to antigens, neutralizing the antigen and increasing antigen clearance through opsonization; and (3) its smaller size enables it to diffuse more readily into intercellular tissue fluids. The disadvantages of IgG compared to IgM are: (1) it lacks multivalency and therefore is less able to agglutinate antigens and (2) it is less able to activate the complement system.

4. (a) See Figure 5-4. (b) Draw as a dimer containing α heavy chains. Add J chain protein and the secretory component. (c) Draw as a pentamer containing μ heavy chains. The μ heavy chain has 5 domains and no hinge region. The extra C_H domain replaces the hinge. Add J chain protein. IgM has additional interchain disulfide bonds joining the pentamer subunits to one another and to the J chain.

5.

Property	Whole IgG	H chain	L chain	Fab	F(ab')2	Fc
Binds antigen	+	Weak +	Weak +	+	+	−
Bivalent antigen binding	+	−	−	−	+	−
Monovalent antigen binding	−	+	+	+	−	−

Property	Whole IgG	H chain	L chain	Fab	F(ab')2	Fc
Fixes complement in presence of antigen	+	−	−	−	−	−
Has V domains	+	+	+	+	+	−
Has C domains	+	+	+	+	+	+

6. (a) Anti-allotype antibodies; (b) Anti-idiotype antibodies; (c) Anti-isotype antibodies; (d) Anti-allotype antibodies; (e) No antibodies will be formed.

7.

	Rabbit antisera to mouse antibody component				
	γ chain	κ chain	IgG Fab fragment	IgG Fc fragment	J chain
Mouse γ chain	Yes	No	Yes	Yes	No
Mouse κ chain	No	Yes	Yes	No	No
Mouse IgM whole	No	Yes	Yes	No	Yes
Mouse IgG-Fc fragment	Yes	No	No	Yes	No

8. The hypervariable regions are located in the V_H and V_L domains. There are 3 hypervariable regions in the V_H domain and 3 in the V_L domain. They comprise the major amino acids of the antigen binding cleft.

9. (a) Domains of approximately 110 amino acid residues in length. Stabilization of domain by intra-domain disulfide bridge formed by two conserved cysteine residues about 60 amino acid residues apart. Immunoglobulin fold (2 antiparallel β-pleated sheets, each composed of 3–4 β strands separated by short loops of variable sequences. (b) These proteins are members of the immunoglobulin superfamily. The domain structure is thought to facilitate interaction between the faces of the β-sheets, allowing members of this family of molecules to bind to each other.

10. The antiserum also contained antibodies to the kappa and lambda light chains. The technician needs to reduce the interchain disulfide bonds with mercaptoethanol and isolate the heavy chain. If the technician immunizes the rabbits with

the heavy chains alone, the rabbit antisera will be specific for the IgG isotype.

11. IgA: 3, 6, 10, 11; IgD: 4; IgE: 2, 6, 9; IgG: 5, 12, 13; IgM: 1, 3, 4, 7, 8, 12, 13.

12.

Immunogen	Animal immunized	Antigenic determinant against which antibodies are produced
IgG from C57Bl/6 mouse	Balb/c mouse	Allotypic
IgG myeloma protein from C57Bl/6 mouse	C57Bl/6 mouse	Idiotypic
IgG from C57Bl/6 mouse	Rabbit	Isotypic

Chapter 6

1. (a) True; (b) True; (c) False: Fab fragments are monovalent and, therefore, cannot crosslink antigens; (d) True; (e) True; (f) True; (g) False: It is qualitative but not quantitative; (h) False: Agglutination tests are more sensitive.

2. Coat a microtiter plate with antigens from HIV. Add serum from a patient suspected of being infected with HIV. Incubate plate. Wash away unbound antibodies. Add a goat anti-human immunoglobulin reagent that has been conjugated with an enzyme. Incubate the plate and wash away unbound antibody. Add substrate and observe for a colored reaction.

3. (a) Use whole bovine serum as the antigen.

(b)

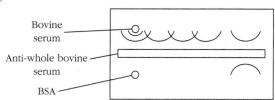

4. A: H1-C1
   B: H2-C2
   C: H2-C1
   D: H1-C2

5. ELISA assay and radioimmunoassay can both be used to determine the concentration of a hapten.

6. A: Fab fragment from an IgG myeloma protein ($\gamma 2\kappa 2$)
   B: γ heavy chain
   C: A mixture of γ heavy and κ light chains
   D: κ light chain
   E: λ light chain
   F: Fc from an IgG myeloma protein ($\gamma 2\lambda 2$)

7. Isolate heavy chains from known immunoglobulin isotypes (μ, γ, α, δ, ϵ). Use the isolated heavy chains to immunize a rabbit and produce antisera specific for each heavy chain class. Test each antisera for reaction with the myeloma protein X. The level of the myeloma protein could be determined by a Mancini radialimmunodiffusion assay or by a more sensitive assay, such as an ELISA.

8. (a) Rocket electrophoresis or Mancini radialimmunodiffusion; (b) ELISA or RIA assay; (c) RIA; (d) Fl-antibody to C3 component; (e) Agglutination of type-A RBCs; (f) Ouchterlony; (g) Fl-antibody to the syphilis spirochete.

9. (a) Antiserum #1 $K_0 = 1.0 \times 10^5$, Antiserum #2 $K_0 = 4.5 \times 10^6$, Antiserum #3 $K_0 = 4.5 \times 10^6$; (b) Each has a valence of 2; (c) Antisera 2 is monoclonal; (d) Antisera 2 would be best since it is a monoclonal, and therefore recognizes a single epitope on the hormone, and is therefore less likely to crossreact with other serum proteins.

10. (a) Tube #1 contained F(ab')$_2$ fragments; (b) Tube #2 contained Fab fragments; (c) Tube #3 contained intact antibody; (d) Tube #4 contained Fc fragments.

Chapter 7

1. (a) False: an HGPRT$^-$ myeloma cell lacks the enzyme to utilize hypoxanthine; (b) True; (c) True; (d) False: hypoxanthine allows cell growth by the salvage pathway; (e) False: the unfused revertant would grow in HAT medium making it impossible to select for the hybridomas.

2. Immortal growth to enable hybridoma to be cultured indefinitely; Ab$^-$ to ensure that the hybridoma only secretes antibody of plasma cell fusion partner. HGPRT$^-$ to ensure that unfused myeloma cells will be unable to grow.

3. You could not select for the hybridoma, since the fused and unfused cells would grow using the denovo pathway.

4. (a) The hybridoma formed by fusing the B lymphoma cells with a human myeloma was to produce a human hybridoma secreting the antibody of the B lymphoma cells. The mice were then immunized with this monoclonal antibody. The second hybridoma was formed by fusing the primed mouse spleen cells with mouse myeloma cells. The purpose of this hybridoma was to produce a monoclonal antibody specific for the idiotype of the antibody on the human B lymphoma cells. (b) To screen for the anti-idiotype monoclonal antibody, the mouse hybridoma supernatents should be tested for their ability to bind to the human monoclonal antibody derived from the B cell lymphoma and with normal human antibodies. The anti-idiotype monoclonal would only be able to bind to the monoclonal derived from the B-cell lymphoma and not with other normal human immunoglobulins.

5. The mouse antibody will be polyclonal and, therefore, will recognize many different epitopes, will have a heterogeneous affinity for the antigen, and will consist of more than one isotype. The monoclonal antibody is homogeneous and, therefore, will recognize a single epitope, will be of a single isotype, and will have a homogeneous affinity for the epitope.

6. If the epitope density on the antigen is very low the monoclonal antibody may not be able to crosslink the antigen to form a precipitate. Because polyclonal antibodies recognize multiple epitopes, crosslinkage of multiple antigens is more likely to happen.

7. Different antigens can have identical or similar epitopes, and therefore a monoclonal antibody to the epitope on one antigen may also bind to the same epitopes on similar antigens.

8. (a) The epitope density may be low and, therefore, inhibit precipitation in an immunodiffusion assay. (b) The Western Blot involves protein denaturation in SDS. It is possible that a conformational epitope that is dependent on the tertiary structure of the protein may be lost. If the monoclonal antibody is to such an epitope, it may now fail to bind. (c) For the same reason cited in (a) above.

9. (a) Western blot: electrophorese the HIV virus antigens, transfer the HIV antigen bands to a suitable filter such as nitrocellulose and then flood the filter with each monoclonal antibody. If both monoclonal antibodies react with the same antigen component, then they may be the same. Immunoadsorption: make an immunoadsorbent column with one monoclonal antibody. Run solution of HIV antigens over the column. Take depleted solution and run over the second adsorption column. If the second column is able to retain the antigen, then the antibodies are different. (b) Sequence the monoclonal antibodies. If the variable regions are the same, then they are the same antibody.

10. $1 = H_{spleen}/L_{spleen}$; $2 = H_{myeloma}/L_{myeloma}$; $3 = H_{spleen}/L_{myeloma}$; $4 = H_{myeloma}/L_{spleen}$. (a) 4 different antigen binding sites; 10 different antibody molecules $1:1$; $2:2$; $3:3$; $4:4$; $1:2$; $1:3$; $1:4$; $2:3$; $2:4$; $3:4$. (b) 2 different antigen binding sites; 3 different antibody molecules $1:1$; $2:2$; $1:2$. (c) 1 antibody molecule $1:1$.

11. The immunotoxin lacks the binding polypeptide of the toxin, and therefore if the antibody is degraded, the toxin will be unable to get into the cell.

4. $500\ V_L \times 4\ J_L = 2 \times 10^3$ Light Chains
$300\ V_H \times 15\ D_H \times 4\ J_H = 1.8 \times 10^4$ Heavy Chains
$2 \times 10^3 \times 1.8 \times 10^4 = 3.6 \times 10^7$ Potential Antibody Molecules.

5. (1) e; (2) c; (3) c; (4) e; (5) b,c,d.

6. (a) Progenitor B cell: no cytoplasmic or membrane staining with either reagent; (b) Pre- B cell: F1-anti μ staining in cytoplasm; no staining on membrane; (c) Immature B cell: F1-anti μ staining in cytoplasm; F1-anti μ staining on membrane; (d) Mature B cell: F1-anti μ and Rh-anti δ in cytoplasm; F1-anti μ and Rh-anti δ on membrane; (e) Plasma cell: F1-anti μ in cytoplasm; No membrane staining but pentameric IgM is being secreted.

7. Somatic mutation generates all three hypervariable regions. In addition, junctional diversity at the heavy chain V-D and D-J junctions and the light chain V-J junction, as well as N-nucleotide additions at the heavy chain V-D and D-J junctions, contributes to additional variability in the third hypervariable region of the heavy and light chains.

8. See table top of p. 548.

9. The κ chain DNA must be in germline configuration because a productive H chain rearrangement must occur before the κ chain DNA can begin to rearrange.

10. Random addition of nucleotides at the V-D-J junctions contributes to H chain diversity within the third CDR but can result in a nonproductive rearrangement if the nucleotide addition does not preserve the triplet reading frame.

Chapter 8

1. (a) False. V_λ and C_κ are located on separate chromosomes and cannot be brought together during rearrangement; (b) True; (c) True; (d) True; (e) True; (f) True.

11. See table below.

2. (a)

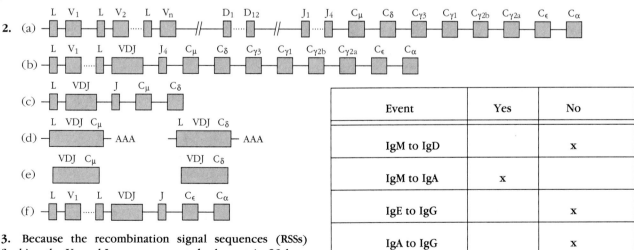

3. Because the recombination signal sequences (RSSs) flanking the V_H and J_H gene segments both contain 23 base pair spacers. According to the 12/23 joining rule, only a RSS with a 12 bp spacer can join with a RSS having a 23 bp spacer.

Event	Yes	No
IgM to IgD		x
IgM to IgA	x	
IgE to IgG		x
IgA to IgG		x
IgM to IgG	x	

8.

Gene	Configurations		
	Possible	Not possible	Reason
Heavy chain, allele 1	R	G or NP	Productive rearrangement of allele #1 is required.
Heavy chain, allele 2	G	R	Allelic exclusion forbids allele #2 from productive rearrangement.
κ chain, allele 1	NP	G or R	Kappa rearranges before lambda—both kappa and lambda alleles need to be nonproductive so that lambda chain genes can rearrange.
κ chain, allele 2	NP	G or R	
λ chain, allele 1	R	G or NP	Productive rearrangement of lambda allele #1 is required.
λ chain, allele 2	G	R	Allelic exclusion forbids allele #2 from productive rearrangement.

11. Liver   B
       Pre-B lymphoma   C
       IgM secreting myeloma   A

Chapter 9

1. (a) True; (b) True
2. (a) S; (b) C; (c) S; (d) C; (e) S; (f) S; (g) C.
3. (a) Strain A; (b) Strain B; (c) Strain A; (d) To introduce parental alleles at all loci except for the selected MHC; (e) To achieve homozygosity within the MHC; (f) To identify progeny that are homozygous bb within the MHC.
4. Liver cells: Class I K^b, K^k, D^b, D^k, L^k, L^b; Macrophages: Class I K^b, K^k, D^b, D^k, L^b, L^k; Class II $IA\alpha^k\beta^k$, $IA\alpha^b\beta^b$, $IA\alpha^k\beta^b$, $IA\alpha^b\beta^k$, $IE\alpha^k\beta^k$, $IE\alpha^b\beta^b$, $IE\alpha^k\beta^b$, $IE\alpha^b\beta^k$.

Transfected gene	MHC molecules expressed on the membrane of the transfected L cells					
	D^k	D^b	K^k	K^b	IA^k	IA^b
None	+	−	+	−	−	−
K^b	+	−	+	+	−	−
A^b_α	+	−	+	−	−	−
A^b_β	+	−	+	−	−	−
A^b_α and A^b_β	+	−	+	−	−	+

6. (a) SJL macrophages will express the following MHC molecules: K^s, D^s, L^s, IA^s; (b) The additional MHC molecules expressed on the transfected SJL cells will be: IE^k, $IE\alpha^s\beta^k$.
7. See Figure 5-16.
8. The polymorphic residues are clustered in short stretches within the $\alpha1$ and $\alpha2$ domains of the class I MHC molecules and within the $\alpha1$ and $\beta1$ domains of the class II MHC molecules. These regions are thought to form the peptide binding groove of the MHC. The clustered distribution is thought to arise by gene conversion of short nearly homologous DNA sequences from unexpressed pseudogenes within the MHC to functional class I or class II genes.
9. (a) Assay 1 indicates the proliferation of the T_H cell population while assay 2 indicates CTL activity. (b) T_H cells in assay 1 recognize IA^k LCM pulsed macrophages. CTL in assay 2 recognize D^d virus infected target cells. (c) Transfect L cells with the IA^k gene and show that the transfected L cells stimulate T_H production of IL-2. You would also need to run a control to show that LCM-pulsed L cells transfected with inappropriate class II genes would not stimulate IL-2 production. You would need to perform a similar transfection experiment to show that the CTL could kill LCM-infected L cells transfected with the D^d gene. (d) The immunized spleen cells came from either the A.TL strain or the (Balb/c × B10.A)F1 since these are the only strains that are both IA^k and D^d.
10. It is not possible to tell. Since the antigen binding groove is identical, both MHC molecules should bind the same peptide. However, the amino acid changes outside the groove may interfere with the TCR recognition of the MHC.
11. Use monoclonal antibodies specific for each MHC haplotype to determine if both strains express the same set of MHC molecules.
12. If RBC's expressed MHC molecules then one would have to perform extensive tissue typing prior to a blood transfusion, and very few individuals would be potential blood donors for a given individual.

Chapter 10

1. (a) False: CD3 is located very close to the TCR and, therefore, will co-precipitate; but the distance of CD4 from the TCR is further and therefore, the two membrane molecules do not co-precipitate; (b) True; (c) True; (d) False. The TCR variable region genes are located on different chromosomes from the immunoglobulin variable region genes; (e) False: The $\alpha\beta$ heterodimer has a single antigen/MHC binding site.

2. Functional $\alpha\beta$ genes from a T_C clone specific for one hapten on an H-2^d target were transfected into another T_C clone specific for a second hapten on an H-2^k target. Cytolysis assays revealed that the transfected T_C cell recognized both hapten/MHC molecule complexes for which the original T_C clones were specific.

3. (a) The $\gamma\delta$ TCR is expressed first during thymic ontogeny. (b) No. Because the δ chain genes are located between the $V\alpha$ and $J\alpha$ gene segments, then a productive rearrangement of the α-chain genes will delete the δ-chain gene segments.

4. See Figure 10-6.

5. The CD3 membrane complex is required for the expression of the TCR and plays a role in signal transduction across the membrane. The CD4 and CD8 accessory molecules increase the avidity of the T cell interaction with class II or class I MHC respectively. Both CD4 and CD8 play an additional role in signal transduction. CD2 plays a role as an adhesion molecule by binding to LFA-3, strengthening the interaction of T_H cells with antigen-presenting cells or T_C cells with target cells. CD2 also plays a role in signal transduction across the membrane.

6.

Property	TCR	Ig
Is associated with CD3	x	
Is monovalent	x	
Exists in membrane-bound and secreted forms		x
Contains domains with β-pleated-sheet structures	x	x
Is MHC restricted	x	
Diversity generated by imprecise joining of gene segments	x	x
Diversity generated by somatic mutation		x

7. (a) The three assumptions were: 1) That the TCR was an integral membrane protein and was, therefore, transcribed on polyribosomes. They, therefore, isolated the polyribosomal mRNA fraction and eliminated the cytoplasmic mRNA. 2) That subtractive hybridization could be used to subtract the B cell mRNA common to the T cell so that only the unique T-cell mRNA remained unhybridized. 3) That the TCR genes undergo DNA rearrangement and, therefore, can be detected by Southern blotting. (b) If they wanted to identify the IL-4 gene they should perform subtractive hybridization using a T_H clone as an IL-4 producer and a T_C clone as a source of

mRNA lacking the message for IL-4. In addition, the gene for IL-4 would not be expected to rearrange, and therefore they could not look for gene rearrangement using Southern blot analysis.

8. See table at the top of p. 550.

9. (a) Exp A thymus donor: Balb/c (H-2^d); Exp B thymus donor, C57Bl/6 (H-2^b). (b) The H-2^b target cells were lysed in experiment B because the MHC of the thymic epithelial cells will determine the MHC restriction of the T cells maturing in the thymus. Only T cells whose TCR recognizes virus presented by H-2^b will be positively selected. (c) The H-2^k target cells were not lysed in either experiment because neither thymus expressed H-2^k MHC, and therefore H-2^k reactive T cells were not positively selected.

10.

T-cell population	Transgene expression	
	H-2^k strain transgenic	H-2^b strain transgenic
CD4$^+$ CD8$^+$ thymocyte (double-positive)	+	+
CD4$^+$ T cell	+	−
CD8$^+$ T cell	+	−

11. See table at the top of p. 550.

12. (a) Since the TCR and CD3 are co-expressed, 70% of the cells will be expressing the TCR. The unstained cells are mostly CD4$^+$8$^+$, TCR$^-$, and a small percentage are CD4$^-$8$^-$, TCR$^-$. (b) You cannot determine how many TC (CD8$^+$) cells are present because some of the unstained cells may be expressing the $\gamma\delta$ TCR. To determine the number of CD8$^+$ cells, stain with a different fluorescent monoclonal antibody.

Chapter 11

1. (a) True; (b) False: It binds to the p55 kD component of the IL-2 receptor; (c) True; (d) False: It binds IL-2 but with a low affinity and, therefore, does not serve to activate the T cell; (e) False: The β subunit is expressed following T_H activation.

2. Only antigen-activated T cells express the high affinity IL-2 receptor and are activated by IL-2.

3. The clone appears to express only the low affinity α subunit of the IL-2 receptor. It may not be able to express the β subunit of the IL-2 receptor, or it may express a mutated form of the β subunit.

4. (a) Clone 1 lacks both subunits of the IL-2 receptor. Clone 2 lacks the p75 subunit of the IL-2 receptor. Clone 3 doesn't secrete IL-2. (b) Transfect genes under active promoters for the p55 and p75 subunits into clone 1 and a gene for the p75 subunit into clone 2, and see if IL-2 binding, anti-Tac staining, and proliferation is restored. Add recombinant IL-2 to clone 3 to see if it restores proliferation.

For use with Question 8 in Chapter 10.

Source of spleen cells from LCM-infected mice	Release of [^{51}Cr] from LCM-Infected target cells			
	B10.D2 (H-2^d)	B10 (H-2^b)	B10.BR (H-2^k)	F$_1$ (BALB/c × B10) (H-2$^{b/d}$)
B10.D2(H-2^d)	+	−	−	+
B10(H-2^b)	−	+	−	+
BALB/c (H-2^d)	+	−	−	+
BALB/b (H-2^b)	−	+	−	+

For use with Question 11 in Chapter 10.

Gene product	Source clone for cDNA	Clone supplying mRNA for subtraction hydridization	Reason
IL-2	a. T$_H$	b. T$_C$	T$_H$ secretes IL-2 and T$_C$ doesn't
CD8	b. T$_C$	a. T$_H$	Only T$_C$ expresses CD8
J chain	d. IgA secreting myeloma	g. IgG secreting myeloma	J chain expressed for dimeric IgA
IL-1	c. Macrophage	f. Neutrophil	Macrophage secretes IL-1 and neutrophil is closely related myeloid cell
CD3	a or b	d or g	Both T$_H$ and T$_C$ express CD3 and B cells don't

5. The TNF-α released by activated macrophages during the acute phase inflammatory response acts on vascular endothelial cells and macrophages inducing secretion of colony stimulating factors. The CSFs act on the bone marrow, inducing hematopoiesis.

6. Two types of cell lines have been important in cytokine research: cell lines that produce high levels of a particular cytokine and cell lines that require a particular cytokine for its growth. The high producing cell lines were especially important prior to cloning of the cytokine genes, enabling early cytokine researchers to obtain higher concentrations of a particular cytokine. The cytokine dependent cell lines enable researchers to determine whether a particular cytokine is present in a supernatent.

Chapter 12

1. (a) False: The indirect hemolytic plaque assay detects both IgM and IgG secreting plasma cells; (b) True; (c) False: IL-4 increases IgE production; (d) True; (e) True; (f) True.

2. (a) Heterogeneous; low affinity; IgM; (b) Homogeneous;

high affinity; IgG; (c) Heterogeneous; low affinity; IgM; (d) Heterogeneous; low affinity; IgG.

3. (a) Use direct hemolytic plaque assay for 1° response (see Figure 12-3a); use indirect hemolytic plaque assay for 2° response (see Figure 12-3b). (b) The direct PFC assay gives the number of IgM secreting plasma cells. Subtract the direct PFCs from the indirect PFCs to obtain the number of IgG PFCs. A = 310 IgM secreting plasma cells and 33 IgG secreting plasma cells; B = 62 IgM secreting plasma cells and 3998 IgG secreting plasma cells; C = 366 IgM secreting plasma cells and 20 IgG secreting plasma cells. (c) Group B illustrates the carrier effect. Only group B received a secondary immunization of both hapten and carrier, and therefore only group B has both memory B cells for DNP and memory T cells for the BSA carrier, allowing class switching from the IgM isotype to the IgG isotype.

4. Activation of virgin B cells requires crosslinkage of the membrane immunoglobulin receptors by antigen together with co-stimulatory IL-1 and IL-4 signals derived from a T$_H$ cell. Additional proliferation and differentiation of the activated B cells is provided by IL-2, IL-4, IL-5, IL-6, IFN-γ, and TGF-β.

Chapter 13

1. The monoclonal antibody to LFA-1 should block formation of the CTL-target cell conjugate. This should inhibit killing of the target cell and, therefore, should result in diminished ^{51}Cr release in the CML assay.

3. The proliferating cell in the MLR is a CD4$^+$ T$_H$ cell. You can prove the identity of the proliferating cell by using F1-anti CD4 monoclonal antibody and Rh-anti CD8 monoclonal antibody to stain the cells. The proliferating cells can be shown to stain with the F1-anti CD4 reagent. As CD4$^+$ T$_H$ cells recognize class II MHC antigen differences on the stimulator cells, they secrete IL-2. It is the IL-2 that stimulates proliferation of the CD4$^+$ T$_H$ cells.

2.

Population 1	Population 2	Proliferation
C57BL/6 (H-2^b)	CBA (H-2^k)	1 & 2
C57BL/6 (H-2^b)	CBA (H-2^k) mitomycin C-treated	1
C57BL/6 (H-2^b)	F$_1$ (CBA × C57BL/6)	1
C57BL/6 (H-2^b)	C57L (H-2^b)	Neither

4.

Property	T$_H$ cell	CTL	Property	T$_H$ cell	CTL
Can make IL-1	−	−	Expresses CD4	+	−
Can make IL-2	+	−	Can respond to IL-1	+	−
Is class I MHC restricted	−	+	Expresses CD3	+	+
Expresses CD8	−	+	Adheres to target cells via LFA-1	−	+
Is required for B-cell activation	+	−	Can express the IL-2 receptor	+	+
Is cytotoxic for target cells	−	+	Expresses the $\alpha\beta$ T-cell receptor	+	+
Is the main proliferating cell in an MLR	+	−	Is the principal target of HIV	+	−
Is the effector cell in a CML assay	−	+	Responds to soluble antigens alone	−	−
Is class II MHC restricted	+	−	Produces perforin molecules	−	+

5.

Source of primed spleen cells	[^{51}Cr] release from LCM-infected target cells			
	B10.D2 (H-2^d)	B10 (H-2^b)	B10.BR (H-2^k)	F$_1$ (BALB/c × B10) (H-2$^{b/d}$)
B10.D2 (H-2^d)	+	−	−	+
B10 (H-2^b)	−	+	−	+
BALB/c (H-2^d)	+	−	−	+
(BALB/c × B10) (H-2$^{b/d}$)	+	+	−	+

6. To determine T$_C$ activity specific for influenza, perform a CML reaction by incubating spleen cells from the infected mouse with influenza infected syngeneic target cells. To determine T$_H$ activity, incubate the spleen cells from the infected mouse with syngeneic APCs presenting influenza peptides, and measure IL-2 production.

Chapter 14

1. (a) False: Immature B cells are tolerized more readily; (b) True; (c) False. Antigenic competition will reduce the response to SRBC; (d) True; (e) True; (f) True; (g) False: TEPC-15 is a myeloma-derived antibody specific for phosphorylcholine. It can serve as an antigen to which anti-idiotype antibody can bind; (h) True; (i) False: Deaggregated antigens induce tolerance more readily because they are less able to be internalized and processed by antigen-presenting cells. It is thought that in the absence of a co-stimulatory signal, a state of tolerance is more readily achieved; (j) True; (k) False: Some T cell tolerance occurs by clonal anergy.

2. Immunize an animal with monoclonal antibody (Ab-1) specific for hepatitis B virus to produce anti-idiotype antibody (Ab-2). Then use the anti-idiotype antibody to immunize other animals. The immunized animals should now be protected against hepatitis B virus.

3. Remove the spleen from the tolerant animal and divide the spleen cells into two aliquots. To one aliquot, remove the T cells by staining the T cells with F1-anti-CD3 and passing the labeled cells through a FACS; the remaining cells in this aliquot include B cells. To the other aliquot, remove the B cells by using F1-anti-μ and passing the labeled cells through a FACS; the remaining cells in the aliquot include T cells. Now culture the B cell aliquot from the tolerant mouse with syngeneic T cells from a normal mouse, and culture the T cell aliquot from the tolerant mouse with syngeneic B cells from a normal mouse. Add antigen A to both cell cultures and see if plasma cells to antigen A are produced by performing a Jerne plaque assay. This procedure should reveal whether the B cells or T cells or both populations are tolerant to antigen A.

4. (a) Paratope: idiotopes within the antigen-binding site of an antibody that are involved in binding to the antigenic determinant (epitope). (b) Epitope: the antigenic determinant that interacts with an antibody or T cell receptor. (c) Idiotope: the set of antigenic determinants within the variable region that comprise the idiotype of an antibody. (d) Agretope: the region on a peptide antigen that interacts with a MHC molecule.

5. (a) Both single and double transgenics carried the anti-lysozyme transgene. Because the anti-lysozyme transgene H and L chains were already rearranged, the developing B cells will not rearrange the other immunoglobulin H and L chain genes and, therefore, will only express the rearranged immunoglobulin of the transgene. (b) Add radiolabeled lysozyme and see if it binds to the B cell membrane using autoradiography. To determine the isotype on the membrane of these B cells, incubate the cells with fluorochrome-labeled antibodies specific for each isotype (e.g., anti-μ, anti-γ, etc.) and see which fluorescent antibodies stain the B cells. (c) So that the lysozyme transgene could be induced by adding Zn^{++} to the mouse's water supply. (d) Isolate B cells and T cells from the transgenic mice using a FACS. Mix the transgenic B cells

with normal syngeneic T cells, and mix the transgenic T cells with normal syngeneic B cells. Transfer each cell mixture to lethally x-irradiated, syngeneic adoptive transfer recipients, and challenge the recipients with lysozyme. See if anti-lysozyme PFCs are generated by using a hemolytic plaque assay with lysozyme conjugated SRBCs.

6. In the Kappler and Marrack experiment, expression of the V$_\beta$17a TCR was assessed in IE$^+$ and IE$^-$ mice. In the IE$^+$ mice the expression of IE on thymic stromal cells resulted in negative selection (clonal deletion) of the self-reactive T cells. In Burkly's experiment IE$^-$ mice were used, and an IE transgene was engineered to an insulin promoter. Therefore, the expression of IE was limited to the pancreatic islet cells, and IE was not expressed in the thymus. As T cells expressing the V$_\beta$17a TCR matured in the thymus of these mice, they were not exposed to IE on thymic stromal cells, and therefore they were not eliminated in by negative selection. When these T cells encountered the IE molecule on a non-antigen presenting cell (in the absence of a co-stimulatory signal) the T cells entered an anergic state.

7. (a) The T cells would not be MHC restricted. Instead T cells bearing receptors specific for antigen alone or antigen associated with non-self MHC might also mature. (b) Self-reactive T cells would be released from the thymus, and autoimmunity could develop.

8. (a) When animals were tolerized with high doses of an antigen, the tolerant state could be transferred to syngeneic mice by transferring simply the tolerant T cells. (b) 1) inability to identify a unique membrane molecule on the T$_S$ cells distinct from known membrane markers on the CD8$^+$ T$_C$ cells 2) inability to identify and characterize unique rearranged TCR genes in T$_S$ hybridomas 3) inability to maintain stable T$_S$ clones capable of mediating suppression 4) inability to clone antigen-specific suppressor factors. (c) 1) absorption of IL-2 by activated T$_C$ cells would deplete the necessary IL-2 from the culture supernatent 2) antagonistic effects of cytokines produced by different T cell subpopulations 3) diversion of the immune response to a different isotype or a different branch of immune activity that was not being monitored and so went undetected.

9. (a) In the H-2^b mice, T cells expressing the transgene will make it through both positive and negative selection in the thymus. In the H-2$^{b/d}$ mice, T cells expressing the transgene will be selected in positive selection but will be eliminated as self-reactive in negative selection. (b) H-2$^{b/d}$ mice were used so that T cells expressing the transgene could make it through positive selection. If H-2^d mice had been used instead, the T cells expressing the transgene would not have matured within the thymus. (c) A CML assay was used in which the CTL cells expressing the transgene were incubated with ^{51}Cr-labeled target cells that expressed L^d molecules.

Chapter 15

1. (a) True; (b) True; (c) True; (d) True; (e) False: Enveloped viruses can be lysed by complement because their outer envelope is derived from the plasma membrane of a host cell; (f) True.

2. Serum IgM is in a planar form in which the Fc-region complement binding sites are not accessible. Only after binding to antigen will the IgM assume a staple form, allowing the Fc complement sites to be accessible.

3. A C3 deficiency is more serious clinically because both classical and alternative pathways are inhibited.

4. The degraded antibody will be less able both to serve as an opsonin and to activate the complement pathway.

5. (a) Initial activation of the classical pathway occurs by antigen-complexed to IgG or IgM antibody while the alternative pathway can be activated by bacterial cell wall components. (b) See Figure 15-1. (c) Both pathways result in MAC pore formation and consequently cell lysis. Both pathways generate anaphylatoxins (C3a and C5a), although only the classical pathway generates C4a. Both pathways generate chemotactic factors (C3a, C5a, and C5b67). Both pathways generate lots of C3b, which serves as an opsonin. Both pathways can lead to viral neutralization. Both pathways can serve to solubilize and clear immune complexes.

6. The C5b67 complex can be released from the membrane and bind to a nearby cell mediating innocent bystander lysis. The regulatory protein S binds to the released C5b67 complex and prevents its insertion into the membrane of a nearby cell.

7. See Figure 15-8.

8. a. <u>4</u> C3b; b. <u>5</u> C1, C4, C2, and C3; c. <u>6</u> C9; d. <u>2</u> C3, Factor B, and Factor D; e. <u>7</u> C1q; f. <u>9</u> C3bBb; g. <u>3</u> C5b, C6, C7, C8, and C9; h. <u>1</u> C3 → C3a + C3b; i. <u>8</u> C3a, C5a, and C5b67; j. <u>10</u> C3a, C4a, and C5a; k. <u>9</u> C4b2b.

Chapter 16

1. (a) False: IgE is increased. (b) False: IL-4 increases IgE production. (c) False: IgE is not able to pass through the placenta like IgG. (d) False: Type III hypersensitivity involves immune complex deposition and mast cell degranulation plays a minor role. (e) False: Most pollen allergens contain multiple allergenic components.

2. (a) Antibodies would crosslink the IgE Fc receptor on the mast cell or basophil membrane resulting in activation and the subsequent degranulation of the cell with the release of mediators inducing vasodilation and smooth muscle contraction. (b) The Fab fragment is monovalent and, therefore, cannot crosslink the IgE Fc receptors. Therefore, the Fab fragment cannot induce degranulation. However, it might block IgE binding to the Fc receptors. In (a) it would make no difference if a person was allergic or not since receptor crosslinkage is independent of specific IgE/allergen. In (b) the Fab fragment might have a beneficial effect to individuals with allergies if it is able to effectively block IgE binding to the Fc receptor without inducing degranulation.

3. Engineer chimeric monoclonal antibodies to snake venom that contain mouse variable regions but human heavy and light chain constant regions.

4.

	Poison oak	Ragweed pollen
Lymphocytes involved	T$_{DTH}$ cells	IgE secreting plasma cells (B cells and T$_H$ cells)
Other cells	Macrophages	Mast cells and Basophils

	Poison oak	Ragweed pollen
Mediators	MIF, IFN-γ (MAF), MCF, lysosomal enzymes	Histamine, leukotrienes, platelet activating factor, eosinophil chemotactic factor
Mechanism	Cytokines released by sensitized T$_{DTH}$ cells recruit and activate macrophages. The activated macrophages release lysosomal enzymes which cause tissue damage.	Mediators released from mast cell and basophil induce smooth muscle contraction and vasodilation

5. (a) Type I hypersensitivity: localized atopic reaction with allergen crosslinkage of fixed IgE on skin mast cells inducing degranulation and mediator release. (b) Type III hypersensitivity: immune complexes of antibody and insect antigens form and are deposited locally, causing an Arthus type reaction resulting from complement activation and complement split products. (c) Type IV hypersensitivity: sensitized T$_{DTH}$ cells release their mediators inducing macrophage accumulation and activation. Tissue damage results from lysosomal enzymes released by the macrophage.

6.

Immunologic event	Hypersensitivity			
	Type I	Type II	Type III	Type IV
Ig-E-mediated degranulation of mast cells	+	−	−	−
Lysis of antibody-coated blood cells by complement	−	+	−	−
Tissue destruction in response to poison oak	−	−	−	+
C3a- and C5a-mediated mast cell degranulation	−	−	+	−
Chemotaxis of neutrophils	−	−	+	−
Chemotaxis of eosinophils	+	−	−	−
Activation of macrophages by IFN-γ	−	−	−	+
Deposition of antigen-antibody complexes on basement membranes of capillaries	−	−	+	−
Sudden death due to vascular collapse (shock) shortly after injection or ingestion of antigen	+			−

Chapter 17

1. 1. f; 2. i; 3. h; 4. j; 5. l; 6. g; 7. c; 8. k; 9. b; 10. a; 11. e; 12. d.

2. (a) EAE is induced by injecting mice or rats with myelin basic protein in complete Freund's adjuvant. (b) The animals that recover from EAE are now resistant to EAE. If they are given a second injection of myelin basic protein in complete Freund's adjuvant they no longer develop EAE. (c) If T cells from mice with EAE are transferred to normal syngeneic mice, the mice will develop EAE.

3. A number of viruses have been shown to possess sequences in common with sequences in myelin basic protein (MBP). Since the encephalitogenic peptides of MBP are known, it is possible to test these peptides to see if they bear sequence homology to known viral protein sequences. Computer analysis has revealed a number of viruses that bear sequence homology to MBP. By immunizing rabbits with these viral sequences, it was possible to induce EAE. The studies on the encephalitogenic peptides of MBP also showed that different peptides induced EAE in different strains. Thus the MHC haplotype will determine which crossreacting viral peptides will be presented and, therefore, will influence the development of EAE.

4. (1) A virus might express an antigenic determinant that cross-reacts with a self component. (2) A viral infection might induce localized concentrations of IFN-γ. The IFN-γ might then induce inappropriate expression of class II MHC molecules on nonantigen presenting cells, enabling T_H activation of self-peptides presented together with the class II MHC molecule. (3) A virus may damage a given organ allowing for the release of antigens that are normally sequestered from the immune system.

5. (a) So that the IFN-γ transgene would only be expressed by pancreatic beta cells. (b) The mice developed diabetes, and there was a cellular infiltration of lymphocytes and macrophages similar to that seen in insulin dependent diabetes mellitus. (c) The IFN-γ transgene induced the pancreatic beta cells to express the class II MHC molecule. (d) A localized viral infection in the pancreas might result in the localized production of IFN-γ by activated T cells. The IFN-γ might then induce the inappropriate expression of class II MHC molecules by pancreatic beta cells as well as the production of other cytokines such as IL-1 or TNF. If self-peptides are presented by the class II MHC molecules, then IL-1 might provide the necessary co-stimulatory signal to activate T cells against the self-peptides. Alternatively, the TNF might also cause localized cellular damage.

6. Increased expression of IL-2 and the IL-2 receptor on T cells may promote T cell activation, resulting in production of other cytokines and possibly leading to various effector functions that might cause tissue damage.

7. Anti-CD4 monoclonal antibodies have been used to block T_H activity. Monoclonal antibodies specific for the high affinity IL-2 receptor have been tried to block activated T_H cells. The association of some autoimmune diseases with restricted T cell receptor expression has prompted researchers to see if it might be possible to use a monoclonal antibody specific for the TCR to block only selective T cells expressing a particular receptor.

Chapter 18

1. (a) True; (b) True; (c) True; (d) True.

2. Attenuated organisms are capable of limited growth within the host cells and are, therefore, processed by the endogenous processing route and presented on the membrane of the infected host cell together with the class I MHC molecule. These molecules are, therefore, more likely to induce a cell-mediated immune response. In addition, because attenuated organisms are capable of limited growth within the host, it is often not necessary to give a second booster with the vaccine. Also, if the attenuated vaccine is able to grow

along the mucous membrane, then the vaccine will be able to induce the production of secretory IgA.

3. The antitoxin was given to inactivate any toxin that might be produced if *Clostridium tetani* infected the wound. The antitoxin was necessary since the child had not been previously immunized and, therefore, did not have circulating levels of antibody to tetanus toxin or B memory cells specific for tetanus toxin. If the child steps on a rusty nail 3 years later, the child will not be immune and will, therefore, require another dose of antitoxin.

4. The Sabin polio vaccine is attenuated and, therefore, is capable of limited growth along the gastrointestinal tract. The Sabin vaccine will induce a secretory IgA response.

5. The amphipathic peptides are most likely to represent T cell epitopes, and the mobile peptides are more likely to represent accessible B cell epitopes.

6. The MHC haplotype of the strain B mice is not able to bind the peptide and present it to the T cells. You could test this hypothesis by transfecting each MHC molecule of the strain A and strain B mice into L cells and then incubate the transfected L cells with the peptide to see if they can activate T cells.

7. A short incubation period, such as that seen with influenza, means that the memory cell response is not effective. Protection against such a pathogen is achieved by maintaining high levels of neutralizing antibody. For pathogens with a longer incubation period, such as the polio virus, high levels of neutralizing antibody at the time of infection are not necessary, and instead the memory cell response is sufficient to afford protection.

8. The attenuated Sabin vaccine can cause life-threatening infection in severely immune suppressed individuals, such as children with AIDS.

Chapter 19

1. (a) There was no killing in system A because the target cell was influenza infected H-2^k, and the CTL was H-2^b restricted. (b) Because the influenza nucleoprotein can be processed and presented by the endogenous processing pathway. (c) Probably because the transfected class I D^b molecule is only able to present peptide 365–380 and not peptide 50–63. (d) These results suggest that a cocktail of several immunogenic peptides would be more likely to be presented by different MHC haplotypes in humans and would provide the best vaccine for humans.

2. (a) The non-specific host defenses include: ciliated epithelial cells, bacteriocidal substances in mucous secretions, complement split products activated by the alternative pathway that serve both as opsonins and as chemotactic factors, phagocytic cells. (b) The specific host defenses include secretory IgA in the mucous secretions, IgG and IgM in the tissue fluids, the classical complement pathway, complement split products, the opsonins (IgM, IgG, and C3b), and the phagocytic cells. Cytokines produced during the specific immune response, including IFN-γ TNF, IL-1, and IL-6, will each contribute to the overall intensity of the inflammatory response.

3. Humoral antibody peaks within a few days of infection and binds to the influenza HA glycoprotein blocking viral infection of host epithelial cells. However, the antibody is strain specific and therefore its major role is in protecting against re-infection with the same strain of influenza. The cell-mediated response peaks about 8 days after infection and serves to kill virally infected self-cells. The CTL response is necessary to eliminate the virus. Unlike the humoral antibody response which is strain specific, the CTL response is able to recognize epitopes shared by different influenza subtypes.

4. (a) The fact that the CTL response is cross-reactive means that it might be possible to induce an immune response to several human pandemic subtypes with a single vaccine. However, because the MHC haplotype determines which peptides are presented to the T cells, it will be necessary to identify immunodominant T cell epitopes for individuals with different MHC haplotypes and then prepare a cocktail of synthetic peptides. (b) The nucleoprotein can serve as a potential vaccine because it will be processed by the endogenous processing pathway and presented together with class I MHC molecules on the membrane of the infected host cell.

5. (a) IA^b; (b) Because the B cell requires the activity of an antigen-specific, MHC-restricted T$_H$ cell for its activation.

6. African trypanosomes are capable of antigenic shifts in its surface glycoprotein, the variant surface glycoprotein (VSG). The antigenic shifts are accomplished as gene segments encoding part of the VSG are duplicated and translocated to transcriptionally active expression sites. Plasmodium evades the immune system by continually undergoing maturational changes from sporozoite to merozoite to gametocyte, allowing the organism to continually change its surface molecules. In addition, the intracellular phases of its life-cycle reduce the level of immune activation. Finally, the organism is able to slough off its circumsporozoite coat after antibody binds to it. Influenza is able to evade the immune response through frequent antigenic changes in its hemagglutinin and neuraminidase glycoproteins. The antigenic changes are accomplished by the accumulation of small point mutations (antigenic drift) or through genetic reassortment of RNA between influenza virions from humans and animals (antigenic shift).

Chapter 20

1. (a) True; (b) False: Bruton's agammaglobulinemia results in a reduction in B cells and an absence of immunoglobulin; (c) False: Phagocytic defects result in recurrent bacterial and fungal infections; (d) True; (e) True; (f) True; (g) True; (h) False: The mice need lymphoid stem cells that are not defective in the recombinase enzyme; (i) False. These children are usually able to eliminate common encapsulated bacteria with antibody plus complement but are susceptible to viral, protozoan, fungal, and intracellular bacterial infections; (j) False: Class II MHC expression is required for T$_H$ activation in humoral immunity as well.

2. (a) The rearranged heavy chains in *scid* mice show deletions of D and or J gene segments. (b) Kappa chain genes are not rearranged because, according to the model of Yancopolis and Alt (discussed in chapter 8), a productive heavy chain gene rearrangement is necessary before light chain gene rearrangement can proceed. (c) Yes. The rearranged µ heavy chain gene would be transcribed to yield a functional M heavy chain. The presence of the functional µ heavy chain would then allow kappa chain gene rearrangement to proceed. (d) The β chain of the TCR would show defective D-J joining so that one or both of the gene segments are deleted during the joining process.

3. (a) SCID-human mice are prepared by implanting portions of human fetal liver, thymus, and lymph nodes into *scid* mice. (b) The fetal liver is used to provide a source of hematopoietic lymphoid stem cells. (c) The human cells are not rejected because the mouse does not have functional immunocompetent T or B lymphocytes. (d) Graft-versus-host disease does not develop in this system because the human T cells mature within the human thymus but are exposed to mouse MHC molecules (expressed on macrophages and dendritic cells that can migrate into the human thymus) and mouse antigens (carried into the human thymus), and therefore the human T cells become tolerant to the mouse antigens during thymic processing.

4. (a) Leukocyte adhesion deficiency results from defective biosynthesis of the β chain component of the integrin adhesion molecules. Since LFA-1, CR3, and CR4 each contain a common b chain, expression of all three molecules is affected. (b) The LFA-1 integrin molecule plays a role in cell adhesion by binding to ICAM-1 molecules expressed on cells. The LFA-1/ICAM-1 interaction is involved in the T$_H$-B cell interaction, in the CTL-target cell interaction, and in the interaction of circulating lymphocytes with vascular endothelial cells during extravasation. (c) Because the LFA-1/ICAM-1 interaction is involved in conjugate formation between the T$_H$ cell and the B cell, B cell activation is diminished and circulating antibody levels are reduced.

Chapter 21

1. (a) False: HIV-2 and SIV are more closely related; (b) False: HIV-1 infects chimpanzees but does not cause immune suppression; (c) True; (d) False: The *nef* gene has an uncertain function and may down-regulate the expression of the structural genes, *gag, pol,* and *env;* (e) True; (f) False: Some CD8$^+$ cells have been shown to be infected by HIV: (g) False: Patients with advanced AIDS sometimes have no detectable serum antibody to HIV: (h) False: The PCR detects HIV proviral DNA in latently infected cells; (i) True.

2. The soluble CD4 is used to bind to the gp120 on the viral envelope and prevent HIV binding to CD4$^+$ cells. The major limitation of this approach is the extremely short serum half-life of the soluble CD4. To overcome this limitation, the CD4 gene is engineered with the constant region gene of human IgG1. The CD4-immunoglobulin hybrid, called an immunoadhesion, now has a longer serum half-life in the range of the IgG1 subclass (expected to approach 21 days in humans).

3. No. In the latency period the virus is not replicating and, therefore, the levels of p17 and p24 decline.

4. An increase in the levels of p24 indicates that HIV infection is progressing from the latent phase into lytic infection. Increased levels of p24 can be used to indicate that an HIV-infected individual is progressing into AIDS.

5. Skin test reactivity is monitored to indicate the functional activity of the T_{DTH} cells. As AIDS progresses and CD4$^+$ T cells decline, there is a decline in skin test reactivity to common antigens.

6. Cell-mediated immunity.

Chapter 22

1. (a) The best possible match is identity in the MHC haplotypes of donor and recipient. (b) There is a 25% chance that siblings will share identical MHC haplotypes. (c) Perform HLA typing using a microcytotoxicity test with monoclonal antibody to class I and class II MHC antigens. In addition, a MLR can be performed mixing mitomycin C treated donor lymphocytes as stimulator cells and untreated recipient lymphocytes as responder cells.

2.

Donor	Recipient	Response	Type of rejection
BALB/c	C3H	R	FSR
BALB/c	Rat	R	FSR
BALB/c	Nude mouse	A	
BALB/c	C3H, had previous BALB/c graft	R	SSR
BALB/c	C3H, had previous C57Bl/6 graft	R	FSR
BALB/c	BALB/c	A	
BALB/c	F_1 (BALB/c $\times$ C3H)	A	
BALB/c	F_1 (C3H $\times$ C57Bl/6)	R	FSR
F_1 (BALB/c $\times$ C3H)	BALB/c	R	FSR
F_1 (BALB/c $\times$ C3H)	BALB/c, had previous F_1 graft	R	SSR

3. (a) Graft-versus-host disease (GVHD) develops as donor T cells recognize alloantigens on cells of an immune-suppressed host. The response develops as donor T_H cells are activated in response to recipient peptide/MHC complexes displayed on antigen-presenting cells. Cytokines elaborated by the T_H cell activate a variety of effector cells including NK cells, CTL, and macrophages which damage the host tissue. In addition cytokines such as TNF may mediate direct cytolytic damage to the host cells. (b) GVHD develops when the donated organ or tissue contains immunocompetent lymphocytes and when the host is immune suppressed. (c) Monoclonal antibodies to CD3 or to CD4 or to the high affinity IL-2 receptor could each be tried to deplete T_H cells from the donated organ or tissue. The rationale behind this approach is to diminish T_H activation in response to the alloantigens of the host. The use of anti-CD3 will deplete all T cells; the use of anti-CD4 will deplete all T_H cells; the use of anti-IL2R will deplete only the activated T_H cells.

4. (a) Based on the microcytotoxicity test, sibling A or sibling C would both be potential donors. (a) Based on the MLR, sibling A is the better donor.

Chapter 23

1. (a) False: Cancer cells do not respond to normal regulatory constraints but their rate of cell division is not necessarily any faster than normal cells. (b) True. (c) True. (d) True. (e) False: Some oncogenic retroviruses do not have viral oncogenes. (f) True. (g) False: LAK cells kill a wide variety of tumor cells and are not specific for a single type of tumor.

2. Cells of the pre-B cell lineage have rearranged the heavy chain genes and express the μ heavy chain in their cytoplasm.

You could perform Southern blot analysis with a Cμ probe to see if the heavy chain genes have rearranged. You could also perform fluorescent antibody staining utilizing methods to stain the cytoplasmic μ heavy chain.

3. (a) Early stage melanoma cells are functioning as antigen-presenting cells and are processing the antigen by the exogenous pathway and presenting the tetanus toxoid antigen together with the class II MHC DR molecule. (b) Advanced stage melanoma cells might have a reduction in the expression of class II MHC molecules or they may not be able to internalize and process the antigen by the exogeneous route. (c) Since the paraformaldehyde fixed early melanoma cells could present processed tetanus toxoid, they must express class II MHC molecules on their surface. (d) Stain the early and advanced melanoma cells with fluorescent-monoclonal antibody specific for class II MHC molecules.

4. Anti-CD3 has been shown to activate T cells. It is hoped

that, as the T cells are activated, it will enhance the anti-tumor response. However, the concentration of anti-CD3 is critical, and it is not known whether the dose of anti-CD3 will lead to T cell activation or to unwanted immune suppression.
5. 1) IFNα, IFNβ and IFNγ enhance the expression of class I molecules on tumor cells and thereby increase the CTL response against the tumor. 2) IFNγ increases the activity of CTL, macrophages and NK cells which each have been shown to play a role in the immune response to tumors. 3) TNFs have direct anti-tumor activity inducing hemorrhagic necrosis and tumor regression. 4) IL-2 activates LAK and TIL cells which both have anti-tumor activity.

Credits

Line illustrations rendered by Network Graphics.

Figure 1-4 From J. R. Goodman, Department of Pediatrics, University of California at San Francisco.

Figure 1-12 From *Immunology: Recognition and Response* edited by William E. Paul, W. H. Freeman and Company, 1991, p. 49. Originally from "How T Cells See Antigen," by H. M. Grey et al., *Scientific American*, November 1989, p. 57. Copyright © 1989 by Scientific American Inc. All rights reserved. Micrograph courtesy of Morten H. Nielson and Ole Werdelin.

Table 2-1 Adapted from Federation of American Societies for Experimental Biology, *Biological Handbooks, Vol. III: Inbred and Genetically Defined Strains of Laboratory Animals*, Pergamon Press Ltd., 1979.

Table 2-3 From J. D. Watson, J. Tooze, and D. T. Kurtz, *Recombinant DNA: A Short Course*. Copyright © 1983 by W. H. Freeman and Company.

Figure 2-7 From J. Darnell, H. Lodish, and D. Baltimore, *Molecular Cell Biology*. Copyright © 1990 by Scientific American Books.

Figure 2-8 From J. Darnell, H. Lodish, and D. Baltimore, *Molecular Cell Biology*. Copyright © 1990 by Scientific American Books.

Figure 3-1b From M. J. Cline and D. W. Golde, "Cellular Interactions in Hematopoiesis," reprinted by permission from *Nature*, 1979, Volume 277, p. 180. Copyright © 1979 Macmillan Magazines Ltd. Micrograph courtesy of Shirley Quan.

Figure 3-5 Adapted with permission from E. R. Unane and P. M. Allen, "The Immunoregulatory Role of the Macrophage," *Hospital Practice*, Volume 22, Issue 4, pp. 87–104. Illustration by Nancy Lou Gahan Makris.

Figure 3-6 From Lennart Nilsson, "Our Immune System: The Wars Within," *National Geographic*, June 1986, p. 718. Copyright Boehringer Ingelheim International GmpH, Stockholm.

Figure 3-8 From A. K. Szakal et al., "Isolated Follicular Dendritic Cells: Cytochemical Volume Antigen Localization, Momarski, SEM, and TEM Morphology," *Journal of Immunology*, Volume 134, 1985, p. 1354. Copyright © 1985 American Association of Immunologists. Reprinted with permission.

Figure 3-9b From J. R. Goodman, Department of Pediatrics, University of California at San Francisco.

Figure 3-10 Adapted from N. K. Jerne, "The Immune System," *Scientific American*, Volume 229, 1973, p. 54. Copyright © 1973 by Scientific American Inc. All rights reserved.

Figure 3-11 From W. van Ewijk. Adapted, with permission, from the *Annual Review of Immunology*, Volume 9, © 1991 by Annual Reviews Inc.

Figure 3-15a Adapted from A. O. Anderson and N. D. Anderson, "Structure and Physiology of Lymphatic Tissues," in *Cellular Functions in Immunity and Inflammation*, edited by J. J. Oppenheim et al., Elsevier Science Publishing Company, Inc., 1987, p. 39.

Figure 3-15b From S. D. Rosen and I. M. Stoolman, *Vertebrate Lectins*, Van Nostrand Reinhold, 1987.

Figure 3-15c From S. D. Rosen, *Current Opinion in Cell Biology*, Volume 1, 1989, p. 913. Reprinted by permission of Current Science.

Figure 3-16 From J. J. Woodruff, L. M. Clark, and Y. H. Chen, reprinted, with permission, from the *Annual Review of Immunology*, Volume 5, © 1987 by Annual Reviews Inc.

Figure 3-17 Adapted from A. Duijvestijn and A. Hamann, *Immunology Today*, Volume 10, 1989, p. 26. Reprinted by permission of Elsevier Science Publishing Company, Inc.

Figure 4-2 Adapted from M. Zanetti, E. Sercarz, and J. Salk, *Immunology Today*, Volume 8, 1987, p. 23. Reprinted by permission of Elsevier Science Publishers.

Figure 4-3 From E. Kabat, reprinted with permission from *Journal of the American Chemical Society*, Volume 76, 1954, p. 3709. Copyright 1954 American Chemical Society.

Figure 4-4 Adapted from M. Sela, "Antigenicity: Some Molecular Aspects," *Science*, Volume 166, December 12, 1969, p. 1365. Copyright 1969 by the American Association for the Advancement of Science.

Figure 4-5 Adapted from M. Z. Atassi, *Immunochemistry*, Volume 12, 1975, p. 423. Copyright © 1975 by Pergamon Press.

Table 4-5 Table from E. A. Kabat, *Structural Concepts in Immunology and Immunochemistry*, 2nd Edition, Holt, Rinehart and Winston. Copyright © 1976 by E. A. Kabat, reprinted by permission of the author.

Figure 4-6ab Adapted from W. G. Laver et al., *Cell*, Volume 61, 1990, p. 554. Reprinted by permission of Cell Press.

Figure 4-7abc Adapted from D. Benjamin, J. Bersofsky, I. East et al., adapted, with permission, from the *Annual Re-*

view of Immunology, Volume 2, © 1984 by Annual Reviews Inc.

Table 4-7   From H. Margalit et al., "Prediction of Immunodominant Helper T Cell Antigenic Sites from the Primary Sequence," *The Journal of Immunology*, Volume 138, 1987, p. 2219. Reprinted by permission.

Figure 4-9   From J. Rothard.

Figure 4-10   From H. M. Grey et al., *Scientific American*, November 1989. Copyright © 1989 by Scientific American Inc. All rights reserved.

Figure 4-14   From B. Heymer, *Immunology of the Bacterial Cell Envelope*, edited by D. E. S. Steward-Tull and M. Davis. Copyright © 1985 by John Wiley & Sons, Inc.

Figure 5-1   Adapted from A. Tiselius and E. A. Kabat, reproduced from the *Journal of Experimental Medicine*, 1939, Volume 69, p. 119, by copyright permission of the Rockefeller University Press.

Figure 5-2a   Adapted from R. R. Porter, *Biochem J.*, Volume 73, 1959, p. 119.

Figure 5-2b   Adapted from J. B. Fleishman, *Archives of Biochemistry Supplement 1*, Academic Press, Inc., 1962, p. 1974.

Figure 5-5a   Adapted from J. Darnell, H. Lodish, and D. Baltimore, *Molecular Cell Biology*. Copyright © 1990 by Scientific American Books.

Figure 5-5b   Adapted from M. Schiffer et al., reprinted with permission from *Biochemistry*, Volume 12, 1973, p. 4620. Copyright 1973 by American Chemical Society.

Figure 5-6   From E. W. Silverton et al., *Proc. Natl. Acad. Sci. U.S.A.*, Volume 74, 1977, p. 5140.

Figure 5-7b   From J. D. Capra and A. B. Edmundson, *The Antibody Combination Site*. Copyright © 1977 by Scientific American Books.

Figure 5-8   From A. G. Amit, R. A. Mariuzza, S. E. V. Phillips, and R. J. Poljak, "X-ray Chrystallographic Analysis of Lysozyme and Fab Fragment of a Monoclonal Antibody Specific for Lysozyme," *Science*, Volume 233, 1986, p. 747.

Figure 5-10ab   From R. C. Valentine and N. M. Green, *Journal of Molecular Biology*, Volume 27, 1967, p. 615. Reprinted by permission of Academic Press Inc. (London) Ltd.

Table 6-2   From V. M. Sarich, "Immunological Time Scale for Hominid Evolution," *Science*, Volume 158, December 1, 1967, p. 1200. Copyright © 1967 by the American Association for the Advancement of Science.

Table 6-3   Adapted from *Manual of Clinical Laboratory Immunology*, edited by N. R. Rose, H. Friedman and J. I. Fahey, American Society for Microbiology, 1986.

Figure 6-5, Figure 6-9, and Figure 6-12   From *Methods in Immunology*, Third Edition; Justine S. Garvey, Natalie E. Cremer, Dieter H. Sussdorf. Copyright 1977 by Addison-Wesley Publishing Co.

Figure 7-2   From R. I. Davidson and P. S. Gerald, *Somatic Cell Genetics*, Volume 2, 1976, p. 165. Reprinted by permission of Plenum Publishing Corporation.

Figure 7-4   From "Antibody-Secreting Clone," *Scientific American*, Volume 143, October 1980, p. 67. Copyright © 1990 by Scientific American Inc. All rights reserved.

Figure 7-6   Adapted from *Genetic Engineering News*, April 1989, p. 5. FIND/SVP © Genetic Engineering News.

Figure 7-11   Adapted from M. Verhoeyen and L. Reichmann, *BioEssays*, Volume 8, 1988, p. 74. Reprinted by permission of Cambridge University Press.

Figure 7-13   Adapted from W. D. Huse et al., *Science*, Volume 246, 1989, p. 1275.

Figure 7-14   Adapted from R. A. Lerner and A. Tramontano, *Scientific American*, Volume 258, p. 66. Copyright © 1988 by Scientific American Inc. All rights reserved.

Figure 8-1   Adapted from N. Hozumi and S. Tonegawa, *Proceedings of the National Academy of Science*, Volume 73, 1976, p. 3628.

Figure 8-10   Adapted from G. D. Yancopoulos and F. W. Alt, adapted, with permission, from the *Annual Review of Immunology*, Volume 4, © 1986 by Annual Reviews Inc.

Figure 9-11a   After original drawing by M. Silver in P. J. Bjorkman et al., reprinted by permission from *Nature*, Volume 329, p. 506. Copyright © 1987 Macmillan Magazines Ltd.

Figure 9-11d   From P. J. Bjorkman and D. Wiley, "Computer-generated Model of the Peptide-binding Site at the Top of the MHC Class I Molecule," in Darnell et al., *Molecular Cell Biology*, 2nd Edition, W. H. Freeman and Company, 1990.

Figure 10-4   Adapted from D. Raulet, adapted, with permission, from the *Annual Review of Immunology*, Volume 7, © 1989 by Annual Reviews Inc.

Figure 10-9   From R. H. Schwartz, "A Cell Culture Model for T Lymphocyte Clonal Anergy," *Science*, Volume 248, June 15, 1990, p. 1349. Copyright 1990 by the American Association for the Advancement of Science.

Figure 10-11   From M. Davis and P. J. Bjorkman, reprinted by permission from *Nature*, Vol. 329. Copyright © 1987 Macmillan Magazines Ltd.

Figure 10-16   From H. von Boehmer, "Self-Nonself Discrimination by T Cells," *Science*, Volume 248, June 15, 1990, p. 1364. Copyright 1990 by the American Association for the Advancement of Science.

Figure 10-17   Adapted from B. J. Foglrop and D. M. Pardoll, *Advances in Immunology*, Volume 44, 1989, p. 207. Reprinted by permission of Academic Press, Inc.

Table 11-5   From Mosman and Coffman, "Two Types of Mouse Helper T-cell Clones," *Immunology Today*, 1987. Reprinted by permission of Elsevier Science Publishers.

Table 11-6   From G. Crabtree, *Science*, Volume 243, 1989, p. 357. Reprinted by permission of the author.

Figure 11-7ab   From "Tumor Necrosis Factor," by L. J. Old, *Scientific American*, May 1988, p. 59. Copyright © 1988 by Scientific American Inc. All rights reserved.

Figure 11-7cd   From L. J. Old, "Tumor Necrosis Factor," *Scientific American*, May 1988, p. 74. Copyright © 1988 by Scientific American Inc. All rights reserved.

Figure 12-4   From N. K. Jerne, "The Immune System," *Scientific American*, Volume 229, July 1973, p. 53. Copyright © 1973 by Scientific American Inc. All rights reserved.

Figure 12-10   From V. M. Saunders et al., "Characterization of the Physical Interaction Between Antigen-Specific B and T Cells," *The Journal of Immunology*, Volume 137, 1986, p. 2395. Reprinted by permission.

Figure 12-11   From W. J. Poo et al., reprinted from *Nature*, Volume 332, p. 378. Copyright © 1988 Macmillan Magazines Ltd.

Figure 13-2   From J. D. E. Young and Z. A. Cohn, *Scientific American*, January 1988, p. 38. Copyright © 1988 by Scientific American Inc. SEM by Dr. Gilla Kaplan, The Rockefeller University.

Figure 13-6   From J. R. Yannelli et al., "Reorientation and Fusion of Cytotoxic T Lymphocyte Granules After Interaction with Target Cells as Determined by High Resolution Cinemicrography," *The Journal of Immunology*, Volume 136, 1986, pp. 377–382. Reprinted by permission.

Figure 13-8a   From J. D. E. Young and Z. A. Cohn, *Scientific American*, January 1988, p. 38. Copyright © 1988 by Scientific American Inc. SEM by Dr. Gilla Kaplan, The Rockefeller University.

Figure 13-8b   From E. R. Podack and G. Dennert, reprinted from *Nature*, Volume 301, p. 442. Copyright © 1983 Macmillan Magazines Ltd.

Figure 13-9a   Adapted from P. J. Peters et al., *Immunology Today*, Volume 11, 1990, p. 38. Reprinted by permission of Elsevier Science Publishing Company, Inc.

Figure 13-14   From J. R. David, *Immunology*, 1970, The Upjohn Company.

Figure 14-1   Adapted from C. G. Romball and W. O. Weigle, reproduced from the *Journal of Experimental Medicine*, 1973, Volume 138, p. 1426, by copyright permission of the Rockefeller University Press.

Figure 14-4   Adapted from H. Cozenza, *European Journal of Immunology*, Volume 6, 1976, p. 114.

Figure 14-6   Adapted from S. Hedrick et al., *Proceedings of the National Academy of Science*, Volume 82, 1985, p. 531. Reprinted by permission of the author.

Figure 14-7   Adapted from N. A. Mitchison, *Proceedings of the Royal Society of London*, Volume 161, 1964, p. 275. Reprinted by permission of The Royal Society.

Figure 14-8   From J. Chiller, "Kinetic Differences in Unresponsiveness of Thymus and Bone Marrow Cells," *Science*, Volume 171, February 26, 1971, p. 813. Copyright 1971 by the American Association for the Advancement of Science.

Figure 14-9   Adapted from R. H. Schwartz, "A Cell Culture Model for T Lymphocyte Clonal Anergy," *Science*, Volume 248, June 15, 1990, p. 1349. Copyright 1990 by the American Association for the Advancement of Science.

Figure 14-11   Adapted from W. C. Sha et al., reprinted from *Nature*, Volume 336, p. 73. Copyright © 1988 Macmillan Magazines Ltd.

Figure 15-2a   From N. C. Hughes-Jones, "The Classical Pathway," *Immunobiology of the Complement System*, Academic Press, 1986. Originally published in H. R. Knobel et al., *European Journal of Immunology*, Volume 5, 1975, p. 78.

Figure 15-2c   From N. C. Hughes-Jones, "The Classical Pathway," *Immunobiology of the Complement System*, Academic Press, 1986. Originally published in J. Tschopp et al., *Proceedings of the National Academy of Science*, Volume 77, 1980, p. 7014.

Table 15-2   From M. K. Pangburn, "The Alternate Pathway," in *Immunology of the Complement System*, Academic Press, 1986.

Figure 15-3   From A. Feinstein, E. Munn, and N. Richardson, *Monographs in Allergy*, Volume 17, 1981, p. 47, S. Karger AG, Basel; and from A. Feinstein, E. Munn, and N. Richardson, *Annals of the New York Academy of Science*, Volume 190, 1981, p. 121.

Table 15-6   From N. R. Cooper and G. R. Nemerow, "Complement-Dependent Mechanisms of Virus Neutralization," *Immunobiology of the Complement System*, Academic Press, 1986.

Figure 15-7a   From E. R. Podack, "Assembly and Functions of the Terminal Components," *Immunobiology of the Complement System*, Academic Press, 1986.

Figure 15-7b   From J. Humphrey and R. Dourmashkin, *Advances in Immunology*, Volume 11, 1969, p. 75. Reprinted by permission of Academic Press.

Figure 15-10   From R. D. Schreiber et al., "Bacterial Activity of the Alternative Complement Pathway Generated from 11 Isolated Plasma Proteins," reproduced from the *Journal of Experimental Medicine*, 1979, Volume 149, p. 870, by copyright permission of the Rockefeller University Press.

Figure 15-11   From N. R. Cooper and G. R. Nemerow, "Complement-Dependent Mechanisms of Virus Neutralization," *Immunobiology of the Complement System*, Academic Press, 1986, p. 155.

Figure 15-12abc   From N. R. Cooper and G. R. Nemerow, "Complement-Dependent Mechanisms of Virus Neutralization," *Immunobiology of the Complement System*, Academic Press, 1986, p. 150.

Figure 16-2   From S. Burwen and B. Satir, *J. Cell Biol.*, 1977, Volume 73, p. 662.

Figure 16-5   Adapted from T. Ishizaka et al., *International Archives of Allergy and Applied Immunology*, Volume 77, 1985, p. 137. Reprinted by permission of S. Karger AG, Basel.

Figure 16-10   From K. Ishizaka and T. Ishizaka, *Asthma Physiology, Immunopharmacology, and Treatment*, K. F. Austen, L. M. Lichtenstein, eds., © 1973 Academic Press.

Figure 17-1   From L. V. Crowley, *Introduction to Human Disease*, Second Edition, © 1988 Boston: Jones and Bartlett Publishers. Reprinted by permission.

Figure 17-2   From J. A. Charlesworth and B. A. Pussell, in *Clinical Immunology Illustrated*, edited by J. V. Wells and D. S. Nelson, Williams & Wilkins.

Figure 17-3   From M. A. Atkinson and N. K. Maclaren, "What causes diabetes?" *Scientific American*, July 1990. Copyright © 1990 by Scientific American Inc. All rights reserved.

Figure 17-8   From V. Kumar et al., adapted, with permission, from the *Annual Review of Immunology*, Volume 7, © 1989 by Annual Reviews Inc.

Figure 17-9   From G. Kroemer and G. Wick, *Immunology Today*, Volume 10, 1989, p. 246. Reprinted by permission of Elsevier Science Publishing Company, Inc.

Figure 17-10b   From N. Sarvetnick et al., *Cell*, Volume 52, 1988, p. 773. Reprinted by permission of Cell Press.

Figure 17-12   From D. Wofsy, *Monoclonal Antibody Therapy*, edited by H. Waldmann, 1988.

Figure 17-13   From G. Murti, Department of Virology, St. Jude Children's Research Hospital, Memphis, TN.

Figure 18-1   Adapted from C. A. Mins et al., *Viral Pathogenesis and Immunology*, Blackwell Scientific Publications, Ltd., 1984.

Figure 18-3   From M. Sanetti, E. Sacarz, and J. Salk, *Immunology Today*, Volume 8, 1987, p. 18. Reprinted by permission of Elsevier Science Publishing Company, Inc.

Figure 19-3   From G. G. Brownlee, in Alan R. Liss, *Options for the Control of Influenza*, p. 47. Copyright © 1986 by John Wiley & Sons.

Figure 19-4   From C. Mins et al., *Viral Pathogenesis of Immunology*, Blackwell Scientific Publishing, Ltd., 1984. Originally published in Wiley et al., reprinted by permission from *Nature*, Volume 289, pp. 373–378. Copyright © 1981 Macmillan Magazines Ltd.

Figure 19-6   From M. E. Ward and P. J. Watt, *Journal of Infectious Diseases*, Volume 126, 1972, p. 601. Copyright © 1972. Reprinted by permission of The University of Chicago Press.

Figure 19-7   From T. F. Meyer, modified, with permission, from *The Annual Review of Microbiology*, Volume 44, © 1990 by Annual Reviews Inc.

Figure 19-10   Adapted from M. F. Good et al., *Science*, Volume 235, 1987, p. 1059.

Figure 19-11b   Adapted from John Donelson, in Alan R. Liss, *The Biology of Parasitism*. Copyright © 1988 by John Wiley & Sons.

Figure 20-2   From R. J. Schlegel et al., reproduced by permission of *Pediatrics*, Volume 45, p. 926, copyright 1970.

Figure 20-3   From R. Kretschmer et al., "Congenital Aplasia of the Thymus Gland," reprinted, by permission of *The New England Journal of Medicine*, Volume 279, p. 1295, 1968.

Figure 20-4   Courtesy The Jackson Laboratory, Bar Harbor, ME.

Figure 20-5   From D. D. Manning et al., reproduced from the *Journal of Experimental Medicine*, 1973, Volume 138, p. 488, by copyright permission of the Rockefeller University Press.

Figure 20-6   From G. D. Yancopoulos and F. W. Alt, *Science*, Volume 241, 1988, p. 1581.

Figure 21-1   Adapted from *Science*, Volume 252, 1991, p. 372. Copyright © 1990 by the American Association for the Advancement of Science.

Figure 21-2a   From R. C. Gallo and L. Montagnier, "The AIDS Epidemic," *Scientific American*, Volume 259, 1988, p. 40. Copyright © 1988 by Scientific American Inc. All rights reserved. Micrograph courtesy of Hans Gelderbloom.

Figure 21-2b   From B. M. Peterlin and P. A. Luciw, "Molecular Biology of HIV," *AIDS*, 2(suppl 1), 1988, pp. S29–S40. Reprinted by permission of Current Science.

Figure 21-5   Adapted from W. C. Greene, reprinted by permission of *The New England Journal of Medicine*, Volume 324, 1991, p. 308.

Figure 21-6   From R. C. Gallo, "HIV — The Cause of AIDS," *Journal of Acquired Immune Deficiency Syndrome*, Volume 1, No. 6, 1988, p. 533. Reprinted by permission.

Figure 21-8   From D. J. Capon and R. H. R. Ward, reproduced, with permission, from the *Annual Review of Immunology*, Volume 9, © 1991 by Annual Reviews Inc.

Figure 21-9   From H. C. Lane and A. S. Fauci, reproduced, with permission, from the *Annual Review of Immunology*, Volume 3, © 1985 by Annual Reviews Inc.

Figure 21-10b   From J. N. Weber and R. A. Weiss, *Scientific American*, October 1988. Copyright © 1988 by Scientific American Inc. All rights reserved.

Figure 21-10a   From R. C. Gallo, "HIV — The Cause of AIDS," *Journal of Acquired Immune Deficiency Syndrome*, Volume 1, No. 6, 1988, p. 533. Reprinted by permission.

Figure 21-14   From D. E. Mosier, "Human Immunodeficiency Virus Infection of Human-PHL-SCID Mice," *Science*, Volume 251, September 15, 1991, p. 791. Copyright © 1991 by the American Association for the Advancement of Science.

Index

Transgenic mice
in allelic exclusion, 169
in clonal anergy, 326–330
in clonal deletion, 326–330
in c-myc expression, 515
in thymic selection, 233–234
Translocation, in B lymphocyte
tumors, 514–515
Transplantation, 487–504
discovery of major histocompatibility complex, 188, 192–193
immunologic basis of graft rejection, 488–492
of bone marrow, 499–500
for severe combined immunodeficiency disease, 453
organ, clinical, 500–501
Trinitrophenyl (TNP), 278
Trypanosomes
antigenic variation in, 435–437
infection by, 435
variant surface glycoproptein of,
435–436
trypanosomiasis, African, 435–437
TSS. See Toxic shock syndrome.
TSTAs. See Tumor-specific transplantation antigens.
T suppressor cells, 58, 320–322
Tuberculin reaction, 238, 310–311
Tuberculosis. See Mycobacterium tuberculosis.
Tumor(s)
B lymphocyte
chromosomal translocations in,
514–515
chemically induced, 516
chromosomal abnormalities
aneuploidy, 508
chromosomal deletions, 508
chromosomal translocations,
507–508
homogeneously staining regions
(HSRs), 512
development of
DNA viruses in, 510, 516, 518–
519
retroviruses in, 511–513
evasion of immune response, 522
antigenic modulation, 523–524
blocking antibody, 522–523
reduction of class I MHC, 524–
525
immune response to
role of humoral antibody, 522
role of macrophages, 521
role of NK cell, 520–521
role of T_C cell, 520
immune surveillance theory, 522
immunotherapy of

cytokine therapy in, 525–528
engineered melanoma cells
immune adjuvants, 525
LAK cells, 527
monoclonal antibody, 149, 528
TIL cells, 528
tumor cell vaccines, 519
malignant transformation, 509
chemical and physical carcinogens, 510
viral transformation, 510
oncogenes, 510, 520
function, 511
conversion of protooncogenes
into oncogenes, 511–512
properties of, 507
transgenic mouse models, 514
Tumor antigens, 515–520
chemically induced, 516
identification using Tum⁻ cell lines,
517
oncofetal antigens, 519
alpha fetoprotein, 519–520
carcinoembryonic, 519–520
oncogene encoded antigens, 520
thymus leukemia antigen, 523
tumor-associated (TAAs), 515
tumor-specific (TSAs), 515
virally induced, 518–519
Tumor necrosis factor (TNF), 50,
202–203, 258
biological activity of, 203, 248,
253, 258, 264
cellular sources of, 50, 248–249,
253, 258
in delayed type hypersensitivity, 379
in graft-versus-host disease, 500
in HIV gene transcription, 475
in inflammatory response, 263
in Leishmania major infection
in malaria, 430
in bacterial septic shock, 265
in bacterial toxic shock, 259, 265,
429
in tumor immunotherapy, 259–
260, 520, 521, 527
toxicity of, 266, 527
Tumor-associated antigens (TAAs), 515
Tumor-cell vaccines, 529
Tumor-infiltrating lymphocytes
(TILs), 528
Tumor-specific transplantation antigens (TSTAs), 516–517

Unanue, E. R., 85, 254

V (variable) genes
in autoimmunity, 393, 401

of immunoglobulins, 161–162
of T cell receptors, 220
rearrangements of, 221–225
somatic mutations in, 181–183
V (variable) regions, 102, 159–160
of antibody heavy chains, 102, 159
of antibody light chains, 102, 159
of T cell receptors, 220–222
Vaccination, history of, 2, 406–408
Vaccine(s)
active immunization, 407–416
AIDS, 478–484
attenuated vaccines, 410
capsular polysaccharide, 412
Haemophilus influenzae, 412
herd immunity, 408
idiotype vaccines, 416, 484
inactivated vaccines, 411, 480
measles vaccine, 407–408
passive immunization, 406–407
polio vaccine, 409
recombinant vaccines, 412, 482
recombinant vector vaccines, 413,
482
synthetic peptide vaccines, 414, 482
toxoids, 412
Vaccinia virus
smallpox vaccine, 125
vectors, 413, 480, 482
Variant surface glyocoprotein (VSG),
of trypanosomes, 435–436
Varmus, H. E., 510
Vascular addressins, 68–70
Vascular cell adhesion molecule-1
(VCAM), 264–265
VCAM-1. See Vascular cell adhesion
molecule-1.
Vector vaccines, 411
vif gene, in HIV, 466–467
Viral vectors, live, 482
Virus(es)
antigenic drift and shift in, 422–
423, 479
DNA, in tumor development, 510
Epstein-Barr. See Epstein-Barr virus.
evasion of host defense, 420–422
immunity to
cell-mediated, 420
humoral, 420
influenza, 421–425
oncogenic, 510
RNA, 513
vpr gene, in HIV, 463–464
vpu gene, in HIV, 463–464
VSG. See Variable surface glycoprotein.

Waksman, B. H., 251
Weaver, C. T., 254
Weissman, I. L., 46